Paediatric Audiological Medicine

Paediatric Audiological Medicine

Edited by

VALERIE E. NEWTON, MSc, MD, FRCP, FRCPCH

Human Communication and Deafness,
The University of Manchester

W

WHURR PUBLISHERS
LONDON AND PHILADELPHIA

First published 2002 by
Whurr Publishers Ltd
19b Compton Terrace, London N1 2UN, England and
325 Chestnut Street, Philadelphia PA 1906, USA

British Library Cataloguing in Publication Data
A catalogue record for this book is available from the British Library.

ISBN: 186156 228 4

Printed and bound in the UK by Athenaeum Press Ltd,
Gateshead, Tyne & Wear

Contents

Contributors

P Axon University Department of Otolaryngology, Head and Neck Surgery, Manchester Royal Infirmary, Manchester, UK.

G Baird Newcomen Centre, Guy's Hospital, London, UK.

FH Bess Vanderbilt University Medical Center, Nashville, Tennessee, USA.

GM Cleator Neurosciences Research Group, Faculty of Medicine, University of Manchester, Manchester, UK.

CWRJ Cremers Department of Otolaryngology, University of Nijmegen, Nijmegan, The Netherlands.

A Davis MRC Institute of Hearing Research, Nottingham, UK.

TG Delap Georgia Ear Institute, Memorial Medical Center, Savannah, Georgia, USA.

J Dodd-Murphy Department of Language, Reading and Exceptionalities, Appalachian State University, Boone, North Carolina, USA.

C Gallaway Centre for Human Communication and Deafness, University of Manchester, Manchester, UK.

M Goldsmith Georgia Ear Institute, Memorial Medical Center, Savannah, Georgia, USA.

MD Graham Georgia Ear Institute, Memorial Medical Center, Savannah, Georgia, USA.

JW Hall III School of Health Professions, University of Florida Health Science Center, Gainsville, Florida, USA.

F Hickson Centre for Human Communication and Deafness, University of Manchester, Manchester, UK.

RW Keith Division of Audiology, University of Cincinnati Medical Center, Cincinnati, Ohio, USA.

PE Klapper Clinical Virology, Central Manchester Healthcare Trust, Manchester, UK.

D Lucas Nuffield Hearing and Speech Centre, Royal National Throat, Nose and Ear Hospital, London, UK.

W Lynas Centre for Human Communication and Deafness, University of Manchester, UK.

G Mencher MRC Institute of Hearing Research, Nottingham, UK.

JC McLachlan University of St Andrews, St Andrews, Scotland.

C Möller Department of Audiology, Sahlgrenska University Hospital, Gothenburg, Sweden.

VE Newton Centre for Human Communication and Deafness, University of Manchester, Manchester, UK.

A Palmer MRC Institute of Hearing Research, Nottingham, UK.

S Palmer Centre for Human Communication and Deafness,University of Manchester, Manchester, UK.

G Parker Central Sheffield University Hospitals, Sheffield, UK.

T Penn Vanderbilt University, Nashville, Tennessee, USA.

P Phelps Royal National Throat, Nose and Ear Hospital, London, UK.

C Powell Mary Hare Grammar School, Newbury, Berkshire, UK.

R Ramsden University Department of Otolaryngology, Head and Neck Surgery, Manchester Royal Infirmary and University of Manchester, UK.

AP Read Department of Medical Genetics, University of Manchester, Manchester, UK.

AM Rothpletz Vanderbilt University Medical Center, Nashville, Tennessee, USA.

RJ Smith Department of Otolaryngology, University of Iowa, Iowa City, Iowa, USA.

S Snashall Department of Audiological Medicine, St George's Hospital, London, UK.

JC Stevens Central Sheffield University Hospitals, Sheffield, UK.

D Toe Renwick College, University of Newcastle, Parametta, Australia.

I Tucker Mary Hare Grammar School, Newbury, Berkshire, UK.

RS Tyler Department of Otolaryngology, University of Iowa, Iowa City, Iowa, USA.

PJ Vallely Neurosciences Research Group, Faculty of Medicine, University of Manchester, Manchester, UK

J Witana Department of Audiological Medicine, St George's Hospital, London, UK.

Foreword

It is now some considerable time since the specialty of audiological medicine was officially established in the National Health Service in the United Kingdom. The government of the day recognized the serious gap in provision for people who were in need of services that were not being provided by the existing specialties. Before the initial onset of training of audiological physicians and the establishment of consultant jobs there were a few centres where this work had been developed, thus providing a base for the development of services. Since those early days the appointment of consultant audiological physicians throughout the United Kingdom moved apace, together with the appointment of academic professorial chairs in selected universities.

This publication is the evidence of the fruits of these years of work here and in other continents. Professor Newton has used her skills to draw on experts from other parts of the world to offer leading articles on their specialist subjects. The book has been ambitious in offering a comprehensive cover of those subjects central to the practice of paediatric audiological medicine, and in including those areas of immediate interest to the educational management of hearing-impaired children.

It was my good fortune, before I retired from the Chair at the University of Manchester, to have been part of the establishment of the work with Professor Ramsden in the development of the Cochlear Implant Programme. Perhaps it is this project that serves to emphasize the necessary inter-disciplinary relationship amongst the several specialties, now recognized in the team approach.

The same can be said for all the work with hearing-impaired children. The reader will gain essential insights into the educational approaches now developed worldwide as well as the systems practised in these islands. The thoughtful articles by Wendy Lynas, Ivan Tucker and Con Powell serve to lay out the issues that are germane to educational selection and practice.

It was the Ewings who set out so much of the basis of good practice in audiology. In their work was the first recognition of the need to identify hearing impairment as early as possible, and of the importance of involving the whole family in the process of early management. Since those days, recognition of the urgency of diagnosis of hearing impairment in the newborn child has opened up new opportunities. The reality now is that it seems within our grasp that the great majority of hearing-impaired babies will be identified much earlier than before.

Perhaps it is in the field of the definition of the cause of deafness that the greater paradox remains. Paediatric audiological medicine has now benefited from the scientific development of gene and chromosomal studies, giving rise to the possibility of such definition, which would have hardly been possible even 10 years ago. Such is the rapid advance in this field. On the other hand, so many problems face the clinician when considering the several adverse perinatal factors. The present teasing out of the significance of the factors during the perinatal period remains an area that will require the collaborative work of the paediatric specialist and the paediatric audiological physician.

This publication has succeeded in setting forth best practice for the clinician, the nature of the various communication difficulties in the clinical setting, and the availability of educational management. The doctors who have been responsible for the development of services will be helped and guided by the information now available on the prevalence of hearing impairment and the changing pattern of the causes of hearing impairment.

We must not lose sight of the fact that we are dependent on our clinical colleagues to operate in the fields of medicine to prevent conditions that are responsible for sensorineural losses in infants. It is now exceedingly rare to see babies handicapped by congenital rubella, or the effect of the rhesus factor. This would remind us of the need to keep close to our medical colleagues, who will directly influence the incidence of pathological conditions

At the time of my retirement from the Chair in 1988, the principles of good practice had been established. Reading this excellent text made me realize how much progress has been made in almost all areas of work.

Ian G Taylor
Professor Emeritus
University of Manchester

Preface

The aim of this book is to provide an up-to-date text for clinicians working in the field of audiology. It has drawn upon the knowledge and experience of experts from various countries and with differing professional backgrounds. The result is a volume that gives coverage to a range of topics relevant to clinical practice.

There are chapters on the development and function of the ear and these initial chapters are well illustrated. Prevalence and causation of sensorineural hearing impairment are given ample coverage with chapters dedicated to a more detailed consideration of specific etiological factors. The importance of a thorough investigation of children to establish the etiology of their hearing impairment is emphasized together with inclusion of their immediate family in the process. The chapter on radiology illustrates the degree to which advances in imaging are now able to assist in the investigative process.

In recent years many advances have been made in discovering the locations of genes causing hearing impairment, and the methods employed and the current extent of knowledge in this area are reviewed. Infective causes are important, as they are potentially preventable. The chapter on infections discusses the epidemiology, pathogenesis and control of a range of intrauterine and post-natally acquired infections, some of which are now becoming less prevalent as a result of immunization initiatives.

The potential exists for adverse perinatal conditions to cause sensorineural hearing impairment. The various conditions to which the neonate may be exposed are described and the question is raised as to whether or not a history of problems around the time of birth is necessarily causative of hearing impairment in an individual child.

Although the book is primarily concerned with sensorineural hearing impairment, otitis media is a major cause of hearing impairment in young children and a chapter is devoted to the diagnosis and management of this condition.

Children suffer from tinnitus with or without an associated hearing impairment and a chapter is devoted to the topic of tinnitus in children. Hearing impairment may be accompanied by a balance disorder and there is a useful chapter on the causes of balance disorders and methods of detecting a balance problem in children. Some children without hearing impairment have problems processing auditory signals. Detecting these children is not always easy and the chapter on this, written by an expert in this field, reviews the tests available and suggests methods of remediation.

The detection of a hearing impairment as soon as possible after the defect has occurred is essential to enable early habilitation to take place. The issues surrounding targeted and universal neonatal screening are covered as well as screening or surveillance at an older age. Methods of detecting a hearing impairment, measurement of the degree of hearing loss and determination of the site of lesion are detailed in two chapters, one of which (Chapter 6) provides two useful case histories.

The chapter on amplification for children illustrates the extent to which there have been improvements in matching provision to the child's needs. The appropriate fitting of hearing aids to young children is essential and the chapter provides information on how this can be achieved. Not all children will, however, benefit from hearing aids and the chapter on cochlear implants indicates how much the outlook for children with a profound bilateral hearing impairment has improved through the advent of this provision. Children with a unilateral sensorineural impairment also have special needs, and the problems experienced by these children and ways in which these can be alleviated are covered in a chapter specifically devoted to this type of hearing impairment.

The ability to communicate is crucial and there are two chapters that consider the development of speech and language in hearing and hearing-impaired children and which include discussion of both oral and signing communication systems. There is one chapter devoted to speech and language disorders in children, which provides the reader with a useful overview.

The psychological effects of a hearing impairment and the educational placement of hearing-impaired children are thoughtfully considered in two further chapters.

Overall the book gives the reader comprehensive coverage of the topics that are considered essential knowledge for those working as clinicians with hearing-impaired children. Further study is guided by including a large reference section.

Valerie Elizabeth Newton
University of Manchester

CHAPTER 1

Developmental anatomy of the ear

JC McLACHLAN

Evolution of hearing

Adult structures are consequences of both developmental and evolutionary processes, and understanding the adult anatomy is greatly facilitated by some insight into both processes (Hildebrand, 1982).

In our marine ancestors (as in modern fish) movement relative to the surrounding water was detected via the lateral line – a trough or channel developed from ectodermal placodes and running along the length of the animal. This channel contained sensory cells, which fired nerve impulses when hairs projecting into the channel were deflected. Fluid movements in the channel were amplified by embedding the tips of the hairs in extracellular structures. Part of the channel sank in from the ectoderm and became isolated to form a labyrinthine structure, capable of determining orientation.

This lateral line system cannot operate effectively in air because the delicate hair cells operate best in a fluid environment. So as terrestriality began to evolve, hearing and detection of movement were both carried out in a sealed fluid-filled pouch (the inner ear) deep beneath the surface.

In water, vibrations have low amplitude and high energy, but in air vibrations have large amplitude and low energy, so they cannot readily pass through intervening tissue. It therefore became necessary to step down the amplitude of airborne vibrations and to transmit them directly to the hearing detection system. Fortunately, the means were at hand to do so. Our early vertebrate ancestors had a rather complex jaw articulation, which had arisen from *ad hoc* modification of the cartilage rods supporting the first and second gill arches. A more direct jaw articulation was associated with terrestriality. This made several elements redundant, and because evolution adapts rather than invents, these jaw elements were pressed into a new role. In amphibians a single bone was employed to transmit sound to the inner ear apparatus. In mammals, three bony elements derived from the first and second pharyngeal arches were incorporated into the hearing apparatus as levers that stepped down the amplitude of vibrations and transmitted them to the sensory apparatus.

The external pharyngeal grooves and corresponding internal pharyngeal pouches were also available for modification as air breathing meant that gills were no longer required. The closely apposed ectoderm and endoderm lying between the pouch and groove formed the eardrum, the external groove formed the auditory meatus, and the internal pouch formed the middle-ear cavity.

The process of ectodermal placode formation followed by invagination from the surface is recapitulated during the course of development. The extracellular structures in which the tips of the lateral line hair cells were embedded are now represented by the tectorial membrane.

Although the hearing apparatus develops to form an integrated structure, it is probably easier in terms of description to follow the development of the components – inner ear, middle ear and external ear – separately. Table 1.1, pages 4–5, is intended to help overcome the illusion of separate development that this may convey, by illustrating how each component is developing compared to the others.

Inner ear

The development of the inner ear has been extensively described (Bast, Anson and Gardner, 1947; O'Rahilly, 1963; O'Rahilly and Muller, 1987). Early in week four, a thickening – the otic placode or placode VII – forms in the ectoderm on each side of the head, at the level of the rhombencephalon (Pearson et al., 1973; Figure 1.1). This is the most marked of a series of four ectodermal placodes, which contribute to the developing nervous system. It forms in close association with the facioacoustic crest or crest VII, one of the streams of neural crest cells which arise from the dorsal aspect of the neural tube.

The placode may develop in response to inductive signals from the underlying brain (Cordes and Barsh, 1994). It has been suggested that, at least in mice, the thickening is relative rather than real, and results from a thinning of the surrounding ectoderm (Verwoerd van Oostrom and Verwoerd-Verhoef, 1981). Later in the same week, the otic placodes invaginate to form pits, which in turn become the otic vesicles (Figures 1.1, 1.2). These lie lateral to rhombomeres 5 and 6. The process of invagination of the pit is not dependent on distant tissue interactions – in isolated placodes in organ culture, invagination takes place as normal (McLachlan and Lamont, unpublished observations). Cell division does not appear to be the underlying factor driving invagination (Meier, 1978a,b; Alvarez and Navascues, 1990).

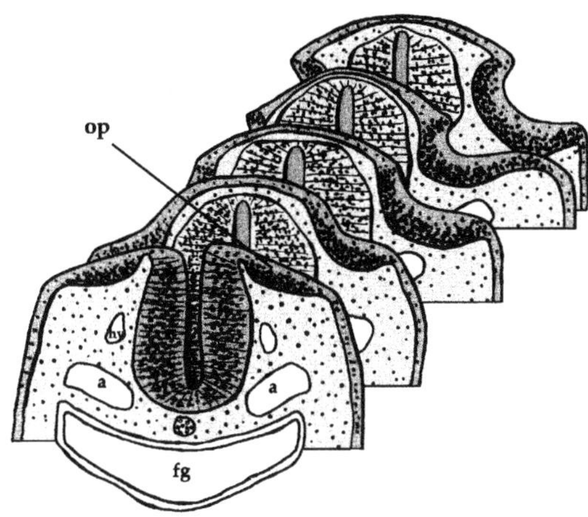

Figure 1.1. Development of otic placodes and pits during Carnegie Stage 11 (approximately 23–25 days after fertilization). Based on O'Rahilly and Müller (1987) and Patten (1953).
fg: foregut. a: aorta. hv: head vein. op: otic placode.

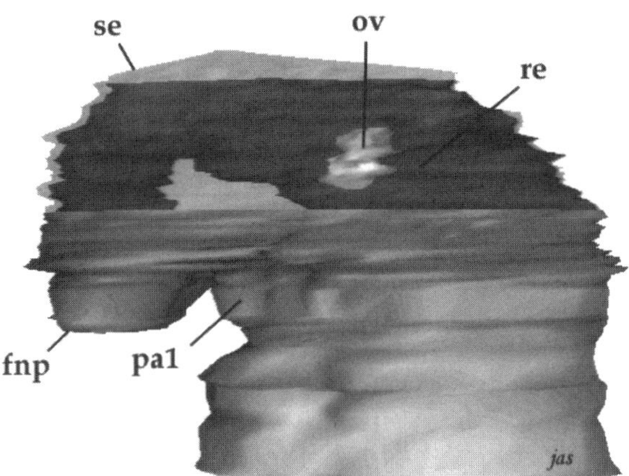

Figure 1.2. Otic vesicle in a Carnegie Stage 12/13 embryo (26–28 days after fertilization). Based on a computer 3D reconstruction of embryo W003/2 from the Walmsley Collection. The 3D model is accessible via http://embryos.st-and.ac.uk.
fnp: frontonasal process. se: surface ectoderm. ov: otic vesicle. re: rhombencephalon. pa1: pharyngeal arch 1.

The morphology of the otic vesicle develops in a complex manner. Three distinct regions will develop (Figures 1.3, 1.4, 1.5(b)). (i) A long process, known as the endolymphatic appendage extends dorsally from the medial aspect. (ii) The dorsal part of the otic vesicle, the vestibular part or pouch, gives rise to the utricle and semicircular canals. (iii) The more

Table 1.1. Comparison of inner, middle and outer ear development over the embryonic period

Carnegic Stage	Time since fertilization	Length	Inner Ear	Middle Ear	Outer Ear
Stage 9	20 days	1.5–2.5 mm	Otic placode first forms in close association to facio-acoustic crest.		
Stage 10	22 days	2–3.5 mm	Otic plate contributes cells to facial neural crest.	The first pharyngeal arch, with associated pouch and groove, begins to form.	
Stage 11	24 days	2.5–4.5 mm	Otic placode sinks about half way in		
Stage 12	26 days	3–5 mm	Otic vesicle nearly complete by end of stage – but not quite detached from surface ectoderm.		
Stage 13	28 days	4–6 mm	Otic vesicle closed. Later, the endolymphatic appendage is recognisable. Blood vessels begin to condense round otocyst.		The dorsal part of the first pharyngeal pouch is in close association with the ectoderm of dorsal pharyngeal groove – forming the precursor of the tympanic membrane.
Stage 14	32 days	5–7 mm	Otic vesicle grows overall, and becomes more oval as cochlear duct begins to be evident.	The tubotympanic recess begins to expand from pouch 1.	
Stage 15	33 days	7–9 mm	Mesenchyme condenses round the otic vesicle. The endolymphatic duct becomes more slender.		
Stage 16	37 days	8–11 mm	The endolymphatic duct becomes longer. Thickenings in utricle wall pressage the semicircular ducts. The acoustic part of crest becomes vestibulocochlear nerve. Vestibular and cochlear ganglia form.	Precartilage condensation of the first and second arch cartilages are present.	Three auricular hillocks appear on each of the first and second arches.

Stage 17	41 days	11–14 mm	The cochlear duct elongates while the walls of the utricle are coming closer together at the forming semicircular canals.	The auditory ossicles are present.	The auricular hillocks are more defined on second arch. The groove between the first and second arch deepens to form the external auditory meatus. The hillocks begin to fuse.
Stage 18	44 days	13–17 mm	The cochlear duct is now L-shaped. The semicircular canals form in the order anterior – posterior – lateral.	The stapes and stapedius can be identified. Bars of pharyngeal arches begin to chondrify.	The auricular hillocks begin to form identifiable parts of the external ear.
Stage 19	47 days	16–18 mm	The cochlear duct is J-shaped. Cartilage begins to form in the condensed mesoderm surrounding the inner ear apparatus.		
Stage 20	50 day	18–22 mm	The cochlear duct has the shape of a cursive J.		
Stage 21	52 days	22–24 mm	The cochlear duct forms a single turn.		
Stage 22	54 days	23–28 mm	The cochlear duct is represented by one and a half turns. The ductus reuniens is visible.		
Stage 23	56 days	27–31 mm	The cochlear duct has a double turn. After stage 23 (the last in the Carnegie series) it will develop the definitive 2.5 turns.	The endodermal lining of tympanic cavity begins to expand to engulf the middle ear bones and the chorda tympani nerve.	The perilymphatic space begins to develop. The meatal plug begins to form. The auricular cartilages appear as condensations.

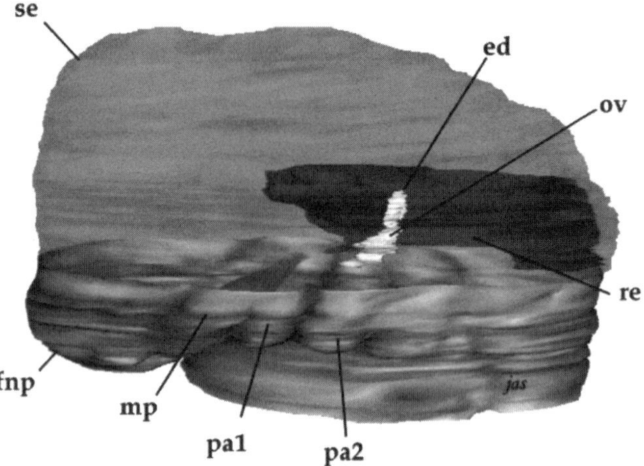

Figure 1.3. Otic vesicle in a Carnegie Stage 15 embryo (33 days after fertilization). Based on a computer 3D reconstruction of embryo W008/1 from the Walmsley Collection. The 3D model is accessible via http://embryos.st-and.ac.uk.
fnp: frontonasal process. se: surface ectoderm. ed: endolymphatic duct. ov: otic vesicle. re: rhombencephalon. pa1: pharyngeal arch 1. pa2: pharyngeal arch 2. mp: maxillary process.

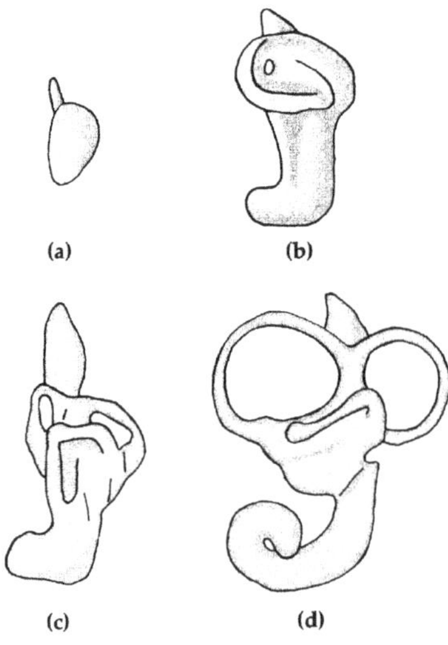

Figure 1.4. Differentiation of otic vesicle into endolymphatic, vestibular and cochlear regions. (a) Approximates to an 8 mm embryo, Carnegie Stage 15, 33 days after fertilization. (b) Approximates to a 15 mm embryo, Carnegie Stage 18, 44 days after fertilization. (c) Approximates to an 18 mm embryo, Carnegie Stage 19, 48 days after fertilization. (d) Approximates to a 23 mm embryo, Carnegie Stage 21, 52 days after fertilization. Scale bar represents 0.5 mm. Based on Keibel and Mall (1912) and Streeter (1918).

ventral part (the cochlear pouch) gives rise to the saccule and cochlea. The terms 'saccule' and 'utricle' have sometimes been applied to the vestibular and cochlear pouches of the otocyst respectively. However, it is probably better to reserve these terms for the definitive later structures.

Endolymphatic system

The most dorsal portion of the endolymphatic appendage expands during week five to form the endolymphatic sac, and the remainder of the appendage elongates to form the endolymphatic duct.

The endolymphatic duct and sac are originally simple, single-lumen structures. However, in the adult, the intraosseus, intermediate part consists of a network of interconnected tubules (Linthicum and Galey, 1981). Studies of fetal specimens indicate that the time of transition between these two states is very variable, ranging from 26 weeks gestation to post-natally, and even differing from right to left (Ng and Linthicum, 1998).

Vestibular pouch

Three flat, mutually orthogonal projections in the form of discs grow out from the vestibular pouch during week seven (Figure 1.4). The tissue of the flat discs will become thinner away from the margins and eventually disappear leaving the rim as the semicircular canal. Each duct has an expanded ampulla at one end. The ventral part of the vestibular pouch becomes the utricle, into which the semicircular canals open.

Cochlear pouch

A long coiled tube, the cochlear duct, begins to elongate ventrally and medially from the cochlear pouch during week five. This will gradually coil during the embryonic period to become the cochlea (Table 1.1 and Figure 1.4). The dorsal part of the cochlear pouch forms the saccule. The connection between the cochlea and the saccule narrows to form an isthmus known as the ductus reuniens. Development of the cochlea is described in more detail in Lim and Rueda, 1992. During week seven, the internal cells of the cochlear duct begin to differentiate to form the organ of Corti (Pearson et al., 1973). By 25 weeks, the organ of Corti shows considerable maturity (Anson and Donaldson, 1981). There is both a radial and longitudinal gradient of development on the organ of Corti (Lim and Rueda, 1992).

However, the cochlear duct forms only a component of the functional hearing apparatus. The duct is surrounded by loose mesenchyme, which is reticular in nature. At about eight to nine weeks after fertilization, a space develops in this loose connective tissue postero-medial to the duct, perhaps

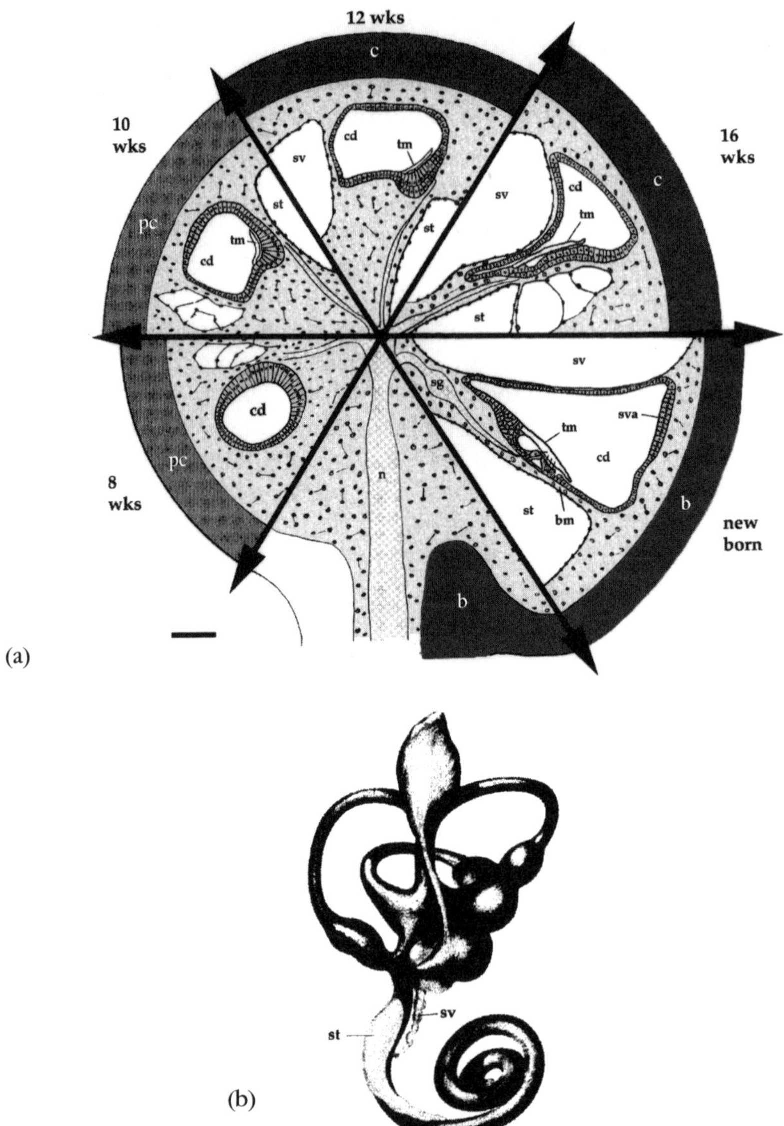

Figure 1.5. (a) Diagram showing development of the cochlear duct, scala tympani and scala vestibuli. The scale bar represents 0.1 mm. The cochlear duct is drawn to approximate scale, but the cartilage and bony surrounds are diagrammatic. Based on Bleischmidt (1961), Keibel and Mall (1912), Patten (1953) and Streeter (1918).
pc: pre-cartilage. cd: cochlear duct. tm: tectorial membrane. st: scala tympani. sv: scala vestibuli. sva: stria vascularis. sg: spiral ganglion. n: nerve.
(b) Median view of the inner ear at about 10 weeks after fertilization, showing the scala tympani and vestibuli in surface view. Modified from Streeter (1918).
st: scala tympani. sv: scala vestibuli.

by coalescence of the reticular spaces (Streeter, 1918; Figure 1.5 (a, b)). This will form the scala tympani. Beginning near the saccule, it gradually extends along the length of the coiled cochlear duct, and thus is coiled itself. Shortly afterwards a similar space, the scala vestibuli, begins to develop on the other side of the cochlear duct. By 16 weeks after fertilization, the scala tympani communicates with the scala vestibuli at the distal tip of the cochlea (at the helicotrema). The ectodermally derived cochlear duct now lies between these two mesodermal spaces, and is sometimes described as the scala media, although this is not a very useful terminology. The fluid filling the scala tympani and vestibuli is known as perilymph; that filling the cochlear duct is known as endolymph, and these are of very different constitution. The scala vestibuli communicates with the oval window, and the scala tympani with the round window. Sound waves are therefore transmitted through the scala vestibuli first, through the helicotrema, and on to the scala tympani, where the round window allows oscillation to persist.

The organ of Corti sits on the basilar membrane between the scala tympani and the cochlear duct or scala media (Figure 1.5 (a)). It develops from the floor of the cochlear duct. An acellular membrane, the tectorial membrane, overlies an epithelial thickening, beginning during the third month. The outer hair cells differentiate from the three outer rows of this thickening, while the inner hair cells arise from a single inner layer. The inner tunnel will form between these, lined by the pillar cells. An outer tunnel also forms beyond the outer hair cells.

The supporting cells in the organ of Corti possess a highly organized cytoskeletal framework. This is extremely important in functional terms because it connects the sensory cells, which detect movement, to the basilar membrane, which vibrates when the ear is exposed to sound waves. The mechanisms by which cytoskeletal organization occurs have been the subject of considerable study, and seem likely to inform wider views on the cytoskeleton (Tucker et al., 1998).

Tissue maturation is comprehensively reviewed in Dechesne (1992). An important conclusion is that there are likely to be periods of particular sensitivity to trauma and teratogenic action in the fetal period, as complex maturation events take place. A variety of transcription factors have been shown to be involved in differentiation of cells of the inner ear (Corey and Breakefield, 1994)

Middle ear

The first pharyngeal pouch elongates and expands to form the tubotympanic recess. Laterally, this expands to form the middle-ear cavity; medially, where it retains its connection to the foregut, it forms the auditory tube (Kanagasuntheram, 1967). Both of these are lined with endoderm. The apposed endoderm and ectoderm between the pouch and the groove will contribute to the tympanic membrane.

Over the next few weeks (up to week eight) the cartilaginous precursors of the middle-ear bones are forming from neural crest cells in the first and second pharyngeal arches. These lie rostral and caudal respectively to the developing inner ear, although this is not often clear in the standard two-dimensional view (Figure 1.3). The malleus and incus are generally described as forming in the first pharyngeal arch, with the stapes forming in the second.

During the later part of pregnancy, the middle-ear cavity expands by means of programmed cell death and resorption into the loose mesenchyme of the pharyngeal arches, so that the middle-ear ossicles become suspended within the cavity. As a result, these are covered with tissue that is sometimes described as being derived from the endoderm that lines the middle-ear cavity. The middle-ear muscles – the tensor tympani attached to the malleus, and the stapedius, attached to the stapes – arise in the mesoderm of the first and second arches respectively. This accounts for their respective innervation by the Vth and VIIth cranial nerves.

The temporal ring develops as membranous bone, which partly surrounds the external auditory meatus and developing tympanic cavity. It has been shown that the relationship between the development of the tympanic ring and the external auditory meatus is a very close one. Loss or duplication of the ring, achieved via retinoic acid treatment or manipulation of Hoxa2 expression, results in corresponding changes to the external auditory meatus (Mallo and Gridley, 1996).

The mastoid antrum will also expand, and air cells will form in late fetal and early post-natal life. These are also lined with endoderm.

External ear

The external auditory meatus forms from the first pharyngeal groove (Figure 1.6 a–c). It becomes occluded during the early fetal period due to overproliferation of the ectodermal lining cells to form what is known as the meatal plug, but normally reopens during later fetal life. The purpose of this phenomenon is unknown. However, in a rather similar situation, the lumen of the gut occludes during development due to proliferation of the epithelial cells, and subsequently recanalizes. It has been proposed that the proliferation of endoderm provides material for the elongation of the gut during development. Perhaps similar considerations apply in the ear – certainly, the external auditory meatus elongates considerably, before and also after birth.

The external ear develops from three pairs of auricular hillocks, which arise on the first and second pharyngeal arches during week five. These

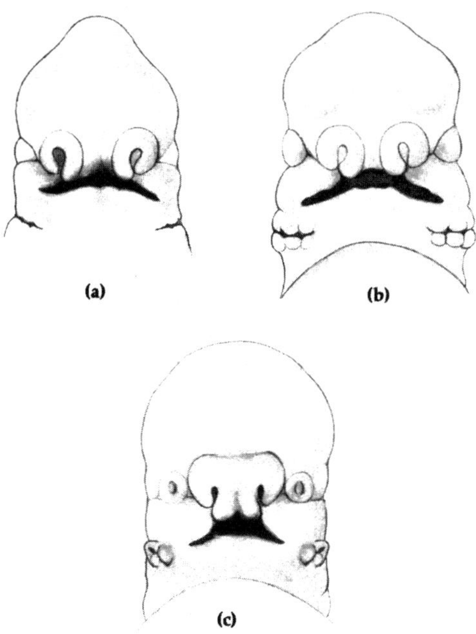

Figure 1.6. Views of face showing development of external ears. (a) Approximates to an 8 mm embryo, Carnegie Stage 15, 33 days after fertilization. (b) Approximates to a 12.5 mm embryo, Carnegie Stage 16, 35 days after fertilization. (c) Approximates to a 21 mm embryo, Carnegie Stage 20, 50 days after fertilization. From McLachlan (1994). Used with permission of Addison Wesley.

form round the first pharyngeal groove (Figure 1.6). As the embryonic stage gives way to the fetal period, these hillocks begin to enlarge, and as they come in contact, gradually begin to fuse to form the pinna or auricle of the external ear.

The external ear begins its development in a position that corresponds to where the neck would be in the adult (Figure 1.6). Differential relative proliferation alters the relative position of the external ear to the adult site. Ears remaining low set may therefore be an external marker of a more serious genetic abnormality of the head and neck region.

Support structures and innervation

In the same way as mesoderm condenses round the brain to give the dura mater, or round the optic cup to form sclera, so it condenses round the inner ear, beginning in week nine. This process has been beautifully illustrated by Bast and Anson (1949). As is also the rule with the optic sclera and the chondrocranium, the ectodermally derived tissues probably induce cartilage formation, ensuring that the support structures are moulded to the form of the sensory structures (Thorogood, 1987). There is a steady progression of interactive stages in the mouse, which probably correspond closely to events in humans (McPhee and Van de Water, 1986; Van de Water et al., 1992). The cartilaginous capsule undergoes growth, requiring that it be hollowed out from the inside as well as expanding in its external diameter (Streeter, 1918). The cartilaginous otic capsule will begin to ossify between the fifth and sixth months of gestation, to form the petrous part of the temporal bone. Prior to ossification, spaces develop around the utricle and semicircular canals, which are continuous with the scala tympani and scala vestibuli. This perilymphatic space is fluid filled, and becomes continuous with the subarachnoid space.

In the cochlear region two openings or windows persist in the bony covering (the oval and round windows) to provide communication between the inner ear and the middle ear, and hence the external ear. The stapes attaches to the oval window, and the malleus to the tympanic membrane so that vibrations of the membrane are transmitted but stepped down in amplitude to the fluid in the perilymphatic space and thence to the cochlea.

Nerves

The otic placode arises in close association with the facioacoustic neural crest. This contributes to the vestibulocochlear nerve and to the vestibular and cochlear ganglion. However, the common ganglial precursor (the statoacoustic ganglion) is of mixed origin, and the otic placode contributes to it by delamination (Van de Water et al., 1992). The statoacoustic ganglion is not necessary for the development of the inner ear in the early stages, but the inner ear derivatives are necessary to the development of the statoacoustic ganglion (Van de Water, 1988). The ganglion is susceptible to the action of nerve growth factor. The cochlear ganglion forms at stage 16, and provides branches to the cochlea, spiralling along with it. The chorda tympani branch of the facial nerve can be also identified at stage 16.

Genes involved in morphogenesis of the hearing apparatus

Genes involved in deafness have been extensively reviewed (Steel, 1995; Petit, 1996; Hughes, 1997; see Chapter 8 in this volume). Many of these are structural and are not involved in the mechanics of morphogenesis. Others again reflect degeneration after the rudiments have formed. Relatively few are morphological in their effect.

The gene *kr,* associated with the ***kreisler*** mutant, is expressed in the neural tube only, but none the less leads to defects in the inner ear (Cordes and Barsh, 1994). The vesicle is displaced, and the endolymphatic duct fails to develop. Vestibular and cochlear structures also subsequently fail to develop. This strongly suggests that *kr* is involved in inductive events between the hindbrain and the surface ectoderm. The action of PAX3 seems to confirm this, because gross cranial defects are observed that also affect inner ear development (Deol, 1966; Goulding et al., 1991; Baldwin et al., 1992; Tassabehji et al., 1992).

PAX3 mutations in humans are the causes of Waardenburg Type I and Type III syndromes. Both PAX3 and the product of the *kr* locus (bZIP) are transcription factors, and stand at the head of inductive cascades. Other transcription factors involved in morphogenetic defects include the zinc finger transcription factor *Gli3,* encoded by the *Xt* locus (corresponding to the mutant *Extra-toes*) in mice (Johnson, 1967; Hui and Joyner, 1993) and Hoxa1 (Lufkin et al., 1991; Chisaka, Musci and Capecchi, 1992). Hoxa1 knockouts cause hindbrain abnormalities and, probably as a consequence, inner ear abnormalities.

PAX3 appears to play a role in the differentiation of melanocytes from neural crest cells (Ryan, 1997). Melanocytes are found in the stria vascularis of the cochlea, and in the dark cells of the vestibular labyrinth, and are involved in endolymph production. The transcription factor MITF is also involved in melanocyte differentiation, and defects in MITF gives rise to Waardenburg Type II syndrome (Moore, 1995). POU domain transcription factors may also be important (Cremers et al., 1995; Ryan, 1997).

Transcription factors are only one link in the inductive cascade. FGF3 also seems to be involved (Mansour, Goddard and Capecchi, 1993), and antisense oligonucleotides or antibodies to FGF3 affect otic vesicle development. The FGF receptor FGFR3 also seems to be involved in the differentiation of hair cells (Peters et al., 1993) and mutations can lead to a variety of hearing abnormalities. In addition, the enzyme histidase, when mutated in mothers, leads to higher levels of histidine, which in turn result in inner ear malformations in the offspring (Kacser et al., 1977).

The above are defects of the inner ear. Hoxa1 transgenics also reveal that the gene affects the middle-ear bones and inhibits development of the pinna (Chisaka et al., 1992). The ligand endothelin-1 has a similar effect when the gene is interrupted transgenically, and the tympanic ring is also affected (Kurihara et al., 1994).

PAX2 is related to deafness but less to the vestibular system (Terzic et al., 1998). In humans, it is strongly expressed in the utricle at eight weeks after fertilization. Murine Pax2 is expressed in regions of the otic capsule that will be neurogenic: in the early otic capsule it is strongly expressed on the medial aspect, near the neural tube, from where the contribution to the acoustic ganglia arises. Later it is expressed in the more ventral parts of the capsule, but not in the endolymphatic region (Nornes et al., 1990). Pax2 null mutants show agenesis of the cochlea and the spiral ganglion (Torres et al., 1996)

Acknowledgements

Three-dimensional reconstruction work was supported by Wellcome Trust Grant number 052185. Particular thanks are due to Julie Scarborough for all her help during the preparation of the manuscript.

Figure Legends

All times given are times after fertilization, not of gestation. For fetal material and embryos from older literature, Carnegie stages are not available. Ages are therefore estimated from lengths, and this is an inexact process.

Chapter 2

Physiology of the auditory and vestibular systems

A Palmer

Introduction

Within the inner ear, embedded in the temporal bone, are the organs of balance and gravity (the vestibular apparatus) and of hearing (the cochlea) as shown in Figure 2.1. The auditory and vestibular systems, along with several other sensory systems, share a common type of receptor cell: the hair cell. Within these various sensory systems, hair cells, by virtue of specialized accessory structures, are sensitive to sound, gravity, water, motion and acceleration. I begin with a description of the operation of the transduction processes (changing mechanical energy into an electrical signal) common to these hair cells and then elaborate on the accessory structures and the central pathways by which the information from auditory and vestibular systems is processed. In both auditory and vestibular systems impairments are often peripheral in origin (conductive and sensorineural) and often associated with vertigo. It is therefore appropriate to provide more detail for the periphery than for central processes.

Hair cell structure and function

Figure 2.2 shows an archetypal hair cell. The hair cell derives its name from the multiple extensions from its apical surface. The longest of these is the kinocilium, a true cilium with (9 + 2) structure. The other extensions (usually about 100 in number), which form several seried rows, are termed stereocilia, but are in fact modified microvilli packed with actin filaments. In both the auditory and vestibular systems there are two types of hair cell (I and II) as shown in Figure 2.2, which differ in shape and, at least in the auditory system, in function. The type I hair cells (inner hair cells in the cochlea) that are more flask-shaped are certainly sensory,

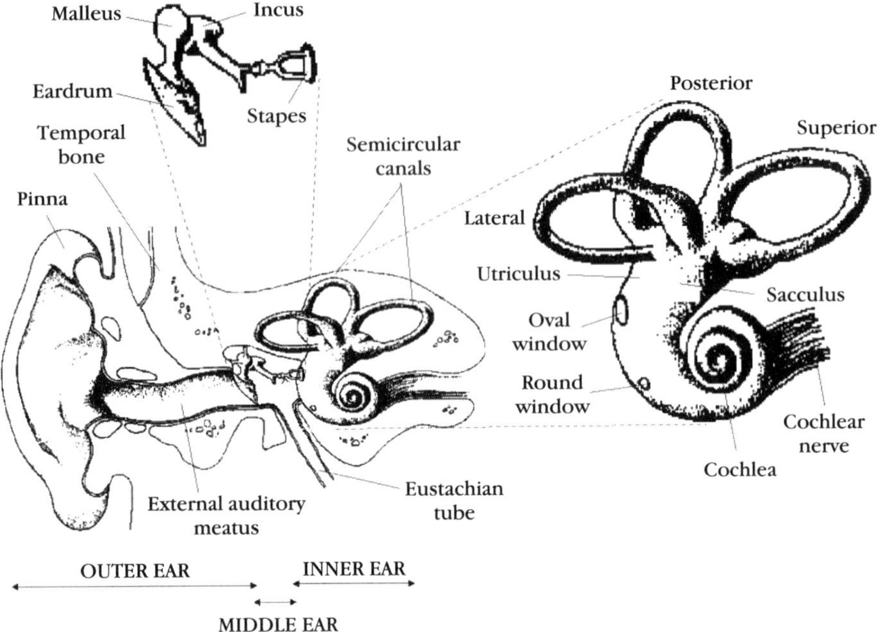

Figure 2.1. The human ear showing the organs of hearing (the cochlea), balance (the semicircular canals) and gravity (the utricle and saccule).

sending information in the form of a pattern of action potentials to the brain via the chemical synapse at their base. The type II hair cells in the cochlea are known as outer hair cells and appear to have a unique specialization that allows them to provide positive mechanical feedback (see later). Hair cells, like other neural cells, have a negative resting potential inside of the order of minus 45 to 60 mV as a result of the usual high-potassium, low-sodium ionic environment (Russell and Sellick, 1978).

The effective stimulus for a hair cell is a deflection of its stereocilia in a specific direction: deflection in the direction of the kinocilium depolarizes (the resting potential becomes less negative) the hair cell, while deflection in the opposite direction hyperpolarizes (the resting potential becomes more negative) the hair cell. Deflections across the line of the stereocilia rows are ineffective (Hudspeth and Corey, 1977). Hair cells in the cochlea lack a kinocilium, but are still directional. Indeed, the presence of the kinocilium is not necessary for hair cell function as it has been shown that the mechanical sensitivity of hair cells in the vestibular system is retained without deflection of the kinocilium (Hudspeth and Corey, 1977). The stereocilia are joined to each other by lateral links and by a link across

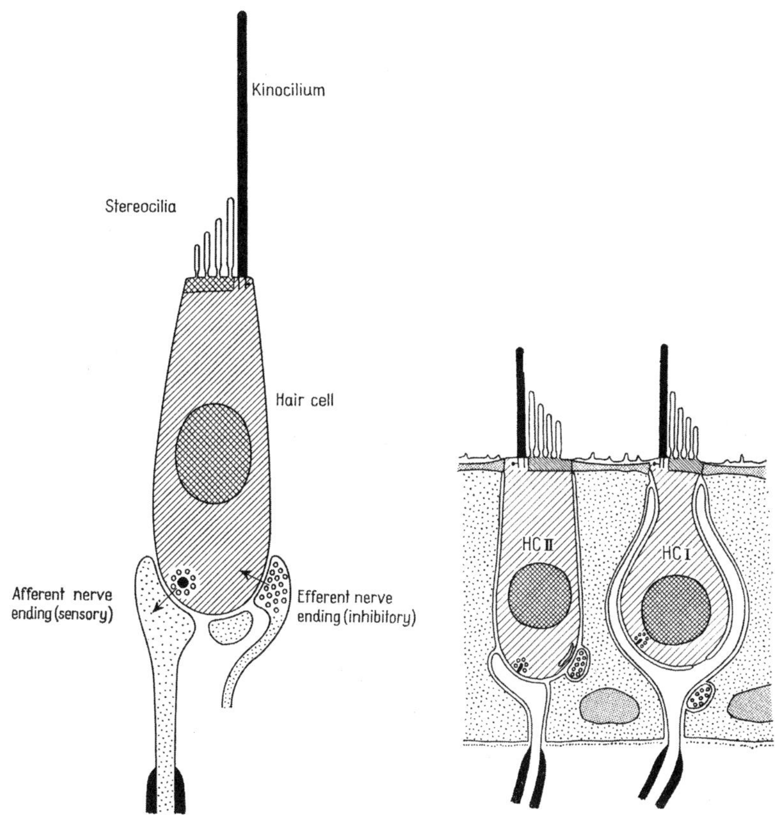

Figure 2.2. The archetypal hair cell. From Flock 1971 with permission.

their tips (the tip link: Figure 2.3), a fine flexible thread that extends from the tip of one stereocilium to the side of the next tallest stereocilium (Pickles, Comis and Osbourne, 1984).

The identification of the tip link led to the development of a model of how the hair cell might transduce the mechanical energy of sound into an electrical signal. The model assumes that a transducer channel sensitive to mechanical distortion is located at one or other end of the tip link. Tension on the tip link when stereocilia are deflected exerts force directly upon the transducer channel, increasing the probability that the transducer channel will be in the open state. Deflection of the stereocilia in the opposite direction increases the probability that the channel will be in the closed state. Auditory transduction needs to employ such direct gating of the transducer channel because auditory hair cells can respond to frequencies of 100 kHz more, which is far too fast for a second messenger to act.

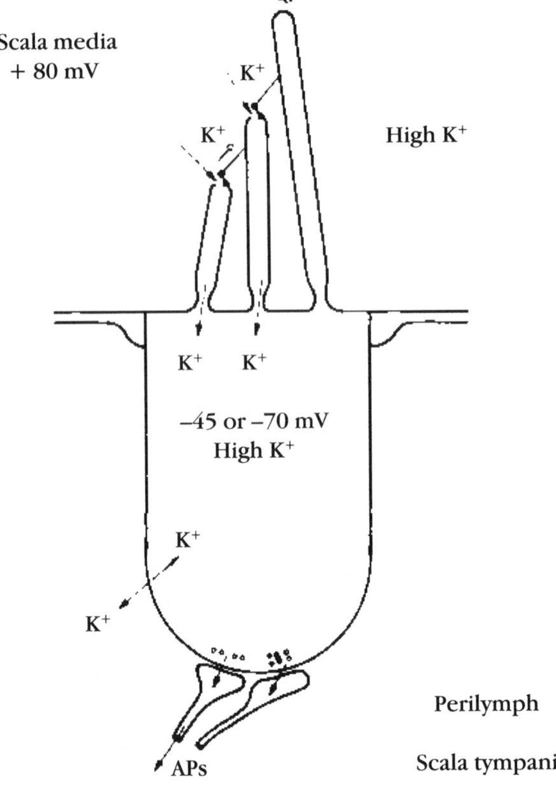

Figure 2.3. The tip link hypothesis of transduction. From Pickles 1988 with permission.

There are about 100 or so transducer channels on a single hair cell (probably one per stereocilium): the opening and closing of these transducer channels as the stereocilia are deflected back and forward causes modulation of the ionic current passing through the top of the hair cell, producing a change in the hair cell intracellular potential. The transducer channels are non-ion specific; however, the top of the hair cell is bathed in a very special fluid called the endolymph, which is akin to intracellular fluid (high potassium, low sodium; see Bosher and Warren, 1978) and the current that flows is therefore made up of potassium ions. The endolymph is produced by the vascular system of the inner ear (the stria vascularis) which contains electrogenic potassium/sodium pumps that not only maintain high potassium and low sodium but also generate a potential in the endolymph (the endolymphatic potential) of about +80 mV (Von Bekesy, 1960). Across the hair cell apical surface there is therefore a large ionic battery (+125 to +140 mV) due to the added effects of the endocochlear potential and the hair cell resting potential. This ionic battery ensures that potassium ions flow into the hair cell when the transducer channels open, despite the fact that the internal and external ionic milieu across the apical surface are similar. The base of the hair cell is bathed in perilymph (very similar to cerebro-spinal fluid) which has the high sodium/low potassium constitution of extracellular fluid and the potassium therefore flows out of the hair cells from the high concentration inside to the low concentration outside.

The model accounts for the asymmetric response to deflection of the stereocilia in opposite directions (larger depolarizations than hyperpolarizations) because only 5–15% of the channels are open in the resting position (Hudspeth and Corey, 1977). Thus, there are more channels available to be opened when the stereocilia are deflected from rest in an excitatory direction than are available to be closed when the stereocilia bundle is deflected in the opposite direction. We know practically nothing about the molecular basis of hair-cell transduction, although there is evidence that a myosin motor is involved in long-term adjustment of the tension of the tip link (Hudspeth and Gillespie, 1994; Solc et al., 1995). The 'tip link' model is widely accepted as the most likely mechanism for auditory transduction, although it has not yet been proven (Hudspeth and Gillespie, 1994).

Depolarization of the hair cell activates voltage-dependent calcium channels in the basolateral membrane of the hair cell increasing the intracellular calcium and resulting in a release of neurotransmitter from the synapse at the hair-cell base, triggering neural action potentials in the afferent neurone. A detailed treatment of the transducer action of cochlear hair cells may be found in Kros (1996).

The auditory system

Transmission of sound to the cochlea

Figure 2.1 illustrates the peripheral parts of the auditory system. The stimuli for the auditory system are vibrations in air, which consist of rapid fluctuations in the pressure above and below atmospheric pressure. These vibrations are channelled into the hearing apparatus via the pinna, external auditory meatus and middle ear. These structures each have characteristic transmission properties that shape the spectrum of the sound in ways that often provide additional perceptual cues. The pinna, for example, alters the spectrum of the sound giving peaks and notches that can be used to determine the sound source elevation (Shaw, 1974; Gardner and Gardner, 1973). The external meatus is a long canal that acts as a tube resonator and, in humans, enhances the amplitudes of sounds of

2 to 4 kHz by 10–20 dB (Shaw, 1974). Sound causes the eardrum (tympanic membrane) to vibrate and this vibration is transmitted to the inner ear via the three small bones (the middle-ear ossicles) that traverse the air-filled middle-ear cavity (the bulla): the malleus, connected to the tympanic membrane, the incus, and the stapes, which inserts into the oval window of the inner ear. The middle-ear cavity is maintained at atmospheric pressure by periodic opening of the Eustachian tube, which connects the middle-ear cavity to the pharynx.

The acoustic impedance of the inner-ear fluids at the oval window is much greater than the impedance of the air. Without some means of matching these acoustic impedances the transmission of sound energy into the inner ear would be very inefficient and most of the energy would be reflected back out again. The middle ear acts as a pressure amplifier and produces a good impedance match and hence efficient transfer of sound energy into the inner ear. This is achieved in three ways. The major contribution arises because the tympanic membrane has a much greater area than the oval window of the inner ear, allowing force to be collected over a wide area and delivered to a small area thus increasing the applied pressure by about 35 times. Further pressure amplification is provided by the lever action, which results from different lengths of the ossicles (1.15x) and by deformation or buckling of the tympanic membrane (2x). Other factors also influence the transmission of sound through the middle ear, and the efficiency of transmission at different frequencies is a major factor shaping the audiogram (see Pickles 1988 for detailed discussion).

Contraction of muscles that connect the malleus and stapes to the middle-ear wall stiffen the ossicular chain reducing the energy transmission. When these muscles are activated by sound it is known as the middle-ear reflex. This reflex may protect the ear against very loud sounds, reduce the interfering effects of internally generated sounds or enhance the detectability of high frequencies (Wever and Vernon, 1955; Zakrisson and Borg, 1974).

Cochlear function

The vibration of the middle-ear ossicles efficiently transfers the airborne pressure variations at the tympanic membrane to the fluids of the inner ear via the oval window at the base of the cochlea. The cochlea consists of a bony tube spiralling around a central core (the modiolus) divided by a central partition (the basilar membrane) along its length. The spiral shape appears to have no functional significance other than keeping the space occupied by the relatively long cochlear duct (30 mm) at a minimum.

The basilar membrane becomes progressively wider along the length of the cochlear duct from the base to the apex. With other differences along the length of the cochlea, this leads to a systematic variation in stiffness of the basilar membrane. Increases in pressure at the oval window cause the round window (which opens directly into the bulla) to move out and decreasing pressure causes it to move in. These alternating pressures across the basilar membrane move it up and down producing a wave-like motion (a travelling wave) which appears to move from the base toward the apex of the cochlea. The passive mechanical properties of the basilar membrane, especially its stiffness gradient, lead to a peak in the amplitude of its vibration occurring near the base of the cochlea for high-frequency sounds, and moving progressively toward the apex for lower-frequency sounds (Von Bekesy, 1960).

The spatial separation of the vibration patterns of the basilar membrane to different frequencies means that the basilar membrane is performing a passive filtering action that can still be measured *post mortem*. However, the most recent measurements of the basilar membrane in living mammals reveal that the range of frequencies causing a particular part of the basilar membrane to vibrate is much narrower, and the vibration amplitude is higher, than can be accounted for by its passive mechanical properties. This suggests that the minute motions of the basilar membrane are locally amplified by some form of active feedback process (see Patuzzi, 1996 for review). A manifestation of the active amplification of the basilar membrane motion is the generation of sound by the organ of Corti, which can be measured using a microphone in the ear canal (otoacoustic emissions; Kemp, 1978). Otoacoustic emissions are used to assess cochlear function because they appear to reflect outer hair-cell activity in a place-specific manner.

A cross-section of the cochlear duct is shown in Figure 2.4a in which it can be seen that, in addition to the basilar membrane, a second membrane (Reissner's membrane) along the length of the cochlea divides the duct into three chambers. This membrane has no mechanical significance but acts as an ionic barrier because the upper and lower chambers (the scala tympani and scala vestibuli, Figure 2.4a) are filled with perilymph whereas the middle chamber (the scala media, Figure 2.4a) is filled with endolymph. On top of the basilar membrane along its length is the organ of Corti that contains the auditory hair cells arranged in four rows topped by the gelatinous tectorial membrane (Figure 2.4b).

In the cochlea there is a single row of inner hair cells (type I) and three rows of outer hair cells (type II). The flask-shaped inner hair cells are surrounded by supporting cells, and are the primary receptor cells; they receive 90–95% of the afferent innervation of the cochlea (Spoendlin, 1972) and so account for most of the activity of the cochlear nerve. Each inner hair cell is contacted by 15 to 20 auditory nerve fibres. The outer hair cells are long and cylindrical in shape, with their lateral walls contacting fluid-filled Nuel spaces. Most of the innervation of outer hair cells is efferent. Sound-induced vibration of the basilar membrane causes a radial shearing motion between the tops of the hair cells and the tectorial membrane, which in turn deflects the stereocilia. The hair cells are oriented so that the most sensitive direction of stereocilia deflection is in the radial direction of the shearing motion.

Currently the active mechanical feedback to the basilar membrane is thought to be from shape changes of the outer hair cells acting as a motor. Outer hair cells isolated *in vitro* change their length in response to electrical stimulation (Brownell et al., 1985) and can also respond to changes within the cochlea caused by sound stimuli by contracting and expanding *in vivo.* These length changes are very rapid (Gale and Ashmore, 1997) and are thought to augment the movement of the basilar membrane on a cycle-by-cycle basis. The enhanced movement of the basilar membrane occurs only over very restricted spatial regions and, being an active process, is highly susceptible to disruption. Loss of the motor function of the outer hair cells is thought to be the common factor in sensorineural hearing impairments with a variety of aetiologies (Patuzzi, Yates and Johnstone, 1989a). Exactly what causes the outer hair cell to change length *in vivo* is not known, and could be mechanical, electrical or chemical changes that occur initially in response to the passive movement of the basilar membrane. The motor that drives this length change is known to be located in the lateral cell membrane, but the identity of the motor molecule is not known.

The structure of the organ of Corti (Figure 2.4b) appears to be specially designed to transmit tiny vibrations of the basilar membrane to the tops of the hair cells with the minimum of losses through absorption by flexible components.

Sharp intracellular microelectrode studies of the responses of cochlear hair cells to tone stimuli have been made *in vivo.* These have revealed that inner hair cells respond to a tonal stimulus with an oscillating potential that follows the low-frequency tone waveforms and a steady potential that lasts for the tone duration (Russell and Sellick, 1978). The steady potential change results from asymmetrical responses to deflection of the stereocilia and, at higher frequencies, is the only component measured (due to the low-pass filtering action of the hair cell membranes). Inner hair cell responses vary between the base and apex of the cochlea, with the oscillating component of the response predominating in apical hair cells, whereas the steady component is the major component in basal inner hair cells (Russell and Sellick, 1978; Cheatham and Dallos, 1993). The oscillating and steady voltage responses in outer hair cells are smaller than in inner hair cells. The voltages measured in both inner and outer hair cells in a healthy *in vivo* preparation, whether steady or oscillating, are as sharply tuned as the vibration pattern of the basilar membrane. A gross electrode placed on, or near, the round window of the cochlea (as in electrocochleography) records several different responses simultaneously: the compound action potential (CAP), the summating potential (SP) and the cochlear microphonic (CM). The SP is the gross correlate of the hair-cell receptor potential change during stimulation (Dallos, Schoeny and Cheatham, 1972). The CAP is the summed activity of the initial, highly synchronized discharges of the auditory nerve fibres. The CM exactly reproduces the waveform of the sound and is thought to represent the summed oscillating receptor potentials of the outer hair cells. The cochlear microphonics recorded from the round window reflect local basal turn outer-hair-cell activity (Dallos and Cheatham, 1976; Patuzzi, Yates and Johnstone, 1989b).

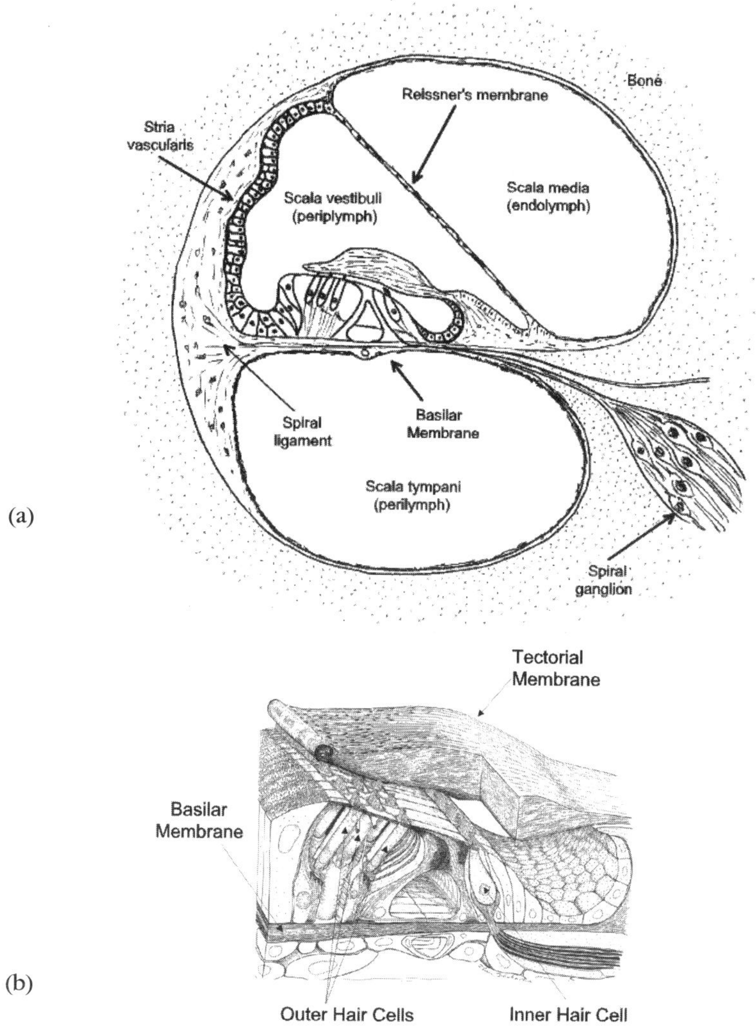

Figure 2.4. (a) Cross section of the cochlear duct. (b) The organ of Corti. From Takasaka 1993 with permission.

The central auditory system

The voltages generated inside the inner hair cells, which are as sharply tuned as the basilar membrane vibration, are responsible for increasing the probability of release of transmitter from the base of the cell into the synaptic cleft, eventually initiating an action potential in the afferent neurone. Inner hair cells connect via the synapses at their base with the dendrites of bipolar spiral ganglion neurones situated in the modiolus at the centre of the cochlea. The axons of these neurones (about 30000 in man) form the auditory nerve that projects to the central nervous system and terminates in the cochlear nucleus in the brainstem (see Figure 2.5). All auditory information passes through this nerve, the responses of individual fibres of which have been extensively studied (see for example Kiang et al., 1965). Auditory nerve fibre responses are stereotypical and relatively simple: each fibre has a rate of spontaneous activity (SR) in the absence of sound (from 0 to over 100 spikes/second) that is increased by sound stimulation of appropriate frequency and level. No inhibitory responses are seen at the auditory-nerve level, but effects reflecting mechanical events in the cochlear may lead to suppression of responses when more than one frequency component is present (Arthur, Pfeiffer and Suga, 1971).

Auditory-nerve fibre responses are as sharply tuned as the basilar membrane vibration pattern and the hair cell voltage responses. The frequency of the lowest threshold is known as the characteristic or best frequency of an individual neurone and reflects the position of its connection to a hair cell along the length of the basilar membrane (Liberman, 1982). A sample of 10 auditory nerve fibre frequency responses are shown in Figure 2.6: such curves are variously known as tuning curves or frequency threshold curves and trace out the limits of frequency and sound level that evoke activity from a single nerve fibre.

Frequency discrimination (hearing the frequency difference between sequentially heard sounds) depends upon the very sharp high-frequency edge of the fibre response areas whereas frequency selectivity (separation of simultaneously present frequency components) depends on the width of the response areas. The sharply tuned region of the nerve fibre response is critically dependent on the active processes that permit sharp basilar membrane tuning, and these are highly susceptible to trauma: the loss of this sharply tuned tip is a common characteristic of sensorineural hearing impairment. The auditory nerve can be thought of as a bank of narrow filters that overlap extensively, spanning the whole hearing range of the animal. The minimum thresholds (at the tuning curve tips) of the most sensitive fibres (high SR) match the behavioural audiogram. Many characteristics of auditory nerve fibre responses are correlated with their SR despite the fact that it appears that both high and low SR fibres appear to derive from the same hair cells: low (<0.5 spikes/second) and medium

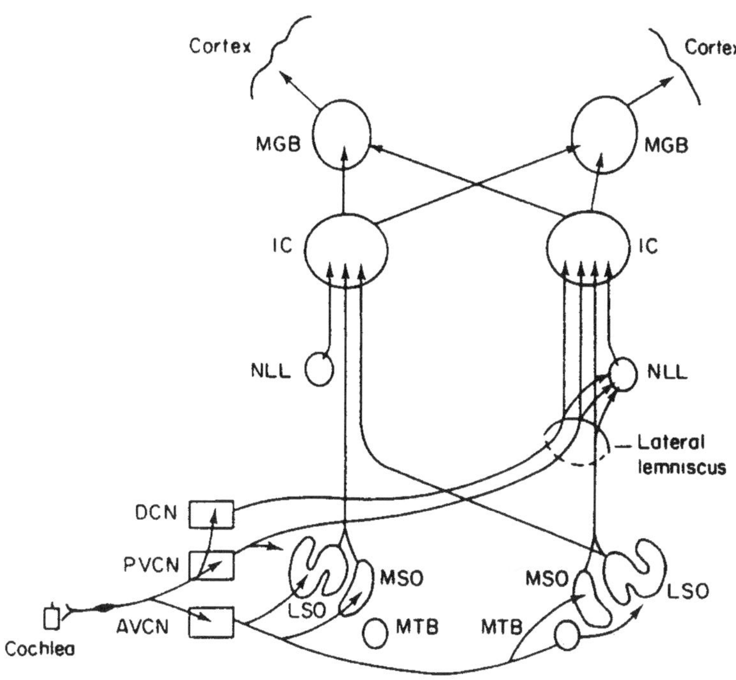

Figure 2.5. The auditory pathway. MGB medial geniculate body, IC inferior colliculus, NLL nucleus of the lateral lemniscus, DCN dorsal cochlear nucleus, PVCN posteroventral cochlear nucleus, AVCN anteroventral cochlear nucleus, LSO lateral superior olive, MSO medial superior olive, MTB medial nucleus of the trapezoid body. From Pickles 1988 with permission.

(0.5 to 18 spikes/second) rates are recorded from thin fibres contacting the modiolar side of inner hair cells, whereas high rates are associated with fibres contacting the side nearest the outer hair cells (Liberman, 1982). Thus, for example, high SR fibres are the most sensitive, low SR fibres are the least sensitive and medium fibres are in between.

As the levels of sounds are raised the discharge rate of auditory nerve fibres increases and in the case of the majority of nerve fibres saturates within about 40–50 dB of threshold (termed the dynamic range). The shape of this rate-versus-level function for high SR fibres is sigmoid, whereas low and medium SR fibres exhibit more extended dynamic ranges. One model for how the auditory system operates over a very extended range of sound level involves optimal combination of the level information provided by fibres with different thresholds and dynamic ranges (for more detailed discussion see Palmer, 1995).

At least two different temporal aspects of nerve fibre discharge are important in shaping the patterns of activity that are sent to the central

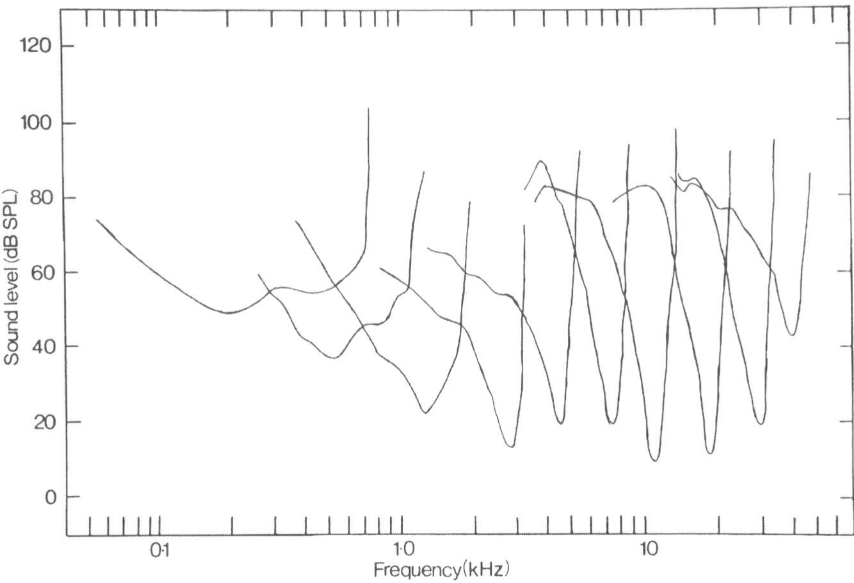

Figure 2.6. Frequency threshold curves from ten nerve fibres in the cat auditory nerve. From Palmer 1987 with permission.

nervous system. The first is a gradual decrease in discharge rate most prominent over the first tens of milliseconds of activation, which is termed *adaptation,* and reflects events occurring at the hair cell synapse (Smith, 1979). The second is a preferred time of occurrence of discharges at discrete phases of low-frequency waveforms. This is termed *phase locking* and enables the waveform of low-frequency sounds (below about 5 kHz in mammals) to be signalled in the fine timing of auditory-nerve fibre discharges (Kiang et al., 1965, Rose et al., 1967). Phase locking is absolutely essential in localizing low-frequency sounds (see below) and may be important in signalling the detailed spectra of complex sounds.

All fibres of the auditory nerve terminate in the cochlear nucleus of the brainstem where the information is reprocessed and passed to higher brain centres via several parallel output pathways, which appear to serve different hearing functions as illustrated schematically in Figure 2.7. The pattern of termination in the cochlear nucleus, and indeed in all other nuclei of the ascending auditory pathway through the brainstem, thalamus and cortex, is ordered according to the origin within the cochlea thus creating a cochleotopic organization spatially across every nucleus (see Merzenich et al., 1977). In most mammals this corresponds to a progressive increase in frequency so it is often known as a *tonotopic organization.*

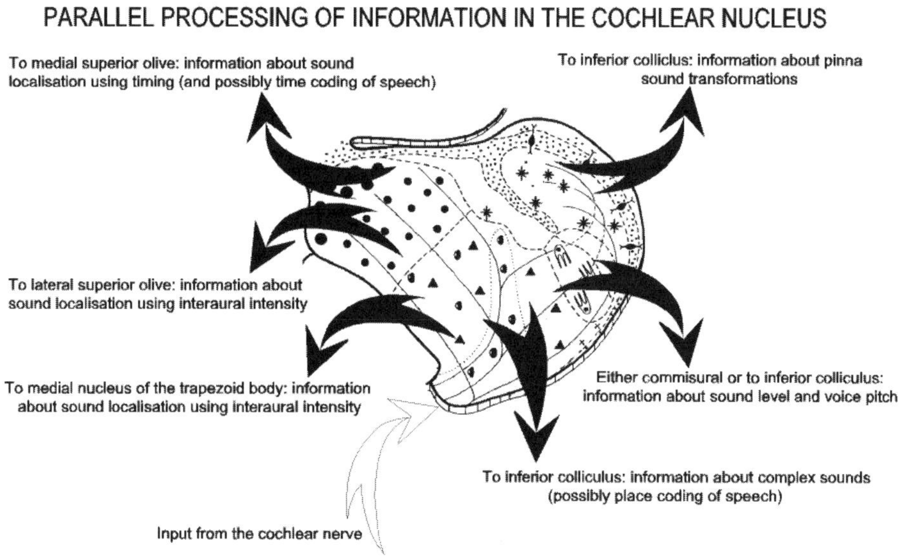

Figure 2.7. The output pathways of the cochlear nucleus complex. Modified from Osen and Roth (1969) with permission.

All aspects of the discharge patterns of auditory neurones show greater variation in central nuclei than in the auditory nerve, often as a result of widespread inhibitory effects. Thus, although sigmoid rate-versus-level functions are found in central nuclei, there is a progressive increase in the proportion and magnitude of non-monotonic rate-versus-level functions (functions that, after an increase to a peak, then decrease with further increase of stimulus level). Phase locking is found at all levels but there is a progressive lowering of the highest frequency at which it occurs to a few hundreds of Hz in the midbrain to a few tens of Hz at the cortex. The simple adaptation pattern of the auditory nerve is also found in central nuclei but more commonly there are temporal discharge patterns in which there is evidence of temporal interplay of excitation and inhibition or only a response to the stimulus onset or offset or both. The discharge characteristics of central neurones are determined by the nature of their input, their intrinsic biophysical properties and their interconnections with other neurones whether excitatory or inhibitory. For a detailed review of central processing see Palmer (1995).

Figure 2.7 shows a highly schematized version of the possible roles for the various output pathways of the cochlear nucleus, which is consistent with much of our current knowledge. Note that four of these pathways seem to be involved in the localization of sounds. The pathway from the dorsal division to the inferior colliculus in animals probably has a role in compensating for pinna and head position. The dorsal division of the cochlear nucleus in man is not so obviously laminar in structure as in other animals and this may reflect the fact that we have an immobile pinna: head and neck position information are still, however, necessary. The pathways from the ventral division of the cochlear nucleus to the superior olivary nuclei in the centre of the brainstem are all high fidelity pathways that preserve the accuracy of individual discharge timings (and hence phase locking). This is essential because in the superior olivary nuclei the signals from both ears are combined.

Cells in the superior olive act as coincidence detectors that transform differences in the time of arrival of discharges from the two ears into a discharge rate code. As a result, sensitivity to interaural time differences (as generated by the spatial position of low-frequency sound sources) is of the order of tens of microseconds. Cells in the lateral superior olive receive the input from one ear via an inhibitory relay, which makes them very sensitive to the difference in the level of the signals at the two ears (a cue for the spatial position of high-frequency sounds). In man, the lateral superior olive is reduced or absent and the medial superior presumably takes its functions. The combined information from the two ears is sent to the inferior colliculus and other higher order nuclei. The remaining pathways from the cochlear nucleus directly to the inferior colliculus, based on their properties, seem most likely to transmit information more specifically about characteristics of complex sounds such as their pitch and spectrum.

All nuclei from the brainstem send inputs to the auditory midbrain nucleus (the inferior colliculus). This provides an ideal opportunity for information such as the spatial position and spectral characteristics to be recombined in various ways. In fact, there are only a few clear examples of emergent properties at the level of the inferior colliculus: most responses such as rate-level responses and frequency and binaural sensitivity seem to be reflections of brainstem processing with the addition of intrinsic membrane properties. One of the most exciting of these emergent properties is the apparent formation of a topographical representation within each iso-frequency sheet of sound modulation frequency.

Neurones at and below the inferior colliculus respond best to a particular modulation frequency. Within the inferior colliculus these best modulation frequencies appear to be arranged in contour-like fashion (Schreiner and Langner, 1988). Such an organization has obvious applications to pitch detection. Surprisingly perhaps, this form of organization is not found above the inferior colliculus in the thalamus and cortex.

A second emergent feature at the inferior colliculus is to the direction of sound source motion (Spitzer and Semple, 1993). This asymmetry in the response to motion in one direction compared to the opposite is also found (possibly more pronounced) at higher levels. For a detailed account of inferior colliculus functional physiology see Irvine (1986) and Caird (1991).

The core projection of the auditory pathway is from the central nucleus of the inferior colliculus, through the ventral nucleus of the medial geniculate body of the thalamus to the primary auditory cortex. In general the responses within this projection are crisp, short latency and sharply tuned. A belt projection from nuclei that surround the inferior colliculus via the medial and dorsal thalamus innervates secondary and belt regions of the auditory cortex. Responses in these belt projection nuclei are less reliable, may be multi-modal, tend to habituate and have long latencies.

The auditory cortex consists of a primary field and a secondary field surrounded by various other secondary fields. Despite detailed study, a full understanding of the processing that requires the auditory cortex is eluding us. Certainly, sensitivity to various aspects of sounds has been sought and found, however, it has not yet been possible to attribute specific functions to these different fields, even though there is topographical organization with respect to a range of stimulus parameters in the primary auditory field (minimum threshold, sharpness of tuning, asymmetry of inhibitory areas and so forth) and the different fields have different rate-level functions, modulation sensitivities and responses to complex sounds (see for review Ehret, 1997).

The overriding impression is currently that neurones are rarely uniquely selective for identifiable features of complex sounds, even when ecologically significant sounds such as species specific calls are used. However, in the bat, a highly specialized animal, specific functions associated with echolocation can be attributed to several secondary cortical areas (Suga, 1988). Recently, it has been suggested that the organization of the auditory cortex may be similar to that of vision in having relatively simple responses in primary auditory cortex and processing more complex sounds in higher order secondary areas (Rauschecker,1998). However, it should be remembered that with the plethora of different processing nuclei in the pathway to the auditory cortex audition might be quite different from vision, which reaches the cortex after only the thalamic synapses. Lesion studies in animals in which the auditory cortex was completely removed did not result in deafness – indeed, it required subtle testing to establish that performance was not completely unaffected. The advent of techniques such as imaging and multiple neuronal recording seem set to advance our knowledge of the cortex rapidly in the next few years.

The vestibular system

The vestibular system is situated in the inner ear and consists of the balance organs (the three semicircular canals) and the gravity organs (the utricle and saccule). Many of the functions of the vestibular organs are accomplished without conscious involvement, such as the reflex adjustment of muscles in the limbs and neck to maintain an upright posture and to keep the head in a vertical position. Another automatic function involves sending signals to the oculomotor system to stabilize the eyes during head movements and thereby to reduce the movement of images of stationary objects on the retina. One function we are aware of is in maintaining balance and providing the sensation of motion and spatial position.

The most comprehensive review of all aspects of vestibular structure and function is still to be found in the somewhat dated Kornhuber (1974).

The semicircular canals

The semicircular canals provide dynamic information about movement (angular acceleration) of the head in three dimensions which allows control of the eye position. To fulfil this function there are three canals in each ear, oriented in planes that are approximately perpendicular to each other (posterior, superior and lateral see Figure 2.1). The canals are filled with endolymph as is the whole of the membranous labyrinth that makes up the inner ear. The loops of the semicircular canals begin and end in the utricle and at one end of each is an enlargement known as the ampulla within which is situated the crista containing the sensory epithelium. The sensory epithelium contains the hair cells whose 'hairs' insert into a gelatinous membrane called the cupula (as shown in Figure 2.8), which tops their apical surfaces and extends completely across the ampulla. The physical characteristics of the semicircular canal end organ are matched to the likely patterns of head movement experienced by the animal (Melville-Jones, 1974).

At rest the fibres from the bases of the semicircular canals hair cells exhibit very high rates of spontaneous discharge that can be up to 200 spikes/second but on average are about 100 spikes/ second (Goldberg and Fernandez, 1971). The fibres fall into two classes with either regular or irregular spontaneous activity, which is correlated with other response properties such as sensitivity (Fernandez and Goldberg, 1971). All of the hair cells in a single ampulla are oriented in the same direction, such that in the lateral canal bending of the hairs toward the utricle is excitatory producing an increase in the discharge rate, whereas in the superior and posterior canals bending away from the utricle is excitatory (Lowenstein and Sand, 1940a; Szentagothai, 1950; Goldberg and Fernandez, 1971).

The displacement of the cupula and hence the stereocilia, as a result of movements of the fluids in the canals, is the effective stimulus for the semicircular canal hair cells. This action comes about because there is very little flow of fluid past the cupula. When the head is rotated the cupula bends over (like a swing door) due to displacement of the endolymph by a combination of inertial and viscous forces. When the head begins to move (accelerates) the inertia and viscosity of the endolymph causes it to push against and bend the cupula. When the rotation is maintained at a constant velocity, elastic restoring forces return the cupula to its rest position by pushing the endolymph through the canal against the viscous forces (over tens of seconds; see Lowenstein and Sand, 1940b). Constant rotational velocity of the head is not a common situation and in fact the semicircular canal output firing rate signals the instantaneous velocity rather than the acceleration per se (Fernandez and Goldberg, 1971; Melville-Jones, 1974).

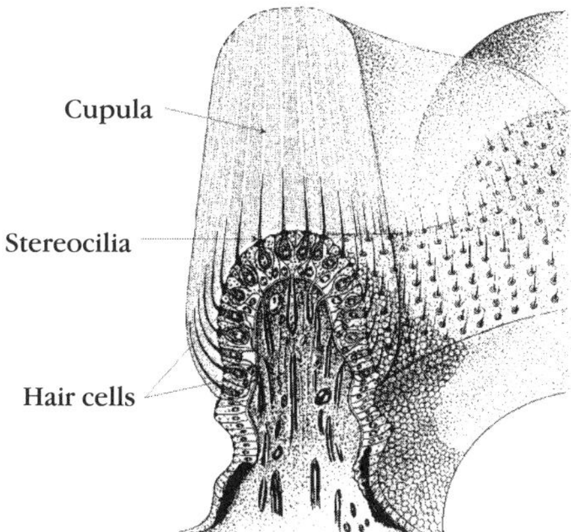

Figure 2.8. The crista and cupula from a single semicircular canal showing the insertion of the stereocilia. From Flock 1971 with permission.

The vestibular apparatus is extremely sensitive, responding at threshold to angular displacements of the cupula of the order of one thousandth of a degree (Melville-Jones and Milsum, 1971; Melville-Jones, 1974). Linear accelerations are not effective in stimulating the canal hair cells because the inertial forces at all points in the endolymph will be equal and in the same direction thus producing no net flow through the canals.

The canals in the two ears make up functional pairs. This is most easily appreciated when considering the lateral semicircular canals that most obviously lie in the same plane. Rotation of the head will cause the endolymph in the lateral canal of one side to flow toward the utricle thereby producing excitation of the hair cells, while simultaneously producing flow away from the utricle on the other side and reducing the activity on that side. The posterior canals form functional pairs with the superior canals on the other side. The brain thus receives complementary signals that the head has moved. The horizontal canals do not respond to rotation about the longitudinal or transverse planes whereas the other canals respond to the resultant vector of movements in all three planes (Lowenstein and Sand, 1940b).

The otolith organs

The otolith organs provide static information about the absolute position of the head in space, which is used to adjust posture. In both the utricle and the saccule there is a thickened area of the wall that is termed the macula and, like the crista of the semicircular canals, contains the sensory epithelia with hair cells. As shown in Figure 2.9, the maculae in both utricle and saccule are covered with a gelatinous membrane known as the otolith into which are embedded crystals of calcium carbonate (otoconia). The macula of the utricle lies approximately in the horizontal plane, whereas that of the saccule is in the saggital plane.

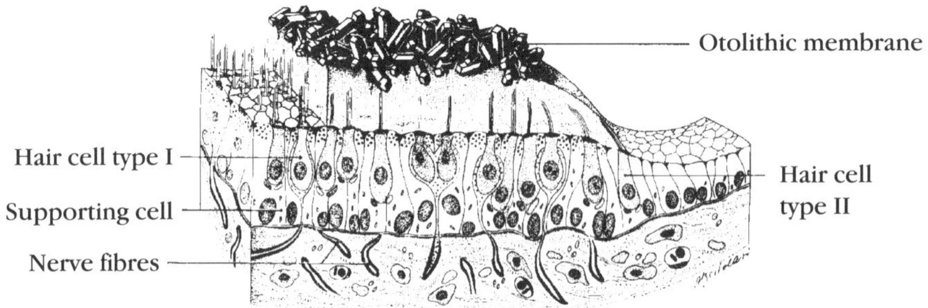

Figure 2.9. A cross section of an otolith organ showing the insertion of the hair cells into the otolith. From Flock 1971 with permission.

When the head is erect the otoliths bear directly down on the hair cells of the utricular macula and therefore do not generate bending or deflection of the stereocilia. Tilting of the head in any direction causes displacement of the otolith under the influence of gravity. This in turn produces a deflection of the stereocilia and an activation of the hair cells. Obviously, the effect of the deflection on the hair cell responses depends upon the orientation of the deflection with respect to the functional polarization of the hair cell. In both utricle and saccule the hair cells are arranged in a very precise topography (Spoendlin, 1966). This is illustrated in Figure 2.10 for both the utricle (2.10a) and saccule (2.10b).

The polarization of all hair cells in the utricular and saccular maculae is oriented towards a marked feature called the striola, which forms a curving border across the middle of the macula. Because of this orientation toward the striola and the fact that the striola curves round through at least 90 degrees, there are hair cells with all possible polarizations and head tilt in any direction will produce characteristic patterns of activity with the discharge from some hair cells increased and from others reduced. Because of the mass of the otolith any acceleration will leave the otolith behind due to inertia and this imbues the otolith organs with sensitivity to linear acceleration: the saccule is sensitive to vertically directed head acceleration. The orthogonal orientation of the two maculae provides information about the direction of the acceleration.

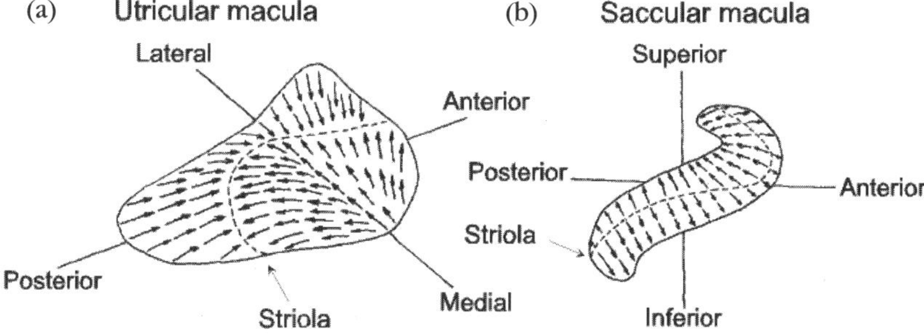

Figure 2.10. (a) Orientation of hair cell polarizations in the utricular macula. (b) Orientation of the hair cell polarisations in the saccular macula. Modified from Spoendlin 1966.

The central vestibular system

All five of the hair cell epithelia in the vestibular system have cell bodies in the vestibular ganglion (Scarpa's ganglion), which is situated near the internal auditory meatus, giving rise to about 20 000 fibres in each vestibular nerve (Rasmussen, 1940). As in the spiral ganglion of the cochlea, these cells are bipolar. The synapses at the base of the vestibular hair cells project to cell bodies in Scarpa's ganglion, and the centrally directed axons project to the vestibular nucleus in the brainstem via the eighth cranial nerve.

The vestibular nucleus consists of four parts: the lateral nucleus, the medial nucleus, the superior nucleus and the inferior nucleus, situated in the brainstem below the floor of the fourth ventricle (see Brodal, 1981 for details of the anatomy). Reflexes that adjust the neck and limb muscles to maintain posture depend primarily on the otolith input, whereas the semicircular canal input is primarily concerned with adjustment of the neck and ocular muscles in the cordination of eye movement with head movement.

The lateral nucleus receives input ventrally from the utricular macular and from the semicircular canals and is a relay for information to the motor centres controlling the eye muscles for the oculomotor reflex and for the limbs and neck muscles for postural control. Input to all parts of the spinal cord from the lateral nucleus is via the lateral vestibulospinal tract, which directly affects the motor neurones supplying the upper and lower limbs (facilitating extensors and inhibiting flexors). The medial and superior nuclei also contribute to the oculomotor reflex and receive input from the semicircular canals. The output from the medial and superior nuclei also contributes to descending pathways to the spinal cord particularly to the neck region via the medial vestibulospinal tracts. This again is part of the reflex that maintains the stability of the retinal image despite movements of the head.

The pathway for controlling the eye position consists of the input from the semicircular canals to the ocular motoneurones via the vestibular nucleus. The eye is moved by only six muscles and the vestibular input acts in a complementary fashion on pairs of these muscles to move the eye (inhibiting one and exciting the other). When the head is moved, the semicircular canals detect this movement and induce an opposite movement of the eyes of the same velocity. While the vestibulo-ocular reflex is continually active it can be switched off voluntarily. The overall sensitivity of the vestibulo-ocular reflex is modulated by input from the cerebellum (Robinson, 1976).

The inferior nucleus receives both otolith and semicircular canal input and its output contributes to both descending systems to the spinal cord for the control of posture and to projections to rostral areas involved in eye position control.

Summary

As a result of a variety of sophisticated accessory structures the auditory and vestibular systems provide sensitivity to a variety of sensory modalities using only a single receptor type: the hair cell. The activation of the hair cell in all cases is achieved by deflection of their stereocilia. The external and middle ears ensure the most efficient transmission of sound energy into the cochlear fluids, whereupon the combination of the structural specializations of the basilar membrane and the motor action of the outer hair cells break up the sound into frequency specific channels. The inner hair cells signal this information to the central nervous system via the cochlear nucleus, which routes information into parallel pathways for further analysis.

In the vestibular system the high rates of spontaneous discharge of the neurones contacting the hair cells provides the possibility of a positive and a negative modulation providing information to the central nervous system. Additionally, the paired semicircular canal inputs from the two sides and the orthogonal arrangement of the otolith organs means that complementary and rich information will reach the central processors whenever the head undergoes angular or linear acceleration. This information is crucial both for maintaining posture via spinal reflex pathways and for stabilizing the visual scene.

CHAPTER 3

Radiological abnormalities of the ear

P PHELPS

Introduction

The management of the hearing-impaired child usually needs imaging of the petrous temporal bone at some stage unless the impairment is conductive and temporary, as from serous otitis media. The advances in computerized imaging that have occurred in the past few years have found many applications in paediatric otolaryngology. The principles of technique that apply to imaging in adults apply equally to the demonstration of head and neck lesions in infants and children. Optimal spatial and density resolution with lowest possible level of patient irradiation and freedom from movement artefacts must be achieved. Limitation of the dose of radiation is particularly important in this age group, and minimal patient movement is hard to obtain.

The middle and inner ears are fully developed at birth, but the temporomandibular joint, external auditory canal (EAC), and mastoid process are not. Post-natal changes in the temporal bone consist of growth and pneumatization of the mastoid process and alteration in the shape of the tympanic ring. Prior to full ossification of the petrous pyramid, the dense bone of the labyrinthine capsule can be clearly identified by plain mastoid views, thus enabling gross developmental abnormalities to be identified without the need for sectional imaging (Figure 3.1). In the middle ear, the ossicles can be shown and, in the neonate, even marrow spaces within them. The mastoid antrum is fully developed at birth but further pneumatization posteriorly occurs only during the first decade of life with the development of the mastoid process. It is not yet clear how much the variable extent of this pneumatization is due to genetic factors or to interference by disease processes such as otitis media. Plain (x-ray) lateral oblique mastoid views show the extent of pneumatization (Figure 3.2), which some

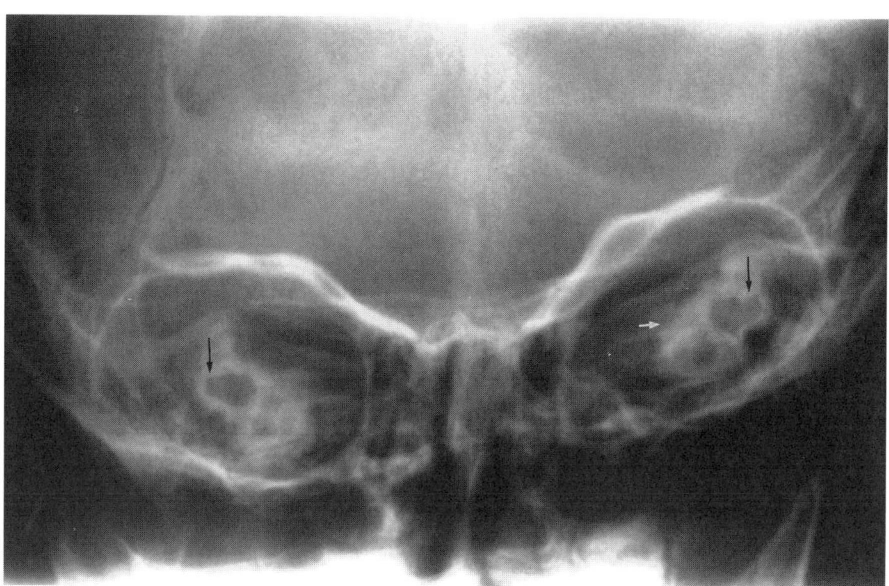

Figure 3.1. Plain perorbital view of congenital deformity of the ear. The black arrows indicate dysplastic lateral semicircular canals. The white arrow shows a narrow internal auditory meatus on one side. Note the normal cochleae.

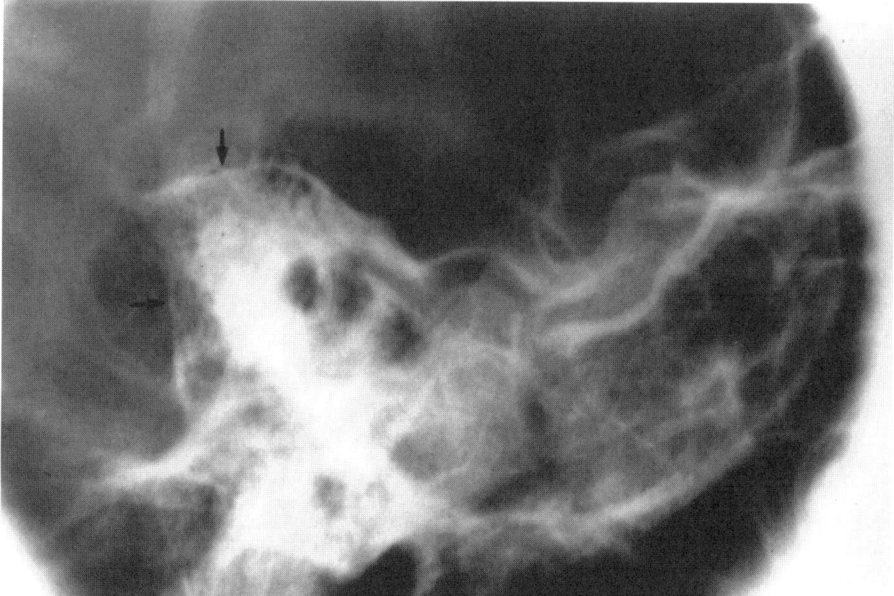

Figure 3.2. Tilted lateral view of the mastoid. The arrows point to the dural and sigmoid sinus plates.

surgeons prefer for pre-operative assessment. Pneumatization can also be assessed by plain skull views, but x-ray examinations are rarely indicated, are inferior to computed tomography (CT) and are no substitute for adequate clinical assessment of the eardrum in inflammatory ear disease.

Computed tomography is now the imaging investigation of choice in most cases because of short scan times, excellent bone detail, and better outlining of soft tissue abnormalities. Only from the point of view of tissue characterization has CT been disappointing and measurements of x-ray attenuation have only a very limited role, for example, for bone dysplasias such as otosclerosis. Careful consideration must always be given to the amount of radiation, especially to the eyes, which should be kept clear of the direct beam whenever possible.

Absence of radiation and some tissue characterization make magnetic resonance imaging (MRI) best for the paediatric age group, although difficulties may occur when there is need for sedation or general anaesthesia. Lack of signal from bone is both a disadvantage and advantage. Because both air and cortical bone appear black on MRI they cannot be distinguished. Generally speaking, MRI does not demonstrate the middle-ear cleft unless it is filled with fluid. Although absence of bony landmarks is therefore a problem, it does mean that soft tissue entities and both normal and pathologic fluids are demonstrated clearly. New MRI techniques such as fast spin echo (FSE) and three-dimensional Fourier transform (3DFT) allow thinner sections to be obtained with high spatial resolution that gives bone detail comparable with that from high-resolution CT. Magnetic resonance angiography (MRA) using the phase contrast or time-of-flight techniques is improving rapidly and replacing conventional angiography in many situations.

Computed tomography

The main examination consists of contiguous axial and coronal sections 2 mm thick at 30° to the anthropological baseline parallel to the roof of the orbit defined on a lateral scout view (Figure 3.3). This is to limit the radiation dose to the eye, because although some slices pass through the orbit, the centre of the globe is not in the direct x-ray beam. The sections are viewed on a wide window setting of 4000 Hounsfield units. If greater detail is required, for instance, for the oval window or incudostapedial joint region, then 1 mm sections are necessary. To optimize resolution, individual sides are reformatted to a 10 cm field of view, a 512 × 512 pixel matrix.

Sections in the axial plane (Figure 3.4) start just below the external auditory canal meatus and show the basal turn of cochlea and round

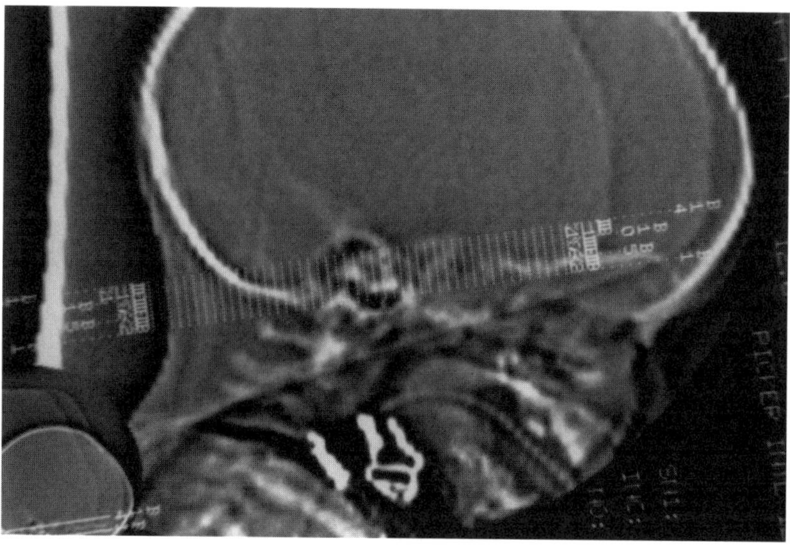

Figure 3.3. Lateral scout view showing the scan planes for a CT examination in the axial plane.

window niche. These sections best show the internal auditory meatus (IAM) and the vestibular aqueduct (VA). The head of the malleus and the body and short process of the incus are also shown at the level of the vestibule. The three parts of the facial nerve canal can be identified, although the axial plane is least satisfactory for the descending portion, which is seen in cross section behind the pyramidal eminence. The small muscles of the middle ear, the tensor tympani in front and the stapedius posteriorly, are best shown in the axial plane with the stapes between them.

Coronal sections

Coronal sections are obtained in head-hanging or chin-up position. Sections are obtained as near as possible in the coronal plane aided by gantry tilt. The radiation dose to the eyes from coronal sections is very low because the eyes are not in the x-ray beam.

The eight most important coronal sections are shown in Figure 3.5. They begin at the level of the carotid canal and curl of the central bony spiral of the cochlea. The malleus is shown well at this level. Further back, the section at the level of the vestibule shows the internal auditory meatus as well as the stapes and oval window. Further back still, at the most prominent part of the lateral semicircular canal, the pyramidal eminence is shown between facial recess and sinus tympani. The descending facial

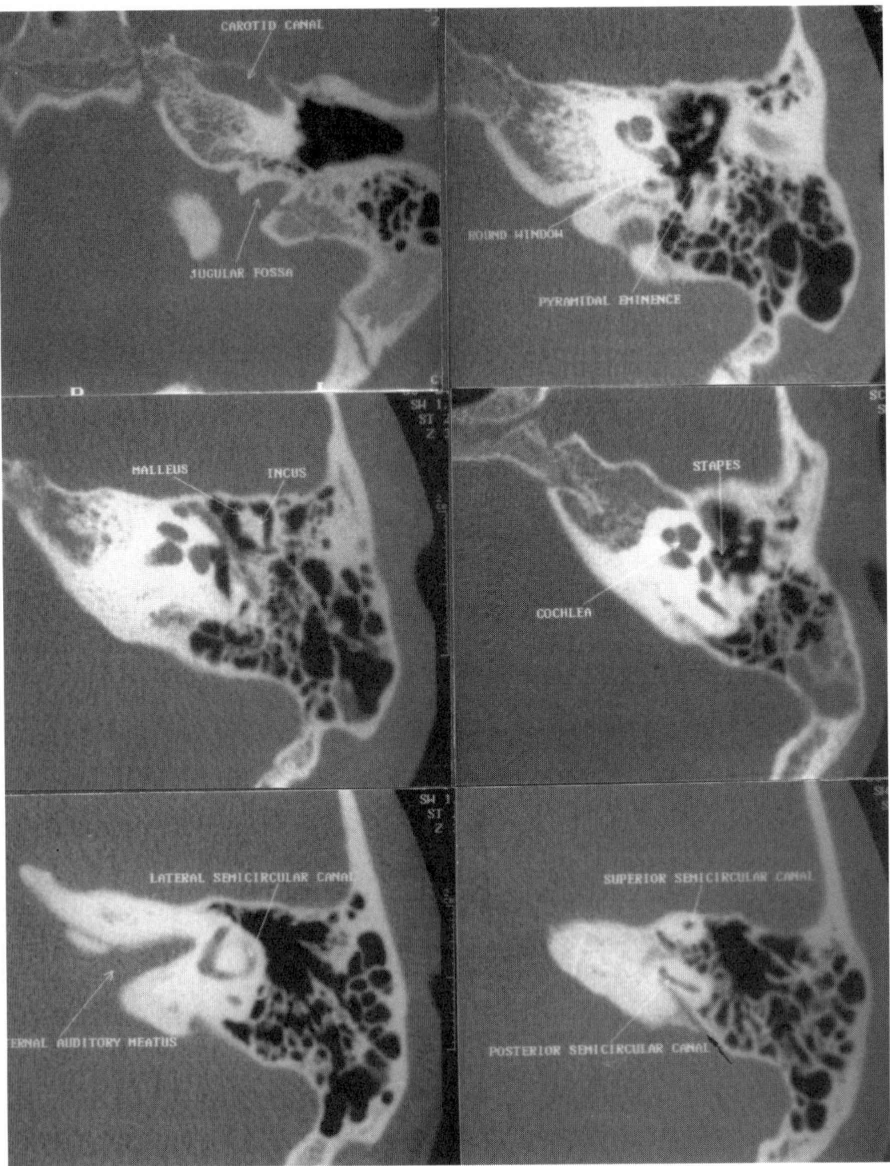

Figure 3.4. Six axial CT sections through the ear extending from the skull base at the level of the carotid canal and jugular fossa through the labyrinth to the superior and posterior semicircular canals in the largest section. The black arrow indicates the external aperture of the vestibular aqueduct.

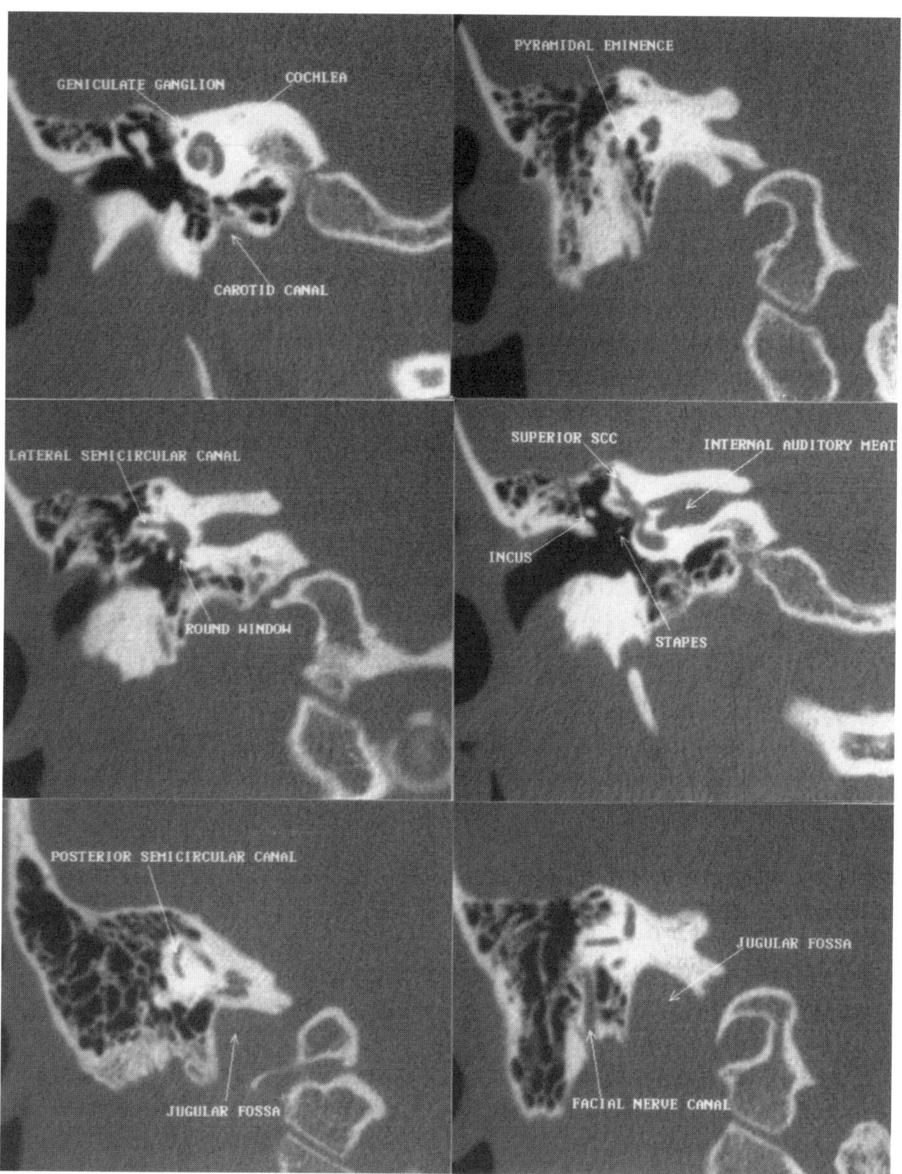

Figure 3.5. Six coronal sections through the ear from the cochlea anteriorly to the posterior semicircular canal.

canal and jugular fossa are assessed, and the examination finishes at the posterior semicircular canal, although further sections may be necessary to show the mastoid antrum and air cells.

Examinations with contrast

Examinations using CT with contrast are now rarely performed because of the availability of MRI, but they may be necessary to view intracranial or extracranial complications of suppurative ear disease, such as extradural or brain abscess.

Reformatted images

These can be obtained from multiple thin contiguous axial sections. Reformatted images can be made in any plane but the quality is always inferior to a direct examination and depends on two factors: (a) the number, thickness and overlap of individual sections and therefore the amount of raw data available for the reconstruction process; and (b) absolute immobility of the patient while the sections are being obtained. Reformatted images in the sagittal plane are helpful to assess a large vestibular aqueduct (see below).

Three-dimensional scanning

Three-dimensional (3D) CT is a relatively new imaging facility available for radiology and has come about due to the advanced capabilities of computer systems. From a series of two-dimensional CT scan slices it is now possible to obtain 3D reconstructions. This can be achieved by manipulating the data obtained from a 2D study with use of specific 3D software computer program.

The full advantages of this imaging technique have not yet fully been explored; however, it has proved to be particularly useful for facial reconstructions due to trauma or to congenital deformities (Figure 3.6). Only recently has 3D CT been used to investigate other more specific anatomy, namely the petrous bone.

The scanning parameters in the 2D plane have a major influence on the quality of the resultant 3D image, including spatial resolution and contrast. An important factor to be taken into consideration when using 3D is the slice thickness and the bed increment of the original study. Obviously, the thinner the slice thickness, the greater the resolution of the 3D image, but this level of resolution comes at a cost – namely, a possible increase in the radiation dose to the patient because the total number of scans in any one plane is increased.

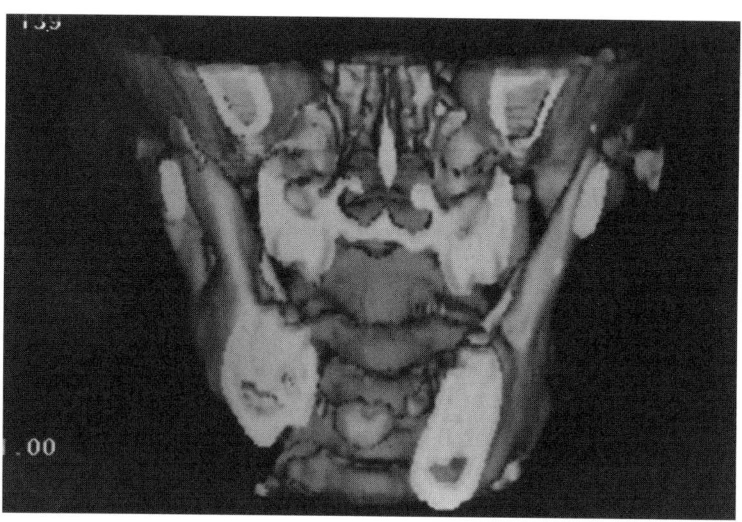

Figure 3.6. 3D reconstruction of the face in a case of hemifacial microsomia.

Magnetic resonance imaging

In the early days of MRI, it soon became apparent that this imaging was better than CT for the investigation of the posterior cranial fossa, because of better soft tissue differentiation, multiplanar capability, and freedom from beam-hardening artefacts. However, because air and bone give essentially no magnetic resonance signal the normal middle ear is not depicted. The fluids of the labyrinth give high signal on T2-weighted sequences, and nerves in the IAM and cerebellopontine angle can be seen as well as the facial nerve in its whole length.

Fast spin echo is a new fast-scanning method that uses spin echoes and altered k-space (collection of raw data) filling. It is designed to provide more conventional spin echo-type contrast in shorter times by the use of repetitive refocusing 180° radio frequency pulses, which means that 8–32 times as much k-space can be filled compared with a traditional spin echo in which one line of k-space is generally completed per resolution time (TR). Each echo is acquired with a different phase encode gradient. The total acquisition time is greatly reduced with FSE, thus enabling a greater number of phase encoding steps to be made. The matrix size can therefore be increased to provide improved spatial resolution and still maintain an acceptable examination time. Thus the latest MRI equipment can give image detail almost on par with that of CT, 2 mm or less thick sections and good contrast between bone, soft tissues, and fluids of the inner ear. The normal cranial nerves in the internal auditory meatus are clearly seen surrounded by the high signal cerebrospinal fluid (Figure 3.7).

The usual 90° pulse of the spin echo sequence provides the highest signal as long as the longitudinal magnetization has almost completely recovered. If shorter TR values are used, the signal becomes weaker, but better signal-to-noise ratios can be achieved per unit time with use of pulse flip angles less than 90°. This is known as gradient echo because the echoes are generated by gradient reversal instead of the subsequent 180° pulse used in spin echo imaging (TE). The ability to use shorter TR makes thin sliced 3D volume practical and although the presentation of 3D data is usually in 2D slices, 3D pictures can be made by post-processing (Figure 3.8).

Magnetic resonance angiography is a new technique that is rapidly replacing conventional angiography. It employs flowing blood as a physiologic contrast medium is a non-invasive technique with no risks for the patient, and can be added to routine MRI study.

Arterial MRA can be accomplished with time-of-flight or phase contrast sequence. Large and medium-sized arteries can be demonstrated, but evaluation of the type and extent of vascular pathology may be upset by altered (non-laminar) blood flow. Arterial MRA has limited use in evaluation of smaller sized vessels.

Venous MRA requires the employment of sequential flow compensated sequences due to the slow blood flow in veins. Venous MRA is optimized by employment of an additional RF saturation pulse below the imaging slices minimizing signal from arterial blood flow. Venous MRA can demonstrate the intracranial venous sinus system and has replaced catheter venography. The contrast enhancing agent gadolinium (Gd) will show any inflammatory lesion due to increased vascularity but will also show increased signal intensity in the facial nerve in Bell's palsy or of the fluids of the labyrinth in labyrinthitis, but its main use is for showing tumours and gadolinium-enhanced T1-weighted images have proved the gold standard for demonstrating all acoustic neuromas large and small. This is a slightly invasive procedure because an intravenous injection is necessary. However, contrast enhancement using gadolinium (DTPA) has tended to replace the T2-weighted sequences. Most tumours show a significant degree of enhancement.

Sections of the temporal bone as thin as 1 mm can be acquired by a three-dimensional Fourier transformation (3DFT) technique using a small receiver coil, a low flip angle with short TR and gradient reversal instead of 180° radio frequency (RF) refocusing. Images in any plane can be formatted from the data acquired in the axial plane. However, some of the earlier gradient echo 3DFT sequences, although giving high signal from fluids at flip angles of around 50°, were very sensitive to flow of fluids

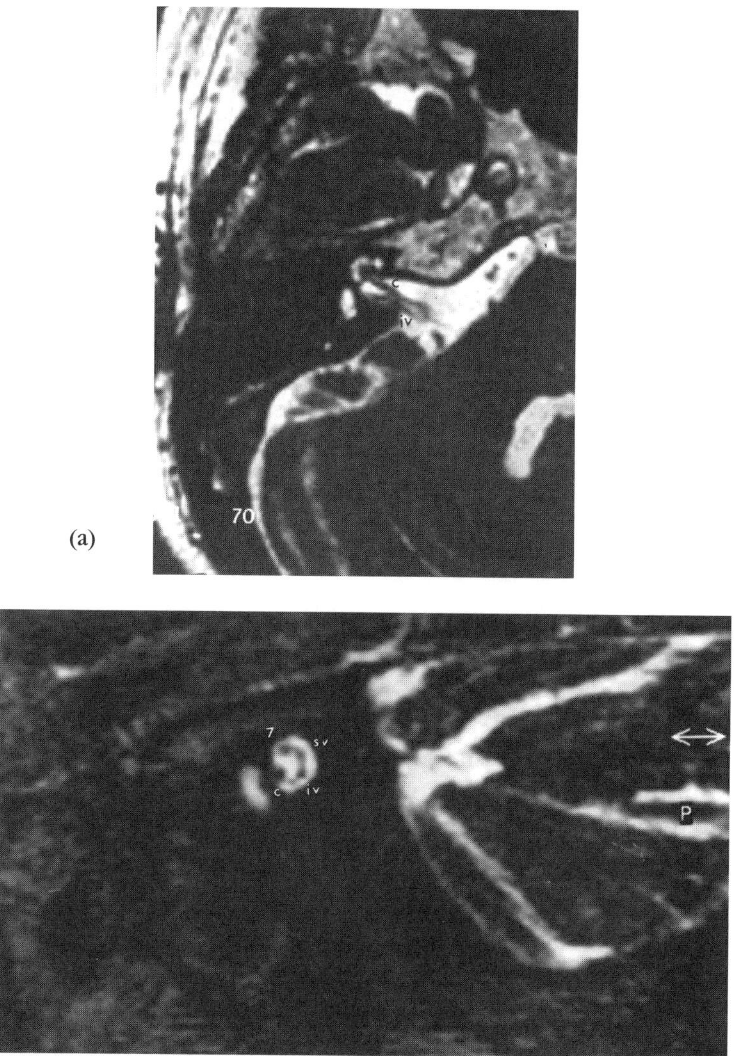

Figure 3.7. a) Thin section T2 weighted MRI in the axial plane b) Thin sagittal sections through the IAM and cerebellopontine angle. C= cochlear nerve; SV= superior vestibular; IV= inferior vestibular; 7= facial nerve. Note the coils of the cochlea on the axial section.

producing artefacts. To overcome this disadvantage Casselman, in 1994, introduced the 3DFT-CISS (constructive interference in steady state) protocol, which ensures that not only the fluid in the membranous labyrinth and IAM, but also the fast-flowing fluid around the brainstem always has a high signal and remains white.

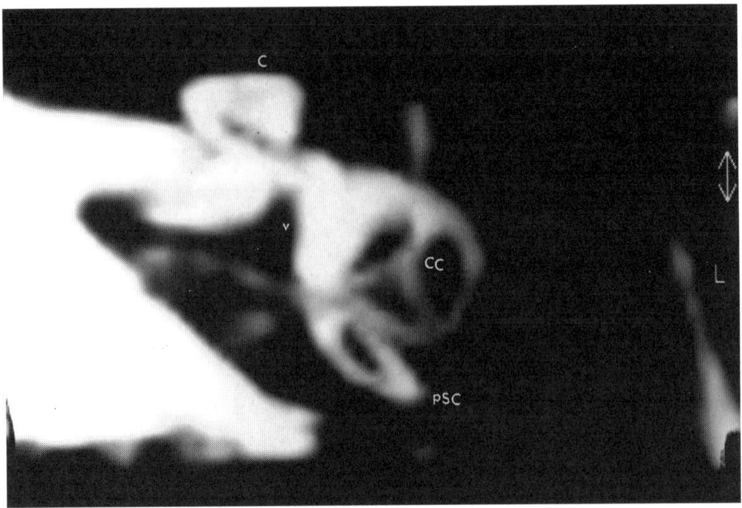

Figure 3.8. 3D MRI of the labyrinth of the inner ear. C= cochlea; CC= crus commune; PSC= posterior semicircular canal; V= vestibule.

Congenital vascular anomalies

The jugular fossa and intrapetrous carotid canal are well shown by CT. Very rarely an ectopic internal carotid artery, or more commonly a large jugular bulb, may appear in the middle ear and cause not only symptoms but problems in differential diagnosis (Figure 3.9) from glomus tumours. An aberrant carotid artery in the middle ear becomes apparent on CT if comparison is made with the course of the normal artery on the opposite side. Vascular anomalies are usually discovered in late childhood or adulthood. The differential diagnosis and their distinction from vascular neoplasms are almost entirely dependent upon radiology. Angiography has been considered the definitive investigation and in many cases is mandatory when there appears to be a vascular mass behind the eardrum. Rare abnormalities are a persistent stapedial artery or an aneurysm of the internal carotid artery. This discussion concerns aberrations in position of the internal carotid artery and jugular bulb.

The anatomy of the jugular bulb is variable, the right usually being larger than the left. Frequently, it extends above the inferior rim of the bony annulus, with or without a bony covering. When the jugular bulb is small it is separated from the floor of the middle ear by a comparatively thick layer of bone, which is usually compact but may contain air cells. Anterior to the bulb is the internal carotid artery. A spur or crest of bone separates the jugular fossa from the carotid canal. When the jugular bulb is very large, it can extend up into the mesotympanum with a thin bony covering, which can easily be damaged at surgery (Figure 3.9). When there is dehiscence of this bony covering, the exposed jugular bulb is at greater risk. The soft tissue mass of a dehiscent jugular bulb is well shown by CT, especially in the coronal plane and the smooth outline of the jugular fossa with no evidence of erosion confirms the nature of this anomaly. Another aspect of the large jugular bulb is encroachment on inner ear structures. The IAM, vestibular aqueduct and posterior semicircular canal may be affected, especially if there is an associated diverticulum from the bulb.

Aberrations in the course of the internal carotid artery through the petrous temporal bone are extremely rare. Normally the artery ascends vertically, medial and anterior to the middle-ear cavity before bending sharply anterior and medially below the Eustachian tube and cochlea; it then passes through the foramen lacerum into the cranial cavity. A thin bony septum separates the artery from the hypotympanum. There is said to be dehiscence in 1% of people, but the true incidence is probably much less than this. If the ascending part of the artery is more posteriorly placed than usual with a very acute bend, it is more likely to be dehiscent, although the spur between the carotid and the jugular bulb remains intact. In more severe aberrations a soft tissue mass will be shown in the middle

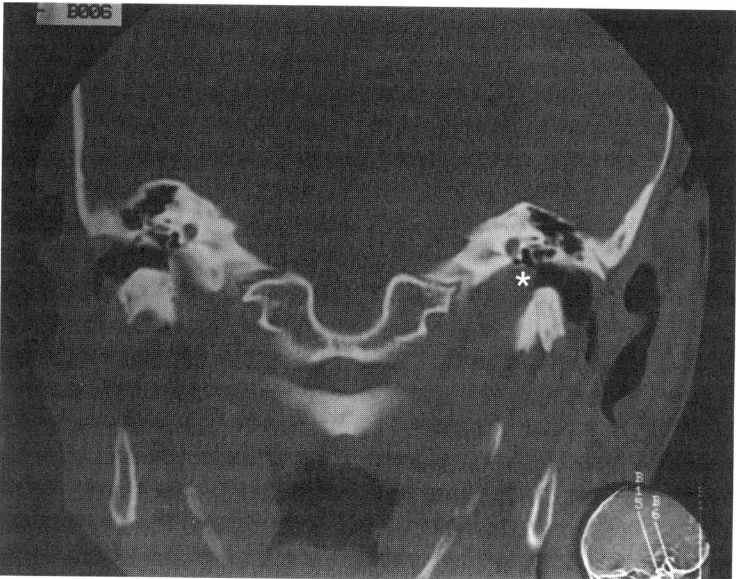

Figure 3.9. Coronal CT section showing high jugular bulb (asterisk) with the round window niche.

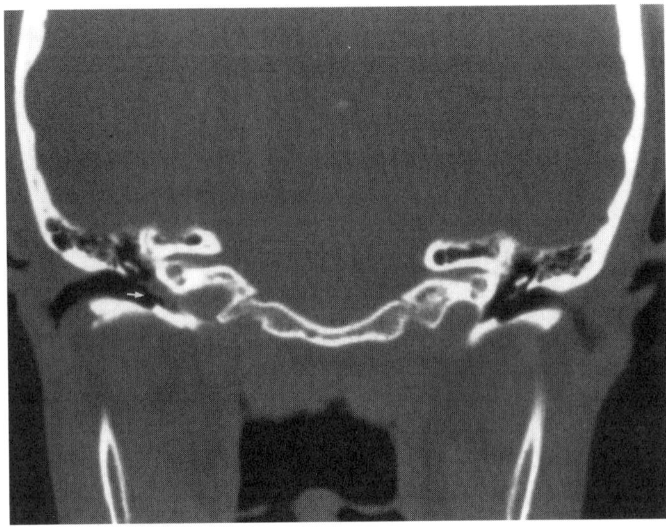

Figure 3.10. Coronal CT section at the level of the cochlea showing an aberrant internal carotid artery in the middle ear (arrow). Note the absence of the normal bony septum between artery and hypotympanum.

ear by CT (Figure 3.10), but the important differentiating feature of coronal CT is absence of the normal carotid canal and a laterally and more posteriorly placed vertical canal. These features need to be confirmed by angiography and no attempt at surgical interference should be made.

Congenital ear deformities

Congenital abnormalities of the ear can be shown in great detail by CT if there is osseous deformity, but MRI is now providing evidence of soft-tissue lesions in some cases and is the imaging investigation of choice for abnormalities of the cranial nerves or their central connections. Unfortunately, affected children are usually referred between the ages of two and four years, when the hearing impairment is first confirmed, and sedation or a general anaesthetic is required for the examination. If, after careful consideration, it is felt that the results of the investigation are unlikely to affect patient management, it may be reasonable to defer the examination until the child can cooperate. In the neonatal period a few sections can usually be obtained after a large feed, and this is recommended for those infants with relevant external deformities or syndromes of which temporal bone abnormalities are a feature. Plain films will also give some information at this stage, when full ossification of the petrous pyramids has not yet occurred, but at a later stage are only really useful for showing the degree of pneumatization.

Congenital abnormalities of the middle and external ear are seen much more often than deformities of the inner ear, although combined deformities occur in 20% of patients. The study of the outer ear relates to the prospects for surgical intervention to improve the sound-conducting mechanism and is mandatory before any exploration of congenital atresia. Surgery is now, however, rarely performed for unilateral lesions, but in bilateral atresias the radiological examination is crucial to indicate the best side for exploration, especially the all-important assessment of the presence, state and size of the middle-ear cavity, but in fact the success of bone-anchored hearing aids has meant that only the most minor deformities of the conducting mechanism now warrant surgical exploration.

Inner ear deformities

Congenital malformations of the bony labyrinth, IAM and vestibular aqueduct, which vary widely in severity from minor anomalies with normal cochlear function to severe deformities that preclude any hearing may be suggested by audiological assessment. Traditionally, two eponyms are enshrined in accounts of congenital hearing impairment and so need to be defined:

- Michel defect: complete lack of development of any inner ear structures (Michel, 1863).
- Mondini defect: a cochlea with one-and-half turns and the apical coil replaced by a distal sac. Although the subject of Mondini's dissection had been completely deaf, the normal basal turn of the true Mondini defect means that some hearing is possible. Mondini's patient also had very dilated vestibular aqueducts (Mondini, 1791; Phelps, 1994).

Line drawings of some examples of labyrinthine deformities are shown in Figure 3.11. A primitive sac with one or more appendages is more common than a Michel deformity.

The semicircular canals may be missing or dilated in varying degree, but the commoner inner ear anomaly, namely a solitary dilated dysplastic lateral semicircular canal, is often associated with normal cochlear function. Dilatation of the vestibular aqueduct often accompanies minor abnormalities of the bony cochlea and vestibule and congenital hearing impairment. The hearing impairment may be fluctuant or progressive, or both. Such is a common feature of Pendred syndrome as well as a true Mondini type of cochlea and MRI shows the accompanying enlargement of the endolymphatic sac and duct (Figure 3.12) (Phelps et al., 1998).

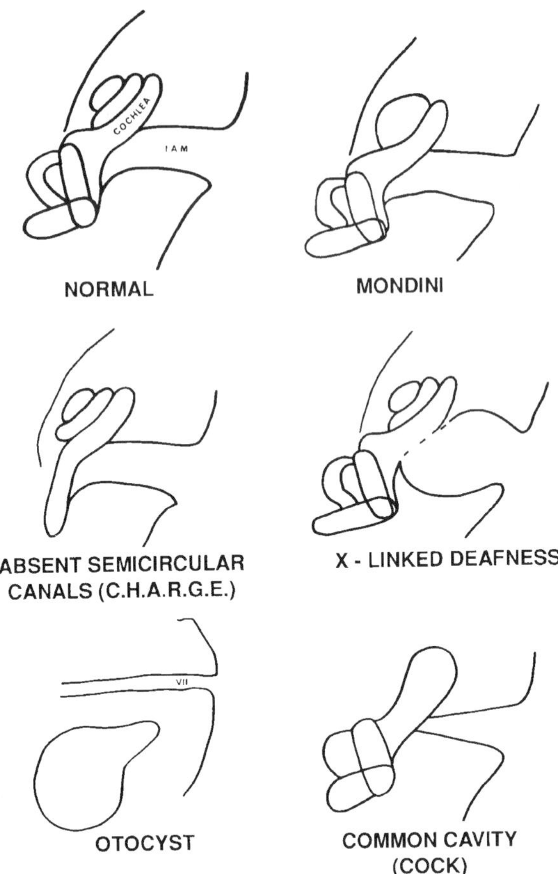

Figuure 3.11. Examples of congenital deformities of the inner ear based on axial CT sections.

Inner ear lesions associated with cerebrospinal fluid fistula

Congenital cerebrospinal fluid fistula into the middle-ear cavity is a rare but potentially fatal condition that is frequently misdiagnosed. When the fistula occurs spontaneously it usually appears in the first five or 10 years of life as:

- cerebrospinal fluid rhinorrhoea, if the eardrum is intact; cerebrospinal fluid passes down the Eustachian tube causing a nasal discharge
- cerebrospinal fluid otorrhoea, if there is a perforation in the eardrum, or if myringotomy has been performed for presumed serous otitis media;

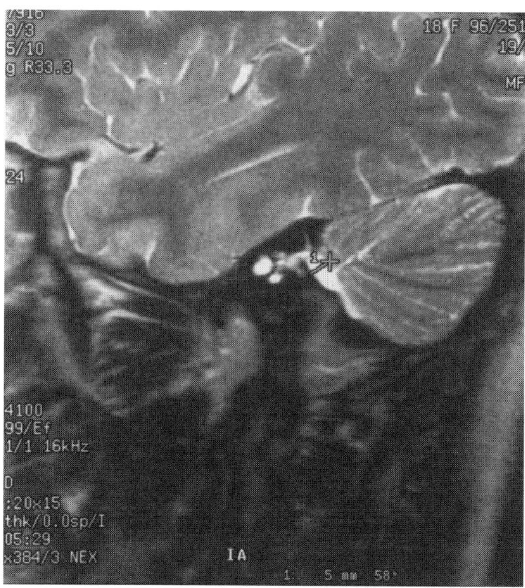

Figure 3.12. Sagittal T2 weighted MRI section showing a large endolymphatic sac measuring 5mm in diameter at its widest part in the posterior cranial fossa, as well as a true Mondini deformity of the cochlea in a case of Pendred syndrome.

- attacks of meningitis that are usually recurrent; at times meningitis is the sole presenting manifestation of a cerebrospinal fluid fistula.

Hearing impairment is usually severe or complete, but it is difficult to diagnose and assess, especially in a young child. It is frequently unrecognized if unilateral. The conductive and sensorineural components of the hearing impairment are also hard to define.

Spontaneous cerebrospinal fluid fistulae from the subarachnoid space into the middle-ear cavity may be classified as perilabyrinthine or translabyrinthine (Phelps, 1986). Those in the very rare perilabyrinthine group, through bony defects close to but not involving the labyrinth, usually have normal hearing initially. The commoner translabyrinthine type is nearly always associated with anacusis, severe labyrinthine dysplasia and a route via the IAM. The labyrinthine deformity is more severe than the type classically described by Mondini, and was first described by Cock in 1838 although it is now usually called the common cavity deformity (Figure 3.11). Evidence of a dilated cochlear aqueduct in these patients is unconvincing. Congenital fixation of the stapes footplate is likely to be associated with a profuse perilymph or cerebrospinal fluid leak after stapedectomy.

The surgical results of stapedectomy for congenital stapedial fixation are not very satisfactory. This certainly applies to males with an X-linked mixed type of hearing impairment and a specific deformity of the inner ear first described in 1991 (Phelps et al., 1991). Deficient bone between the fundus of the bulbous IAM and the basal turn of the cochlea precludes the insertion of a multi-channel electrode as the deficient bone would almost certainly mean that the electrode would enter the IAM rather than staying in the cochlear duct.

Middle ear deformities

Radiology of congenital deformities of the middle and external ear relates almost exclusively to the prospects of improvement of conductive hearing impairment. The size and shape of the middle ear cavity is the most import-ant assessment to be made, especially if there is atresia of the EAM (Figure 3.13).

In the majority of unilateral atresias with associated deformity of the pinna but no other congenital abnormality, there is normally formed mastoid with good pneumatization and the middle-ear cavity is of relatively normal shape. Even in the most severe deformities there is rarely complete absence of the middle ear and usually at least a slit-like hypotympanum can be shown lateral to the basal turn of the cochlea. The middle-ear cavity may be reduced in size by encroachment of the atretic plate laterally, by a high jugular bulb inferiorly or by descent of the tegmen superiorly. In craniofacial microsomia and mandibulofacial dysostosis, the attic and antrum are typically absent or slit like, being replaced in varying degrees by solid bone or by descent of the tegmen.

If the middle-ear cavity contains air, its shape and contents are relatively easy to assess. Frequently, however, the middle ear in congenital abnormalities contains undifferentiated mesenchyme, a thick glue-like substance that is radiologically indistinguishable from soft tissue or retained mucus. Thin bony septa may divide the middle ear cavity into two or more compartments.

The course of the second and third parts of the facial nerve depends on normal development of the branchial arches. The greater the deformity of the petrous bone the more marked is the tendency for the facial nerve to follow a more direct route out into the soft tissues of the face. Exposed facial nerves in the middle-ear cavity are the most common abnormalities recorded at surgery for congenital malformations. Usually the Fallopian canal is dehiscent but the descending segment may also be exposed, and overhang of the facial ridge with absence of the second genu is a usual finding in the Treacher Collins syndrome, making access to the oval window difficult for the surgeon. A short vertical segment of the facial

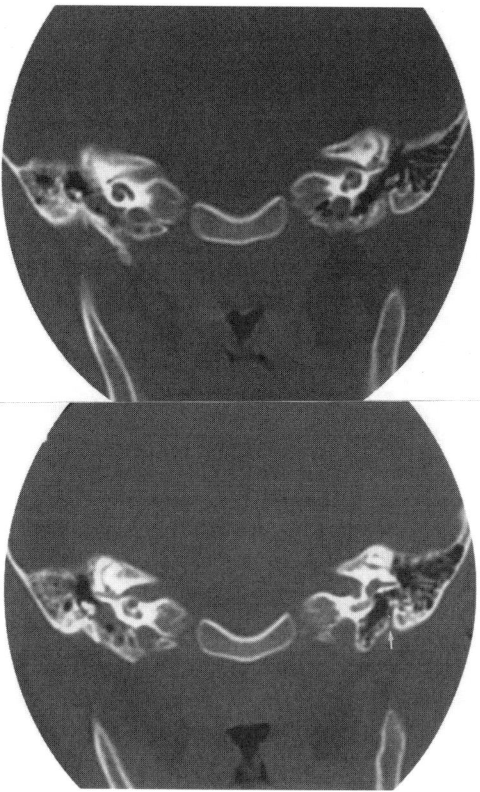

Figure 3.13. Typical bilateral congenital atresia of the external meati. Note the anterior position of the descending facial nerve canal at the level of the oval window shown on these two coronal CT sections.

canal and high stylomastoid foramen mean that the nerve turns forwards into the cheek in a high position (Figure 3.14).

In the pre-operative radiological assessment the descending facial canal and its relationship to other structures must be demonstrated, preferably in lateral and coronal sections. Axial CT sections will show the descending canal in cross-section and identification is less certain. Grossly displaced nerves that cross the middle ear cavity are more difficult to identify.

Ossicles

A normal ossicular chain is rarely found when there is atresia of the external ear, but complete absence of the ossicles is also unusual. In most cases at least some vestige of the ossicular chain is evident. The ossicles are often thicker and heavier than normal or, less frequently, thin and spidery. They

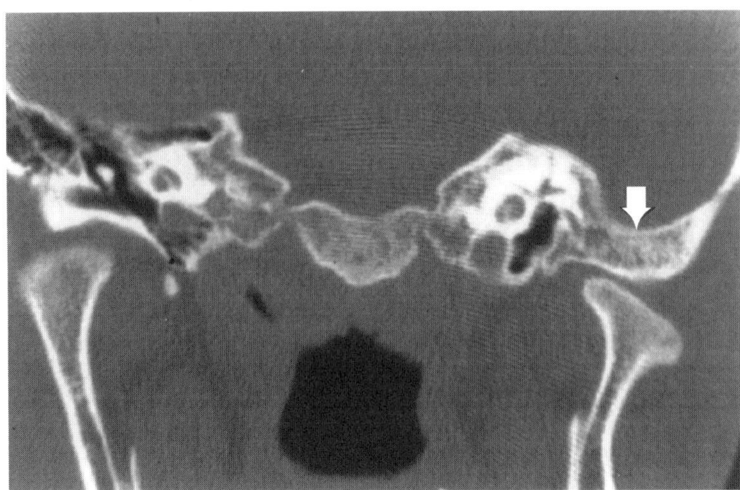

Figure 3.14. Coronal CT section at the level of the cochlea showing gross descent of the tegmen (arrow), deformity of the temperomandibular joint and absence of the ossicles in a typical case of hemifacial microsomia.

may be fixed to the walls of the middle-ear cavity by bosses of bone, but the more usual deformity discovered at surgery is a fusion of the bodies of the malleus and incus. The ankylosis varies in degree and may be bony or fibrous. The radiological recognition of this ossicular union is difficult but is, in any case, not of great practical importance, and an irregular lump of bone in the middle-ear cavity usually represents an ossicular mass.

Because of the partial or complete replacement of the tympanic membrane by a bony plate, the handle of the malleus is not surprisingly the part of the chain that is most often abnormal and most easily recognized. If the handle is absent, the 'molar tooth' appearance of the ossicles will no longer be evident in the lateral projection, and a triangular appearance of the ossicular mass will be seen. Often, the handle of the malleus is bent towards the atretic plate to which it may be fixed and this gives a typical L-shaped appearance to the ossicular mass. A slit-like attic so typical of Treacher Collins syndrome or an overhanging facial ridge may obstruct the free movement of the ossicular chain.

External auditory meatus

In congenital deformities of the external ear, the EAM may be narrow, short, completely or partially atretic or it may in an abnormal direction. It often slopes towards the middle ear and in such cases it may be curved in two planes, becoming more horizontal at its medial end. The obstruction in atresia may be due to soft tissue or bone but usually both are involved. The tympanic bone may be hyperplastic, (rarely) deformed or absent.

The so-called atretic plate may therefore be composed partly of a deformed tympanic bone and partly of downwards and forwards extension of squamous temporal and mastoid bones, in which case it may be pneumatized.

Syndromes

It is not intended to discuss the radiological features of syndromic ear deformities except for the commonest and most important.

Hemifacial microsomia

Meatal atresia and middle ear abnormalities are almost constant findings and there may be descent of the tegmen to or even below the lateral semicircular canal (Figure 3.14). Occasionally, some hyperplasia of external ear structures and of the tympanic bone occurs, but the mastoid is hypoplastic and unpneumatized. The middle-ear cavity is usually small being encroached upon by the tegmen and thick atretic plate. The ossicles in such cases are absent or hypoplastic and an ossicular mass is displaced laterally far from the oval window. This is only seen in cases of facial microsomia a condition which is not exclusively unilateral (Phelps et al., 1983). If bilateral, there is always considerable dissymetry between the two sides. This dissymmetry distinguishes the syndrome from Treacher Collins syndrome with which it has often been confused in the past. There is no hereditary factor in hemifacial microsomia. It is the most common of the craniofacial syndromes.

Treacher Collins syndrome (Mandibulofacial dysostosis)

Ear abnormalities in Treacher Collins syndrome are symmetrical and characteristic although they may vary in severity. The mastoid is unpneumatized and the attic and antrum are reduced to slit-like proportions (Figure 3.15). Atresia of the EAM is a less constant feature and in 50% of the patients the meatus may be patent although it tends to be curved, running upwards in its lateral part. Ossicular abnormalities are common and, in nearly all the operated ears in our series, the facial nerve followed a more direct path with opening out of the bends. It usually appeared at surgery as an overhanging facial ridge (Phelps et al., 1981).

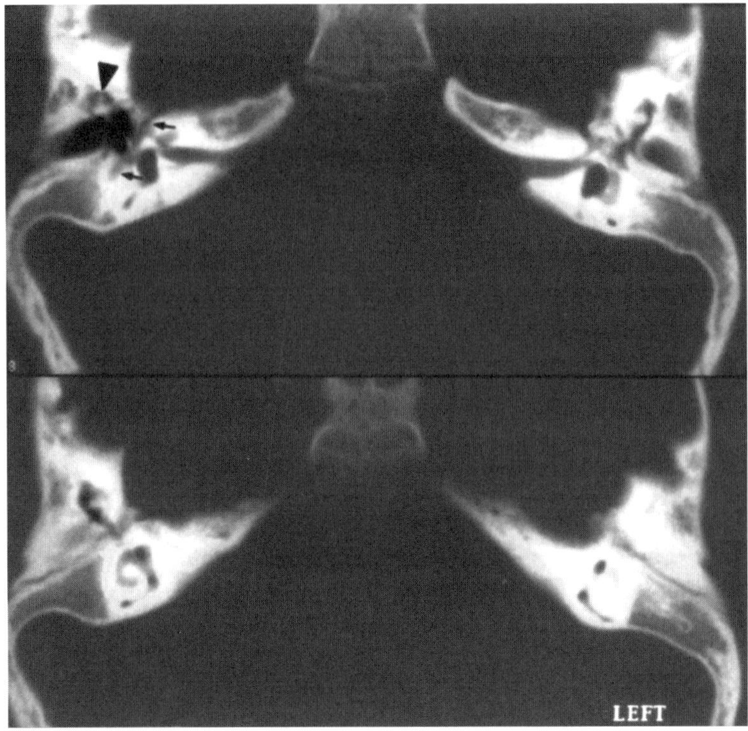

Figure 3.15. Axial CT section of a typical case of Treacher Collins syndrome. Note the small middle-ear cavities and ossicular mass (arrowhead) as well as the overhanging facial ridge (arrows).

Branchio-oto-renal syndrome

Pedigrees of families with this distinctive syndrome indicate an autosomal dominant disorder with a high degree of penetrance. Any of the following anomalies may be present: auricular deformities, pre-auricular pits or sinuses, branchial fistulae or clefts, external meatal atresia and conductive or mixed hearing impairment. Lachrymal duct aplasia occurs rarely, but urinary tract anomalies are common. The base of the skull and petrous pyramids are somewhat distorted in this syndrome. Generally speaking, the petrous pyramids are short and point upwards at their medial end, giving an upwards and backwards slant to the internal auditory meatus (IAM), which appears rather short and bulbous. There is often dysplasia of the lateral semicircular canal, but of more importance is the small cochlea. This seems to have a reduced number of turns, but this is not a true Mondini-type deformity (Figure 3.16). The middle-ear cavities are usually of reasonable size and air-containing, although bony atresia of the external auditory meati may occur. The malleus and incus are usually affected and the stapes, often with

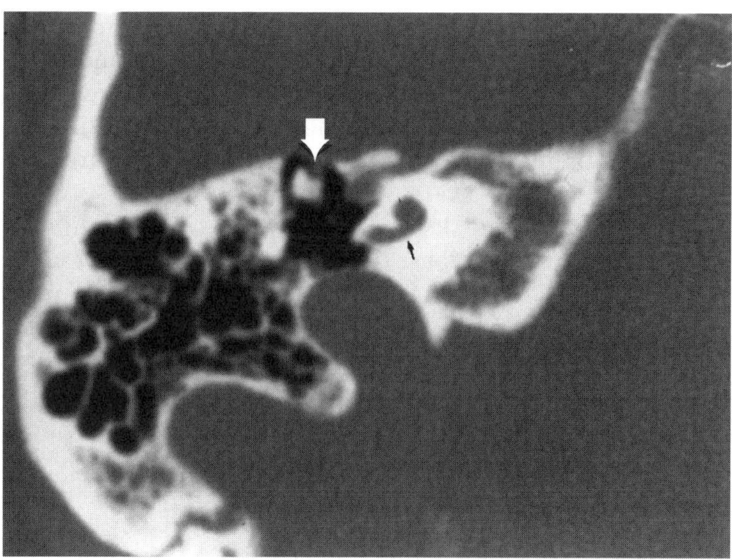

Figure 3.16. Axial CT section of the temporal bone in a patient with BOR. Note the reduced cochlea (arrow) and the ossicular mass attached to the anterior wall of the middle ear.

one crus only and fixation in the oval window, which may appear to be absent. The ossicles also appear to be more anteriorly situated than normal. In theory such cases with a conductive hearing impairment should be amenable to surgical improvement of the sound conductive mechanism, but unfortunately the results have been disappointing (Slack and Phelps, 1985).

The CHARGE association

In 1981 Pagon et al. applied the acronym CHARGE to an association of congenital defects that includes coloboma, heart disease, atresia of the nasal choanae, retarded development or CNS abnormalities, or both, genital hypoplasia and ear anomalies. There are now several published reports of the external ear malformations and hearing impairment in CHARGE association. The most characteristic feature is absence of the semicircular canals (Dhooge et al., 1998).

Bone dysplasias

Hearing impairment is a common childhood feature of the rare congenital generalized bony dysplasias. Only a brief account of the radiological features of osteogenesis imperfecta and of the dysplasias with increased bone density is given here.

Hearing impairment in osteogenesis imperfecta tarda may be conductive, sensorineural or mixed. The radiological appearance consists of demineralization in the labyrinthine capsule indistinguishable from otospongiosis but, in contrast to otospongiosis, which only affects the capsule, deficient ossification occurs in other sites in the petrous pyramid.

The osteopetroses are a group of uncommon genetic disorders that are characterized by increased skeletal density and abnormalities of bone modelling. Common to all of these disorders is a proclivity for involvement of the calvarium and skull base. An associated constellation of neurotological symptoms may result, presumably secondary to bony encroachment on the cranial foramina. Sectional imaging of the petrous temporal bones shows generalized sclerosis and narrowing of the IAM (Figure 3.17). Encroachment by bosses of bone in the attic may also be revealed.

Otitis media

Acute otitis media is essentially a clinical diagnosis and imaging is not usually required. Persistence of the inflammatory process leads to mastoiditis with breakdown of the cell walls. Clouding of the mastoid air cells on otitis media makes the assessment of cell wall breakdown difficult. Computed tomography and MRI should be used for the more serious complications such as petrositis and labyrinthitis. Extradural and subdural empyemas, meningitis, cerebral abscess, lateral sinus thrombosis and

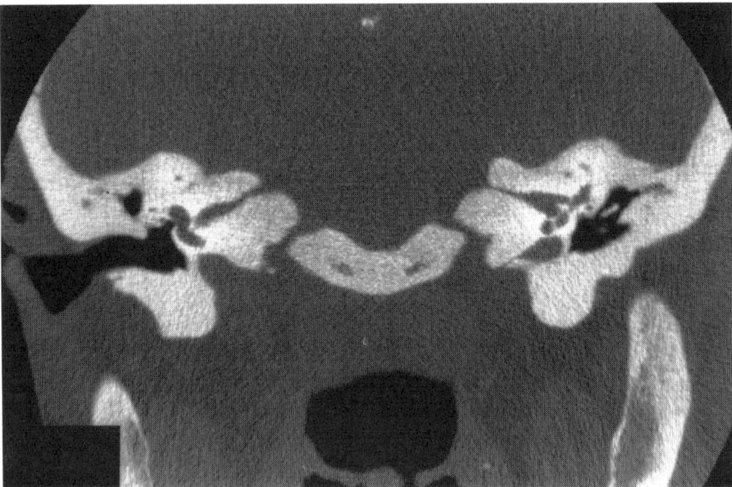

Figure 3.17. Coronal CT section of temporal bones in a case of Engelmann's disease. The periphery of the otic capsule cannot be distinguished from the surrounding sclerotic bone of the rest of the petrous pyramid.

otitic hydrocephalus are complications of otitis media needing CT and MRI studies with contrast enhancement.

Labyrinthitis ossificans, the end result of suppurative labyrinthitis, while associated with complete or almost complete anacusis, has important implications with regard to cochlear implants. Obliteration of the basal turn of the cochlea or round window niche are relative contraindications for cochlear implants (Figure 3.18).

Cholesteatoma

A cholesteatoma (epidermoid) may arise almost anywhere in the cranial cavity or skull base, usually presenting in adulthood. Congenital cholesteatoma of the middle-ear cavity develops behind an intact eardrum in the absence of a history of otitis media and has no demonstrable connection with the external auditory meatus. Since otitis media is very common in early childhood it is probable that many middle-ear cholesteatomas behind an intact eardrum, and mostly in the anterosuperior quadrant, are acquired lesions. Often large cholesteatomas are associated with small perforations of the eardrum and well-pneumatized mastoids.

It has been proposed that the congenital middle-ear cholesteatomas develop from epidermoid cell rests, found in most foetal ears at the junction of the Eustachian tube with the middle ear. There appear to be

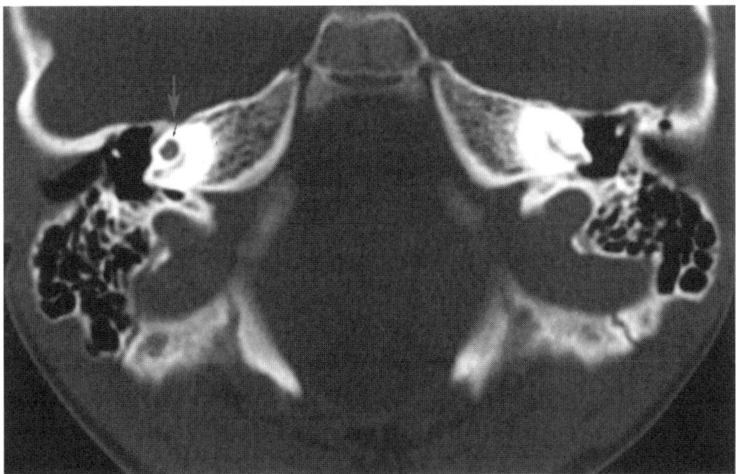

Figure 3.18. Labyrinthitis ossificans. There is partial calcific obliteration of the coils of the cochlea shown on this axial CT section. On one side the distal coils seem to be patent (arrow).

two groups of patients, each with a distinct clinical presentation, that correlate well with the surgical outcome. Anterior lesions are seen in younger patients, with minimal hearing impairment. The disease is less aggressive with less involvement of the ossicles and mastoid cavity. Such lesions can be excised *in toto* through the transcanal procedures and do not recur.

Patients with lesions in the posterior quadrant or diffusely involving the middle-ear cleft appear to have more extensive disease. They are older with moderate conductive hearing impairment. The majority of lesions cause erosion of the ossicles and extend to the mastoid. Total eradication of the disease requires some form of mastotympanic procedure. Computed tomography is the best method of confirming the localized nature of small congenital cholesteatomas in the anterior mesotympanum (Figure 3.19). It is most important to make the correct diagnosis at an early age and to back up good otoscopy with imaging. Although the morphology of a small cholesteatoma in a predominantly air-containing middle ear is fairly characteristic, little can be achieved by CT if the cholesteatoma fills the middle-ear cleft or blockage of the Eustachian tube leads to a secondary serous otitis. Theoretically, a small cholesteatoma should be distinguishable from serous otitis on MRI scans using multiple protocols. In practice, this tissue differentiation is unlikely, although MRI will distinguish cholesteatoma from cholesterol granuloma if the mass is sufficiently large and homogeneous.

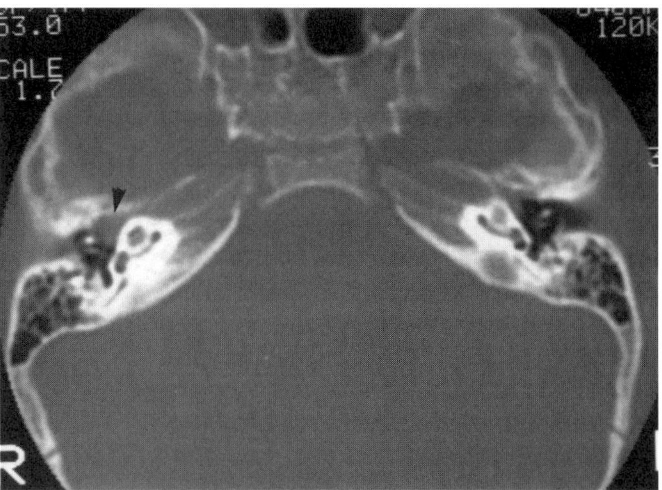

Figure 3.19. Small cholesteatoma in the anterior mesotympanum of a 3-year-old child shown on an axial CT scan (arrowhead).

Neoplasms

Rhabdomyosarcoma is the commonest aural neoplasm of childhood. Facial palsy and the features of acute otitis media usually precede the appearance of a polyp through an eardrum perforation. Bone destruction is an early feature and should be demonstrated by thin section CT. Intracranial extension occurs rapidly with this tumour. Magnetic resonance is the imaging investigation of choice to show the soft tissue mass. Predominantly adult benign tumours such as acoustic neuromas may rarely occur at an early age, especially in neurofibromatosis. The definitive imaging investigation as in the adult is gadolinium-enhanced MRI.

Langerhans cell histiocytosis (X) is a tumour-like condition of unknown pathogenesis characterized by massive infiltration of histiocytes and widespread ragged bone destruction. Presentation may be with a soft tissue mass in the external auditory meatus, but persistent aural discharge is the commonest manifestation of histiocytosis in the head and neck. Plain skull views will show bone destruction of the skull base and typical 'geographic' erosions in the skull vault. Computed tomography allows particular assessment of bone involvement, whereas MRI better demonstrates soft tissue and intracranial lesions (Figure 3.20).

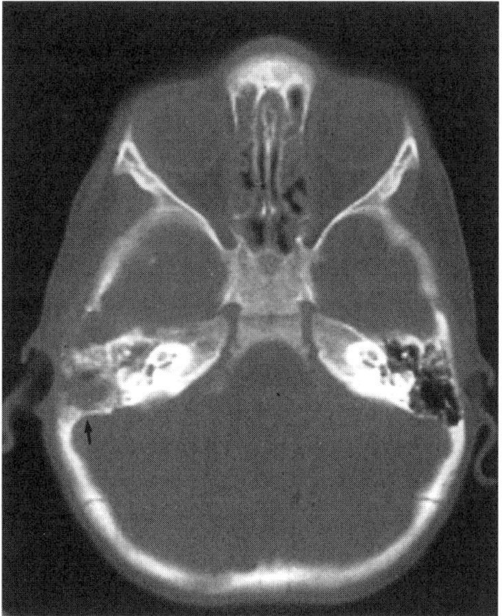

Figure 3.20. Axial CT of the skull bone of a child showing extensive erosion of the mastoid and lateral wall of the skull by histiocytosis.

Temporal bone trauma in children

The labyrinth of the inner ear, the hard bone of the labyrinthine capsule and the middle ear and ossicles are all fully formed at birth. The bony part of the external auditory meatus formed from the tympanic ring, the mastoid process and the articular fossa of the temporomandibular joint, only develop fully during childhood and thus the superficially situated facial nerve is vulnerable to injury. Fractures of the temporal bone in children are similar to those occurring in later life and are usually classified as longitudinal and transverse. The longitudinal fractures are much the commonest and usually follow a characteristic path parallel to the long axis of the petrous pyramid, from the squamous temporal across the roof of the external meatus and middle cavity, then along the anterior aspect of the petrous bone towards the foramen lacernum. A fracture line is often apparent on the lateral skull view. Injury to the facial nerve usually occurs in the region of the genicular ganglion or the second intratympanic part. Longitudinal fractures are shown best by thin section axial CT, but preferably further sections in the sagittal plane, with reformatted views are needed to show the fracture in two planes. Transverse fractures, which run across the long axis of the petrous pyramid, are less common. Generally the impact is exerted over the occipital or frontal area. This causes compression of the skull in an AP direction and a fracture, often visible on plain frontal views, that usually runs from the jugular fossa and across the IAM and/or the labyrinth. Such an injury causes a 'dead ear' and sometimes this can be confirmed by the presence of air in the labyrinth shown by axial CT sections.

The skull of a small child is elastic, and inward compression of the convex surface of the skull can result in extensive lines of fractures that do not fit the above classification. Moreover, in spite of CSF otorrhoea or rhinorrhoea, which seem to be common in children, a temporal bone fracture may not be demonstrated by even thin section high resolution CT. Most cases of traumatic CSF otorrhoea stop spontaneously within two weeks and rarely require surgical intervention, but unfortunately a persistent or recurrent CSF leak is a common cause of recurrent meningitis (Figure 3.21). If a hairline fracture cannot be demonstrated by CT, then an intrathecal contrast agent or isotope studies should be used to try and show the route of the leak.

A conductive hearing impairment following trauma is usually the result of bleeding into the middle-ear space. If the hearing impairment persisting after the haemotympanum has resolved then an ossicular disruption or

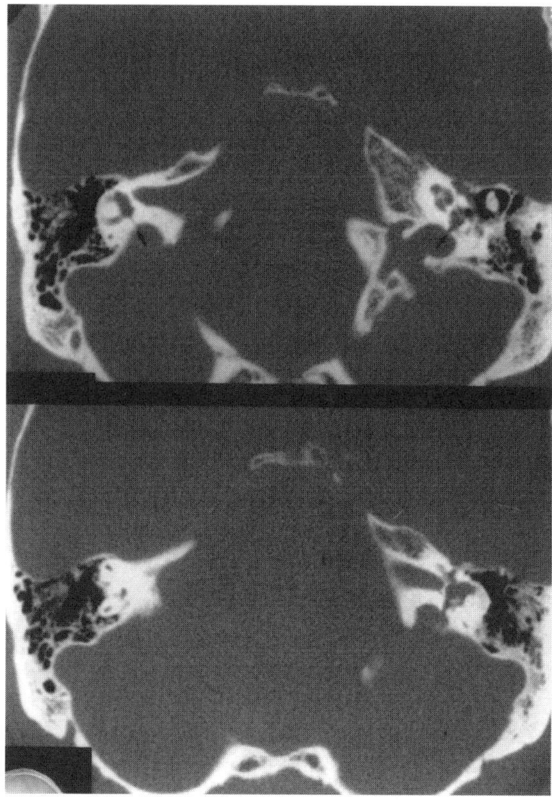

Figure 3.21. Bilateral transverse fractures through the petrous pyramids shown by axial CT. Typically the fracture lines pass from the jugular fossae to the vestibules (arrows).

fracture needs to be considered and if possible demonstrated by imaging. Unfortunately the commonest type of disruption between incus and stapes cannot be depicted reliably by CT, but the second commonest, namely complete dislocation of the incus, usually up into the attic, is well shown by axial and coronal CT. The incus is the most vulnerable of the three ossicles to dislocation because of its situation, suspended precariously between the malleus and stapes. It is believed that reflex contraction of tensor tympani and stapedius muscles in response to a severe blow on the head in childhood may result in dislocation which goes undetected at the time of the accident and is revealed as a unilateral conductive hearing impairment in later life.

Imaging prior to cochlear implantation

As well as providing a 'road map' for the surgeon and revealing potential hazards like a high jugular bulb, CT is important for revealing inner-ear pathology that may make insertion of an electrode array difficult or impossible. The commonest such abnormality is labyrinthitis ossificans, of otogenic or meningitic origin, the result of a suppurative otitis interna (Figure 3.18). Magnetic resonance imaging may also be indicated to confirm fibrosis by absence of the normal high signal from fluids on the T2-weighted sequence; MRI is also indicated in congenital lesions where there is any question of there being an absence of the cochlear nerve (Figure 3.22).

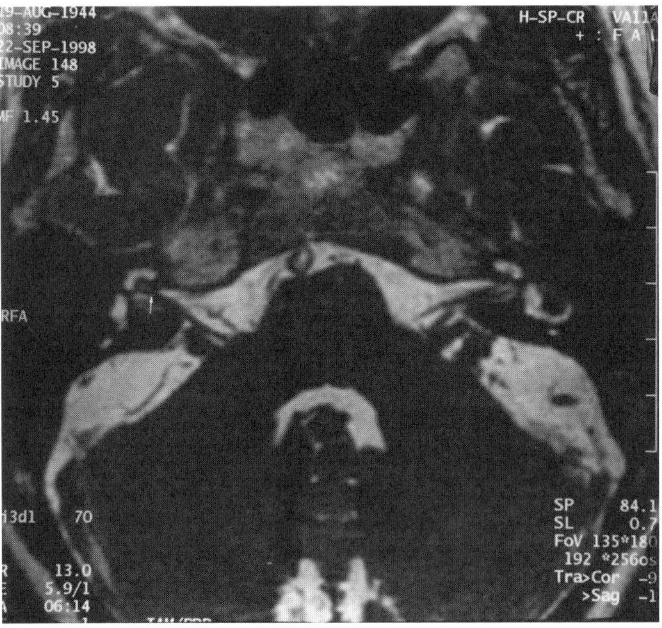

Figure 3.22. Normal axial MRI section showing the cochlear nerve in the IAM (arrow).

CHAPTER 4

Epidemiology of permanent childhood hearing impairment

A DAVIS AND G MENCHER

Introduction

Hearing impairment is the most frequent sensory impairment in humans, with significant social and psychological implications. In the UK, about 800 children are born each year with a significant permanent hearing impairment (Davis, 1993a). It is likely that the greatest impact of hearing impairment upon a child is on the acquisition of language and development of communication, which in turn can lead to poor literacy skills (see, for example, Bench and Bamford, 1979; Conrad, 1979; Levitt, McGarr and Geffner, 1987; Gallaway, Nunes and Johnston, 1994; Gregory, 1995). It is also likely that other areas of development will be affected, for example educational achievement (Powers, 1996), mental health (Laurenzi and Monteiro, 1997), self-esteem (Batchava, 1993), and long-term employment opportunities (Gregory, Bishop and Sheldon, 1995). However, despite these difficulties it is possible that, given adequate support, their impact may be reduced. For example, language development may be enhanced through the use of language support programmes, residual hearing may be used effectively through adequate amplification (hearing aids or cochlear implants), and providing family support through educational services, audiology services and social services. Evidence increasingly shows that such a support programme, used in tandem with early identification procedures – such as universal neonatal hearing screening – is more beneficial the earlier it is embarked upon by the families of hearing-impaired children (see, for example, Yoshinaga-Itano et al., 1998). It has also been recommended in the NDCS guidelines of good practice (1994): 'early detection and management of hearing impairment will help to lessen the impact of the condition on the child's social, emotional, intellectual, and linguistic development. The child and family will benefit from such early detection and management.' In the light of the impact that hearing impairment can have on children and their families, the importance of epidemiological studies cannot be underestimated, because they can provide information concerning the etiology of hearing impairment, the groups within a population who are most at risk, and the overall prevalence of hearing impairment. In this chapter we will focus on permanent childhood hearing impairment (PCHI). However, hearing impairment is not easy to classify. It is necessary to take into account not only the severity of the hearing impairment, but also the pathology and ontogenesis of the impairment. These factors will be the main focus of the chapter.

Definitions used in epidemiological studies

Epidemiology is the study of how often diseases occur in different groups of people and why. Epidemiological information may be used to 'plan and evaluate strategies to prevent illness and as a guide to the management of patients in whom disease has already developed' (Coggon, Rose and Barker, 1993). Sancho et al. (1988) use the term 'epidemiology' to refer to 'the study of the distribution and determinants of hearing disorders in a population, and the application of the knowledge obtained to the prevention and amelioration of hearing problems'. A population study is the primary methodology for gathering information. The word 'population' in this case refers to the whole collection of units from which a sample may be drawn, but not necessarily to a population of people. For example, it may be a collection of hearing aid clinics or schools for the deaf. The sample is intended to give results that are representative of the population as a whole. If the population under study is people, the term *cohort* may be used. A cohort is that component of a population born during a particular period and identified by period of birth, so that its characteristics (such as prevalence of childhood hearing impairment, or age at first hearing aid fitting) can be ascertained as it enters successive time and age periods. If an epidemiological study follows a cohort and studies the group at several different intervals, the project is called a cohort study. A cohort study can be a follow-up study, a prospective study, or a longitudinal study. A cohort study is essential for understanding change over time and the impact of services.

Another key term associated with epidemiology is *incidence*. This refers to the number of new instances of a specific condition (such as hearing impairment from meningitis) occurring during a certain period in a specified population. The incidence rate is the rate at which this occurs per standard population, for example 10 new cases per year per 100 000 children. The term *prevalence* is often confused with incidence. However, these are not the same thing. Prevalence is the total number of instances within a given population at a specific time in which a specific condition (for example, Pendred syndrome) is present. In the case of hearing impairment, prevalence may be described as 'the proportion of individuals with a defined type of hearing impairment in a specified population cohort' (Sancho et al., 1988). Accordingly, the prevalence rate is the number of individuals who have the condition or attribute divided by the population at risk at a point in time.

When attempting a prevalence study, if there are n children with hearing impairment in the study and the whole population is N, then the prevalence rate is (n × 100/N)%. In this case we must be sure that the n hearing-impaired children really come from all the birth cohorts of children represented by the population of N and that there is a co-terminosity of n and N in terms of geographical boundaries. It is quite common to either underestimate n (because not all children with a given condition have been found) or to confuse populations (often because of migration of children into or out of particular districts). A population study is one in which the sample is carefully selected for representativeness of the whole population.

The importance and difficulty of estimating prevalence

One of the most important functions of the collection of epidemiological information is in order that it may be used in planning preventative and rehabilitative services for hearing-impaired children. The paucity of data on the prevalence and causes of childhood hearing impairment worldwide is exacerbated by the great difficulty in interpreting the data; perhaps leading to the variability in prevalence rates seen from study to study. These variations may be due in part to a number of factors: the criteria used to define hearing impairment, adoption of different operational definitions, or use of incompatible methodologies. The importance of having agreed definitions for epidemiological studies, such as the ones outlined in the previous section, can be seen to be of paramount importance. Studies also tend to be cross-sectional and based on retrospective ascertainment rather than from longitudinal studies in well-defined geographical areas. The problem of not using a common definition across studies can be seen to hinder estimates of prevalence rates as well as hindering investigation of possible risk factors and etiologies of hearing impairment. This, in turn, has implications for the planning of service provision. Figure 4.1 presents the commonly used definitions for the various types of hearing impairment.

Given the variety of types of hearing impairments presented in Figure 4.1, it can easily be understood why there may be some confusion when attempting to define prevalence and/or incidence. However, the problem is compounded even further when various generalized categories for the etiology (cause) of the hearing impairment and the pattern of the hearing impairment are taken into consideration. Temporary hearing impairment (usually, but not always a conductive hearing impairment) can be treated and corrected by medical or surgical intervention. Such an impairment is often short-lived and of a mild nature. On the other hand, permanent hearing impairment cannot be treated by surgical or medical intervention and results in a permanent hearing impairment ≥ 40 dB HL. Both temporary and permanent hearing impairments can be unilateral (one ear only has either a greater than 20 dB hearing impairment through 500, 1 000 and 2 000 kHz or one frequency exceeding 50 dB, with the other ear normal) or bilateral (a greater than 20 dB hearing impairment through 500, 1 000 and 2 000 kHz or one frequency exceeding 50 dB in both ears). A unilateral situation is, of course, asymmetrical. However, in studies of hearing, the term asymmetrical hearing impairment specifically refers to a greater than 10 dB difference between the ears in at least two frequencies, with the pure-tone average in the better ear exceeding 20 dB HL. Finally, both temporary and permanent hearing impairments can be progressive. That is, there is a deterioration greater than or equal to 15 dB in the pure-tone average within a ten-year period.

Historically, the convenient figure of one per 1 000 for sensorineural hearing impairment has often been quoted (Fraser, 1976). Further estimates of the prevalence of childhood hearing impairment (worldwide) vary in the literature from 0.5/1 000 to 1.5/1 000 births (see, for example, Newton, 1985; Das, 1990; Feinmesser, Tell and Levi., 1990; Pabla, McCormick and Gibbin, 1991; Davis and Wood, 1992; Parving, 1993; Fortnum and Davis, 1997). Note that the terms used are *sensorineural deafness* and *hearing impairment.* Not only are these different words but they also represent different things. The term 'deaf' is generally associated with the most extreme form of hearing impairment, in which there is no response to auditory stimuli in excess of 120–125 dB at any frequency. This condition is practically never seen and is considered very rare. Hearing impairment, on the other hand, primarily refers to a series of descriptive terms that define the decibel level at which an individual responds to sound (see Figure 4.2). Hearing impairment is also defined by the frequency range the person can hear. That is, a low-frequency range is < 500 kHz; a mid-frequency range is 500 to 2 000 kHz; a high-frequency range is 2 000 to 8 000 kHz; and an extended high-frequency range is > 8 000 kHz. The pattern of the frequencies is also important with some fairly self explanatory terms such as u-shaped, low-frequency ascending, flat, and high-frequency sloping, used as descriptors of the responses plotted on an audiogram.

Sensorineural: related to disease/deformity of the inner ear/cochlear nerve with an air-bone gap less than 15 dB averaged over 0.5, 1 and 2 kHz

Conductive: related to disease or deformity of the outer/middle ears. Audiometrically there are normal bone conduction thresholds (less than 20 dB) and an air-bone gap greater than 15 dB averaged over 0.5, 1 and 2 kHz

Mixed: related to combined involvement of the outer/middle ears and the inner ear/cochlear nerve. Audiometrically greater than 20 dB HL in the bone conduction threshold together with greater than or equal to 15 dB air-bone gap averaged over 0.5, 1 and 2 kHz

Sensory: a subdivision of sensorineural related to disease or deformity in the cochlea

Neural: a subdivision of sensorineural related to a disease or deformity in the cochlear nerve

Central: sensorineural hearing loss related to a disease or deformity central nervous system rostral to the cochlear nerve

Figure 4.1. Definitions of the various types of hearing impairment.

Average hearing level: the level of the thresholds (in dB HL) measured in the better hearing ear at 0.5, 1, 2, 4 kHz
Mild: average hearing level 20–39dB HL
Moderate: average hearing level 40–69 dB HL
Severe: average hearing level 70–94 dB HL
Profound: average hearing level +95 dB HL

Figure 4.2. Definitions of hearing impairment in dB levels.

Prevalence of hearing impairment

Prevalence of hearing impairment in the US

Carney and Moeller (1998), reported that, in 1990, 21 in every 1000 children in the US under the age of 18 (2.1%) had some degree of hearing impairment (NIH, 1993) and approximately one in every 1000 is born with a profound hearing impairment. (0.1%). The hearing impairment in one-third of the hearing-impaired children is thought to result from damage to the inner ear (NIH, 1993). Nearly one in 1000 children suffer from early onset sensorineural hearing impairment severe enough to impede normal language acquisition; thus it follows that severe and profound bilateral, sensorineural hearing impairment affects approximately one in 1000 children. Approximately 90% of children with severe to profound sensorineural hearing impairment have parents with normal hearing (Northern and Downs, 1991). A later estimate of prevalence in the US in a study by Yoshinaga-Itano and colleagues (1998) suggests that the prevalence of bilateral and permanent hearing impairment is between 1.2 and 5.7 per 1000 live births. For milder degrees of bilateral hearing impairment, early estimates report six in 1000 live births (Matkin, 1984). A later report by Bess, Dodd-Murphy and Parker (1998) identified a prevalence of 5.4% for minimal sensorineural hearing impairment in school children in his study – that is one in 20 of his sample exhibited an impairment of greater than 25 dB in the speech frequency range.

In a national population-based cross-sectional health and nutritional survey of over 6000 children aged from six to 19 years, interviews and audiometric testing at 0.5 kHz through to 8 kHz were used to study the prevalence of hearing impairment in the group (Niskar et al., 1998). The results showed that 14.9% of children had low-frequency or high-frequency hearing impairment of at least 16 dB HL, 7.1% had a low-frequency impairment of at least 16 dB HL, and 12.7% had high-frequency hearing impairment of at least 16 dB HL. The majority of conductive hearing impairment was shown to affect the low frequencies, whereas the majority of sensorineural hearing impairment affected the high frequencies. The findings suggest that more children suffer with unilateral than with bilateral hearing impairment, and with a high-frequency hearing impairment more than with a low-frequency impairment. The researchers recommend that audiometric screening in schools should include low- and high- frequency testing to detect hearing impairment. If this is carried out it is suggested that hearing impairment may be detected at an earlier age and thus intervention may prevent further hearing impairment by maintaining residual hearing and enhance educational achievements.

Most of the hearing impairments identified in the Niskar et al. (1998) study were unilateral and mild in severity. Unilateral hearing impairment can affect speech perception, learning, self-image and social skills (Anderson, 1992). Mild hearing impairments, both unilateral and bilateral, can affect children in classrooms where they may have difficulty perceiving and understanding speech sounds. A child with a mild hearing impairment might require intervention such as speech therapy and even possibly hearing aids (Tharpe and Bess, 1999).

Prevalence of hearing impairment in the UK

General studies

According to published figures, for the general population of the UK prevalence rates are 1–2 per 1 000 for severe/profound hearing impairment (see, for example, Newton, 1985; Parving, 1985; Peckham, 1986). Various studies have been carried out in the UK to ascertain accurate prevalence rates; however, there has been considerable disagreement between the rates established. Such variation may be explained by population differences, for example regional variation, different target age groups, success of ascertainment, degree of hearing impairment included in the sample; as well as the method used to collect information: for example, ascertainment, prospective, longitudinal, and the reliability and range of the data collected. This can be best illustrated by outlining some of the studies.

Pabla et al. (1991) concluded a prevalence rate of 0.55/1000 for children born in the Nottingham area from 1981–5, for children with a bilateral hearing impairment greater than 40 dB. Data included family history, medical examination, and audiological testing (distraction test, pure-tone audiometry and electrical response audiometry, and tympanometry). However, a further study in the same region (Davis and Wood, 1992) reported a prevalence rate of 1.2%. Their sample included all children born between 1983 and 1986 who had a sensorineural or mixed hearing impairment of greater than 50 dB HL. Data from this study included records from a hearing assessment centre, NICU records, and records from a targeted screening programme, and hearing assessments. Davis et al. (1995) reported a prevalence of hearing impairment of 1.2 per 1000 live births per annum in Nottingham, Sheffield and Oxford for children born between 1983–8. Hearing impairment included bilateral sensorineural or mixed, and at least 40 dB HL. Moderate hearing impairment (40–69 dB HL) accounted for 50% of these, severe (70–94 dB HL) for 23%, and profound (greater than 95 dB HL) for 27%. A family history of childhood sensorineural hearing impairment was evident in 25% of the children and 32% had spent time in a neonatal intensive care unit (NICU). Similar studies have been carried out in the Manchester area (Newton, 1985; Newton and Rowson, 1988; Das, 1990). These studies identified a prevalence rate of between 0.8/1000 and 1.2/1000 for bilateral sensorineural hearing impairment greater than 25 dB. Audiological, ophthalmic and medical examinations were performed and family history and medical records were also used as sources of information upon which these prevalence rates were based. It is clear from the variability of the prevalence rates obtained in these various studies that care needs to be taken in the definition of hearing impairment for such investigations. Variation in sample populations, hearing levels included in the study, as well as fluctuating numbers of children with hearing impairment are all factors that lead to such variation in prevalence figures.

The Trent ascertainment study

Epidemiological studies have largely been based on small populations (Davis and Wood, 1992), often using just clinic-based lists or registers where information about all levels of severity were not available (see, for example, Martin et al., 1979; Newton, 1985; Das, 1988; Dias, 1990; Shui, Purvis and Sutton, 1996; Sutton and Rowe, 1997). However, an extensive study of epidemiology of permanent childhood hearing impairment (PCHI) has been carried out in the Trent Regional Health Authority (Fortnum et al., 1997). In this study it has been shown there are substantial differences in prevalence over districts in the UK and in the risk profiles of different populations. Prevalence rates of 1.3/1 000 for both acquired and congenital permanent hearing impairment were reported. For congenital hearing impairment alone, the prevalence rate was 1.1/1 000.

All children with a permanent hearing impairment of 40 dB HL or greater in their better ear, averaged over 0.5, 1, 2 and 4 kHz, who had been born between 1 January 1985 and 31 December 1993 and were living within the boundary of Trent Regional Health Authority at the time of data collection (June–September 1995), were included in this study. Sources of information included the Education Database, the Community Audiology and Child Health Database, the Neonatal Screening Database, audiology and medical records, and hearing aid records.

The data collected were divided into two main groups: congenital hearing impairment and acquired hearing impairment. The congenital group consisted of those children presumed to have had a pre-natal or perinatal hearing impairment. The acquired group included those whose hearing impairment came later in life due to disease, progressive hearing impairment or late-onset hearing impairment where there was evidence that the child may have been able to hear at an earlier stage. Table 4.1 shows the prevalence rates ascertained for the Trent Region divided into the two groups for three severity bands: moderate (40–69 dB HL), severe (70–94 dB HL), and profound (95+ dB HL) hearing impairment.

Calculations of prevalence in the UK

Taking the prevalence estimates derived from the Trent region (Fortnum et al., 1997) and data for the number of live births, it is possible to calculate the number of children who may be expected to be hearing-impaired for the whole of the UK. As Table 4.2 indicates, we might expect to find approximately 1 000 hearing-impaired children in the UK per annual birth cohort with at least a moderate hearing impairment, with just under 84% having a congenital hearing impairment.

Given the estimated number of children born with PCHI in the UK, the need for an early identification programme to reduce the impact of those impairments is clear. Undoubtedly this has contributed to a decision by the government of the UK to develop such a programme by the year 2002. Ultimately, a universal newborn screening programme should enable a more precise appraisal of the prevalence of hearing impairment, provide a more accurate etiological picture, and provide for earlier audiological and educational intervention programmes to be established.

Table 4.1. The prevalence (per 100,000 children) of three broad severity categories of Permanent Childhood Hearing Impairment (PCHI) as a function of onset (congenital versus acquired) for the 1985–90 birth cohort in the Trent Region

	Severity (dB HL)	Prevalence per 100000	95% CI
Congenital	40–69	64	56–73
	70–94	23	19–29
	95+	24	20–30
Acquired	40–69	9	7–12
	70–94	5	3–8
	95+	7	5–10

Table 4.2. The estimated number of children with permanent childhood hearing impairment (PCHI) in the UK per annual birth cohort.

Severity of hearing impairment (dB HL)	All PCHI	Congenital PCHI
40	998	840
50	825	675
60	608	480
70	443	353
80	353	278
90	263	210
95	233	180
100	180	135
110	83	68
120	30	23

Prevalence of hearing impairment in Europe

Martin et al. (1981) performed an ascertainment study of hearing-impaired children in the European Community (nine countries) who were born in 1969 and eight years old at the time of the study, and who had a hearing impairment of at least 50 dB HL. They found a prevalence rate of 0.9 per 1 000. They also reported that 29% of the children had additional disabilities, and a conductive hearing impairment was present in 7% of the cases. Feinmesser et al. (1990) identified a slightly higher prevalence rate of 1.18/1 000 in the population of children born in Jerusalem between 1968 and 1985, whose bilateral sensorineural hearing impairment was greater than 55 dB.

Prevalence of hearing impairment in UK has also been compared with that in Denmark (Davis and Parving, 1994) where differences and similarities between Denmark and England for PCHI were assessed. The severity profile of the hearing impairment, risk factors, and the age of identification were examined. The criteria for inclusion in the study were the presence of valid hearing thresholds across the frequencies 0.5, 1, 2, 4 kHz that indicated a bilateral hearing impairment of a sensorineural or mixed type of greater than or equal to 40 dB HL in the better-hearing ear. Data collected included NICU attendance, family history of PCHI, and age of identification. Children were divided into the categories of congenital or acquired hearing impairment. Prevalence of all permanent sensorineural and mixed childhood hearing impairments per 100 000 children in the birth cohort 1982–88 were calculated and are shown in Table 4.3.

Table 4.3. Prevalence of all (congenital and acquired) permanent sensorineural and mixed childhood hearing impairments per 100000 children in the birth cohort 1982–88 for Denmark and England

Country	40–130 dB HL	70–130 dBHL	95–130 dB HL
Denmark	145	86	54
England	121	64	37
Denmark and England	127	69	41

Prevalence of congenital sensorineural and mixed childhood hearing impairment per 100 000 children in the birth cohort 1982–88 were also calculated and are shown in Table 4.4. Results indicated a prevalence of 1.3 per 1 000 by the age of five years, approximately 90% of hearing impairment reported was congenital. It can be seen that there were significantly more severely and profoundly hearing-impaired children in Denmark than in England. When risk factors were investigated it was found that significantly more congenitally hearing-impaired children had a

NICU history in England (33%) than in Denmark (17%). The number of hearing-impaired children with a family history of hearing impairment differed significantly between the two countries: in England 27% indicated a family history, whereas in Denmark this figure was 40%.

The median age of first appointment for hearing assessment was 12 months. The age of identification did not differ between the two countries for severely or profoundly hearing impaired children, but there was a significant difference between them for the age of identification of children with a moderate hearing-impairment (40–69 dB HL) with a non-NICU history. The median age of identification in England was 18 months and in Denmark it was 30 months. For those with a NICU history the figures were 11 months in England and 20 months in Denmark. It can be seen from this study that more than 50% of the congenitally hearing-impaired children were identified before the age of one year. While this is a good improvement from the last estimate of three years, indicated by Martin et al. (1979), it falls below the recommended target, to identify all children with hearing impairment between six and 12 months of age.

Table 4.4. Prevalence of only congenital sensorineural and mixed childhood permanent hearing impairment per 100000 children in the birth cohort 1982–88 for Denmark and England

Country	40–130 dB HL	70–130 dBHL	95–130 dB HL
Denmark	134	80	52
England	110	54	30
Denmark and England	116	60	36

In addition to studies that compare the various aspects of childhood hearing impairment in Denmark and England, further work by Uus and Davis (2000) centres around the same issues in Estonia. Based on data gathered as a retrospective study at the only two service locations for hearing-impaired children in the country, it was found that the median age for confirmation of the presence of hearing was 46 months whereas the median age for the first hearing aid fitting was 57 months (see Table 4.5). Uus and Davis also reported that the prevalence of hearing impairment in Estonia (172 per 100 000) was higher than that of England (121 per 100 000) and that of Denmark (145 per 100 000). Furthermore, detection, and thus intervention, occurred significantly later.

The hearing impairments reported were primarily sensorineural (91.5%) and conductive (8.5%). It was also noted that 18.6% of the Estonian children have a progressive hearing impairment. Congenital impairment accounted for 88.3% of the cases, while 8.5% were known

Table 4.5. The average age of identification and hearing aid fitting (birth cohort 1985–90) in Estonia

Severity of hearing impairment	Mean age of identification (in months)	Mean age of hearing aid fitting (in months)
Moderate	65.5	73.2
Severe	37.7	48.3
Profound	25.3	40.5
Total	46.4	57.0

acquired hearing losses. The remaining 3.2% were unknown. In comparison to the data from Estonia, results from the Trent study indicated approximately 84.2% congenital hearing impairments compared to approximately 15.8% acquired for the UK.

Finally, when the etiology of the hearing impairments in Estonia was considered, it was found that 36.3% were of a genetic origin. Pre-natal and perinatal factors, including NICU and low birth weight were present in 20% of the children. Meningitis was the largest single post-natal factor (8.5%). However, one-third (34.3%) of the children had a hearing impairment of unknown origin.

It is possible to see from the data presented by this study that it may not be possible to generalize the findings of one study regarding prevalence to other geographical areas or, for that matter, to other birth cohorts. For that reason epidemiological studies at the local level should be considered necessary to determine needs when planning for service provision.

Prevalence rates around the world

From data collected in previous studies where maximum ascertainment from several sources has been achieved, it may be possible to calculate prevalence rates around the world. Table 4.6 illustrates the estimated global prevalence of PCHI including acquired disorders, while the following table (Table 4.7) shows the estimated global prevalence of OME and other associated forms of childhood hearing disorders.

Risk factors

Sensorineural hearing impairment can lead to problems with communication, academic performance, psychosocial behaviour and emotional development (Bess and McConnell, 1981; Davis, Johnsson and Kornfeld, 1981; Davis 1990; Karchmer, 1991; DeVilliers, 1992; Holt, 1993). It can also affect the family and society, causing tension and disruption, social isolation and a breakdown in

Table 4.6. Estimated numbers (000s) of children aged 0–19 years with permanent childhood hearing impairment (PCHI) including acquired hearing losses

Region	Total population	Number of children aged 0–19 years	Mild PCHI 20dB HL + unilateral	Moderate PCHI 40dB HL + bilateral	Profound PCHI 95dB HL + bilateral
World	6 228 254	2 494 649	14 967	3 317	73
More developed	1 277 963	348 653	2 091	463	108
Less developed	4 950 291	2 145 996	12 875	2 854	665
Africa	856 154	468 169	2 809	622	145
Latin America	522 962	217 452	1 304	289	67
North America	305 881	86 941	521	115	26
Europe	523 749	131 351	787	174	40
Oceania	30 967	10 425	62	13	3
Asia	3 691 579	1 485 029	8 910	1 975	460

Table 4.7. Estimated numbers (000s) of children aged 0–19 years with OME and other associated forms of childhood hearing disorders

Region	Persistent OME	Persistent OME and hearing loss	Tinnitus	Moderate speech in noise problem	Severe speech in noise problem
World	254 454	99 785	104 775	266 927	37 419
More developed	35 562	13 946	14 643	37 305	5 229
Less developed	218 891	85 839	90 131	229 621	32 189
Africa	47 753	18 726	19 663	50 094	7 022
Latin America	22 180	8 698	9 132	23 267	3 261
North America	8 867	3 477	3 651	9 302	1 304
Europe	13 387	5 250	5 512	14 043	1 968
Oceania	1 063	417	437	1 115	156
Asia	151 472	59 401	62 371	158 898	22 275

social communication and interaction (Davis, 1988; Maliszewski, 1988; Bess and Paradise, 1984). Early identification and (re)habilitation are essential to try to avoid these various potential complications.

One method of early identification of any pathology involves targeting those considered at risk for the problem and applying some sort of screening device to pinpoint those individuals who actually have it. Risk, in this case, refers to the probability that an event will occur, for example that a child will have a hearing impairment.

Notable risk factors that have been associated with hearing impairment include: family history of permanent hearing impairment (present since childhood in at least one of the following family members: parent, sibling, grandparent, great-grandparent, aunt, uncle, nephew, niece, cousin), length of stay in NICU, respiratory distress syndrome, neonatal asphyxia, hyperbilirubinaemia, craniofacial anomalies and retinopathy of prematurity (Kountakis et al., 1997; Mencher, 2000). Borg (1997) has suggested that the total number of risk factors (as indicated by the total length of stay in NICU and the time the baby receives assisted ventilation) are the best predictors of hearing impairment of perinatal origin and that premature babies are more vulnerable than full-term babies. In order to make some sense of the various factors that may be at the root cause of hearing impairment, and to assist in early identification of the problem, a systematic listing of common etiological factors has been developed. This list is called the high-risk register for hearing impairment.

The best known register for helping to identify hearing impairment is the Joint Committee on Infant Hearing High Risk Register (JCIH, 2000). It consists of a list of indicators by which a neonate or infant can be judged to be 'at risk' for sensorineural and/or conductive hearing impairment (Figure 4.3). This list should provide the basis for referral for audiological evaluation, which should take place between three and six months of age.

There have been a number of studies that test the effectiveness of the high-risk register (Thompson and Folsom, 1981; Stein, Clark and Kraus, 1983; Elssan, Matkin and Sabo, 1987; Halpern, Hosford-Dunn and Malachowski, 1987; Swigonski et al., 1987; Mauk et al., 1991; Watkin, 1991). In general, these studies suggested that between 30% and 50% of children would not be detected using such a register. It should be noted, however, that most of the studies reported here were based upon previous versions of the register and the current version may be a better device than its predecessors. Nevertheless, it is clear from such studies that a high-risk register needs to be supplemented by additional measures. One such measure might be a targeted neonatal hearing screening primarily directed toward children on the register. However, as already indicated, it is likely that a significant number of neonates with congenital hearing impairment are not in the high risk group, and therefore may be missed by targeted screening. An alternative appears to be to introduce universal neonatal hearing screening. Guidelines for good practice, which are similar to those of the US Joint Committee on Infant Hearing (JCIH), have been drawn up by the National Deaf Children's Society in the UK (1994). These set targets for age of identification. The first is to detect 80% of bilateral congenital hearing impairment in excess of 50 dB HL within the first year of life and 40% by the age of six months. A second target is to ensure that by the age of one year all children will have benefited from either a formal screen or a specific surveillance procedure to assess their risk of hearing impairment.

For use with infants (birth–28 days)

1. family history of hereditary childhood sensorineural hearing impairment
2. *in utero* infection (e.g. CMV, rubella, syphilis, herpes, toxoplasmosis)
3. craniofacial anomalies
4. birth weight less than 1500 grams
5. hyperbilirubinaemia at a serum level requiring exchange transfusion
6. ototoxic medications
7. bacterial meningitis
8. Apgar score of 0–4 at one minute and 0–6 at five minutes
9. mechanical ventilation lasting 5 days or more
10. stigmata associated with a syndrome known to include sensorineural and/or conductive hearing loss

For use with infants 29 days–2 years when health conditions develop that require rescreening

1. parent concern regarding hearing, speech, language, and/or developmental delay
2. bacterial meningitis and other infections associated with sensorineural hearing loss
3. head trauma associated with loss of consciousness or skull fracture
4. stigmata associated with a syndrome known to include sensorineural and/or conductive hearing loss
5. ototoxic medications
6. recurrent or persistent otitis media with effusion for at least three months

For use with infants (aged 29 days–3 years) who require periodic monitoring of hearing

1. family history of hereditary childhood hearing loss
2. *in utero* infection
3. Neurofibromastosis Type II and neurodegenerative disorders

Indicators associated with conductive hearing loss include:

1. recurrent or persistent otitis media with effusion
2. anatomic deformities an other disorders that effect Eustachian tube function
3. neurodegenerative disorders

Figure 4.3. Joint Committee on Infant Hearing High Risk Register for identification of hearing impairment (1994).

Following the JCIH (1994) report on risk factors, it was noted that the majority of children on the register will actually fall into three larger categories:

- a stay of 48 hours or longer in NICU;
- a family history of permanent childhood hearing impairment; and
- craniofacial anomalies (Davis and Wood, 1992).

Subsequently, in a further study of these elements, Davis and Wood (1992) studied children falling into four categories:

- those with no high risk factor;
- graduates from the NICU;
- those with a family history of hearing impairment; and
- those with a syndrome associated with hearing impairment.

These groups were divided into congenital, progressive and acquired. Davis and Wood acknowledged that meningitis-induced profound hearing impairment accounts for a large proportion of children with profound hearing impairment overall. The main conclusions reached from the study were:

- Approximately one in 900 children have a bilateral 50 dB HL hearing impairment or greater.
- NICU babies are at least 10 times more likely to have a significant bilateral sensorineural or mixed hearing impairment than non-NICU babies, who have neither family history of hearing impairment nor a syndrome noticeable at birth.
- The prevalence of substantial other problems in addition to hearing impairment, was approximately 35%. Approximately 70% of the NICU babies had substantial other problems.

In the later Trent study (Fortnum et al., 1997) it was reported that 59% of the congenital PCHI have one or more of the three larger risk factors (history of NICU for 48 hours or longer – 29%; family history of PCHI – 31%; craniofacial abnormality noticeable at birth – 12%). When a stay in the NICU and/or a family history have been taken into account for those children with multiple categories, the craniofacial group declines in size to only to 3.7%, indicating that the first two categories are the major risk factors for permanent childhood hearing impairment. For children identified in the Trent study who had spent time in the NICU, the proportion of 'acquired' cases was 12%, compared to 10% for those with a family history, and 22% for those with no risk factors at all.

In summary then, it has been reported (Davis and Wood, 1992) that children with a history of admission to a neonatal intensive care unit (NICU) have a much increased risk of hearing impairment over children with no risk factors. Other reports also show that there is a high proportion of mild to moderate hearing impairment among children who have attended NICU (Davis et al., 1995). Babies attending NICU suffer many complicating factors, and it is often hard to judge, therefore, which of those factors may be causal in the resulting hearing impairment. In general, although there is a specific high-risk register for hearing impairment it does appear as though the items on that list may be reasonably combined into three larger categories, which may be used to describe those with an increased risk of hearing impairment. The groupings are considered to be of major importance when planning services for identification of hearing impairments detectable at or around birth. They are:

- admission for 48 hours or longer to a neonatal intensive care unit (NICU);
- a family history of permanent hearing impairment arising in childhood; and
- the presence of craniofacial abnormality (CFA).

These risk factors can also be used when targeting specific groups for neonatal hearing screening. Over half of the babies with detectable hearing impairment might be identified if all those with at least one of the above risk factors were screened within a screening programme that had a sensitive test and high coverage (Davis et al., 1995; Sutton and Rowe, 1997).

Etiology

Before embarking on a detailed discussion of the various etiologies of hearing impairment, there are two very important terms that must be defined. All etiologies fall into one or the other of these two groups:

- Congenital hearing impairment: hearing impairment considered by examination of the case history to be present and detectable using appropriate tests at or very soon after birth.
- Acquired hearing impairment: hearing impairment acquired post-natally, or of late onset, or of progressive nature, which, on the basis of case history, was not considered to be present and detectable using appropriate tests at or very soon after birth.

The frequency of occurrence of some causes of hearing impairment has changed over the past 30 years, and further changes will occur with the implementation of new ways of preventing hearing impairment. For example, in the US rubella and bacterial meningitis have been greatly reduced though vaccination programmes. In addition, hyperbilirubinemia, once the major cause of cerebral palsy and approximately 7–10% of congenital hearing impairment, is now nearly a thing of the past with the introduction of photosynthetic lights in the NICU and *in utero* exchange transfusions.

On the other hand, since the 1960s, medical advances have ensured that more premature, asphyxic and low-birth-weight babies now survive, leading to a greater proportion of NICU babies with hearing impairment. Thus, hereditary factors, CMV and babies who have attended NICU are now the main causal factors for hearing impairment in children. Babies who have attended NICU may typically experience several of the high-risk criteria listed by the Joint Committee on Infant Hearing: low birth weight, low Apgar score, and mechanical ventilation lasting five days or more. NICU babies may also experience other identified risk factors such as exposure to ototoxic medications and bacterial meningitis. Children with *in utero* infections such as CMV, rubella, herpes, syphilis and toxoplasmosis, as well as those with craniofacial anomalies or syndromes known to be associated with sensorineural or conductive hearing impairment (such as Down's syndrome), are frequently admitted to the NICU for associated problems. Roizen (1999) suggests that in the period 1983–92 in the US, the percentage of children with hearing impairment identified by NICU admission increased, with 19% being of low birth weight and 8% having perinatal factors.

It is clear that over the past 25 years there have been changes in the proportion of children in each broad etiological group (less rubella, more prematurity, possibly more genetic), specific determination of the etiology of any given hearing impairment continues to be difficult. The major etiological classification system suggested by Davidson, Hyde and Alberti (1989) has been used in most recent studies. The categories are:

- genetic;
- pre-natally acquired;
- perinatally acquired;
- post-natally acquired;
- craniofacial anomalies;
- other; and
- missing.

Unfortunately, however, the major problem with most studies is that children do not always have an ascribed etiology. There are reports of 30% to 50% of unknown origin (Parving, 1984; Newton, 1985; Davis and Wood, 1992). In the Trent study, 41% of children did not have an identifiable etiology. Nevertheless, it is possible to impute etiology from other data such as medical notes. For the Trent study, such a step reduced the percentage who had no etiological information to approximately 25% (Table 4.8).

Table 4.8. Classification of aetiological groups for children with PCHI in the Trent region born between 1985–93 (n=653), and separated into congenital (n=556) and acquired (n=97) hearing impairment

Category	Overall % (imputed)	Congenital %	Acquired %
Genetic	44.7	48.2	24.7
Pre-natal	4.0	4.0	1.0
Perinatal	16.7	17.6	11.3
Post-natal	6.0	0	41.2
CFA	2.5	2.9	0
Other	2.0	1.0	3.0
Missing	24.6	25.7	18.6

Pre-natal factors

Pre-natal factors often cause sensorineural hearing impairment. They can result from genetic anomalies, infection or maternal drug therapy.

Genetic hearing impairment

At least half of all cases of permanent childhood hearing impairment are known to have a genetic cause (Reardon, 1992). Further, studies have shown that between 30% and 50% of childhood hearing impairment of an unknown etiology are presumed to be genetically based (Parving, 1984; Newton, 1985; Davis et al., 1995, Parving, 1996). It has been estimated that the common 35delG mutation in the Connexin-26 gene accounts for 20% of all genetic childhood hearing impairment (Kelley et al., 1998). Parker et al. (1999) investigated childhood hearing impairment from a genetic perspective, specifically with reference to Connexin-26 and the 35delG mutation. The families of 526 hearing-impaired children (aged 4–13) were sent questionnaires asking about their experience of clinical genetics, and they also participated in clinical assessment and molecular sampling. Results pointed toward a definitive relationship between non-syndromal hearing impairment and autosomal dominant, autosomal recessive and sporadically based hearing impairment. The authors recommend a specific protocol to be used for the investigation of permanent childhood hearing impairment. The protocol contains specific mechanisms to explore the probability of a genetically based hearing problem. It is clear that recent advances in genetic technology will allow genetic causes to be more readily identified in the future.

Approximately 30% of genetic hearing impairment is syndromal (Bergstrom, Hemenway and Downs, 1971; Reardon and Pembrey, 1990). There are currently approximately 170 chromosomal disorders and 400 syndromes of single gene or unknown etiology that have hearing impairment as an associated feature. It has been estimated that 10% of all disease-associated gene mutations can cause some degree of hearing impairment (McKusick et al., 1994); indeed, estimates of the proportion of genetically related hearing impairment have varied from 23% (Das, 1990), to 30 % (Peckham, 1986), to 39.7% (Fortnum and Davis, 1997) up to 50% (Reardon, 1992).

Syndromal hearing impairment can be sensorineural, due to structural anomalies of the auditory system. An association of hearing impairment in children with syndromes should not be overlooked as it can be important in determining prognosis and intervention measures as well as for estimating the recurrence risks in the family (Mueller, 1996). Chromosomal abnormalities may occur, either during meosis or mitosis, resulting in too much or too little genetic material. Examples of this, which can result in hearing impairment, include Down syndrome, Patau syndrome, Edward syndrome and Turner syndrome (Northern and Downs, 1991).

The majority of non-syndromal genetic hearing impairment is prelingual, inherited in an autosomal recessive way and is extremely heterogeneous. Autosomal recessive hearing impairment is the most common form of genetic hearing impairment, accounting for 40% of profound deafness (Gerkin, 1986). In recessive inheritance, both parents – although not exhibiting the trait – carry a defective gene. There is therefore a 25% chance of the child inheriting both genes and manifesting the genetic disorder, and there is also a 50% chance that the child will become a carrier for that disorder and not manifest the disorder. Such disorders include: Usher syndrome, Cockayne syndrome, Pendred syndrome, Jervell and Lange-Nielsen syndrome, Hurler syndrome and Alstrom syndrome (Gibbin, 1988). Numerous non-syndromal recessive hearing impairment genes have been localized. Autosomal recessive inheritance is thought to account for approximately 15% of the cases.

X-linked inheritance accounts for approximately 2–3% of the inherited hearing impairments (Fraser, 1976; Rose, Conneally and Nance, 1977). A more recent review suggests that a constant 5% of congenital male hearing impairment is the result of X-linked recessive inheritance (Bitner-Glindzicz et al. 1994). X-linked hearing impairment, which is sex linked, is probably not present at birth but develops in early infancy. The main characteristic of this type of inheritance is that it affects males only, because they inherit only one X chromosome – if this carries the affected gene, hearing impairment will be inherited. Examples of X-linked syndromes include Hunter syndrome, Alport syndrome and Norrie syndrome.

Autosomal dominant non-syndromal hearing impairment usually becomes manifest post-lingually, either because it is congenital and progressive or because it has late onset, however factors such as infection and noise exposure need to be considered in these cases. Further, hearing-impaired children of hearing-impaired parents are often identifiable at birth. In dominant inheritance, only one parent need exhibit the trait. When that is the case, there is a 50% chance of the child inheriting the gene and manifesting the genetic disorder, usually as a high-frequency bilateral hearing impairment. If both parents exhibit the trait, there is a 75% chance of the child manifesting the disorder. Examples of autosomal dominant syndromes include: Marshall-Stickler syndrome, Waardenburg syndrome and Treacher Collins syndrome.

Audiological characteristics of genetic hearing impairments

There have been various attempts to classify and describe hearing impairment. For example, Gorlin (1995) divided genetic sensorineural hearing impairment into nine audiometric types. Autosomal dominant could be congenital severe, congenital low frequency, progressive low frequency, mid frequency, high frequency progressive or unilateral. Autosomal recessive could either be congenital severe to profound or congenital moderate. X-linked stood alone as X-linked congenital and was not subdivided.

Non-syndromal hearing impairment has also been classified according to audiogram shape (for example, Lui and Xu, 1994; Parving and Newton, 1995). The more established audiogram profiles are sloping (loss greater at high frequencies), ascending (loss greater at low frequencies), U-shaped (loss greater at middle frequencies), and flat (all frequencies falling within a narrow range). It is difficult to distinguish patterns of genetic hearing impairment from the confounding effect of age-related hearing impairment, which is common in a normal population (Martini et al., 1996). However, this has been attempted by Martini et al. (1996) who have found that dominant inheritance was strongly associated with a sloping audiogram profile, which also equates to the dominant high frequency progressive type identified by Gorlin. Martini et al. also stated that profound, early-onset hearing impairment is most likely to be recessive. Genetic hearing impairment is generally symmetrical (Langenbeck, 1935). Recessive forms are usually profound and present at an early age, whereas dominant types are less severe but progressive (Fraser, 1976).

Infections

Infections are considered to be the main cause of pre-natally acquired hearing impairment. In the 1970–80s, congenital rubella was the single most common reported cause of sensorineural hearing impairment, accounting for 16–22% of cases of hearing impairment in babies (Martin et al., 1981, 1982; Parving and Hauch, 1994). This figure has been reduced dramatically by the introduction of rubella vaccination (Tookey and Peckham, 1999). Lower rates have now been reported: 10% by Newton (1985), and 5% by Das (1996). If infected during the first month, there is a 50% chance of developing rubella defects. This risk declines throughout pregnancy to an approximately 6% chance in the fifth month and beyond. Problems associated with congenital rubella include learning disability, heart disease, cataracts, microcephaly, hepatomegaly, splenomegaly, bone lesions, purpura, glaucoma, and hearing impairment (Gerkin, 1984). The hearing impairment is usually severe to profound sensorineural hearing impairment, with the mid-frequencies being the most effected (Wilde et al., 1990). Rubella infection may also result in middle-ear anomalies that cause a conductive hearing impairment (Anvar, Mencher and Keet, 1984). Hearing impairment is the most common permanent manifestation and affects 68% to 93% of children with congenital rubella. Roizen (1999) notes that the SNHL is most frequently profound and bilateral, affects all frequencies equally, and is progressive in some cases.

Other infections such as toxoplasmosis (Gerkin, 1986) and cytomegalovirus (CMV) can also result in sensorineural hearing impairment. These together may account for approximately 15% of children with congenital hearing impairments (Davidson, et al., 1989). Other studies have suggested that CMV may account for 2.5% to 3.0% of sensorineural hearing impairment (see, for example, Das, 1996; Newton, 1985). Usually hearing impairment is manifest by the age of two in babies who have been infected, although its onset may be later and the hearing impairment may be progressive. Roizen (1999) has observed that cytomegalovirus infection occurs in 2.2% of all newborns, making it the most common intrauterine infection. Fowler et al. (1997) investigated 307 children with asymptomatic congenital CMV infection and found that 7.2% had sensorineural hearing impairment, 3% of which was unilateral, and 4% severe to profound hearing impairments. Peckham et al. (1987) had previously suggested that children with congenital CMV represented approximately 12% of all children with congenital sensorineural hearing impairment.

Maternal drug therapy

Maternal drug therapy during pregnancy can also contribute to congenital hearing impairment. Some substances may permanently injure or destroy the hair cells of the cochlea resulting in a SNHL. For example, alcohol, streptomycin, quinine and chloroquine phosphate may destroy neural elements of the inner ear. Use of thalidomide can cause damage to structures of the middle and inner ear (Strasnick and Jacobson, 1995). The loss is usually triggered by the ingestion of ototoxic drugs during the first trimester, with damage to the auditory system occurring especially in the sixth or seventh week. Conductive hearing impairment can result from ototoxicity, primarily as a result of ossicular malformations of the middle ear. Exposure to some drugs causes irreversible SNHL, and other drugs cause a hearing impairment that can be reversed once the drug is stopped. Of particular note are loop diuretics, aminoglycosides and alcohol (resulting in foetal alchohol syndrome). A hearing impairment due to ototoxicity is usually bilateral and symmetric, but may be of any degree of severity. Such a hearing impairment is usually progressive, with the high frequencies affected first.

Perinatal factors

Perinatal factors have been associated with approximately 20% of sensorineural hearing impairment in developed countries, generally resulting in elevated high-frequency thresholds (Das, 1996). These include prematurity, anoxia, kernicterus, trauma, apnoea and cyanosis, hyperbilirubinaemia, severe neonatal sepsis, rhesus incompatibility, and low birth weight (Razi and Das, 1994). The incidence of perinatal factors resulting in hearing impairment has been estimated by various studies. Such estimates range from lower estimates of 2.8% (Das, 1996) and 6.1% (Fortnum and Davis, 1997), to higher estimates of 9% (Parving and Hauch, 1994), 11.6% (Thiringer, 1984), 13.5% (Newton, 1985) and 14% (Feinmesser, Tell and Levi, 1986).

Problems associated with prematurity, such as anoxia, hyperbilirubinaemia, increased bacterial and viral infections, treatment with ototoxic drugs and low birth weight are thought to cause hearing impairment (see, for example, Bradford et al., 1985; Veen et al., 1993). Indeed, Veen concluded that in their study of 890 five-year-olds who had had very low birth weight or had been very premature, the prevalence of sensorineural hearing impairment was 15 times higher than the average Dutch population of five- to seven-year-olds. The incidence of sensorineural hearing impairment in infants with a birth weight of 1500 g or below is estimated to be between 3% and 10% (see, for example, Newton, 1985). In this group of infants it is hard to identify the precise cause of hearing impairment due to the sheer numbers of possible complications such infants may experience. However, it has been suggested that hearing impairment in this group may be caused by bilirubin toxicity, anoxia, exposure to ototoxic drugs, incubator noise, apnoeic spells, pre-natal viral infection, or intracranial haemorrhage (see, for example, Gerkin, 1986; Gibbin, 1988).

Post-natal factors

It is possible for post-natal causes of hearing impairment to be genetic, such as familial sensorineural hearing impairment, or syndromes with delayed onset of hearing impairment. However, the main post-natal causes are non-genetic, such as meningitis, head injury, measles, and ototoxic agents. Otitis media would be included here even though, in and of itself, it is an uncommon cause of permanent hearing impairment, because it may delay the detection of permanent hearing impairment. Parving (1993) reported an incidence of 15% for post-natal causes for hearing impairment. Feinmesser et al. (1986) and Newton (1985) reported lower rates of approximately 4.6%.

Bacterial meningitis is a serious infectious disease both in the neonatal period and throughout childhood. It is also the most common cause of post-natally acquired hearing impairment. For children who survive meningitis there are often sequelae, which include learning and speech and language disabilities, hydrocephalus, motor abnormalities, vestibular deficits, psychosis, hyperactivity, visual and sensorineural hearing impairments. Reports have indicated that acquired hearing impairment represents 9.5% of the total childhood hearing-impaired population, with 6.5% of these being caused by meningitis (Davis et al., 1995). Meningitis has also been found to be the cause in 16% of children with a profound hearing impairment. Gerber (1990) reported that the most severely deafened children in the study were the product of a meningitis illness and, when they studied the most severely deafened children at a local programme for the hearing impaired, the children were primarily the product of a meningitis illness. In recent years children who have lost their hearing to meningitis have been considered the best candidates for cochlear implants due to their previous experience with language and their total loss of any auditory neural function.

Fortnum and Davis (1993) reported an average incidence of 16/100 000 with the overall mortality incidence per 100 000 being 1.8. However, Fortnum and Davis (1997) reported considerable variation in the incidence rate with age of onset (see Table 4.9).

Meningitis-induced hearing impairment is often bilateral, severe or profound and rapid at onset. Clinical and experimental studies have shown that the loss results from direct damage to the cochlea, but it may be exacerbated by additional cochlear damage resulting from any ototoxic drugs used to treat the disease (Francois et al., 1997). The incidence of post-meningitic hearing impairment varies from 6% to 31% depending on the type of meningitis and type of hearing impairment included (see for example Martin, 1982; Fortnum and Hull, 1992; Fortnum and Davis, 1993; Das, 1996).

Table 4.9. Incidence rate for meningitis in relation to age

Age of Onset	Incidence Rate (Per 100 000)
0–28 days	37.2
1–11 months	115.5
12–9 months	28.5
5–16 years	2.8

Evaluation of the etiology of hearing impairment

Every child with hearing impairment should be evaluated to determine the cause of the impairment. Medical measures that can be taken include history of pregnancy, labour, delivery, medical history, family history and physical examinations. History of meningitis, NICU attendance, hearing impairment in other family members may also indicate possible causes. If these factors are not present, the most likely cause may be genetic or infection. The identification of a cause can be extremely helpful in determining a successful intervention strategy for the child.

Concluding remarks

From the information presented in this chapter, it is reasonable to suggest that the prevalence of significant bilateral hearing impairment is approximately 1.3 per 1000 in the UK. This is in close agreement with the 1.38 per 1000 figure international average presented by Mencher (2000). Further, evidence has been presented here with respect to the numbers of children in each of the sub-categories such as mild, moderate and severe hearing impairments and regarding the various etiologies for those impairments. What has been presented is based, for the most part, on solid well-defined epidemiological research. However, therein lies a problem. Generally, this type of epidemiological research is based on the notion that if one takes a large enough slice or section of a population and accounts for all the possible variables (economic, social, political, health, and so forth), it is possible to extrapolate from the results and make statements about the entire population. A similar approach, of course, is to take several different slices of the test population and interpolate between them. However, in either case, the resulting analysis provides a best estimate of the true state of the entire population. In the case of hearing impairment, as has been evident throughout this chapter, there are many slices of the population and the results are usually comparable – but not always. Thus, we currently have best estimates, but not an exact figure with respect to all aspects of hearing impairment in children. Hopefully, that is going to change.

The advent of universal infant hearing screening will offer a unique opportunity to view the entire paediatric population from birth. Within a few short years, because of the accuracy of the testing instruments and procedures, it will be possible to tell more precisely how many babies are born with a hearing impairment and of what type (mild, moderate, severe or profound). New developments in genetics may permit us to precisely determine which children have hearing impairments that are the product of a dominant, recessive or X-linked gene. New developments in medicine will not only go a long way toward eliminating some of the major causes of hearing impairment, but will permit us to be more specific in diagnosing etiology. In short, there are going to be some very important and rapid changes in our data with respect to hearing impairment in children as we currently know and understand it, and in terms of how the future database will appear.

The early identification associated with universal screening will also lead to earlier intervention. Both the child and society will benefit from such an effort in terms of increased communication, better educational status, greater economic opportunity and productivity, and maximum use of skills. It is not beyond the realm of possibility that improved devices and surgical technique could lead to cochlear implants for younger children with milder hearing impairments than are now deemed appropriate.

CHAPTER 5

Behavioural tests of hearing

F HICKSON

Introduction

Historically, behavioural tests of hearing assessment preceded electrophysiological techniques. However, each has a role in the audiology clinic of today. Behavioural tests can not only demonstrate that the ear and auditory pathways are processing the sound but the child can be observed to respond to sound due to high level cortical processing. Strategies have been developed and refined over many years for structuring the conditions that optimize the elicitation of responses appropriate to the child's developmental status. Such responses can be to stimuli with specific acoustic parameters, thus giving detailed information about a child's complex auditory function. Electrophysiological techniques can give reliable information without high-level processing being required by the child and can offer information complementary to or independent of behavioural tests. In particular electrophysiological techniques can offer information where behavioural responses are not sufficiently reliable for the assessment of hearing, as in the case of very young babies and some children with severe learning difficulties.

Behavioural observation audiometry

Behavioural observation audiometry refers to a technique formerly used in the assessment of babies aged up to six months, whereby changes in state of activity of the child were observed and judged as to whether they were in response to sound stimuli. Usually broad-band and high-intensity stimuli are most likely to produce behavioural responses in such young children. Unfortunately this meant that the assessment was not frequency specific and prediction of thresholds of hearing from the results was unreliable. Furthermore there was variability in judgement of responses between testers, and testers could have a high rate of misinterpreting random movements as responses in control trials with no auditory presentations (Moncur, 1968). Thus behavioural observation audiometry is a very questionable technique, particularly since the advent of electrophysiological techniques. However, in some circumstances it may the most appropriate technique available. It has been found to be the second most informative test for children with profound learning disability, after the auditory brainstem response, in a study by Gans and Gans (1993) where a test protocol was implemented, although this did not include otoacoustic emissions.

Behavioural observation audiometry should not, however, be considered a low-technology option for hearing assessments: Gans (1987) recommends that systematic scoring, without observer bias, be obtained using video recordings of the procedure with presentation of sound and no-sound trials whereby, on play-back, the observers score the behaviour of the child but are denied knowledge of the details of the stimulus or whether a stimulus was presented. Indeed, Bench and Boscak (1970) suggested automation of the technique because the number of trials needed to get a reliable estimate of the probability of true and false positive responses is so high. Automated systems for assessing the motor responses of young babies have, however, been found to be much less reliable than electrophysiological techniques for screening the hearing. Fortunately, as babies mature their behavioural responses can be reliably assessed and can normally be used to test hearing in a structured clinical setting such as in the distraction test.

The Distraction Test

This test has been developed from the 'Distracting Test' described by Ewing and Ewing in Manchester in 1944. It involves attracting and releasing the child's attention with a play activity, the presentation of a series of frequency-specific auditory stimuli outside the child's visual field, and observing the child's response of turning towards and localizing the sound source. This form of testing may be used in a screening programme or as part of a hearing assessment to quantify hearing impairment in children from about the age of six or seven months. Children usually begin to inhibit their responses to this technique quickly from the age of 12 months, although the test may be used beyond this age with some difficulty.

The test arrangement

The testing is performed in a quiet, sound-treated room arranged as shown in Figure 5.1. Care is taken to ensure that there are no reflective surfaces or shadows cast that might cause a child to turn to for reasons other than hearing the auditory stimulus. Background noise should not exceed 30 dB (A).

The test involves two trained professionals, the distractor and the assistant, plus the child and one parent (or other adult). The child sits half way along the parent's lap supported at the waist.

Test method

Examination of the child should be made to see if the child can physically make a head turn sufficient to show a response and can be visually distracted. Usually this can be observed while the history is being taken but with some handicapped children it will be necessary for preliminary tests to be carried out – for example, testing the child's ability to visually follow a moving object in an 180° arc from side to side.

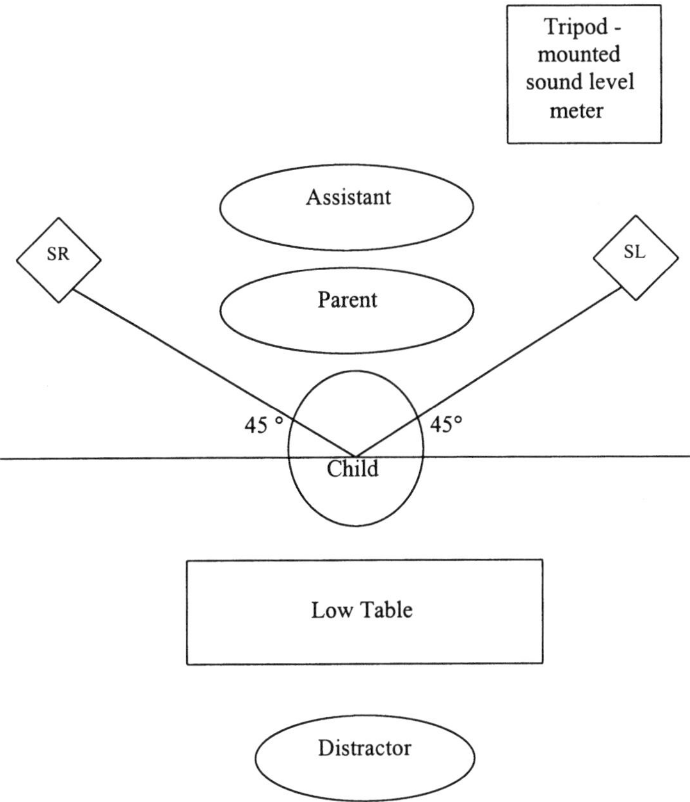

Figure 5.1. Test arrangement for the Distraction Test.
SR: Stimulus on right; SL: Stimulus on left.

The distractor usually kneels or sits behind a low table facing the child. The distractor uses toys to engage the child's attention forward and then, by reducing the play activity, releases the child's attention prior to introduction of the stimulus. Pauses in distracting should not be so long that they allow the child's gaze to wander, and care must be taken not to distract in a manner that is so interesting that the child does not turn although the sound has been heard. The distraction activity can be modified to suit the child's abilities. Visually-impaired children can be distracted using tactile (stroking) stimuli or dimmed room lights, and a light source, such as an otoscope, can be used to control the child's attention. The assistant introduces the auditory stimuli on either side as indicated below:

- One metre from the child's ear to enable the sounds to be presented at the ear at 30 dB (A). If a child has poor head control or needs some support in sitting then sometimes the test is started at a distance of about 15 cm from the ear.
- At an angle of 45° on either side behind the child to avoid visual cues being given.
- On a level with the child's ear as this makes it easier for the child to localize.
- For up to 5s at the initial intensity levels and then raised if the child does not respond.

The high-frequency rattle is often presented first. This is because the more problematic hearing impairments usually involve high frequencies and, with young children, it is advisable to try to obtain important information about hearing at these frequencies first. However, if a child is known to have a hearing impairment, it may be better to start with a low-frequency stimulus in order to observe a positive response at this stage of the test.

When presenting the stimuli, care has to be taken to avoid presentation in a predictable alternating manner and to avoid inadvertent sensory information that might cue the child to the presence of the stimulus. Examples of such information include shadows or reflections and the sight or sound of the assistant moving. If the child turns and localizes the sound source accurately this is recorded as a response. It is the distractor's role to assess whether or not a turn was in response to the stimulus or for other reasons such as visual cues or competing auditory stimuli, or if it was a random check, and whether or not there was correct localization of the sound source. The distractor needs to be able to observe the child's face as this may give clues that a stimulus has been heard prior to localization, for example, a look of recognition such as widening of the eyes or a smile prior to turning. Care must be taken not to maintain eye contact with the child, which may fix his/her attention forward, so it is better to concentrate the gaze a little below the eyes. The distractor must be careful not to glance towards the stimulus and give cues of its presence and location. In some cases, where the child has poor head control or is visually-impaired, the test may be modified so that repeatable responses such as eye turns or reaching for the stimulus may be accepted.

If a response is obtained the intensity is measured using the dB (A) weighted scale on a tripod-mounted sound level meter with the 'fast' response of the meter in order to observe and record the peaks in intensity of the stimulus. The intensity, type and side of the stimulus producing the response are recorded. If the child does not turn then the sound is made at a higher intensity. This can be done in two ways: either by coming closer to the child's ear or by raising the intensity of a sound from the same distance of one metre. The advantage of the latter method is that one is much less likely to give unintentional clues to the presence of the stimulus or assistant. Errors in replicating the distance when measuring sound intensity also have smaller effects at this larger distance. However, the disadvantages are that one might not be able to produce sufficiently high intensity for some hearing-impaired children to hear at that distance and some sounds will lose their frequency specificity at higher intensities (for example, sibilant /s/).

If, when the sound is raised in intensity, the child turns and localizes the source, the intensity at which the response was obtained is measured on a sound level meter and the response noted. If there is no response at maximal intensity the child is given a tactile or visual clue to see if this elicits a turning response. If so, this suggests that the child's state of arousal is appropriate for the test but that he has not heard the auditory stimuli. The maximum level at which the child failed to respond to the auditory stimulus is measured and recorded (for example 'NR (no response) at 90 dB (A)').

Control trials in which all conditions of testing are met other than making the sound should help the distractor to decide if the child is turning genuinely to the stimuli or is turning for some other reason. If there is random 'checking' behaviour by the child this may be stopped by one of these ploys:

- releasing the child's attention without presenting a stimulus until the checking ceases;
- keeping a toy in view to attract the child's attention forward (i.e. providing a more interesting distraction in front);
- the distractor and assistant changing places.

Any localization difficulties should be noted during the test as these difficulties may indicate a difference in hearing level between the two ears, although children with severe and profound bilateral hearing impairment may have difficulty localizing generally (Cosgrove and Hickson, 1996).

Test stimuli

Frequency-specific auditory stimuli are used to test high, mid and low frequencies separately. This is necessary to measure hearing impairment in those instances where auditory sensitivity differs over the speech frequency range, for example those with a 'ski-slope' or 'U-shaped' hearing impairment. Specification of spectra of frequency-modulated (FM) warble tones is variable among the different manufacturers of signal generators but is generally preferable to mechanically produced sounds, in terms of increased frequency specificity (Figure 5.2).

High-frequency stimuli

- The Manchester high-frequency rattle (available from the School of Education, University of Manchester). This contains frequencies from about 6 kHz to above 20 kHz (Figure 5.3).
- Repetitive sibilant /s/. When correctly produced, this contains audible frequencies from about 3 kHz to 10 kHz (Figure 5.4). It loses frequency specificity when the sound is raised due to the noise of the increased airstream (Figure 5.5).
- Warble tones centred at 3 kHz or 4 kHz. These give more frequency specificity than the two previous stimuli but young babies might be less responsive to warbles because of their narrow bandwidth.

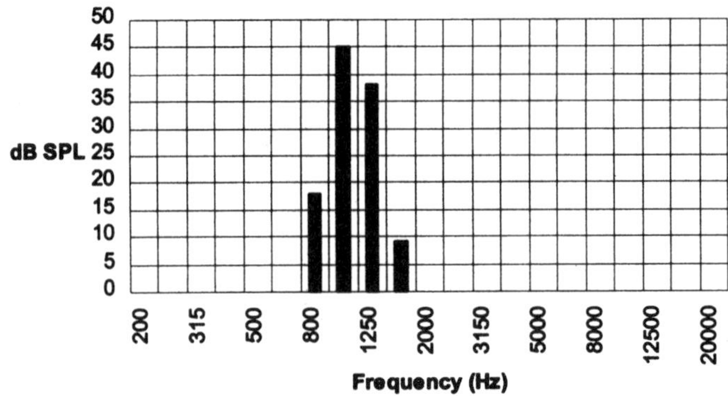

Figure 5.2. Spectrum of a frequency-modulated warble tone, centred at 1kHz.

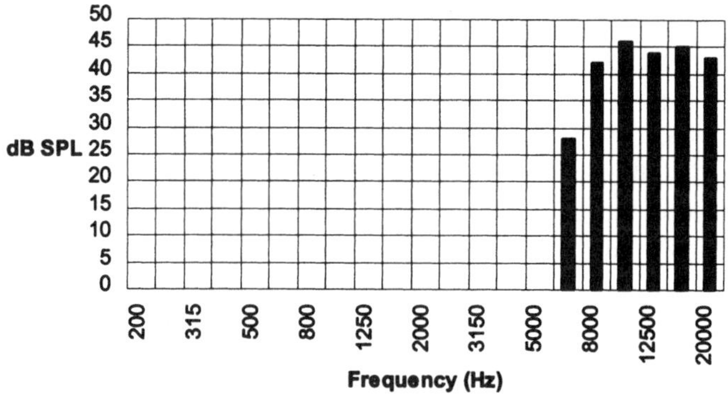

Figure 5.3. Spectrum of Manchester high-frequency rattle.

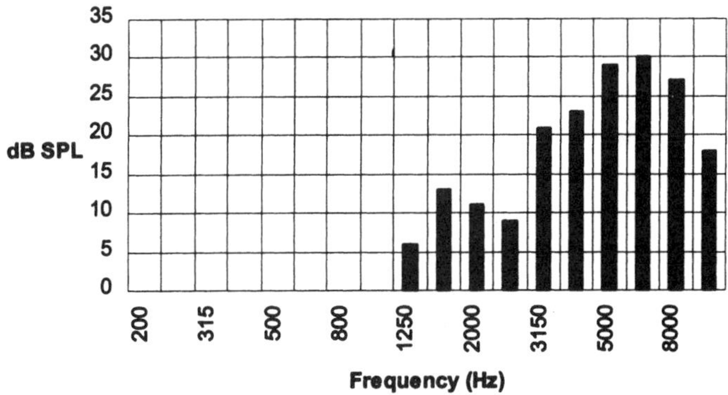

Figure 5.4. Spectrum of sibilant /s/ at low intensity.

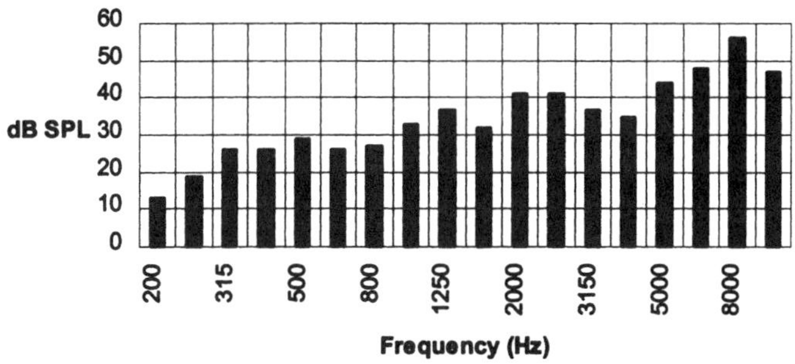

Figure 5.5. Spectrum of sibilant /s/ at raised intensity.

Middle-frequency stimuli

- 'G' chime bar (about 10 cm or 11 cm in length). This produces frequencies around 1600 Hz when struck with the knuckle or soft hammer (Figure 5.6). Impact energy is problematic if the chime is hit with a hard striker such as a hammer or fingernail, as the signal then becomes broad band. (Figure 5.7).
- Warble tones centred at 1 kHz or 2 kHz. These may be used and are more frequency specific than other stimuli (Figure 5.2).

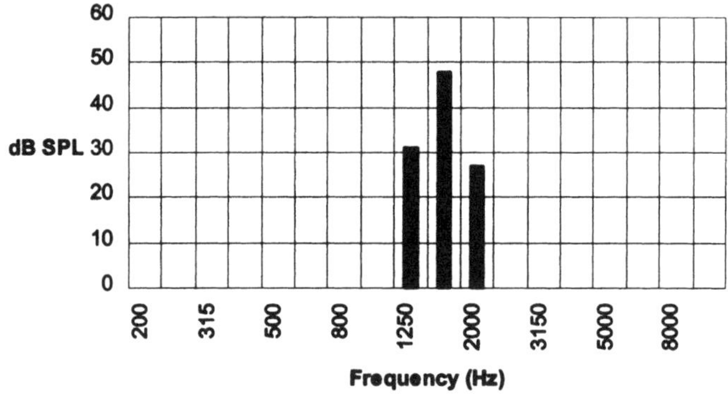

Figure 5.6. Spectrum of "G" chime bar (struck with knuckle).

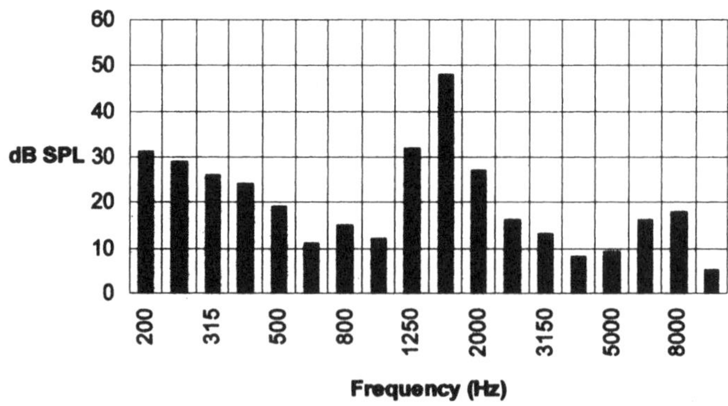

Figure 5.7. Spectrum of "G" chime bar (struck with hard hammer).

Low-frequency stimuli

- Humming sound. This is a continuous voiced low-frequency sound produced with the lips closed (Figure 5.8). A little intonation in the voice makes a more attractive sound but care is needed that this does not produce intensity fluctuations. The continuous nature of the voicing in this stimulus reduces intensity fluctuations which can be present at the initiation of each voicing in other voiced stimuli such as in a repetitive /oo/ stimulus or mumbled speech.

- Warble tones centred at 500 Hz or 250 Hz. Warble tones are more frequency specific than other low-frequency stimuli.
- 'C' chime bar (about 17 or 18 cm in length). This produces frequencies around 512 Hz when struck with the knuckle or soft hammer. The problems with this stimulus are the same as for the middle-frequency 'G' chime.
- /baba/. This can be used if a high intensity stimulus is required though it does contain mid- and high-frequencies.

Additional stimuli

A drum or tambour may be used if there is no response to the stimuli described earlier and may be used to test for an auro-palpebral reflex. Such stimuli contain broad bands of frequencies.

The auro-palpebral (blink) reflex (APR)

Examination is often made for the presence or absence of an auro-palpebral reflex whenever the responses in the Distraction Test are at raised intensities. This is usually done by introducing a /ba/ sound near the ear at high intensities. A small screen or the assistant's hand should be placed over the assistant's mouth to prevent tactile elicitation of the reflex. Usually the sound is first introduced at about 80 dB (A). If there is no corresponding blink the sound is made at a higher intensity; if there is a reflex, it may be useful to find the APR threshold by testing at lower intensities although habituation may soon occur. The reflex threshold is

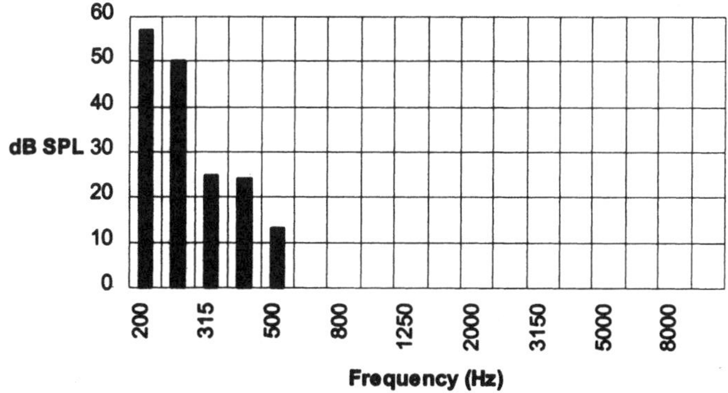

Figure 5.8. Spectrum of humming sound.

thus obtained, or if no reflex is obtained at the highest level introduced without a response the level is measured and the response or no response level recorded. The test is carried out on each side separately. It provides limited information about hearing levels. A reflex present at 'normal' levels of about 80 dB to 100 dB (A) does not exclude a hearing impairment because the child may have a cochlear hearing impairment with accompanying loudness recruitment and/or hearing that varies in sensitivity across frequencies.

Use of the Distraction Test

The Distraction Test has been the basis of health visitor screening of infants in the UK at the ages of seven to eight months. Some babies with a hearing impairment have been found to pass the screen and, in some instances, this has been attributable to poor test techniques. McCormick (1983) was able to show an improvement in test reliability when the testers were given refresher courses. With the onset of neonatal screening, using electrophysiological techniques, fewer babies have their hearing impairment detected using the Distraction Test (Wood, Davis and McCormick, 1997). However, neonatal screening is not yet universal in many geographical regions. Furthermore, even where universal neonatal screening is in place coverage may not be complete. Also, not all prelingual hearing impairments are present in the neonatal period. The Distraction Test thus remains an important tool in identification of hearing impairment although vigilance is necessary to ensure that the standard of test technique using this tool is high.

The Distraction Test can also be useful in the measurement of hearing thresholds. In children with very poor thresholds it enables sounds to be presented at very high intensities in the sound field due to the close proximity of the sound source to the child's ear. The ability to introduce a visual or tactile stimulus is helpful in differentiating the hearing-impaired child from one who has not responded for other reasons. The use of warble tones gives the test stimuli the same frequency specificity as those used in visual reinforcement audiometry.

Visual reinforcement audiometry (VRA)

This procedure enables hearing thresholds to be measured in young children whereby a head turn, in response to hearing a sound stimulus, is reinforced by a visual reward. Localization of the sound stimulus is not required and, indeed, the stimulus and the reinforcer may be spatially separated. Visual reinforcement audiometry is usually possible from the age of six months. The test is applicable up to an age of two or three years, at which point children quickly inhibit responses. Habituation reduces the number of signals that can be used to determine threshold levels and the older the children the more quickly they tend to habituate. Primus and Thompson (1985) and Thompson, Thompson and McCall (1992) showed that two-year-olds habituated their responses more quickly than one-year-olds.

The test arrangement

Testing is usually carried out by two testers using two rooms arranged as depicted in Figure 5.9 but, if necessary, the test can be performed in one room only and with a single tester. The visual reinforcer is placed next to, or on top of, the loudspeaker but can be separated. When they are close to each other, localization of the sound may facilitate the turn to the reinforcer. Primus (1992) has shown that the VRA response is not contingent upon localization but that the performance in the test was affected by localization of the sound. More infants were conditioned and the number of trials needed for conditioning were fewer when the visual reinforcer and sound source were adjacent than when they were separated.

The loudspeakers may be placed at angles of 45, 60 or 90° from the child. The distance of the loudspeakers from the child's ears was investigated by Magnusson, Borjesson and Axelsson (1997). In one arrangement the loudspeakers were placed upon movable arms and positioned 15 cm from each ear. In the other arrangement the loudspeakers were placed 50 cm to 70 cm from the child. Real ear sound pressure measurements

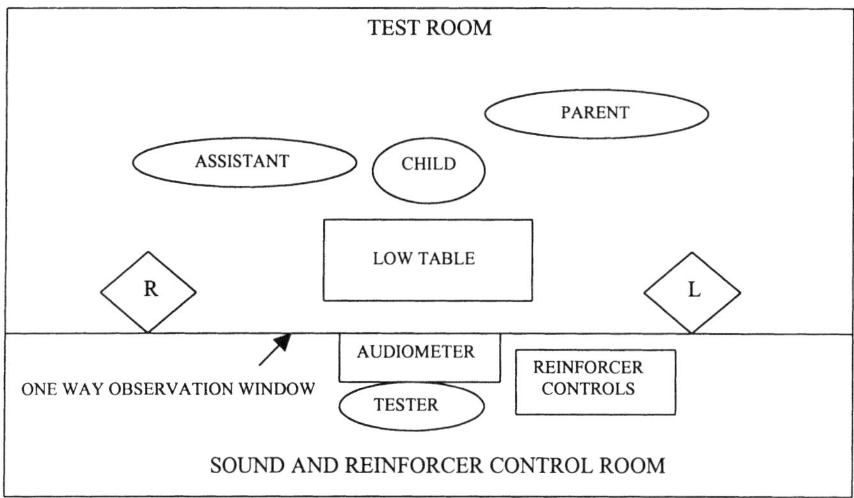

Figure 5.9. Test arrangement for Visual Reinforcement Audiometry.
R: Right loudpeaker and adjacent reinforcer.
L: Left loudspeaker and adjacent reinforcer.

were made and compared between the two positions. Predictably, it was found that in the 15 cm position the measurements were very variable due to slight head movement whereas the more distant positioning of 50 cm to 70 cm was found to be more consistent but variations increased again at a distance of 1 m. However, the International Standard ISO 8253 requires that the loudspeaker distance be at least 1 m. This suggests that clinicians should carefully calibrate their VRA clinic and be aware of the magnitude of fluctuations for their own particular acoustic conditions.

Reinforcers that are commercially available include revolving lights, toys with eyes that light up, and puppets that illuminate, and there is increasing use of video displays.

The signal may be introduced through insert earphones, as shown in Figure 5.10 and when these are employed the signals can be pure tones and calibration in dB HL. The earphones are placed in the ear canal using a foam tip or, if the child wears hearing aids, they may be attached to the earmould. Insert earphones enable more precise information to be obtained about individual ear thresholds than may be obtained using loudspeakers. Masking may be used, the narrow band noise being introduced at specific sensation levels in one earphone whilst the signal is applied through the other.

Test method

The test involves conditioning a child to respond with a turn to a visual reinforcer to a sound introduced from a loudspeaker in the sound field or

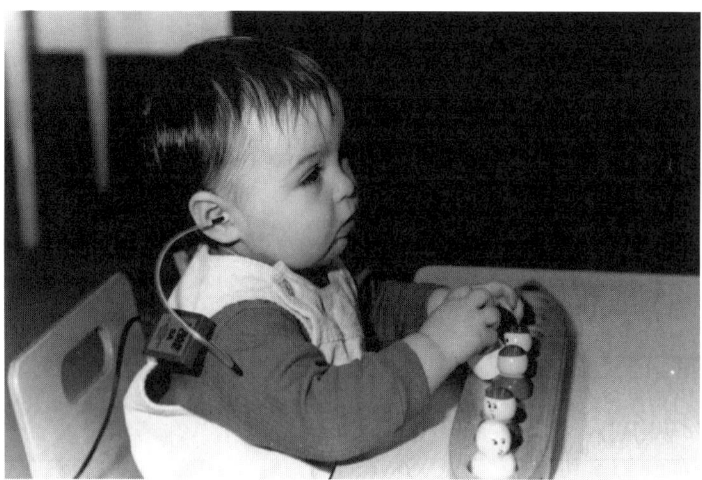

Figure 5.10. Use of insert earphones.

through earphones or a bone vibrator. The sound and visual reinforcer are initially introduced together with the assistant pointing out the reinforcer, if necessary, at this stage. When the child begins to anticipate the visual reinforcement, the sound is introduced alone and an appropriate turning response is rewarded subsequently with the visual reinforcer. Children unable to turn their head or unable to see the visual reinforcer will need to have their hearing assessed using other methods.

Before introduction of the test signal the child's attention is kept in a forward position by the use of play activity. This can be phased out before the sound is introduced or maintained, if necessary, depending upon the child's attentional behaviour. If there are two testers, one in the test room and one in the adjacent room, then agreement between the two as to whether or not a response was a true one may increase the validity of the testing procedure. Computer control of signal level and time period for scoring a response can add objectivity to the test execution and storage of false positive responses (in control trials) can be used in computer decision-making algorithms (Widen, 1993).

Test signals

Visual reinforcement audiometry may be performed using frequency-modulated warble tones usually centred at frequencies of 0.5, 1.0, 2.0, 3.0 and 4.0 kHz, or narrow-band noise can be used if the tones fail to elicit a response. The filter roll-off of most audiometric narrow bands is, however, usually very gradual giving a much wider bandwidth than desirable. The duration of the signal is usually about 2 seconds. The intensity of the sound in a particular clinic, at a particular location where a child is normally seated for testing, may be calibrated using a sound level meter fitted with octave or one-third octave band filters and the dial reading on the audiometer pre-calibrated to read in dB SPL.

Habituation of the response

Habituation of the response was studied by Primus and Thompson (1985) in relation to the number of reinforcers and breaks in the test sessions. Two reinforcers led to more responses than one before habituation and a 10-minute break in the session led to a minimum of five additional responses in the rest of the session for one-year-old but not two-year-old children. Culpepper and Thompson (1994) investigated the effects of reinforcer duration of 0.5, 1.5 and 4.0 seconds on the response behaviour of 60 pre-term two-year-olds using a 50 dB HL bandpass noise stimulus. They found that significantly slower rates of habituation were obtained when the duration of the reinforcer was 0.5 seconds compared with 4.0 seconds. It was thought that decreasing the duration would be particularly helpful in increasing the duration of testing opportunities in children at the older end of the VRA age range.

Visual reinforcement operant conditioning audiometry (VROCA)

Visual reinforcement operant conditioning audiometry involves conditioning the children to press a bar on hearing a sound, the button activating a visual reinforcer. When this test was compared with VRA in two-year-olds, it was found that it was easier to condition the child to VRA than to VROCA (Thompson, Thompson and Vethivelu, 1989).

The Performance Test

This test was described by Ewing and Ewing (1944) and is appropriate for the assessment of hearing of children of a developmental age of two-and-a-half years upwards or until co-operation with pure-tone audiometry is achieved. In its earliest form the signals were a voiced /go/, a sibilant /s/ and other consonants presented in the sound field but now warble tones may be used and ear specificity obtained using insert earphones. In older children, where there is doubt about the child's ability to do an audiogram or willingness to accept headphones, then it is often advisable to start with a sound field performance test in the first instance.

In performance tests the child is conditioned to perform a simple action in response to a sound stimulus. The response required is often to put a peg in a board or ring on a stick or a similar simple action each time the sound is heard. Toys that demand more advanced skills, such as those with assorted shapes that have to be put into a particular hole, are generally unsuitable as they tend to distract the child's attention from listening to the sound signal.

In the initial conditioning process, the child should be given both visual and acoustic cues to the presentation of the sound stimulus in order to facilitate compliance without dependence on hearing sensitivity. The test thus does not depend on hearing or language for co-operation in the procedure; rather it depends on the child's ability to inhibit his or her response until the stimulus has been detected.

Test method

The child is conditioned from in front to respond with the required action to either presentation of warble tones or voiced /go/ at moderate levels of intensity. Care is taken to ensure that the child is watching the tester's finger on the warbler interrupter or tester's face, respectively, in this initial stage. However, once it has been established that the child can wait before responding, the tester goes behind, out of the child's visual field. At this position the stimulus is presented at progressively lower intensities with variable inter-stimulus intervals and with the child facing forward. The intensity of the stimulus is dropped after each positive response. If the child fails to respond at a reduced intensity the tester progressively raises the intensity of the stimulus until a response is obtained and then intensity is measured.

If high intensity levels are required then it is advantageous to produce the sound nearer to the child, but a small screen or the tester's hand should be used in front of the tester's mouth to prevent tactile information reaching the child. Such a method should elicit responses that indicate the threshold of hearing of the child in the sound field. This will reflect hearing of the better-hearing ear or both, if equivalent. Without insert or headphone presentation it is not possible to ascertain ear-specific information due to transmission and diffraction of the stimuli from one side of the child to the other with little or no attenuation.

If there is no response at maximum level, the child is given an additional visual clue to see if this elicits a response and, if so, the level of response is measured and recorded. No response at 100 dBA would be recorded as 'NR at 100 dBA'. For children who have responded to visual cues but failed to hear the most intense signal, it is advised that one attempt to progress to pure-tone audiometry whereby higher intensity stimuli may be used to obtain thresholds. Pure-tone audiometry may begin with a low-frequency stimulus (such as 0.25 or 0.5 kHz) to optimize the possibility of the child hearing the stimulus. Transition to this technique may be facilitated by conditioning the child to tactile stimuli by holding the bone conductor on the child's hand before progressing to insert or headphones. For a child who wears hearing aids, conditioning may be carried out in the sound field whilst the child wears aids and then taken out for threshold measurements. In addition, aided sound field thresholds may be obtained.

Test signals

Frequency-modulated warble tones are the preferred option as they have good frequency specificity and can be used to test low-, mid- and high-frequency hearing. The transition from warble tones to pure-tone audiometry might also be easier than from other sounds. If warble tones are used, low-, mid- and high-frequency information is sought, usually from tests at centred at 1, 4 and 0.5 kHz. Stimulus durations of 1 second to 3 seconds are recommended as in pure-tone audiometry (BSA, 1981) with variable inter-stimulus intervals. Use of variable inter-stimulus intervals is essential to ensure that the child is not merely performing the task independent of hearing.

If warble tones are not available or a less abstract signal is needed by the child, the low-frequency live voiced /go/ and high frequency sibilant /s/ may be used. The /go/ and /s/ threshold information may be supplemented by a test using a mid-frequency warble tone centred at 1 kHz. Some testers omit the initial consonant of /go/ when reaching the lowest intensity levels. This helps reduce the high-frequency consonant content of the signal but some initial high-frequency formant energy will still be present.

The high-frequency /s/ stimulus is most frequency specific when the air stream from the mouth is least, as shown in Figure 5. 4. For higher intensities it is advantageous to be closer to the child's ear rather than increasing the air stream. For such close proximity, however, a small screen or the tester's hand must be placed in front of the tester's mouth to prevent tactile cues alerting the child to the sound stimulus.

It is also important that, when using the /go/ or /s/ in testing any child with the performance test, thresholds of hearing may only be obtained when the whole face is out of vision of the child as in Figure 5.11. Even if the child only sees part of the face, a very small muscle movement may be sufficient to indicate that the stimulus has been uttered, and thus the procedure is no longer valid.

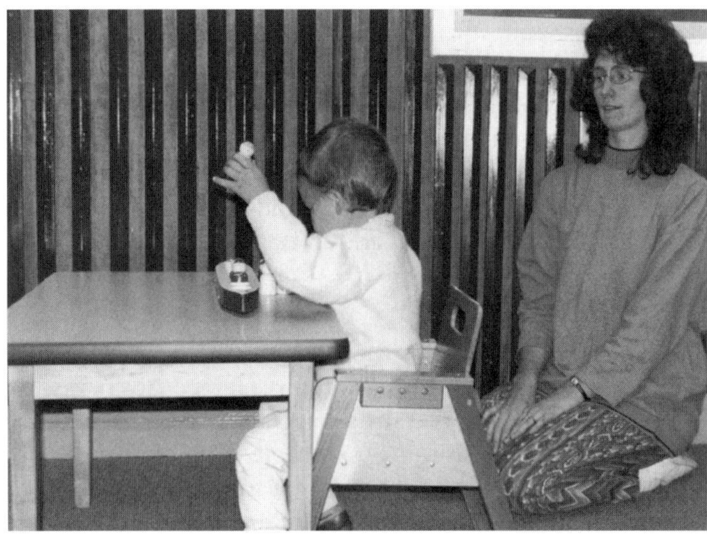

Figure 5.11. Test arrangement for threshold responses in the Performance Test.

Pure-tone audiometry

The conventional technique for obtaining frequency-specific and ear-specific information about a person's hearing is pure-tone audiometry using supra-aural headphones, bone conduction and masking. There are recommended procedures such as the British Society of Audiology Recommended Procedures (BSA, 1981, 1985, 1986) and results relate to an international baseline of average normal hearing for adults (ISO 389, 1991). This technique may be adapted for use with children and results may be interpreted from some children as young as two-and-a-half years old. There is no standard for the interpretation of results in children and hence there is a range of acceptance of the limit of normality that ranges from about 15 dB HL to 30 dB HL in clinical and screening practice.

The adaptations to the adult procedure that facilitate compliance in young children include the use of insert earphones and the use of the conditioning process and play-type of response of the performance test. Indeed, pure-tone audiometry is often introduced as a gradual transition from the performance test and thus termed 'play audiometry'. Care must, however, be taken that no visual cues are present when thresholds are being measured: children, especially hearing-impaired children, are remarkably adept at detecting inadvertently presented visual information, such as movement of the tester, when the interrupter is being pressed.

Insert earphones (Figure 5.12) are less cumbersome and may be accepted more readily than headphones. Furthermore they facilitate more transcranial attenuation of the sound source to the non-test ear than headphones and prevent the collapse of the ear canal, which may occur with supra-aural headphones. Another acceptable transition from sound-field measures to pure-tone audiometry may be made by the use of the bone conductor before ear-specific air conduction procedures are attempted. Indeed, for children with severe or profound hearing impairment, bone conduction offers a tactile stimulus in the low frequencies with which the child may be conditioned to respond. Thus at the age of about two-and-a-half to three years old one may obtain air conduction and/or unmasked bone conduction thresholds. Neilsen and Olsen (1997) found that it was possible to obtain six thresholds from nearly 75% of children from the age of three years, by which one could obtain air conduction information at three frequencies for each ear unless the minimum values of transcranial attenuation are exceeded and the results confounded by cross hearing. Alternatively, or in addition, one or two unmasked bone-conduction thresholds may be attempted at this age if the child has a bilateral hearing impairment, in order to determine if there is a sensorineural element present, although the possibility of the thresholds being perceived by tactile rather than auditory sensations increases at the higher intensity levels – especially the low frequencies (Brasier, 1974). Thus tympanometry may offer more reliable ear-specific information about middle-ear function at this age.

Where minimum transcranial attenuation figures for headphone or insert earphone thresholds have been exceeded, or where ear-specific bone-conduction thresholds are desired, masking of the non-test ear is required but co-operation with this technique will depend partly on the cognitive developmental level of the child and some may not co-operate reliably until the age of seven years (Tucker and Nolan, 1984).

The technique used for masking should be a plateau technique (Hood, 1960) or a formula method (Studebaker, 1985), the former being practised in Britain with the Recommended Procedure of the British Society of Audiology (BSA) (1986). The task may be made more acceptable and easier for the child to co-operate with if terms such as 'whistle' and 'the sea' are used for the tone and the masker respectively, remembering that instructions may be inaudible when the masker has been introduced but that an instruction to 'listen for the whistle' with the visual attention of the child, and accompanied by gesture, may facilitate a correct response to the test tone rather than confusion with the masker.

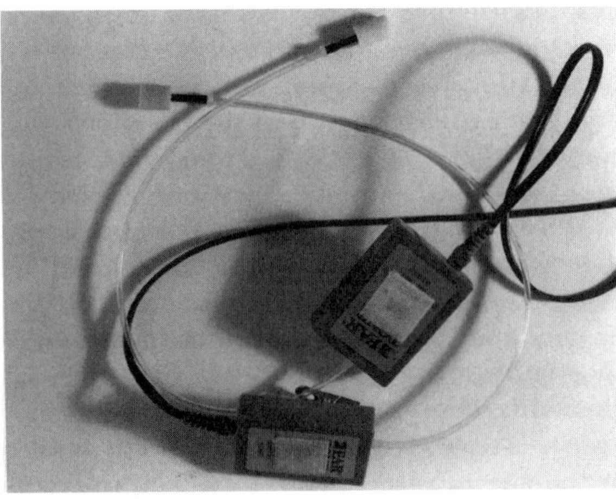

Figure 5.12. Insert earphones.

Non-organic hearing impairment

The elevation of thresholds above organic thresholds may occur when testing some children, either subconsciously or consciously on their part. In most cases over seven years old this presents as a moderate-severe bilateral sensorineural hearing impairment with no relevant medical history (Tucker and Nolan, 1984). Occasionally it may present as a unilateral hearing impairment, often severe or total with no shadow results from the non-test ear for unmasked thresholds. In both cases it is the role of the audiologist to try to determine the true organic thresholds in order to manage any underlying hearing impairment appropriately.

There are several methods to determine organic thresholds in the presence of a non-organic pathology, most of which entail distracting the child's attention away from the loudness of the signal to some other task such as in an ear-pointing technique for bilateral cases where the child concentrates on lateralizing the sound, as described by Nolan and Tucker, (1981). Speech audiometry, using pre-recorded word lists such as the AB Word List (Boothroyd, 1968) may also be helpful if a child is asked if he or she knows the words to be presented and repeated and the intensity is surreptitiously reduced in order that the level required for discrimination of speech may be compared with normal values. For unilateral non-organic hearing impairments, the Stenger Test should give organic thresholds for pure tones with relative ease due to the listener being unaware of sound being present in the admitted normal ear if louder sounds are perceived in the opposite ear (Newby, 1964).

Auditory discrimination of speech

Testing of auditory discrimination of speech has high face validity in the assessment of young children. Although speech discrimination is not a frequency-specific function it illustrates a prime function of hearing in the developing young child and can correlate highly with hearing sensitivity in normally hearing and mildly or moderately hearing-impaired children. Increasingly there has been an interest in testing children's hearing of speech since the use of cochlear implants in young children (Snik et al., 1997) when, as for severely and profoundly hearing-impaired, conventionally aided children, threshold testing is a poor predictor of a child's ability to discriminate speech. Developments in the field of speech discrimination have been in the use of technological devices for the presentation and response mode of tests to improve signal replicability and facilitate compliance appropriate to the child. In particular, spoken responses are generally avoided when assessing auditory discrimination to eliminate the confounding variability of children's articulation patterns.

The Co-operative Test

The Co-operative Test, first described by Ewing and Ewing (1944) is suitable for children with the normal linguistic development level of an eighteen-month-old child or above. Usually, other tests requiring a greater receptive vocabulary are more appropriate to the normally linguistically developing child by the age of two-and-a-half years.

In this test the child is required to carry out instructions in response to simple verbal commands. The object is to record the minimum intensity required for the comprehension of simple verbal instructions.

The stimuli for the co-operative test are voiced instructions and thus contain a wide range of frequencies. Results of the test are not frequency specific. Usually three different instructions are used. The instruction may be 'give it to Mummy' (or 'give it to Daddy') or 'give it to Teddy' or 'put it in the box', for example.

A peg, or similar small toy, is handed to the child and the instruction is given. It is often important for the tester to hold on to the peg until the command has been given otherwise the child may pre-empt the command and deposit the peg elsewhere. Further pegs and instructions are given at conversational voice levels, in random order and initially in front of the child to ascertain his comprehension and co-operation in the procedure.

If the child fails to respond, the tester should ensure that the child is watching the tester's face and help the child carry out the commands in the first few instances. If the child seems uncertain, it may be also appropriate to raise the intensity of the voice slightly to about 60 dB (A). Many children with temporary conductive hearing impairments can do this test if the commands are given at a sufficient intensity level.

For a child who co-operates, the test should proceed by preventing lip reading by covering the tester's mouth or going behind the child, as in the Performance Test (Figure 5.11), and reducing the intensity of commands until the child fails to respond and then increasing them until he or she responds again. The lowest intensity at which the child consistently discriminates the commands correctly without visual cues is then measured. For a child with normal hearing and speech discrimination ability the threshold for the co-operative test will be at 35–40 dB (A). Failure to discriminate without lip reading or a tendency to look for visual information should be noted as indicators of hearing impairment.

For some children, who owing to shyness inhibit their responses, other methods within the child's limited receptive vocabulary may be necessary, such as in McCormick's Four-toy Eye Pointing Test.

The Toy Discrimination test (McCormick, 1977)

By the age of two-and-a-half years old, the receptive vocabulary of children has grown to include many nouns that can be represented in toy form and used in a test involving discrimination of pairs of similar sounding words such as /tree/ and /key/. The toy test uses seven such pairs of words so that consonant discrimination of young children can be tested. Administration of the test, using live voice, has been detailed by McCormick (1977). Presentation of a digitized recording of the speech stimuli via a loudspeaker can also be used in the IHR-McCormick Automated Toy Discrimination Test whereby predictions of average better-ear thresholds can be made from the results of this test (Ousey et al., 1989). This version of the test uses an algorithm to vary the intensity of presentation according to the child's responses. A portable digital screening version of the test, the 'Parrot', allows the tester to choose the presentation level (Shaw, 1997).

For children with less-developed language, or those who inhibit their finger-pointing response, the McCormick Four-toy Eye Pointing Test may be used.

McCormick's four-toy eye pointing test (1988)

In this test, two pairs of the McCormick Toy Discrimination Test items are spaced apart on a low table in front of the child who is asked where the items are, in random order, initially at conversational levels of intensity. Observation of the child's eye movements by the tester is made and the intensity of the voice reduced, visual cues are obliterated by covering the tester's mouth, until threshold levels of 80% correct discrimination are achieved. Details of this test, to ensure avoidance of pitfalls, are given by McCormick (1988).

The E2L toy test

For children with very limited knowledge of the English Language an E2L (English as a second language) toy test has been devised (Bellman and Marcuson, 1991), using everyday English vocabulary, found to be familiar to young children from Bengali/Sylheti speaking families in London, UK. This test is also available in a portable digital version and is appropriate for several groups of children with limited knowledge of the English language.

The Manchester Picture Vocabulary Test

This test, developed by Watson (1957), using language found to be familiar to five-year-olds, involves a pointing response to pictures. Owing to changes in children's receptive vocabulary with time this test was updated in 1984 (Hickson, 1987) and is currently undergoing further revision and digital recording of the stimulus.

The Three-Interval, Forced Choice Test of speech pattern contrast perception (the THRIFT test)

For older children, with cognitive skills of eight years of age or more, Boothroyd's THRIFT test gives a detailed examination of a child's discrimination ability (Boothroyd, 1986). This tests abilities such as auditory discrimination of place of articulation, intonation pattern and consonant voicing, which is useful in the assessment of hearing-impaired children. The test is computer controlled with the option of a visual presentation of the speaker and with a touch screen for the child to select his or her response.

Such technological devices enable controlled replication of the speech stimulus at known intensities and thereby increase the reliability of the test. Pre-recorded or computer-generated material can also be presented using headphones or insert earphones to give ear-specific information (Arlinger and Billermark, 1997).

Conclusion

Hearing assessment, using the methods described in this chapter, can be used to determine frequency-specific hearing thresholds and speech discrimination ability of young children by observation of the child's behaviour in response to sound. Such behaviour is observed within a structured clinical context and in response to defined acoustic stimuli from which a child's auditory function for the real world might be predicted.

CHAPTER 6

Neurodiagnostic paediatric audiology

J HALL III AND T PENN

Introduction

Historical overview

Audiology as a profession, and formal audiological assessment as a clinical service, date back only to the middle of the twentieth century. As we enter the twenty-first century, however, the profession and the techniques available to evaluate auditory function have advanced remarkably. Our knowledge of the auditory system – from the cochlea to the cortex – has also expanded exponentially, especially within the past 20 years. Application of computer-based technology for assessment, coupled with the newly identified principles of auditory neuroscience, are perhaps most obvious in neurodiagnostic paediatric audiology. That is, the thorough description of type, configuration, and degree of hearing impairment in children from the perinatal period onward. Our audiological armamentarium extends far beyond the simple audiogram. Hearing screening of newborn infants within hours after birth is rapidly becoming the universal standard. Differentiation of 'type of hearing impairment' includes not only conductive, sensorineural and mixed hearing impairments. It is now possible to distinguish sensory from neural, and among the latter even inner versus outer hair-cell dysfunction. Fortunately, paediatric audiology is by no means limited to the definition of peripheral hearing impairment, as we really hear with our brain as much as our ears. Behavioural and electrophysiological measures are available for evaluating the central auditory pathways. Indeed, there is unprecedented research and clinical interest in the assessment of central auditory nervous system function with sophisticated techniques and technology, such as the mismatch negativity (MMN) response and functional magnetic resonance imaging (fMRI). In this chapter, we provide a summary of these exciting trends in neurodiagnostic paediatric audiology.

An updated cross-check principle

Over 25 years ago, Jerger and Hayes (1976) defined a fundamental clinical guideline for the audiological assessment of children – 'the cross-check principle'. In an era when behavioural audiometry was relied on almost exclusively in paediatric hearing assessment, the authors presented a compelling argument for the evaluation of children with a test battery consisting of behavioural audiometry, impedance measurements, and the auditory brainstem response. Jerger and Hayes (1976) supported their argument with ample clinical evidence. A quarter of a century later, it is time to revise and update the cross-check principle, especially for paediatric assessments as otoacoustic emissions (OAEs) are now an integral component of the paediatric diagnostic test battery. As noted in Table 6.1, OAEs have earned a unique and valued complimentary clinical role along with these other time-tested audiological procedures.

Diagnostic paediatric audiology in the era of universal newborn hearing screening (UNHS)

The importance of hearing integrity within the first three to four years after birth for normal acquisition of speech and language has long been appreciated (see, for example, Lenneberg et al., 1965). During this sensitive period, speech and language will almost always develop rapidly and normally if the auditory and language regions of the brain are adequately stimulated by sound and, especially, the sounds of communication. Unfortunately, by the time hearing impairment in infancy and early childhood is suspected, audiologically evaluated, and appropriately managed, two or more of these communicatively important years have elapsed and the child has lost an enormous developmental advantage. The rationale for early identification of and intervention for hearing impairment in infants, then, is to optimize language and communication development. During the 1960s, an international collection of papers revealed increasing interest in hearing screening of young children (see, for example, Froding, 1960; Downs and Sterritt, 1964; Feinmesser and Tell, 1976). At the time, however, screening was conducted with behavioural techniques that lacked adequate sensitivity and specificity in the hands of the average audiologist. Early identification of infant hearing impairment was altered dramatically by the discovery of the auditory brainstem response (ABR) by Jewett and Williston (1971) and a subsequent paper by Hecox and Galambos (1974) describing the clinical application of ABR in auditory assessment of infants and young children. As clinical experience accumulated, and screening equipment, techniques and strategies were modified, test performance improved steadily and automated techniques were introduced (for example, Gorga et al., 1987; Hall, Kileny and Ruth, 1987).

Table 6.1. Summary of diagnostic audiologic techniques and strategies appropriate for children as a function of age (ages are approximate). Techniques are arranged with the most important first, but a test battery approach is always advisable. Otoacoustic emissions are now a required component of the diagnostic pediatric audiologic test battery.

Birth to 4 Months

Auditory brainstern response (ABR)

- latency-intensity functions for click stimuli
- analysis of interwave latencies (cochlear vs. retrocochlear status)
- threshold estimation for frequency-specific stimuli (tone bursts)
- threshold estimation for bone-conduction stimuli (as indicated)

Otoacoustic emissions (OAEs)

- distortion product OAEs *or* transient evoked OAEs
- verify cochlear hearing impairment
- rule out auditory neuropathy

Immittance measurement

- tympanometry to assess middle-ear status
- acoustic reflexes to estimate hearing impairment

Behavioural audiometry (if feasible)

- behavioural observation audiometry (BOA) in the sound field (not ear specific)
- evaluate responses to pure tone and speech signals

5 to 24 Months

Behavioural audiometry

- visual reinforcement audiometry (VRA)
- evaluate ear-specific responses (with earphones)
- estimate pure tone thresholds for speech frequencies
- estimate speech signal thresholds

Otoacoustic emissions (OAEs)

- distortion product OAEs *or* transient evoked OAEs
- verify cochlear hearing impairment
- rule out auditory neuropathy

Immittance measurement

- tympanometry to assess middle-ear status
- acoustic reflexes

(contd)

Table 6.1. (contd)

Auditory brainstem response (ABR)

- essential if behavioural audiometry findings are inconsistent, incomplete or inconclusive
- latency-intensity functions for click stimuli
- analysis of interwave latencies (cochlear vs. retrocochlear status)
- threshold estimation for frequency-specific stimuli (tone bursts)
- threshold estimation for bone-conduction stimuli (as indicated)
- sedation usually required

24 to 48 Months

Behavioural audiometry

- visual reinforcement audiometry (VRA), tangible reinforcement conditioned audiometry (TROCA), visual reinforcement conditioned audiometry (VROCA) or conditioned play audiometry
- evaluate ear-specific responses (with earphones)
- estimate pure tone thresholds for audiometric frequencies (250 to 8000 Hz)
- estimate speech signal thresholds
- measure word recognition scores (i.e., speech discrimination)

Otoacoustic emissions (OAEs)

- distortion product OAEs *or* transient evoked OAEs
- verify cochlear hearing impairment
- rule out auditory neuropathy

Immittance measurement

- tympanometry to assess middle-ear status
- acoustic reflexes to confirm hearing impairment

Auditory brainstem response (ABR)

- only if behavioural audiometry findings are inconsistent, incomplete or inconclusive
- latency-intensity functions for click stimuli
- analysis of interwave latencies (cochlear vs. retrocochlear status)
- threshold estimation for frequency-specific stimuli (tone bursts)
- threshold estimation for bone-conduction stimuli (as indicated)
- sedation required

Otoacoustic emissions (OAE) were discovered in 1978 (Kemp, 1978) and, within several years, were used in newborn hearing screening (see, for example, Johnsen, Bagi and Elberling, 1983; Johnsen et al., 1988). Experience with OAEs in newborn hearing screening has led to major modifications in equipment design and, more recently, lower failure rates. Both OAEs and AABR techniques are now endorsed for newborn hearing screening (Joint Committee on Infant Hearing, 2000; European Consensus Conference, 1998; American Academy of Pediatrics, 1999).

The trend toward universal newborn hearing screening (UNHS) has led predictably to a demand for paediatric diagnostic audiological assessment of infants within months after birth. Infants who do not pass the hearing screening at birth must, within one or two months, undergo diagnostic audiological testing to confirm and define hearing impairment so that intervention can be initiated no later than six months. Yoshinaga-Itano and colleagues at the University of Colorado have reported initial findings of an ongoing definitive investigation of the benefits of early intervention on language abilities of children with hearing impairment (Yoshinaga-Itano et al., 1998). The findings of this very thorough and detailed study (at least through 1998) are summarized in Table 6.2. It is clear from this investigation that the definition of 'early' intervention for hearing impairment is younger than six months of age. Secondary to the marked positive influence of early intervention on language acquisition are clear academic, cognitive, social and economic benefits (National Institutes of Health, 1993). Early intervention is entirely dependent, however, on prompt and accurate definition of hearing impairment as soon as possible after birth.

The paediatric test battery

Electrophysiological measures

Aural immittance (impedance) measures are an important part of the basic audiometry test battery. Immittance is a term derived from the terms for two related techniques for assessing middle-ear function (impedance and admittance) – techniques that have been applied clinically since 1970. Briefly, the external ear canal is sealed with a soft rubber probe tip. The probe tip is connected to a device that produces a tone, which is delivered toward the eardrum. Middle-ear impedance or admittance is calculated from the intensity, and other physical properties (such as phase) of the tone in the ear canal. A middle ear (tympanic membrane and ossicular system) with low impedance (higher admittance) more readily accepts the acoustic energy of the probe tone, whereas a middle ear with abnormally high impedance (lower admittance) due, for example, to fluid within the middle-ear space tends to reject energy flow. Thus, impedance (admittance) characteristics of the middle-ear system can be inferred objectively with this technique and related to well-known patterns of findings for various types of middle-ear pathologies.

Table 6.2. Selected features and findings of a study of the language benefits of early intervention (within 6 months after birth) by Yoshinaga-Itano and colleagues at the University of Colorado.

Methodology

- Subjects were 150 hearing-impaired children (72 whose hearing losses were identified between birth and 6 months and 78 identified later).
- Intervention included amplification and ongoing individualized family-oriented communication/language intervention strategies implemented within 2 months after identification.
- Demographic characteristics for subjects in the early and later identified groups were carefully documented, including:
  - ✓ gender
  - ✓ ethnicity
  - ✓ mother's education
  - ✓ medicaid status
  - ✓ degree of hearing loss (all subjects had congenital, bilateral, sensorineural hearing loss)
  - ✓ mode of communication (oral only, or oral and sign language)
  - ✓ multiple handicaps
  - ✓ cognitive ability (quantified with a cognitive quotient)
  - ✓ age at data collection (between 13 and 36 months)
- Children underwent a comprehensive developmental evaluation (Minnesota Child Development Inventory, or MCD1) which included standardized scales for expressive (54 items) and comprehension-conceptual (67 items) language function. Language status was summarized by a composite language quotient (LQ).

Findings and Conclusions

- Children with hearing loss who were identified by 6 months after birth showed significantly better expressive and receptive language skills (higher LQs) than later identified children.
- The effect of age of identification was found across all of the demographic variables (noted above).
- The benefits of early identification were found for all degrees of hearing impairment, from mild to profound.
- There was no significant difference in language performance among four groups of later-identified subjects (from 7 to 25 months of age). That is, the benefits of early identification occur only before 6 months (early intervention = < 6 months).
- For children with hearing impairment, the first 6 months after birth are very important, even critical. For children with congenital hearing impairment of any degree, language can develop on a normal schedule if intervention is begun by 6 months.

Source: Yoshinaga-Itano C et al. (1998). Language of early- and later-identified children with hearing loss. Pediatrics 102 (5): 1161–1171.

Tympanometry is the dynamic recording of middle-ear impedance as air pressure in the ear canal is systematically increased or decreased. The technique is a sensitive measure of tympanic membrane integrity and middle-ear function. Compliance (the reciprocal of stiffness) of the middle ear, the dominant component of immittance, is the vertical dimension of a tympanogram. Tympanometry is very popular clinically because it requires little technical skill and only several seconds of time; it is an electrophysiological (as opposed to behavioural) method that does not depend on the co-operation of the patient, and it is a very sensitive index of middle-ear function. Tympanometric patterns, in combination with audiogram patterns, permit differentiation among and classification of middle-ear disorders. The most clinically widespread approach for describing tympanograms was first reported in 1970 by James Jerger.

The stapedial muscle within the middle ear is the smallest muscle in the body. Measurement of contractions of the middle-ear stapedial muscle to high sound intensity levels (usually 80 dB or greater) is the basis of the acoustic reflex. Acoustic reflex measurement is clinically useful for estimating hearing sensitivity and for differentiating among sites of auditory disorders, including the middle ear, inner ear, eighth cranial nerve and auditory brainstem. The afferent portion of the acoustic reflex arc is the eighth cranial nerve. There are complex brainstem pathways leading from the cochlear nucleus on the stimulated side to the region of the motor nucleus of the seventh (facial) nerve on both sides (ipsilateral and contralateral to the stimulus) of the brainstem. The efferent portion of the arc is the seventh nerve, which innervates the stapedius muscle. The muscle then contracts, causing increased stiffness (decreased compliance) of the middle-ear system. The small change in compliance that follows stapedius muscle contraction within 10 ms is detected by the probe and immittance device, much as compliance changes are detected during tympanometry. Acoustic reflex measurement is very useful clinically because it can quickly provide objective information on the status of the auditory system from the middle ear to the brainstem. Distinctive acoustic reflex patterns for ipsilateral and contralateral stimulation and measurement conditions characterize middle ear, cochlea, eighth nerve, brainstem and even facial nerve dysfunction.

Otoacoustic emissions

Otoacoustic emissions are low-intensity sounds produced by the cochlea in response to an acoustic stimulus (see Hall, 2000 for review). A moderate intensity click, or an appropriate combination of two tones, can evoke outer hair cell movement or motility. Outer hair cell motility affects basilar membrane biomechanics, resulting in a form of intracochlear energy amplification, as well as cochlear tuning for more precise frequency resolution. The outer hair cell motility generates mechanical energy within the cochlea, which is propagated outward, via the middle-ear system and the tympanic membrane, to the ear canal. Vibration of the tympanic membrane then produces an acoustic signal (the OAE), which a sensitive microphone can measure.

There are two broad classes of otoacoustic emissions: spontaneous and evoked. Spontaneous otoacoustic emissions (SOAEs), present in only about 70% of persons with normal hearing, are measured in the external ear canal when there is no external sound stimulation. A significant gender effect for SOAEs has been confirmed with females demonstrating SOAEs at twice the rate of males. Evoked otoacoustic emissions, elicited by moderate levels (50 to 80 dB SPL) of acoustic stimulation in the external ear canal, are generally classified according to characteristics of the stimuli used to elicit them or characteristics of the cochlear events that generate them.

Distortion-product otoacoustic emissions (DPOAEs) are produced when two pure-tone stimuli at frequencies f1 and f2 are presented to the ear simultaneously. The most robust DPOAEs occur at the frequency determined by the equation 2f1-f2, whereas the actual cochlear frequency region that is assessed with DPOAE is between these two frequencies, and probably close to the f2 stimulus for recommended test protocols (Hall, 2000). Transient evoked otoacoustic emissions (TEOAEs) are elicited by brief acoustic stimuli such as clicks or tone bursts. Although there are distinct differences in the methodology for recording DPOAEs versus TEOAEs, and the exact cochlear mechanisms responsible for their generation are also different, each type of evoked OAE is now being incorporated into routine auditory assessment of children and adults, including newborn hearing screening (Hall, 2000). As with ABR, devices permitting automated OAE measurement and analysis, and designed primarily for newborn hearing screening, are now available from a variety of manufacturers. Most of these devices are hand held and very simple to operate. A recent report of accumulated experience with OAE screening of over 50 000 babies confirmed a failure rate of approximately 10%, with a final false-positive failure rate of less than 2% (Vohr et al., 1998).

The use of OAEs in paediatric diagnostic assessment is, perhaps, more valuable and powerful than any other application in children or adults. Why are OAEs a necessary component of the modern paediatric test battery? The answer is their remarkable sensitivity and specificity. As discussed in detail in Chapter 2, OAEs are the product of highly metabolic activity of outer hair cells. Virtually any possible insult to the cochlea, including even subtle disruptions in blood flow to the stria vascularis, will be reflected by OAE changes. There is no more sensitive measure of cochlear function. Otoacoustic emissions are almost entirely sensory and 'pre-neural'. Their measurement does not depend on the functional status of any synapses, nor the rest of the auditory system. This site specificity is a distinct clinical advantage for a component of a diagnostic test battery. In addition to these two essential features – sensitivity and specificity – OAEs are electrophysiological, requiring no behavioural response from the paediatric patient.

These fundamental features of OAEs take on very practical everyday importance in paediatric audiology. Most audiological management of children is predicated on the premise that the hearing impairment is sensory, affecting the cochlea. By definition, audiologists are responsible for evaluation and diagnosis of all types of auditory impairment. Conductive hearing impairment, however, is traditionally treated medically or surgically by physicians. Although the audiologist is integrally involved in the detection of eighth nerve (retrocochlear) and central auditory nervous system dysfunction, treatment (if available) is most often a team effort, which may or may not include the audiologist. Determining whether the hearing impairment is sensory or neural (or some combination) depends very much on results of OAE measurement. If the hearing impairment is sensory, then the audiologist is the professional with primary responsibility for implementing and co-ordinating management with amplification, and a complement of habilitation or rehabilitation strategies and techniques. Otoacoustic emissions are now part of the standard-of-care for paediatric audiology. This serious clinical conclusion is amply supported by diverse OAE applications that are reviewed in this chapter. In short, OAEs are not simply a handy or convenient procedure for assessing auditory function but, rather, an essential component of the test battery. They can play a pivotal and critical role in decisions regarding audiological or medical management of auditory impairment. The clearest example of this role is in patients with suspected 'auditory neuropathy'.

Auditory brainstem response (ABR)

Auditory evoked responses are electrophysiological recordings of responses to sounds. With proper test protocols, the responses can be recorded clinically from activation of all levels of the auditory system, from the cochlea to the cortex (see Hall, 1992 for review). Among these responses, the ABR (often referred by neurologists as the brainstem auditory evoked response or BAER) is applied most often clinically. The ABR is generated with transient acoustic stimuli (clicks or tone bursts) and detected with surface electrodes (discs) placed on the forehead and near the ears (earlobe or within external ear canal). Using a commercially available, computer-based device, it is possible to present rapidly (for example, at rates of 20 to 30 per second) thousands of sound stimuli and to average reliable ABR waveforms in a matter of minutes.

Extensive research has shown that the ABR wave components arise from the eighth cranial nerve and auditory regions in the caudal and rostral brainstem. Wave I unquestionably represents the synchronously stimulated compound action potentials from the distal (cochlear end) of the eighth cranial nerve. Wave II may also arise from the eighth nerve, but near the brainstem (the proximal end). Waves I and II are generated by structures ipsilateral to the ear stimulated. All later ABR waves have multiple generators within the auditory brainstem. Wave III, which is usually prominent, is generated within the caudal pons, with likely contributions from the cochlear nuclei, the trapezoid body, and the superior olivary complex (Hall, 1992). The most prominent and rostral component of the ABR – wave V – is thought to arise in the region of the lateral lemniscus as it approaches the inferior colliculus, probably on the side contralateral to the ear stimulated.

In ABR waveform analysis, the first objective is to assure that the response is reliably recorded. Minimally, two replicated waveforms should be averaged. If the response is not highly replicable, modifications in the test protocol should be made, and then potential technical problems must be considered and systematically ruled out. When a replicable response is confirmed, absolute latencies for each replicable wave component, and relative (interwave) latencies between components, are calculated in milliseconds, and usually compared with appropriate normative data. When applying the ABR in newborn hearing screening, waveform analysis is typically limited to the identification of a reliable wave V component within the expected latency region for a newborn infant. There are now automated ABR (AABR) devices on the market designed specifically for newborn hearing screening by non-professional testers (Hall, 1992). With these devices, stimulus presentation and response analysis is under the control of computer-based algorithms and statistical criteria. Data for one automated ABR system (the ALGO-2 device from Natus, Inc.) confirmed failure rates as low as 2% in a healthy baby population, and only 4% for an intensive care nursery infant population (Stewart et al., 2000).

Electrocochleography

For over 30 years, electrocochleography (ECochG) has been applied in the assessment of peripheral auditory function. Traditionally, ECochG has been performed for intraoperative monitoring of cochlear and eighth nerve status and in the diagnosis of Ménière's disease. More recently, the value of ECochG techniques and principles in paediatric audiological assessment has become appreciated, especially for the diagnostic assessment of infants with suspected 'auditory neuropathy'. Optimal ECochG waveforms are recorded from a small needle electrode placed through the tympanic membrane onto the promontory, although tympanic membrane and, to a lesser extent, ear canal electrode locations are also clinically useful. Stimulus and acquisition parameters for recording ECochG have been well defined for decades (see Hall, 1992). The three major components of the ECochG are the cochlear microphonic (CM), the summating potential (SP), and the action potential (AP). The CM and SP reflect cochlear bioelectric activity, whereas the AP is generated by synchronous firing of distal afferent eighth nerve fibres, and is equivalent to ABR wave I.

Cortical auditory evoked responses

More than a dozen subtypes of auditory evoked responses can be recorded beyond the brainstem, from auditory regions of the thalamus, hippocampus, internal capsule and cortex. Prominent among them in clinical audiology are the auditory middle latency response (AMLR), the auditory late response (ALR), the P300 response, and the mismatch negativity (MMN) response (Hall, 1992). In fact, cortical auditory evoked responses were reported as early as the 1930s and, with the exception of the MMN, all of the above responses were well described before the ABR was even discovered. Cortical auditory evoked responses are characterized by longer latencies (100 to 300 ms) than ECochG and ABR because they arise from more rostral regions of the auditory CNS and are dependent on multi-synaptic pathways. Amplitudes of the cortical responses are considerably larger (two to 20 times larger) than those of the earlier responses because they reflect activity evoked from a greater number of neurons. Measurement parameters are distinctly different for the cortical versus cochlear or brainstem responses. For example, stimulus rate must be slower and physiologic filter settings lower. As a rule, stimulus intensities are moderate, rather than high. Cortical evoked responses are best elicited with longer duration, and therefore frequency-specific, tonal stimuli, rather than the click stimuli that are optimal for evoking ECochG and ABR. The analysis time must, of course, extend beyond the expected latency of the response (>300 ms) for the cortical responses. Recording electrode sites also are different for the cortical responses, with more emphasis on scalp sites over the hemispheres and less concern about electrode sites near the ears.

The AMLR consists of a prominent positive voltage (labelled Pa) component in the 25 to 30 ms region. When recorded with electrodes located over the temporal-parietal region, the AMLR is generated by pathways leading to the primary cortex and from this region of the temporal lobe. The AMLR is reasonably reliable in children, as well as adults. It is thus a good selection for electrophysiological assessment of higher level auditory CNS function in patients at risk for or undergoing evaluation of neurological disease or dysfunction involving the thalamus or primary auditory cortex. The P300 response is recorded using what is typically referred to as the 'oddball paradigm'. Two types of stimuli are used. One – the frequent stimulus – is presented frequently in a very predictable manner. The other – the rare or deviant stimulus – is presented infrequently and pseudorandomly. The rare stimuli account for less than 20% of the total stimuli presented. The patient is instructed to ignore the frequent stimuli and to attend to the rare stimuli. The waveform for the frequent stimulus is essentially an auditory late response consisting of a positive peak of 5 to 10 mV within the 150 to 200 ms region. In contrast, the waveform averaged from the attended rare stimuli is characterized normally by a large positive peak in the 300 ms region, hence the term 'P300 response'. Presumed generators of the P300 response include regions of the medial temporal lobe (hippocampus) that are important in auditory attention.

One limitation of the P300 response paradigm is the requirement for patient's conscious attention to the rare stimulus. This requirement may preclude measurement of the P300 response in patients for whom objective, electrophysiological information on higher level auditory CNS function is most desired, such as infants, children with language-learning disorders, children with attention deficit disorder, and brain-injured adults. Another cortical response – the MMN – offers a potential solution to this clinical dilemma. The MMN is also recorded to frequent and rare (deviant) stimuli, although the distinction between the two types of stimulus is very small. For example, if the two types of stimulus differ along the frequency domain, the P300 response might be elicited by 1 000 (frequent) versus 2 000 Hz (rare) tones, whereas the MMN might be elicited by 1000 versus 1 200 Hz tones, or even speech sounds, such as /da/ versus /ga/. The MMN is thought to be generated before conscious perception by the neuronal mismatch in the brain created when the repetitive frequent stimuli are followed by an acoustically different deviant stimulus. Importantly, the MMN does not require attention to the stimuli. Rather, the patient can be sleeping or involved in some non-auditory task (such as watching a silent movie). Another clinical advantage of the MMN is the wide range of stimulus possibilities, including rather complex speech signals. It is likely that the MMN will soon be incorporated into clinical assessment of auditory CNS function in varied populations of children and adults.

Behavioural measures

Peripheral auditory assessment

Description of behavioural audiometric techniques and strategies is beyond the scope of this chapter. There is a substantial literature on the strategies and protocols for diagnostic paediatric assessment (for example Northern and Downs, 1991; Gerber, 1996; Hall and Mueller, 1997). A general outline of age-appropriate approaches for paediatric audiometry was summarized in Table 6.1.

Central auditory assessment

In the infant years of the profession of audiology, Mylkebust (1954) noted that 'hearing is a receptive sense . . . and essential for normal language behaviour' (p. 11), and noted that 'the diagnostician of auditory problems in children has traditionally emphasized peripheral damage. It is desirable that he also include considerations of central damage' (p. 54). He also explained that 'central deafness [central auditory processing disorder] is a deficiency in transmitting auditory impulses to the higher brain centres while receptive aphasia [language disorder] is a deficiency in the interpretation of these impulses after they have been delivered' (p. 153). During this era, Bocca, Calearo and Cassinari (1954) reported that surgically confirmed central auditory system pathology could be detected with sufficiently sensitive audiological procedures. These pioneering observations and studies have since been validated by many clinical investigations. There are now a variety of behavioural and electrophysiological techniques for the assessment of peripheral and central auditory system function, including central auditory processing disorders (CAPD). The term CAPD is used to describe a deficit in the perception or complete analysis of auditory information due to central auditory nervous system dysfunction, usually at the level of the cerebral cortex (Hall, 1999). Central auditory processing takes place before language processing or comprehension.

The evaluation and management of CAPD is well within the scope of audiological practice, and an accepted clinical activity within the field of communicative disorders as defined by the American Academy of Audiology and the American Speech-Language-Hearing Association. Audiologists are in the business of evaluating hearing and managing non-medical hearing impairments. Each level and specific structure within the auditory system – from the external ear to the temporal lobe – contributes to the sense of hearing. The ear is certainly no more important in hearing than the brain. As indicated by a patient's history, complaints, and preliminary test findings, the audiologist should evaluate comprehensively central, as well as peripheral, auditory function. Lacking training or experience in assessment of central auditory nervous system function, the audiologist would be well advised to refer the patient to a colleague who is experienced in CAPD assessment.

Appropriate assessment and management of CAPD is rapidly approaching a 'standard of audiological care', in view of the professional recognition and definition of CAPD (for example, ASHA, 1996) the availability of a variety of test procedures, accessible treatment strategies and programmes, and the growing number of audiologists prepared to provide all necessary services to patients with CAPD. A patient presenting with indicators for retrocochlear auditory dysfunction – by history, symptoms, or audiological signs – is promptly referred for neurodiagnostic assessment and multidisciplinary management. Similarly, the paediatric or adult patient with risk factors and/or audiological evidence of central auditory dysfunction should promptly undergo the next level of diagnostic evaluation, with multidisciplinary management as indicated.

Central auditory processing disorder assessment is carried out with a battery of behavioural tests that have proven sensitivity to central auditory dysfunction. One battery of audiological tests is summarized in Table 6.3. If a peripheral hearing impairment (unilateral or bilateral) is discovered, medical or audiological management is initiated, and further CAPD assessment is postponed. Typically, however, peripheral auditory function is normal and the CAPD test battery is conducted. Due to age and time constraints, and to avoid a redundancy of information, not all of these procedures are usually applied with each patient. Behavioural CAPD tests are administered first. The overall goal is to measure reliable performance for each ear on a series of speech audiometry procedures. These include a dichotic word test (dichotic digits or the staggered spondaic word test), a dichotic sentence test (the dichotic sentence identification test or, for younger children with poor reading skills, the competing sentences test), a speech-in-competition test (the synthetic sentence identification test with an ipsilateral competing message) and reliable performance with binaural stimulation on one or more non-speech measures, such as the pitch pattern sequence and duration pattern sequence tests.

Auditory evoked responses are recorded if specifically requested by the referring person, or if we have any concerns about the reliability or questions about the interpretation of behavioural test performance. Central auditory processing disorders findings are analysed in comparison to age-corrected normative data. Minimal criteria for confirmation of CAPD are scores that are below the age-corrected normal region (below 2.5 standard deviations from the mean) for one or both ears for at least two different procedures in a child with normal peripheral auditory test findings.

In constructing a CAPD test battery, it is wise to rely on procedures that are not apt to be influenced by linguistic, cognitive or attentional disorders. Interpretation of CAPD tests is most straightforward when deficits are unilateral, which confirms that the patient understood the task and that the outcome was not due to a linguistic, cognitive or attentional disorder. A pronounced unilateral abnormality, specifically a marked left-ear deficit, is one of the most common patterns of CAPD test battery findings in our experience. Another rather definite CAPD test battery pattern is when reduced performance is apparent only on difficult (versus easier) portions of a test. This finding also implies an auditory versus linguistic, cognitive or strictly attentional explanation for the child's poor performance. Other important features of a clinically feasible CAPD test battery are:

- resistance to the influence of even slight peripheral auditory dysfunction;
- the availability of adequate age-matched normative data; and
- professionally produced tape-recorded or compact disc recorded test materials.

Earlier concerns about the usefulness of CAPD assessment with rudimentary procedures lacking these criteria were justifiable. Now, however, clinical feasible and commercially available procedures are available for children and adults (Hall, 1999).

Neurodiagnosis of auditory dysfunction

Definition of hearing sensitivity

The first and essential step in confirmation of hearing impairment is the estimation of hearing sensitivity. A sizeable proportion of newborn infants who do not pass hearing screening, and also older children suspected of hearing impairment, will have hearing sensitivity within normal limits bilaterally throughout the frequencies important for speech perception and acquisition. For children whose developmental age is greater than about six months, definition of hearing sensitivity may be made with behavioural audiometry, at least for the better-hearing ear (Table 6.1). Electrophysiological techniques (OAEs and ABR) should be considered routinely, however, for ear-specific hearing assessment and to confirm incomplete, inconclusive or inconsistent behavioural findings. Applied in combination, these electrophysiological techniques permit reasonably accurate frequency-specific and ear-specific estimation of the configuration and degree of hearing sensitivity loss, and confirmation that the

Table 6.3. Examples of behavioural audiologic procedures for the evaluation of auditory processes. Sources of test materials are listed below. NV = a nonverbal procedure.

Process	Procedure
• sound localization and lateralization	no clinical procedures are currently available (research is underway)
• auditory discrimination	Goldman Fristoe Woodcock Test of Auditory Discrimination in quiet
• auditory pattern recognition	pitch pattern sequence test (NV); duration pattern sequence test (NV)
• temporal aspects of audition	Auditory Fusion Test-revised (NV); dichotic digits; staggered spondaic word (SSW) test; dichotic sentence identification (DSI);
• auditory performance decrements with competing signals	synthetic sentence identification with ipsilateral competing message (SSI-ICM); paediatric speech intelligibilitiy (PSI) test; Goldman Fristoe Woodcock Test of Auditory Discrimination in noise
• auditory performance decrements	time-compressed word test; filtered word test with degraded acoustic signals

All behavioural CAPD test materials are available in analogue or digital tape or CD format from:

- AUDiTEC of St. Louis, 2515 S. Big Bend Blvd., St. Louis, MO, USA. 63143–2105
- Psychological Corporation
- Precision Acoustics, 411 NE 87th Avenue #B, Vancouver, WA 98664, USA. (360–892–9367)
- CD 1.0 and 1.1. Available from: Richard Wilson, PhD, Audiology-126, VA Medical Center, Mountain Home, TN 37684, USA

hearing impairment is cochlear (sensory), rather than secondary to middle-ear or neural dysfunction. As implied earlier, with the expansion of UNHS and the demand for defining hearing status of infants, there is increased interest among clinical audiologists in electrophysiological auditory assessment with OAEs, and ABR measurement with tone burst and bone conduction stimuli. These topics are reviewed in considerable detail in numerous journal articles and textbooks (for example Hall, 1992; Hall, 2000).

Differentiating among sites of auditory dysfunction

There are at least three principles of paediatric hearing assessment today that contribute to accurate description of auditory status and, therefore, lead to a rational and evidence-based strategy for effective management. First, a test-battery approach is essential in the evaluation of hearing in children of any age. With the advent of newborn hearing screening there is increased demand for diagnostic audiological assessment of infants under the age of four months. That is, infants who do not pass a hearing screening at birth require follow-up evaluation within months to confirm and define the hearing impairment so that intervention can begin before six months after birth. This initial description of the type and degree of hearing impairment for each ear is based typically on electrophysiological procedures (see Table 6.1). This information is essential for determining whether hearing aids are indicated and, if so, the specifications of the hearing aid selection and fitting. Reasonably accurate electrophysiological estimations of auditory thresholds for three or four data points within the speech frequency region permit precise 'prescriptive' hearing aid selection and fitting (Mueller and Hall, 1999), even in infants as young as two to three months. The hearing aid fitting will later be adjusted and refined as the hearing impairment is better defined with behavioural audiometry (Table 6.1). Although electrophysiological measures of auditory function are invaluable during infancy, only behavioural measures truly reflect a child's hearing status.

Second, the audiological evaluation should lead to a differentiation of the type of hearing impairment, the general site of lesion, and along with other medical studies, a diagnosis. Examples of types of hearing impairment include conductive (middle-ear dysfunction), sensory (cochlear dysfunction), neural (eighth cranial nerve and/or central auditory nervous system), or combinations of these types. Thus, in addition to estimation of hearing thresholds, the objective of audiometry in infants must provide accurate information on the site of dysfunction within the auditory system. The importance of diagnostic paediatric assessment is easily appreciated by considering the distinctly divergent management approaches taken with three clinical entities all presenting with elevated (abnormal) auditory thresholds for air-conducted signals, but otherwise very different patterns of auditory findings. Middle-ear disease or malformation can be identified by abnormal immitance findings, and better auditory thresholds for bone- versus air-conduction stimulation with either ABR or pure-tone audiometry. Prompt identification of middle-ear disease with proper referral can lead to successful medical management and eliminate the need for amplification. A variety of paediatric diseases are associated with cochlear dysfunction. Some are among the Joint Committee on Infant Hearing (JCIH, 1994) risk indicators.

Diagnosis of the cause for sensory hearing impairment may require radiological studies and laboratory tests. Audiological findings for otoacoustic emissions and ABR and pure-tone audiometry for older children can almost always confirm a sensory hearing impairment and even differentiate between outer and inner hair-cell dysfunction. Amplification, rather that medical therapy, is the most common management strategy for a pure sensory deficit. Management is radically different for a third and recently described clinical entity – 'auditory neuropathy' – which is described in more detail in the next section. Comprehensive diagnostic audiometry for a small proportion of infants with hearing impairment shows normal cochlear function. Based on ABR or behavioural measures, the hearing impairment may initially appear to be sensory in nature. Yet OAE recordings are normal, confirming cochlear outer hair-cell integrity. Complete medical diagnostic workup typically yields the diagnosis of a disorder secondary to neurological dysfunction, such as cerebral palsy or developmental delay. Although children with auditory neuropathy are most often graduates of the intensive care nursery, there are reports of auditory neuropathy in the well baby population. One of the most common risk factors for auditory neuropathy is hyperbilirubinaemia. Audiological management is markedly different for auditory neuropathy versus more common sensory hearing impairment. Since cochlear function may be intact with auditory neuropathy, a hearing aid or cochlear implant is not immediately indicated and, in fact, is clearly contraindicated. Most children with this pattern of audiological findings are candidates for multidisciplinary diagnostic evaluations in a child development centre setting. Management strategies are highly variable depending on the exact auditory and neurological findings (Hall, 2000).

Third, auditory measures used for diagnostic assessment must be age appropriate. All auditory responses in early childhood are affected to some degree by either peripheral and/or central auditory system maturation, and vary as a function of age. Even electrophysiological findings must be interpreted with reference to age-appropriate normative data. For behavioural audiometry, however, the actual procedures used and the entire test strategy are highly dependent on a child's developmental age (see Table 6.1). In the hands of an inexperienced audiologist, or without full appreciation of the most age-appropriate test approach, sophisticated behavioural audiometry test procedures may yield an unreliable and invalid reflection of hearing status. Serious mismanagement of paediatric hearing impairment can result.

Auditory neuropathy

Introduction

The appreciation of the constellation of auditory findings now called 'auditory neuropathy' was due exclusively to routine application of OAEs in patients – in particular infants and young children – at risk for neurological dysfunction. In the early 1990s, as OAEs were initially incorporated into the paediatric audiological test battery in leading clinical centres throughout the world, an unusual pattern of auditory findings was independently reported by investigators around the world (Table 6.4). OAEs have clearly altered our approach for assessment and management of paediatric hearing impairment. This general pattern of findings is now well recognized, but strategies for management of auditory neuropathy, and our understanding of the long-term outcome for these children, is still developing. Auditory neuropathy is practically defined as abnormal ABR findings, and often absent or abnormal behavioural responses to sound, with cochlear integrity. Cochlear function in auditory neuropathy can be documented electrophysiologically with OAE and/or with the cochlear microphonics of the ECochG.

Assessment of auditory neuropathy

Children with neurological disease or dysfunction are, as expected, at greater risk for auditory neuropathy. The diagnosis of some of the more common etiologies is not often made by the time the first audiological signs of auditory neuropathy are recorded. Indeed, at the time the audiological assessment is first completed, often during the neonatal period, there may be no suspicion of neurological dysfunction. The audiological evidence of auditory neuropathy may initiate referral to medical specialists, which will ultimately lead to a definitive diagnosis. An approach for detection of auditory neuropathy is shown schematically in Figure 6.1. Otoacoustic emissions play an essential role in the diagnostic process. If OAEs are absent, then the outcome of the audiological diagnostic assessment leads to either medical management (for example, for middle-ear

Table 6.4. Published reports (arranged chronologically) of patients with normal OAEs and abnormal ABR findings, a pattern consistent with broadly defined auditory neuropathy.

Author (s), year	Comments
Lutman et al, 1989	case report of 11-year-old child with normal OAE and unilateral SNHL by ABR
Prieve et al, 1991	33-year-old with severe-to-profound unilateral SNHL and normal TEOAE
Baldwin & Watkin, 1992	infant with normal TEOAE and abnormal ABR
Katona et al, 1993	3-month-old infant with OAE and CM but profound SNHL by ABR and behavioural findings
Konradsson, 1996	four apparently healthy children (4 and 7 years old) with severe to profound SNHL (ABR and behavioral audiometry) and normal TEOAE
Laccourreye et al, 1996	3-year-old child with normal TEOAE and profound SNHL
Starr et al, 1996	10 children and young adults with OAE and CM but abnormal ABRs; detailed neurologic findings
Stein et al, 1996	4 infants with normal TEOAE
Watkin, 1996	infant with normal TEOAE and abnormal ABR
Deltenre et al, 1997	3 children with normal OAE and CM and abnormal ABRs and behavioural audiograms
Parker et al, 1997	7 patients with normal TEOAE and abnormal ABR (taken from a large series of children)
Psarommatis et al, 1997	two case reports of infants with normal TEOAE and abnormal ABRs
Berlin et al, 1998	5 infants with TEOAEs and CM (in ABR), but absent click-stimulus ABRs
Bachmann & Hall, 1998	case report of infant with Maple syrup urine disease with normal DPOAE and abnormal ABR
Cullington & Brown, 1998	case report of premature infant (history included jaundice and asphyxia) with Mondini dysplasia with normal TEOAE and profound SNHL behaviourally
Starr et al, 1998	4 children with neurologic disorders with normal OAEs and temperature-related ABR abnormalities
Wood et al, 1998	7 infants with normal TEOAE and abnormal ABR screening results
Miyamoto et al, 1999	4-year-old with normal OAE and SNHL who received cochlear implant
Rance et al, 1999	20 infants and young children with ECochG CM but absent click-stimulus ABRs

disease) and/or audiological management (for example, hearing aid selection and fitting). The presence of OAEs, in the context of abnormal ABR findings, is a sign of auditory neuropathy. Auditory brainstem response assessment at this stage is essential. The ABR, including wave I, is dependent on synchronous firing of afferent eighth nerve fibres in the region of the spiral ganglion secondary to synaptic activation by the inner hair cells. Inner hair-cell dysfunction will, to some extent, elevate ABR thresholds. Normal interwave latencies are a reflection of intact retrocochlear pathways. Audiological follow-up assessments with 'the inner hair cell pattern' should continue until behavioural thresholds and speech audiometry findings are recorded. Evaluation of auditory neuropathy requires a finely tuned diagnostic approach, using a variety of techniques for selectively assessing function of specific regions within the auditory system. Diagnosis in auditory neuropathy is quite challenging as clinical presentations are highly varied. In fact, the diagnostic process in auditory neuropathy should be ongoing until hearing status is completely described electrophysiologically and behaviourally, medical diagnosis is reached, and effective medical and audiological management is initiated. Management of auditory neuropathy is also extremely challenging, and a multidisciplinary team approach is necessary. During the first months after detection of auditory neuropathy it is wise to monitor audiological status until a pattern of findings emerges. Experience has shown that follow-up audiological assessment for some children with initial evidence of apparently severe auditory dysfunction will later show normal hearing sensitivity, or audiometric contraindications to amplification. Hearing aid fitting would, in such children, be inappropriate and possibly harmful. Although amplification may be withheld, other management steps can and should be initiated, including referral for comprehensive neurological, developmental and communication evaluation, and neuroradiological workup. Other appropriate referrals include genetics, otolaryngology and speech-language pathology.

Illustrative case reports

Case 1

Estimation of hearing sensitivity. A 2;3-year-old child was referred to the Audiology Service from an audiologist in an outlying community for estimation of hearing sensitivity and recommendations for audiological management. The child's parents and physician were concerned because 'he was talking very little'. According to the paediatrician, the patient had no history of recurrent otitis media and no major illnesses. At age 1;5 years, tympanometry in the paediatrician's office showed a type-C pattern,

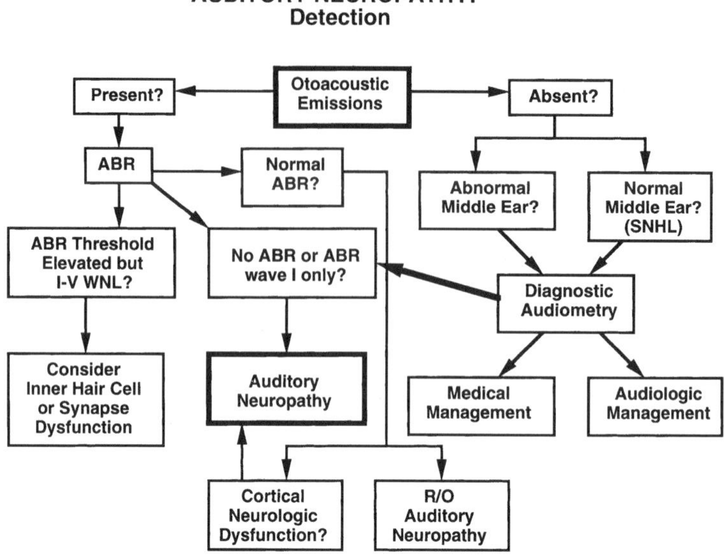

Figure 6.1. A strategy for identification of auditory neuropathy. As a sensory (versus neural) auditory measure, OAEs play a key role in the identification and diagnosis of auditory neuropathy. ECochG components, especially the cochlear microphonic (CM) are also useful in the identification of auditory neuropathy.

although pneumatic otoscopy confirmed mobile tympanic membranes. The patient was evaluated by a speech-language pathologist. Treatment included speech therapy and sign language. The speech-language pathologist expressed concern about possible hearing impairment.

An ABR for hearing assessment was scheduled for the next week at a local otolaryngology clinic. At that time, an attempt to sedate the child with chloral hydrate was unsuccessful. An ABR assessment under sedation was completed one month later at the same clinic. Inspection of the waveforms from this assessment confirmed that a reliable response was observed bilaterally for click stimuli at an intensity level of 85 dBnHL, with absolute and interwave latency values within normal limits. According to the formal report of the assessment 'wave V was tracked down to 25 dBnHL bilaterally, suggesting neural synchrony and probable normal hearing thresholds bilaterally for at least the 1 000 to 4 000 Hz range. OAEs and play audiometry are recommended.' According to our review of the waveforms, however, a very small amplitude and questionable response was observed only for 65 dBnHL click stimulation. There was no clear ABR for lower intensity levels bilaterally. Behavioural hearing assessment in two months using VRA yielded a speech awareness threshold at 20 dBnHL in the sound field. The patient did not accept earphones, and responses could not be conditioned to pure-tone signals (Figure 6.2). The mother then met with a representative from the state parent-infant programme and was encouraged to pursue amplification on a trial basis. She enrolled her son in a pre-school programme for hearing-impaired children. The audiologist managing the child, however, advised against hearing aid use stating that 'all of our test results suggest normal hearing and no hearing impairment at all, therefore I cannot confidently put hearing aids on the child at this time.' The possibility of central auditory dysfunction was raised at this visit. In addition, the parents were urged 'to return for repeat attempts at a pure-tone audiogram. They understand that it will take multiple visits before we complete the puzzle.' The otolaryngologist agreed with this recommendation.

One month later (at age two years) the mother consulted another local audiologist for a second opinion. Again, only sound field testing could be carried out as the child refused to wear earphones. Responses to speech signals and 500 Hz and 1 000 Hz warble-tone signals were observed only for intensity levels of 40 to 50 dBnHL (Figure 6.2). Attempts to obtain conditioned responses were unsuccessful. This audiologist interpreted his findings as consistent with a moderate to moderate-severe hearing impairment, and recommended repeat behavioural audiometry prior to hearing aid fitting. The parents then returned to the paediatrician to discuss their child's hearing status and management. A referral was then made to our clinic.

Auditory brainstem response assessment was carried out with the patient sedated (chloral hydrate) and sleeping. The protocol used for measurement of the ABR with click and tone-burst stimulation has been described in detail previously (for example, Hall, 1992; Hall and Mueller, 1997). Left-ear click stimulation at 95 dBnHL produced a reliable response with waves I, III, and V clearly observed (Figure 6.3). Interwave latency values were within normal limits. A wave V was detected at 85 dbnHL but not at 75 dBnHL. A reliable ABR was also observed for tone-burst stimulation at 500 Hz, 1000 Hz, and 4 000 Hz (Figure 6.3) but the minimal intensity levels producing a wave V component varied among these frequencies. Auditory brainstem response findings for right-ear click and tone-burst stimulation are illustrated in Figure 6.4. All interwave latencies were within normal limits for the click and 4 000 Hz stimuli. ABR 'thresholds' again varied as a function of the stimulus. The reconstruction of an audiogram with ABR data is shown in Figure 6.5. The symbols in this figure do not represent hearing thresholds. Rather, they indicated the minimum intensity level (in 10 dB increments) producing a clear and reliable ABR wave V. Actual thresholds would be expected to be approximately 10 dB better than these levels (Hall, 1992). While the patient remained sleeping, DPOAE measurement was conducted over a test frequency region of 2 000 to 8 000 Hz (Figure 6.6). No DPOAE activity was detected for either ear. These ear- and frequency-specific ABR findings provided unequivocal evidence of bilateral peripheral auditory dysfunction that differs in degree and configuration between ears. DPOAE data confirmed a sensory hearing impairment. The ABR results were consistent with normal brainstem auditory function. We recommended immediate hearing aid selection and fitting based on these ABR findings.

Comments

Without newborn hearing screening, delayed identification and intervention of hearing impairment is commonplace, even for children with concerned parents and a well-meaning paediatrician. Behavioural audiometry is insufficient for early (before six months) identification and intervention. Postponing intervention until behavioural findings are conclusive and complete will result in unacceptable delays. Specifically, decisions on the need for amplification, and hearing aid selection and fitting, simply cannot be made with fragmentary audiological findings – speech awareness thresholds and only sound field findings. Although not adequate for hearing aid selection and fitting, the previous behavioural findings for this case, such as the speech awareness threshold of 20 dBnHL and the sound field responses to pure-tone signals, were consistent with subsequent definition of auditory status by ABR.

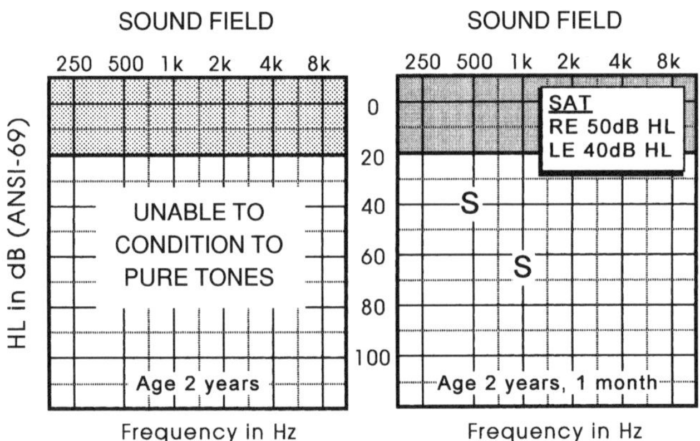

Figure 6.2. Findings from two previous behavioural audiometric assessments for a 2-year-old boy (Case 1) with speech-language delay, and suspected of having hearing impairment by his parents. Neither assessment yielded ear-specific nor frequency-specific information on hearing sensitivity.

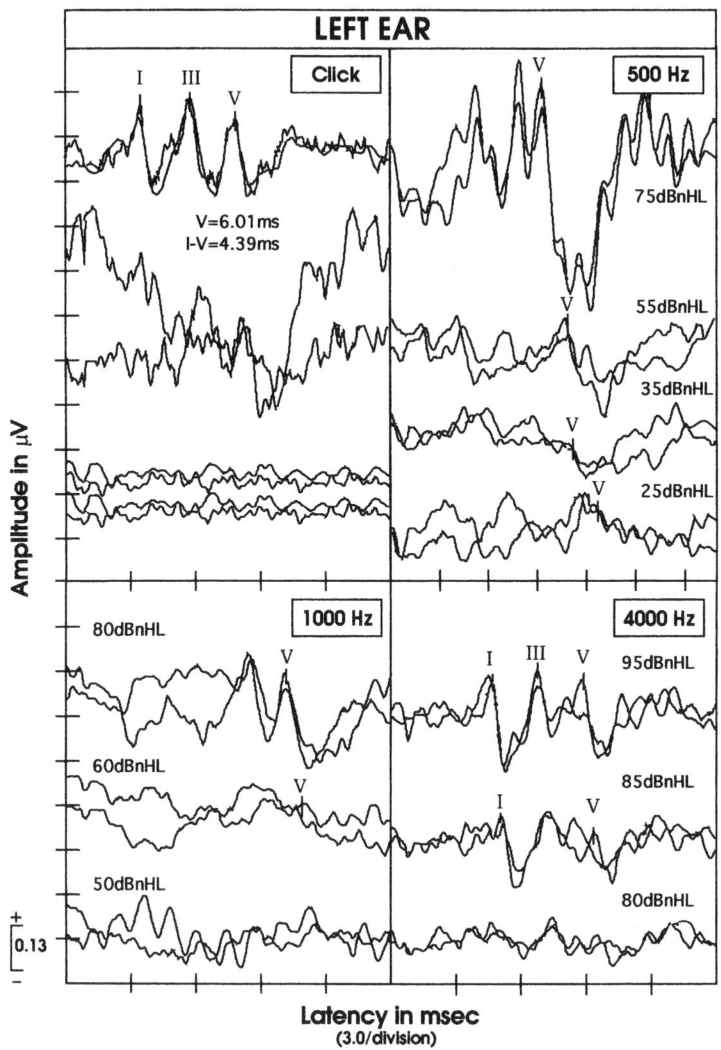

Figure 6.3. Response to left-ear click and tone-burst stimulation.

Frequency-specific ABR findings are essential for timely and appropriate audiological management of infant hearing impairment. For this case, the initial ABR was performed by audiologists in an otolaryngology clinic. However, measurement and interpretation of ABR findings in children requires expertise above and beyond that required for neurodiagnostic ABR applications in adults.

Finally, parents are typically accurate observers of their children's behaviour. Their persistent concerns about unresponsiveness to sound,

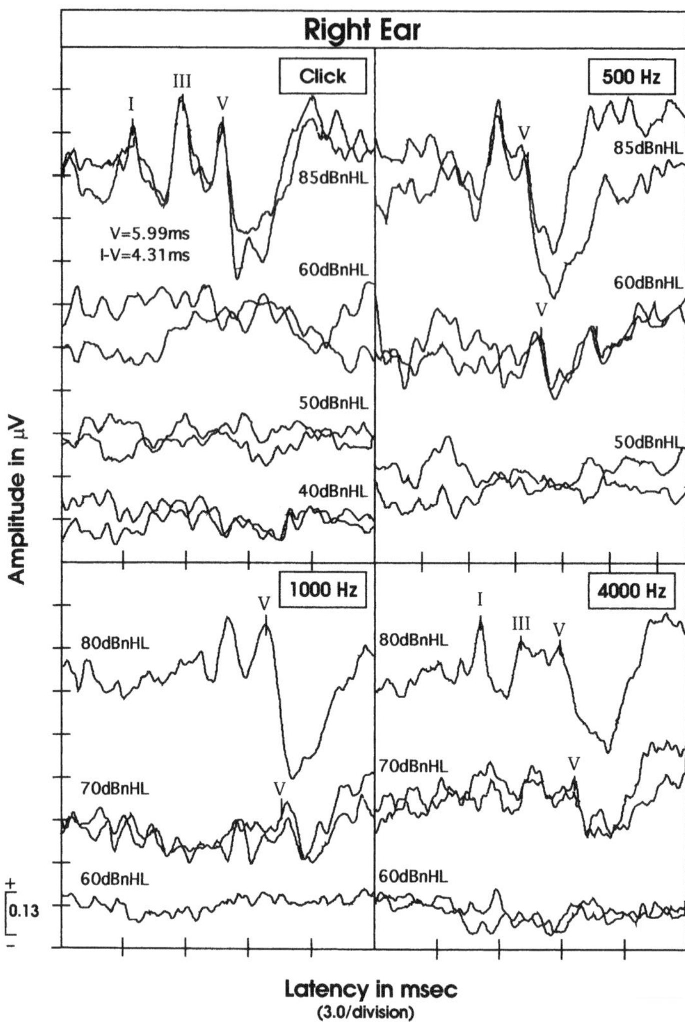

Figure 6.4. Auditory brainstem response findings for right-ear click and tone-burst stimulation.

and speech-language delay require prompt and thorough audiological assessment using the most age-appropriate test strategy likely to yield conclusive ear- and frequency-specific findings.

Cases 2 and 3: identification of auditory neuropathy

The patients were twin girls born at 29 weeks gestational age but otherwise healthy. Before discharge from the nursery, each child underwent

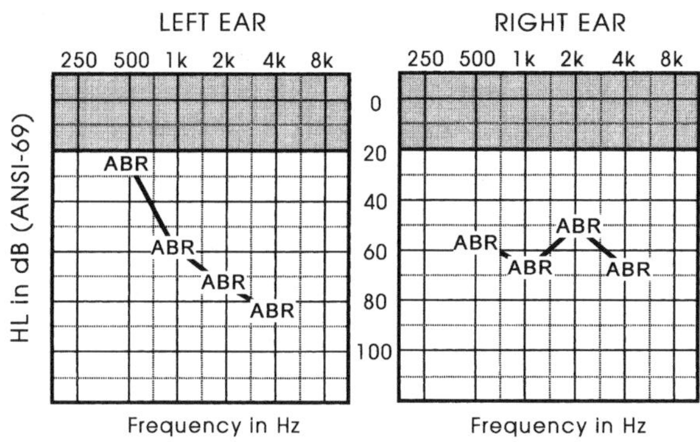

Figure 6.5. The reconstruction of an audiogram with ABR data.

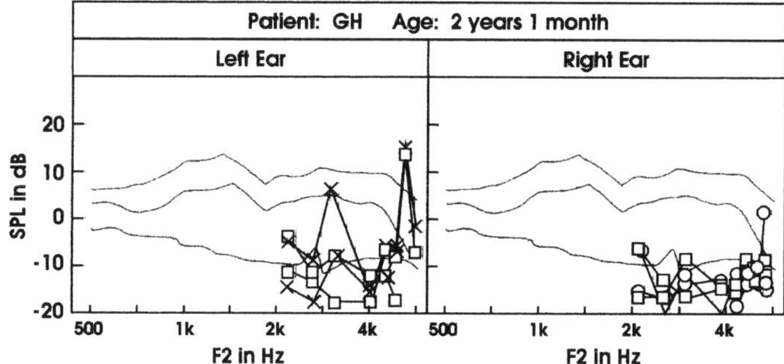

Figure 6.6. Measurement of DPOAE over a test frequency region of 2 000 to 8 000 Hz.

newborn hearing screening with automated ABR (ALGO 2 by Natus, Inc) due to the risk factor of low birth weight (<1500 g). Twin HP (Case 2) passed the hearing screening bilaterally. Twin RP (Case 3), however, yielded a refer outcome for her left ear. In compliance with clinic hearing screening programme policy, the infant (RP) failing the hearing screening unilaterally was recalled for follow-up audiometry within four months after birth. Since HP accompanied her sister to the follow-up visit, both twins underwent ABR and OAEs on that day. Follow-up ABR results for the infant passing the hearing screening bilaterally are illustrated in Figure 6.7. A well-formed ABR was reliably recorded with left- and right-ear click stimulation at intensity levels of 75 dBnHL, and down to 20 dBnHL. Interwave latency values were within an age-appropriate normative region. With the patient still sleeping naturally, DPOAE measurement was conducted over a test frequency region of 2 000 to 8 000 Hz (Figure 6.8). Distortion-product otoacoustic emission amplitudes were normal with an adequately low noise floor. The patient (HP) returned with her sister at one year for additional follow-up with behavioural audiometry. As seen in Figure 6.9, her responses to narrow-band and speech stimuli were within normal limits, although tympanometry suggested middle-ear dysfunction. In view of this finding, OAE measurement was not conducted on this test date.

Follow-up audiometric findings for twin RP were distinctly different. Auditory brainstem response assessment at three months yielded no clear wave V, even at maximum intensity level (Figure 6.10). Single polarity (rarefaction and condensation) click stimuli did, however, produce robust cochlear microphonic (CM) activity, evident within the initial portion of the waveforms as large amplitude periodic waves of opposite polarity for the two stimulus polarities. Predictably, DPOAEs were normal for this infant (Figure 6.11). In combination, the absence of an ABR wave V with obvious CM components and OAE activity offers clear evidence of cochlear integrity and neural auditory dysfunction . . . the hallmark of auditory neuropathy. Follow-up audiometric findings at one year of age for Case 3 are shown in Figure 6.12. Behavioural responses were observed with sound-field presentation. The speech awareness threshold (SAT) for Case 3 was 20 dBnHL (equivalent to her twin's SAT). The responses to narrow-band noise signals were slightly depressed relative to the normal region, and to twin HP's responses. Nonetheless, behavioural audiometry on this test date effectively ruled out the presence of serious peripheral hearing impairment. Tympanometry was consistent with middle-ear dysfunction bilaterally. Otoacoustic emission measurement, therefore, was not attempted. We did not complete ABR assessment at this date because sedation would have been required. Given the behavioural evidence of no more than a mild hearing impairment in the better-hearing ear, an ABR with sedation was not considered necessary. Findings for a previous sedated ABR assessment of twin RP at nine months, however, were identical to the initial ABR at three months (ECochG CM activity and no apparent ABR wave V). Subsequent to the four-month audiological assessment, twin girl RP was referred to a child development centre for a thorough neurological, speech-language, and developmental work-up with normal findings reported.

Comments

Auditory neuropathy in the infant population is readily apparent with the combined use of OAEs and ABRs. The classic pattern for auditory neuropathy was illustrated by Case 3 (twin RP). Most cases of auditory neuropathy demonstrate other sensory or motor deficits, or general developmental delay. Although RP was grossly normal developmentally at age one year, she will be followed closely to verify that speech-language and cognitive functioning progresses normally.

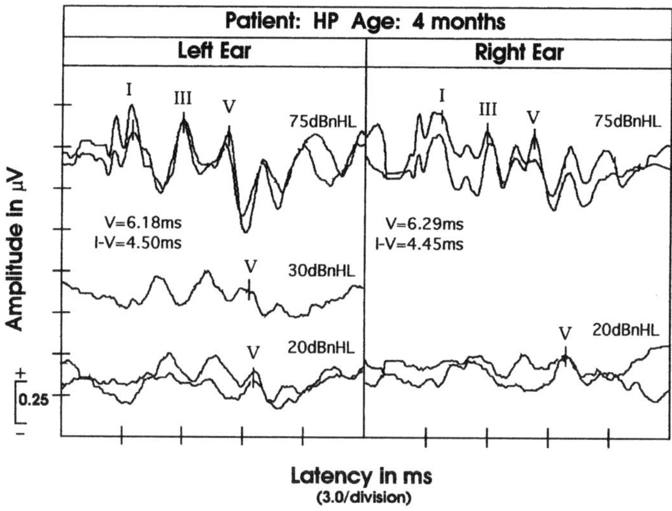

Figure 6.7. Follow-up ABR results for the infant passing the hearing screening bilaterally.

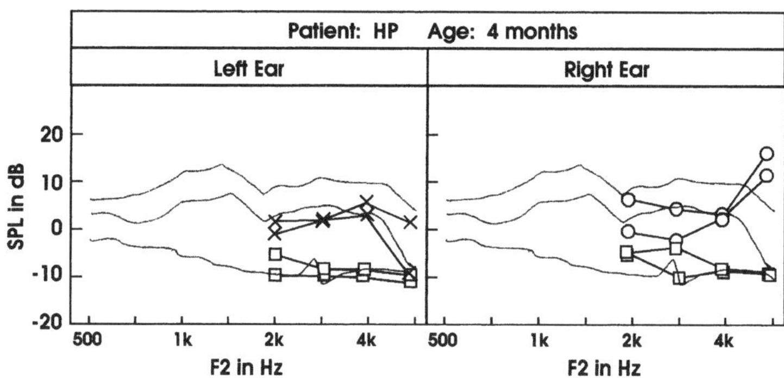

Figure 6.8. Measurement of DPOAE conducted over a test frequency region of 2 000 to 8 000 Hz.

Otoacoustic emissions applied in isolation do not contribute to the detection of auditory neuropathy. Both of these cases (2 and 3) passed the equivalent of an OAE screening. Auditory brainstem response for Case 3, however, clearly documented auditory dysfunction affecting the central nervous system.

Otoacoustic emissions are an essential component of the paediatric test battery for confirmation of sensory (versus neural) hearing impairment. Our clinical experience confirms a principle of paediatric diagnostic audiology . . . neither amplification nor cochlear implantation should be

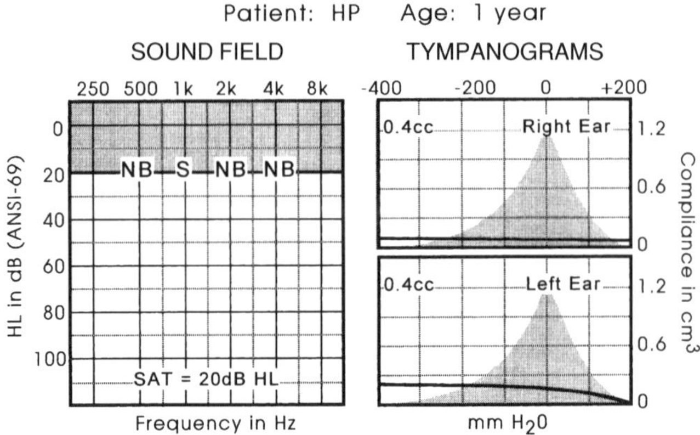

Figure 6.9. Responses to narrow-band and speech stimuli.

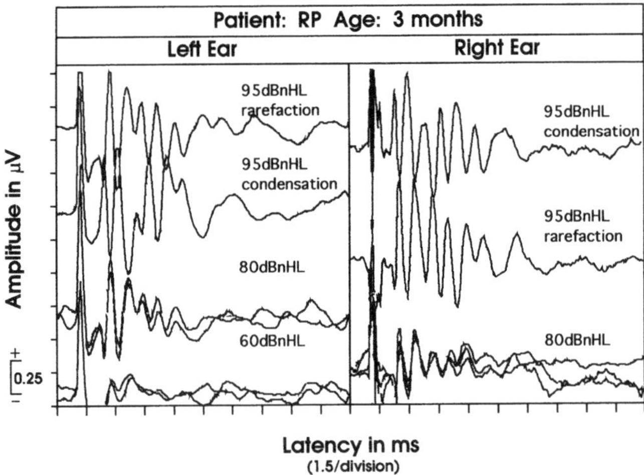

Figure 6.10. Auditory brainstem response at three months.

considered until OAE measurement is completed, and the absence of OAEs confirmed. In some patients, as illustrated by Case 3, the absence of an ABR is not associated with severe-to-profound sensorineural hearing impairment but, rather, a specific form of neural auditory dysfunction. Management with hearing aids or cochlear implants should be deferred until valid OAE findings confirm a sensory hearing impairment. For older infants who are at greater risk for middle-ear dysfunction (such as otitis media), illustrated by the twins, OAEs may play a more limited role in the differentiation of sensory versus neural auditory dysfunction. In such

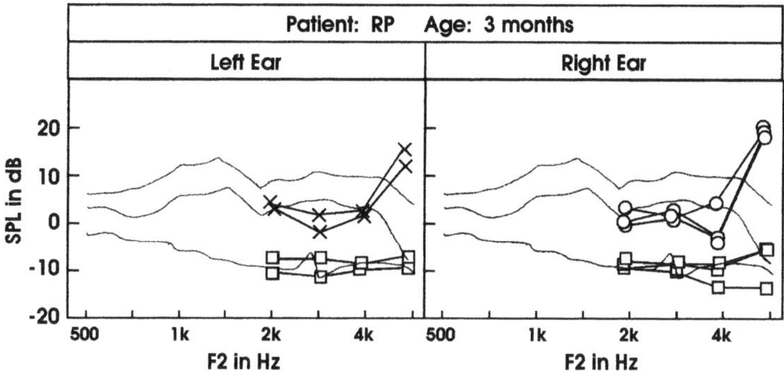

Figure 6.11. Measurements of DPOAEs for twin RP.

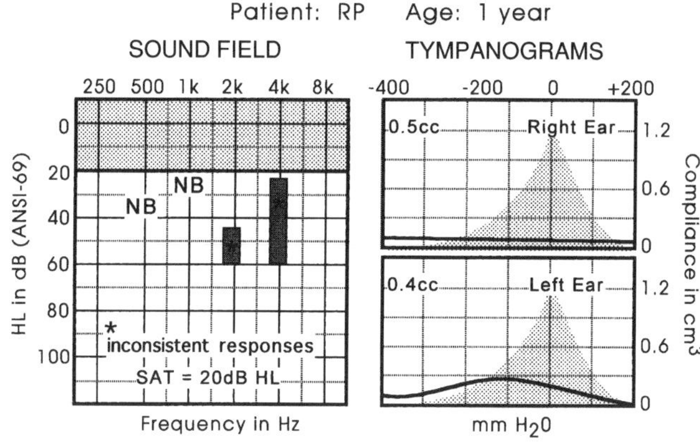

Figure 6.12. Follow-up audiometric findings at one year of age for Case 3.

cases, ECochG techniques may provide information on sensory status necessary for appropriate audiological management.

After the screening: database management, tracking, and follow up

Newborn hearing screening is of no value if the final outcome is not early identification of permanent hearing impairment in infants and young children and intervention. Hearing screening is the first step in a challenging clinical process that, for infants with hearing impairment, often continues throughout childhood. Important components of a comprehensive newborn hearing screening programme were summarized in the 1999 American Academy of Paediatrics statement. With a screening failure in the nursery, the initial follow-up visit is often a secondary screening, either in the hospital or within weeks after discharge. A diagnostic paediatric audiology assessment to confirm and define hearing impairment is scheduled after the refer outcome for the final screening. Although this assessment will be performed by audiologists, it is scheduled by or following consultation with the child's primary care physician. By definition, early intervention is initiated within four to six months after birth (see Table 6.2). Therefore, the diagnostic paediatric assessment should be conducted within two to three months after the final screening failure (or by two to three months of chronological age relative to term birth), so that intervention (including amplification) can occur within the first six months after birth. Another practical reason for scheduling the diagnostic assessment early is to avoid the need for sedation, at least for this first session.

Assessment of hearing in children

There is a substantial literature on the strategies and protocols for diagnostic paediatric assessment (see, for example, Northern and Downs, 1991; Gerber, 1996; Hall and Mueller, 1997). Age-appropriate paediatric hearing assessment techniques are summarized in Table 6.1. For some infants failing the hearing screening, diagnostic assessment will rule out a hearing impairment and the child will require no further audiological management, unless there is a risk factor for progressive or delayed-onset hearing impairment. Hearing impairment will be confirmed, however, for a proportion of infants. It is this small but significant group that requires the prompt and diligent efforts of the child's family and a team of professionals, including the audiologist, primary care physician, speech-language pathologist, and often medical specialists (otolaryngologists, geneticists, paediatric neurologist). The many critical details involved in the management of infant hearing impairment are far beyond the scope of this chapter.

Concluding comment

Universal newborn hearing screening is rapidly becoming a reality. The resulting early identification of, and intervention for, infant hearing impairment will yield unprecedented communicative, academic, cognitive and economic dividends. Effective programmes for early identification of, and intervention for, hearing impairment are highly dependent, however, on a well co-ordinated multidisciplinary strategy involving paediatricians, other medical specialists, audiologists, nurses, parents, parent-infant specialists, hospital administrators, and personnel in state departments of health and education. Professionals in all of these disciplines will be required to update their knowledge and clinical skills to meet the challenges of UNHS. Perinatologists will play a critical role in the successful implementation of UNHS and the enhanced outcome of the many thousands of hearing-impaired babies born each year.

CHAPTER 7

Screening and surveillance

JC STEVENS AND G PARKER

Introduction

In the absence of an effective hearing screen the detection of permanent childhood hearing impairment (PCHI) can be delayed by as much as two to three years. Even with screening programmes in place considerable delays can occur. This is illustrated in Figure 7.1 where the cumulative age of confirmation of PCHI from a recent major UK study is shown (Fortnum and Davis, 1997).

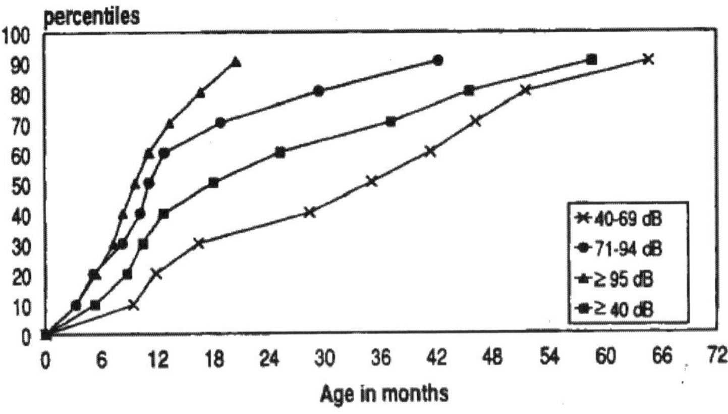

Figure 7.1. Age of confirmation of permanent hearing impairment (Fortnum and Davis, 1997).

The lack of an effective screen has also limited knowledge of the age of onset of hearing impairment in early life, as most studies to date have had to rely mainly on retrospective analysis of case studies, for example Newton (1985) and Fortnum and Davis (1997). These studies have indicated that the majority of PCHI is probably present at birth.

There is also the question of why is it important to detect PCHI at an early age. There is evidence that early diagnosis with effective management can improve the outcome for language development for those children with PCHI (Markides, 1986; Ramkalawan and Davis, 1992; Yoshinaga-Itano et al., 1998). Effective early hearing screening would therefore appear to be an essential part of any child health programme. Until recently the only universal method used in the first year of life was the infant distraction test (IDT). Its implementation is variable between countries and, as will be discussed later, its effectiveness in practice has been brought into question. More recently methods have become available for testing hearing at birth. This has led to the introduction of targeted neonatal screening of babies considered to be at high risk of hearing impairment and in some areas to universal screening at birth. However, as previously noted, not all PCHI is present at the time of a neonatal screen, and systems to detect acquired hearing impairment need to be part of an overall screening and surveillance programme.

It is also important to determine which types of hearing impairment a screening programme should aim to detect. Whereas there is agreement on the detection of PCHI of moderate or greater degree, there is less agreement on the need to detect unilateral hearing impairment, temporary hearing impairment or mild hearing impairment.

The chapter will start by considering the principles of screening. It will then consider the implications of the prevalence of different types of hearing impairment and the rationale for targeted neonatal screening. The alternative methods of universal screening in the first year of life will then be described. This will be covered in detail as this is the most important age to detect PCHI. Later screens carried out at two years and school entry will then be considered.

Principles of screening

Ten principles of screening were laid out by Wilson and Jungner (1968). These have been considered by Haggard and Hughes (1991) in a review of screening children's hearing and more recently by Davis et al. in the critical review of the role of neonatal hearing screening in the detection of congenital hearing impairment (Davis et al., 1997).

Haggard suggested four further principles that were also included in the review by Davis et al. In summary these principles, adapted for hearing impairment in a similar manner to that by Davis et al. (1997), can be stated as:

1. The condition (hearing impairment) should be an important health problem.

2. There should be an accepted treatment – i.e. an acceptable means of habilitation for those identified by the screen.
3. Facilities for assessment, diagnosis and treatment should be available.
4. The hearing impairment should be recognizable at an early stage.
5. There should be a suitable test for use as the screen.
6. The test should be acceptable to the parents and to the child.
7. The natural history of the condition should be known and understood.
8. There should be an agreed policy on whom to treat.
9. The cost of case finding (including all consequential costs of the screening programme) should not be disproportionate to overall healthcare costs of care for the hearing-impaired child.
10. Case finding should be seen as a continuous process.
11. The incidental harm should be small compared to the overall benefits.
12. There should be guidelines on how to explain results to parents with appropriate support.
13. All hearing screening arrangements should be reviewed in the light of changes in demography, epidemiology and other factors.
14. Costs and effectiveness of hearing screening should be examined on a case-type basis to maximize the effectiveness and benefit for each type before considering overall costs, effectiveness and benefit.

Current knowledge of principles 1, 2, and 7 is presented elsewhere in this book. In summary, hearing impairment is an important health problem as it can affect the quality of life in several ways. Language development and the ability to communicate are affected with subsequent effects on educational achievement, social development and employment prospects. Condition 2 is satisfied for bilateral PCHI of moderate or greater level as there is an effective treatment in terms of amplification by using a hearing aid or the use of cochlear implantation in some cases of profound hearing impairment. For unilateral PCHI, mild PCHI and temporary hearing impairment, there is less evidence of the effectiveness of treatment and there is a range of views on whether a screen should aim to detect these cases. Evidence so far published indicates that the majority of PCHI is present at birth. Under condition 7, knowledge of the age of onset of hearing impairment is one of the most important factors when selecting which screen to implement. As more neonatal screening programmes are implemented, knowledge, not only of the age of onset, but also the rate of progression of hearing impairment, will improve.

Principles 3, 8, 10, 12 and 13 relate to the quality of implementation, which is outside the scope of this chapter. Clearly good implementation of these principles is needed if any screen is to be successful. The chapter will therefore focus on principles 4, 5, and 6, which relate to the test method, and principles 9, 11 and 14, which relate to cost, effectiveness and benefit.

Prevalence of hearing impairment

The prevalence of hearing impairment is discussed at length in Chapter 4. A prevalence of 1–2 per 1 000 is generally reported in European studies, depending on population selection, definitions and methodology (Martin, 1982; Parving, 1983). Using results drawn from the Trent Ascertainment Study (Fortnum and Davis, 1997) the overall prevalence for permanent bilateral childhood hearing impairment ≥ 40 dB HL was estimated to be 1.33 per 1000 live births (1 in 750 children), with equivalent figures of 1.10 per 1000 (1 in 900) for hearing impairment >50 dBHL, 0.59 per 1000 (1 in 1700) for hearing impairment >70 dB HL and 0.31 per 1 000 (1 in 3 200) for hearing impairment >95 dB HL. The prevalence of bilateral PCHI ≥ 40 dBnHL that is present at the time of a neonatal screen is reported as 1.12 per 1 000 by Fortnum and Davis (1997).

Davis et al. (1997), in reviewing the current literature, reported yields of 1–1.5/1 000 from universal neonatal hearing screening (UNHS). This is consistent with a high proportion of PCHI being present at the time of the UNHS. Lutman et al. (1997) and Mason et al. (1998) also reported only a small number of cases with documented evidence of late-onset progressive hearing loss in ascertainment studies of field sensitivity following targeted neonatal screening. However, a longitudinal study of an 'at risk' group by Stevens and Webb (1997), where all babies had both neonatal and follow-up tests, reported a much higher proportion of acquired PCHI.

Figure 7.2 (p. 150) compares the prevalence of PCHI with that of other conditions for which screening programmes are currently available or under consideration.

Rationale for targeted screening

The development of techniques for testing newborns, in conjunction with the awareness of an increased risk of hearing impairment in graduates from neonatal intensive care units, first led some centres to introduce screening of these babies (Alberti et al., 1983; Galambos, Hicks and Wilson, 1984). Davis and Wood (1992) provided epidemiological evidence that has further led to the concept of key factors for permanent hearing impairment, which might be suitable for defining an 'at risk' population. Assuming that such a population can be readily identified, this then allows the screening of a targeted group, which is likely to provide a high yield of cases.

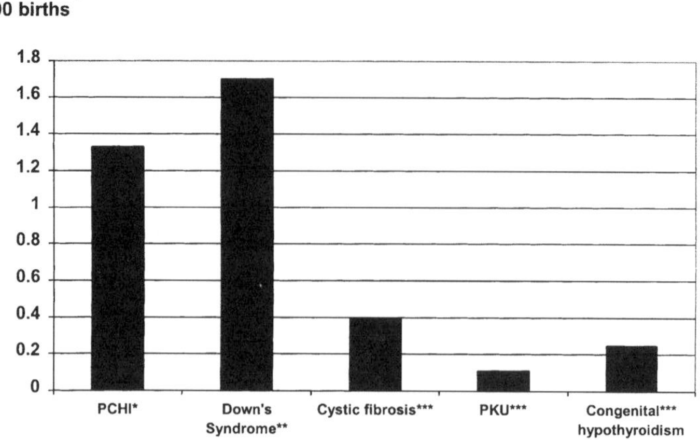

Figure 7.2. Graph to show relative prevalences of PCHI; Down's Syndrome; cystic fibrosis; PKU; primary persistent congenital hypothyroidism. * Davis et al., 1997; ** Howe et al., 2000; *** Pollitt et al., 1997.

Davis and Wood (1992) collected data on 89 children, born between 1983–86, attending the Children's Hearing Assessment Centre, Nottingham, UK and fitted with a hearing aid. One of their most significant findings was that babies, who were admitted to a neonatal intensive care unit (NICU) for more than 48 hours, were 10.2 (95% CI 4.4–23.7) times more likely to have a permanent hearing impairment >50 dB HL than those who did not undergo intensive care, assuming no other predisposing factors.

In fact, three key risk factors were described:

- a history of admission to NICU >48 hours;
- a family history of early childhood deafness;
- a syndrome associated with hearing impairment, for example, a craniofacial anomaly such as cleft palate.

It was estimated that 50% of all children with bilateral hearing impairment >50 dB HL had one or more of these three factors. This was further explored in the more extensive Trent Ascertainment Study (Fortnum and Davis, 1997). Retrospective information on relevant key risk factors was analysed for 653 children born between 1985 and 1993, resident in the Trent Health Authority, with PCHI ≥ 40 dB HL. Of those designated as having congenital impairment, 29% (95% CI 25–33%) had a history of NICU/SCBU admission >48 hours, 31% (95% CI 26–35%) had a positive family history and 12% (95% CI 9–15%) had a craniofacial anomaly. Overall, 59% of the children had one or more of these risk factors. Other factors of lesser significance included ethnicity, with Asian children having an increased risk of 2.5 relative to the non-Asian population and socio-economic group, with an increased risk in those designated as coming from 'struggling' households. There were no statistically significant differences in the distribution for different severities of hearing impairment. Sutton and Rowe (1997) reported broadly similar risk factors in a population of children with sensorineural hearing impairment, but in addition highlighted maternal age over 35 years to be significant.

The feasibility of targeting the 'at risk' group for hearing screening, however, also depends on the ease of identification of each factor. Although admission to NICU and the presence of a craniofacial anomaly can be readily highlighted for inclusion in a screening programme, accurate identification of babies with a relevant family history is likely to prove more difficult (Wood, Farnsworth and Davis, 1995).

From the figures in the Trent Ascertainment Study, Fortnum and Davis (1997) estimated that, in practice, the yield from a targeted screen using the three factors noted above would be 50% or less. The cost of such a programme would depend, in part, on the proportion of the population fulfilling the screen selection criteria. Davis and Wood (1992) found that 5.9% of all births in the Nottingham Health District were admitted to NICU >48 hours, although the percentage may be as high as 12% in other districts. A further study (Wood et al., 1995) estimated a positive family history of childhood deafness in 4.5% of the birth cohort. The large-scale Wessex UNHS study (1998) reported that, of over 25 000 neonates screened, 8.1% (5.1% from the post-natal wards and 3.0% from the special care units) fulfilled high-risk criteria for PCHI.

The implementation of targeted screening programmes in practice is discussed later in this chapter.

Screening in the first year of life

Potential methods and opportunities

In order to produce a satisfactory method of screening the test must be acceptable, non-invasive, reliable, be simple and quick to perform and have a high sensitivity and specificity (relating to principles 5, 6, 11 and 14). There are many physiological responses to sound that might be used for a hearing screen in the first year of life. They originate at different levels of the auditory pathway, from responses of the cochlea up to responses involving the central nervous system. It is important to note that all of these tests check the function of only part of the auditory pathway. None are actually a complete test of hearing. However, as most pathology of the auditory pathway occurs at the cochlear level, it is possible to use most of these physiological responses as potential methods for screening.

Any screening method must determine that there is sufficient hearing present for the child to learn normal language. This means that responses should be obtained to quiet levels of sound (around 40 dBnHL or below) or it must be shown that the test can demonstrate that hearing is present at this level. Many of the physiological responses only occur at high sound levels and so are not useful as a screen (such as heart rate and respiration rate changes). Those that have proved able to meet the above criteria at some point in the first year of life can be grouped under:

- otoacoustic emissions from the cochlea;
- electrical responses of the early auditory pathway;
- behavioural responses.

The actual use of these methods in practice depends on such practicalities as the baby being in a suitable state for the screen to be carried out efficiently and effectively. The first two methods require that the baby is quiet and still. The best opportunity for this is in the first 2–3 months of life, which has the added benefit of the earlier detection of PCHI. Of the electrical responses from the early part of the auditory pathway, the click-evoked auditory brainstem response has proved to be the most effective for use as a screen to date. With the need to carry out follow-up tests, the screen needs to be done soon after birth and at the latest by about four weeks of age.

Behavioural responses can be used at birth but the levels of sound required to elicit them are high and it is not until around eight months of age that responses can be readily obtained to the required low levels of sound. At birth, reflex movement of head and body have generally been used with the baby supine, whereas at eight months the reflex turning of the head towards a sound source is used (the infant distraction test (IDT)).

In summary, the practical screening options in the first year of life are otoacoustic emissions or the ABR soon after birth (or a combination of the two) and the infant distraction test at eight months of age. Behavioural responses soon after birth are a further possible method but a high stimulus level has to be used. Each method will now be considered in detail.

Neonatal screening

The last 15 years have seen many studies carried out on the use of these methods (for example, otoacoustic emissions: White et al., 1994; Watkin, 1996; Lutman et al., 1997; Stevens and Webb, 1997; Wessex UNHS trial, 1998; auditory brainstem response: Hyde et al., 1991; Stevens et al., 1991; Galambos, Wilson and Silva, 1994; Hall, 1996; Mason et al., 1997; Stevens and Webb, 1997; auditory response cradle: Davis et al., 1991; Tucker and Bhattacharya, 1992). It is difficult to carry out studies due to the low incidence of PCHI and the need to follow-up large numbers of children. A review of these studies has been compiled by Davis et al. (1997) and the reader is referred to this document for more detail.

Otoacoustic emissions

In 1978 Kemp recorded the presence of acoustic energy emitted from the ear in response to sound (Kemp, 1978). Studies have shown (Kemp, 1998) that these emissions originate in the cochlea and relate to some biomechanical process associated with normal hearing. The important property for screening is that otoacoustic emissions can only be recorded when a region of normal cochlear function is present. All types of otoacoustic emission are recorded by the placement of a probe into the ear canal. The probe contains one or more miniature loudspeakers to generate the stimulus and a microphone to record the sound in the ear canal.

Classification

Otoacoustic emissions are normally classified by the method of recording. The transient evoked otoacoustic emission (TEOAE) is the response to a short transient of sound. A typical stimulus and response in a baby is shown in Figure 7.3(a). The response is also commonly viewed in the frequency domain as shown in Figure 7.3(b). The response is small compared to the acoustic stimulus presented to the ear and has a sound level around the threshold of hearing.

Recording method for TEOAE

As the response is below the background noise levels a technique known as averaging is used to detect it. This is achieved by adding many hundreds of responses together. The response is also filtered to remove unwanted low- and high-frequency components. To minimize the chance of the response being an artefact (for example, a mechanical echo of the

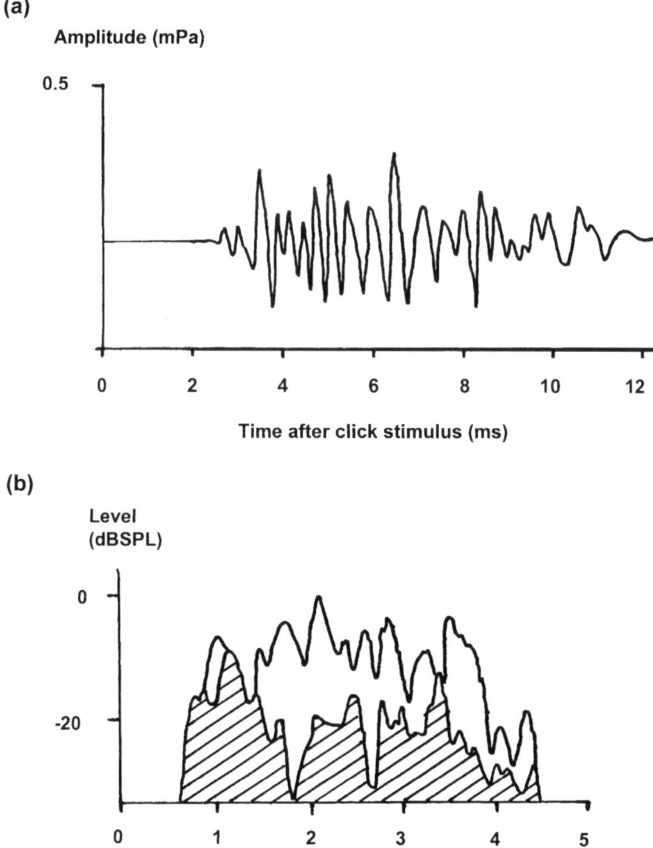

Figure 7.3. Typical neonatal TEOAE response displayed in (a) the time domain and (b) the frequency domain. The response shown is the non-linear component between 2.5 and 12.5ms post stimulus. In (b) the shaded area is the noise component.

stimulus) it is normal to only consider the part of the response that is not proportional to the stimulus (the non-linear component). High continuous background noise levels (for example, an incubator fan, air conditioning, or a computer cooling fan) will prolong the test time or can make it impossible for the test to be carried out. A test room with noise levels below 35 dBA SPL should be used.

Properties of TEOAE and screen pass criteria

The TEOAE is unique to the individual ear although the recording is dependent on the probe characteristics. There is a large variation in both amplitude and waveform between individuals. As noted, the presence of a TEOAE indicates a region of normal cochlear function. Its absence could be for one of many reasons, poor recording conditions, too small an amplitude to record, the presence of outer-ear or middle-ear disease. The frequency spectrum of a typical neonatal TEOAE was shown in Figure 7.3(b). This frequency range can vary between babies with normally hearing ears, some will only give a narrow range of emission frequencies whilst others will produce a broad range. These factors lead to the following typical choice for a pass criteria when using TEOAE as a neonatal screen.

- The presence of a response in a limited number of frequency bands, for example in two half-octave bands from half-octave bands with centre frequencies at 1.5, 2, 3 and 4 kHz.
- A high response to background noise ratio, for example, the response is 6 dB or more above the background level.
- The amplitude is in the physiological range.
- There is a low chance of artefact from the stimulus.

Transient evoked otoacoustic emissions recorded in babies are generally larger and contain higher frequencies than those recorded in adults. In adults studies indicate that the region 1–2 kHz is the most important for the presence of an OAE.

Otoacoustic emissions are not normally present when the hearing impairment is greater than about 30 dB HL (Bonfils and Uziel, 1989).

The distortion product otoacoustic emission (DPOAE) is the other type that has found application in screening. The stimulus consists of two tones at different frequencies. Sounds at other frequencies (called distortion products) at very low sound levels can be recorded. There is a wealth of evidence (Kemp, 1998) that these sounds reflect the properties of a non-linear process associated with outer hair-cell motility. For clinical measurements the distortion product $2f_1$-f_2 is normally recorded at a number of frequency pairs f_1, f_2. The correlation between audiometric threshold and DPOAE amplitude is weak and it is not possible to use the DPOAE amplitude to predict hearing threshold with any accuracy except to say that it is inside or outside normal limits (Kemp, 1998).

Auditory brainstem response (ABR)

Choice of ABR

It is possible in adults to record electrical responses from the auditory pathway from the cochlea to the cortex. In babies, at low stimulus levels used for screening, the cortical responses are difficult to record and the early potentials have therefore been used. The non-invasive requirement restricts measurement to potentials that can be recorded on the skin surface. The result is that the auditory brainstem response has become the method of choice in babies. The ABR records the electrical activity occurring in the first 10–12 ms after the stimulus. The so-called 'wave V', which is recorded at around 8 ms to click stimuli in neonates, is the most prominent wave at low sound levels. A typical neonatal ABR response is shown in Figure 7.4. The wave III and V complex (Figure 7.4) is normally used together with the later slow wave (SN10) to determine whether a response is present.

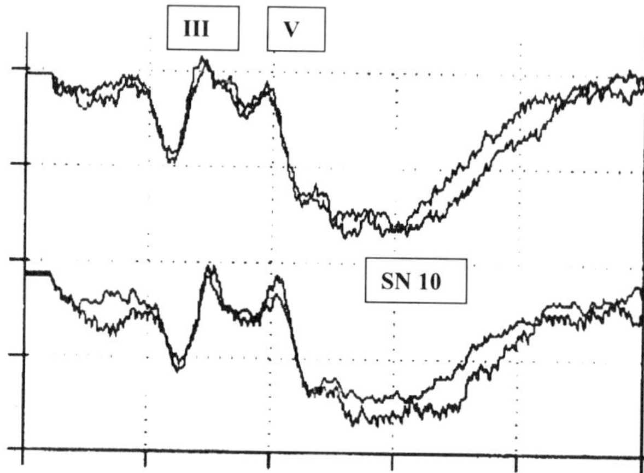

Figure 7.4. Typical ABR waveforms at 50dBnHL (top) and 40dBnHL (bottom) stimulus levels from neonatal screening, showing waves III, V and SN10. The small divisions on the axes are 0.25 μV (vertical) and 4ms (horizontal).

Choice of stimulus and limitations of ABR for screening

For screening, a click stimulus is normally used as it gives the maximum response amplitude. However, it stimulates the whole of the cochlea. This limits the test as it only possible to infer from the result that there is a region of normal hearing. The relationship between the click ABR threshold and pure-tone threshold in adults with different degrees of hearing impairment is shown in Figure 7.5 (Stapells and Oates, 1997). The click ABR is also therefore only a limited measure of hearing. However, as with OAE it is sufficient to detect the majority of clinically significant hearing impairments.

Absence of a response can be due to several factors apart from a raised hearing threshold. Poor recording conditions may affect the detection of the response and any factor that affects the nature and amplitude of the ABR response (such as delayed maturation) should be taken into account.

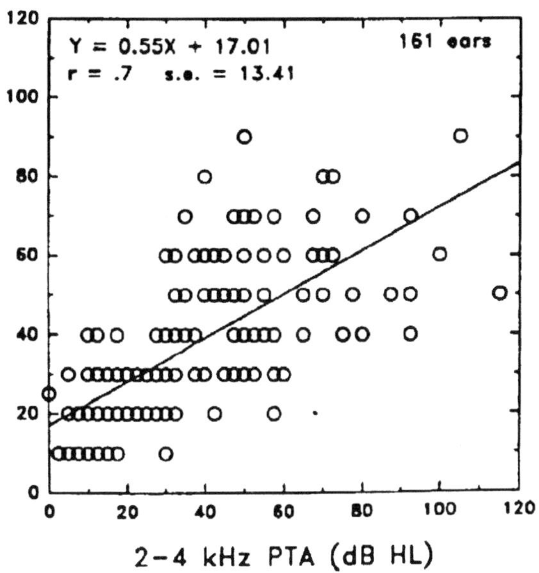

Figure 7.5. Relationship between the click ABR threshold (vertical axis dBnHL) and pure-tone threshold in adults (161 ears with sensorineural hearing impairment) (Stapells and Oats, 1997).

Recording method

The ABR response is less than one microvolt in amplitude. Like the otoacoustic emission the averaging of many responses is required to detect the response above the background electroencephalogram. A good electrical and acoustic environment is required. Protocols for good practice should be followed (for example, Stevens et al., 1999) to avoid errors being made. As with TEOAE, pass criteria should include the conditions of a recognizable physiological response, high repeatability and the absence of artefact.

An electrical response from the post-auricular muscle (PAM) can also be recorded around 15 ms after the stimulus. The response is very dependent on muscle state and is not always present. However, if the response is present, it can be used in place or in addition to the ABR response in screening. On occasions, when a baby is too restless for an ABR to be recorded, it may be possible to obtain a PAM response.

Automated OAE and ABR for screening

Due the fact that a waveform is recorded for both OAE and ABR, it is possible to include in the equipment a mathematical algorithm that can be used to give a measure of the confidence of the presence of a response. As well as determining a measure of the confidence in the response, the algorithms can also check for potential artefacts and that the response is within the physiological range. Several examples have been incorporated into clinical instruments. Their efficacy has been demonstrated in a number of trials (Mason et al., 1998; Brass et al., 1994) and it is likely that their use in screening will increase.

There is variation amongst the automated equipment being currently manufactured as to whether the complete ABR/OAE response is stored or not. One of the advantages of both ABR and OAE over the infant distraction test (IDT) for screening is that a record of the response is available and can be reviewed at a later stage. If screening equipment does not record the full response this advantage will then be lost.

Head and body movement

The third method that has been tried in practice involves the measurement of chest wall movement, head movement and general body movement to sound. The Cribogram (Simmons, 1974) and the auditory response cradle (ARC) (Bennett, 1975) were two attempts to use this method. Both require the use of high sound levels to evoke responses. Evaluation studies for the ARC have been reported by Tucker and Bhattacharya (1992) and by McCormick, Curnock and Spavins (1984).

Neonatal screening protocols

As will be discussed later, Universal Neonatal Hearing Screening has been recommended in consensus statements in the US and Europe (NIH, 1993; EEC, 1998). The statements also recommend using a hospital-based system as it offers a unique accessibility to a high proportion of babies with the potential to achieve a high coverage. This is the model that will be described here. However, in communities where the majority of babies are not born in large maternity units a different model may be more appropriate.

Universal neonatal hearing screening (UNHS)

Transient evoked otoacoustic emissions, DPOAE and AABR are all being used for UNHS. The TEOAE or DPOAE methods do not require the use of electrodes resulting in lower disposable costs and a less invasive procedure. However, the pass rate for OAE methods is reduced in the period up to 24 hours following birth. The NIH document recommends that a two-stage process be adopted with TEOAE being used on all babies and ABR (or AABR) being used on those babies who do not pass OAE to increase the specificity. The document also notes that some centres are using ABR screening alone and encourages sites to continue these programmes. There are also centres that have successfully used TEOAE only, achieving a high screening programme specificity by re-testing those babies not passing in hospital in a screening clinic at around four weeks of age. A typical hospital-based screening model is shown in Figure 7.6.

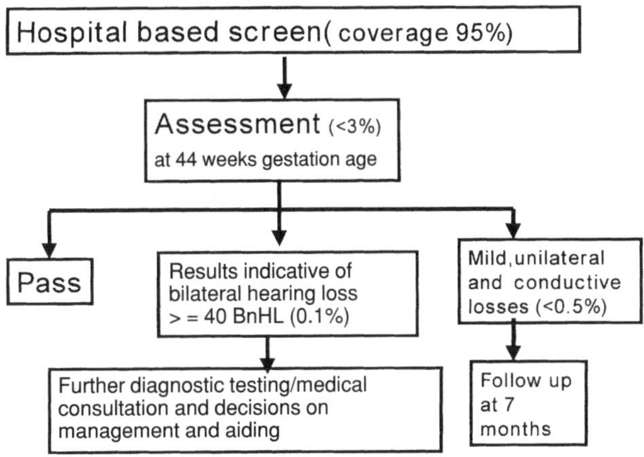

Figure 7.6. Outline of a typical hospital based UNHS screening programme.

Method for NICU

A separate protocol is also adopted in many centres for the testing of babies admitted to NICU. There is some evidence that a small proportion of NICU babies with PCHI will pass OAE, although they would fail an ABR screen (Parker et al., 1999). Babies developing hyperbilirubinaemia requiring exchange transfusion are particularly at risk. Rance et al. (1999) have also reported a series of babies with the similar anomalous combination of raised ABR thresholds in conjunction with recordable OAEs. The pathology is assumed to be 'central' (proximal to the cochlea) and categorized as 'auditory neuropathy'. Audiological outcome in such cases has been found to be variable (Parker et al., 1999; Wood et al., 1998) and presents a dilemma with regard to aiding decisions. Many programmes have therefore adopted the practice of carrying out ABR on all long stay NICU babies.

Targeted neonatal hearing screening

A protocol for a targeted neonatal hearing screen (TNS) requires the implementation of a well-controlled questionnaire. Typically midwives will be asked to check for family history and refer cases to the programme. Medical staff will be asked to refer on any baby that fits the high-risk criteria. In some centres a simple criteria of >48 hours in NICU is used for this risk group. Targeted neonatal hearing screening involves much smaller numbers than universal screening. Given the preferred use of ABR in long stay NICU babies and the higher specificity of ABR in the NICU group, most TNS programmes use ABR on all babies.

Follow-up of neonatal hearing screening

Assessment of hearing following failure to pass a neonatal screen involves a range of tests. The click ABR test is extended to include the use of tone pip stimulation to give more frequency-specific thresholds (Stapells and Oates, 1997). An alternative method using modulated test tones is currently being evaluated (Lins et al., 1995; Rickards et al., 1994). The conductive component of any hearing loss can be estimated by using bone conduction ABR (Webb, 1993; Yang, 1993). This may be supported by the use of the ABR latency-stimulus intensity function and high-frequency tympanometry. Otoacoustic emission testing is important on all babies who fail the ABR screen to check for auditory neuropathy. Information may also be obtained from behavioural observation and parental observation.

Screening at eight months using the infant distraction test

Ewing and Ewing (1944) first described the infant distraction test (IDT) – a behavioural test, suitable for use in babies over six months up to a developmental age of around two years. Its introduction as a universal screen varies from country to country. By the 1960s, this test had been adopted throughout most of the UK as a universal hearing screen, usually performed by health visitors around six to nine months – the so-called 'health visitor distraction test' (HVDT). It was also adopted in many other European countries but has not been introduced, for example, in the US. The methodology is described in Chapter 5.

Unfortunately, almost as soon as the HVDT was introduced, concerns began to emerge regarding its effectiveness at detecting PCHI (Boothman and Orr, 1978). Inaccuracy of the test became the prime suspect when it was realized that less than 50% of children with bilateral PCHI >50 dB HL were being diagnosed by the age of three years (Martin, 1982). It emerged that only 10% to 20% of cases with apparently congenital hearing impairment were generally being identified by the screen (McCormick, 1983). In fact, age at diagnosis was not dissimilar to that in the US, where no screen equivalent to the HVDT was employed (NIH, 1993). It was felt that the screen might even have delayed diagnosis in some cases due to false reassurance.

During the 1980s efforts were made to improve the performance of the HVDT in the UK, by use of calibrated warblers and emphasis on training, particularly headed by McCormick (1983) in Nottingham. An improved sensitivity of 86% was subsequently reported in this area (McCormick, 1990), but Wood, Davis and McCormick (1997) also provide evidence of the difficulty of maintaining this quality of service over the time span of a decade. Fonseca et al. (1999) surveyed the routes of identification for 104 children with congenital PCHI in nine UK centres. Although the HVDT correctly identified 23 cases, a further 20 remained undetected. It was concluded that unreliability of the HVDT was a significant factor in failure of the service to meet NDCS (1994) targets for early identification. Data from the more extensive Trent Ascertainment Study (Fortnum and Davis, 1997) indicated an overall test sensitivity of only 65% (PCHI ≥ 40 dB HL), ranging from 54% for moderate to 80% for profound impairments.

Davis et al. (1997) provides a comprehensive review of the performance of the HVDT, as practised in the UK, in terms of its ability to screen for PCHI. The following key points are summarized as follows:

- Coverage is estimated to be in the range of 80% to 95%, but may fall to around 60% in urban areas, and may be particularly low in Asian populations.
- A wide range of sensitivities are reported (18% to 88%), being generally higher for severe/profound impairment and affected by training, socioeconomic and ethnic factors in the population screened.
- The relatively high referral rate, generally around 5% to 10%, has resource implications.
- The incremental yield for the HVDT was found to be at best 40% when acting as the primary screen, but fell to around 25% when used in combination with a well-run targeted neonatal screen.
- Median age of identification via the HVDT was estimated as 12 to 20 months for PCHI ≥ 40 dB HL, but is likely to be lower for the more severe impairments.
- In summary, for a typical district of 4 000 births per year, one would expect four or five cases of PCHI ≥ 40 dB HL of which one or two might be identified by the HVDT, despite generating 160 to 280 referrals.

One of the reasons for the poor specificity of the HVDT is likely to be the relatively high incidence of fluctuating hearing loss due to OME in the population at the time of screening (Haggard and Hughes, 1991).

Although there is evidence of the impact of persisting OME on language development and behaviour in older children (Chalmers et al., 1989; Bennett and Haggard, 1999) it is hard to justify a single screen in the first year of life for the identification of such a fluctuant condition. Moreover the benefits of intervention, especially in such a young age group have not yet been established (Haggard and Hughes, 1991; Maw, 1995).

Efforts to improve the performance of the HVDT include the use of more automated methods and, in order to improve the specificity of the HVDT, a higher pass level. Although universal neonatal screening is likely to become the universal pre-school screen, it has been stressed (McCormick, 2000) that it is important to maintain quality and confidence in the HVDT in those areas where it remains the primary screen (McCormick, 2000).

Surveillance methods

A survey of current practice in the UK indicated that health visitor surveillance (HVS) played a role in identification of PCHI in around two-thirds of districts (Davis et al., 1997). This may be in the form of unstructured enquiry or using a parental questionnaire, most often based on the 'Hints for Parents' sheet (McCormick, 1983). Action is based on parental or professional concern. Health visitor surveillance is often used in conjunction with not only other hearing screens, but also assessments of language development. Some indication of performance was provided by the Health Technology Assessment survey of practice (Davis et al., 1997), which estimated a referral rate of around 10% and a yield for bilateral PCHI of around 4 per 10 000 children for HVS, although information on age of detection was limited.

Dissatisfaction with the HVDT, has led to some districts abandoning this form of screen completely. In 1989, the HVDT screen in West Berkshire in the UK was replaced by a vigilance programme, incorporating a questionnaire completed by the health visitor (HVQ) in conjunction with parents when the baby reaches eight months (Sutton and Scanlon, 1999). The performance of the HVDT and the HVQ for babies born since 1984, was audited and compared. The overall sensitivity of the HVQ for detection of PCHI (>50 dB HL), was similar to that of the HVDT (39%, compared with 42%). The HVDT was found to be slightly more effective for moderate degrees of impairment. The coverage for the HVQ was estimated at 87% and the referral rate from the screen to be 3%. It was concluded that the vigilance programme performed as well, but no better than the HVDT in terms of detecting significant hearing impairment. Although the cost of the HVQ was less, there was little justification for changing from one poor screen to another.

Cost and effectiveness of screens in the first year of life

This chapter has so far focused on the methodology of each of the screening options in the first year of life and how they relate to screening principles 4, 5 and 6. Screening principles 9, 11 and 14 will now be considered. These relate to the cost, effectiveness and benefit of the screening programme.

In deciding which policy to adopt in the first year of life the cost, effect and benefit (or disbenefit) of each option of screening policy would ideally be known. The costs should include health service costs, costs to the family and costs to society.

Costs

The cost of UNHS in the UK to the health service has been reported at around £14 per infant screened (at 1994 prices, Stevens et al., 1998) or around £17 at year 2000 prices. This figure represented the cost difference between no screen and UNHS, including the follow up of false positives. Davis (1997) compares this UK figure to those from programmes in the US, noting that it falls in the middle of the range. In the same survey (Stevens et al., 1998), the cost of universal IDT was reported as £24.50 at 1994 prices. This figure is currently being revised to take into account slightly lower overheads giving a figure at 2000 prices of around £27.

Effectiveness of screens

The effect of UNHS can be measured in terms of yield. The yield of any screen is affected by the coverage and the sensitivity of the screen. Studies on the performance of UNHS have necessarily been limited due to the size of the study required (typically 1 000 babies required per case identified). The majority of studies have therefore been carried out on an at risk (AR) population. Obtaining follow-up data has also proved difficult, and very few studies have complete follow-up data as a result. Davis et al. (1997) summarized the results from such studies. The Wessex trial (Wessex, 1998) represents the only randomized controlled trial amongst these studies. The protocol used TEOAE followed by AABR. The yield for PCHI for the neonatal screen was 1.2/1 000 (confidence intervals 0.8–1.7) which is close to the expected prevalence of 1.12/1 000 (Davis et al., 1997). Davis also reports the other large source of data on UNHS in the UK where the yield was 1.5–2/1 000 (Watkin, 1996). Results from the US (for example, White and Vohr, 1994) generally give higher yields but often include cases of milder hearing impairment. Results from 'at risk' studies (for example, Lutman et al., 1997; Mason et al., 1998) suggest that the field sensitivity of both the OAE and ABR should be high, although there is evidence of a significant number of cases of acquired hearing impairment as noted earlier (for example, Stevens et al., 1997). Davis et al. (1997), reviewing the available data, suggests a value nearer to 80% for the expected programme sensitivity when using OAE, ABR or a combination of the two.

The results of evaluation studies on the auditory response cradle have been variable. Tucker and Bhattacharya (1992) reported considerable success with the ARC detecting 18 babies with a permanent hearing impairment out of 6 000 tested. However, McCormick et al. (1984) found less encouraging results in an NICU population. The incremental yield of the IDT in the UK was discussed earlier with a best figure of around 40%, falling to around 25% in the presence of a well-run targeted neonatal screen. These figures are much lower than those for UNHS using TEOAE or ABR.

Cost per case

In calculating the true cost effectiveness of a screen the true effect (marginal yield) is the difference between the yield that would exist with a screen in place and that with no screen in place. In the first year of life the yield with no screen in place might be expected to be around 20% using data from the ascertainment study by Fortnum and Davis (1997). For UNHS the marginal yield might therefore be expected to be around 60%, allowing 20% for the no-screen yield. Using a figure of 1.12/1 000 for the prevalence at the time of UNHS and a cost per infant of £17 gives a cost per case of £25 000 at year 2000 prices. However, one of the benefits of UNHS is the earlier detection of hearing impairment and it can be argued that the background yield should be based not on the first year of life but on that which occurs in the first few months of life. This would give a marginal yield closer to 80% and a cost per case of around £20 000. This may seem a large figure but it is not (referring to principle 9) disproportionate to the overall costs of care for the hearing-impaired child.

The cost per case for universal IDT screen is of the order of £60 000 at year 2000 prices based on the cost of £27 noted above and a yield of 40% or 0.45/1 000. However the true effect of the screen, as noted above, is the difference between the yields with a screen in place and without a screen in place. Using an estimate for this of 25–30% gives a true cost per case of £80 000 to £96 000. The figure is also much higher in the presence of a well-run targeted neonatal screen where it was noted earlier that the yield of the universal IDT then becomes around 25%. Even if the cost could be reduced to be similar to those currently reported for UNHS, the cost per case remains much higher than UNHS because of the poor reported yield.

In conclusion, the published evidence on cost and effectiveness indicates that the most cost-effective screen that achieves an acceptably high yield is UNHS. UNHS also has the benefit of an earlier diagnosis compared with IDT. This evidence has reinforced the conclusion in the NIH consensus document, which recommended that universal screening for hearing impairment be carried out before three months of age and was the basis for similar statements made in the European consensus statement on neonatal hearing screening.

Finally, it is important to consider the harm that a screen can produce (principle 11). Reports to date indicate that the degree of anxiety raised by UNHS is very limited (Watkin et al., 1998). However, there remains the potential to cause concern to parents particularly with false positive results. Programmes should ensure that follow-up of false positives is quick and efficient.

Screening after the first year of life

Intermediate screens (18 months – school entry)

Increasing effort is being made to detect PCHI in the first year of life, but evidence indicates that currently around 40% of children with PCHI (≥ 40 dB HL) are still not being correctly identified until after the two years of age (Fortnum and Davis, 1997). This proportion may rise to over 60% for those with moderate degrees of impairment (40–69 dB HL) (Fortnum and Davis, 1997). In the past, a variety of methods were often employed by health visitors or clinic doctors in an attempt to screen hearing in this age group. These included speech discrimination tests such as Kendal or McCormick toy tests, or performance tests using warble tones or voiced sounds ('go/ss').

Haggard and Hughes (1991) reviewed the evidence relating to intermedi-ate screens and found that practice was highly variable, often with a lack of clear objectives and quality control. There were few usable data on sensitivity, specificity or incremental yield and no comparison between alternative arrangements. Identification of children with previously undetected, acquired or progressive permanent hearing impairment is obviously desirable, but the number of such cases would be relatively very small compared to the large number of children with conductive hearing impairment in this age group. A single screen could not determine which cases were transient, so that specificity would inevitably be low. It was concluded that there was no justification for an intermediate screen.

The 'Health for all Children' surveillance programme (Hall, 1996), recommends that 'no attempt should be made to undertake a universal screening test of hearing after the age of 7–9 months, until the child goes to school.' Most districts now operate a reactive system for this age group, referring for an audiological assessment, in cases where there is parental or professional concern regarding hearing or speech development, a history of repeated ear infections, upper airway obstruction or developmental or behavioural problems. There is also compelling evidence to support testing of the hearing of all children following bacterial meningitis (Fortnum and Davis , 1993).

School entry screening

The first attempts to test hearing in school in the UK date back to the 1920s when the 'whispered-voice' test was introduced, followed later by gramophone audiometry. In the 1940s screening pure-tone audiometry became available and was introduced as a universal screen throughout virtually all districts over the next 20 years (HMSO, 1975) and continues to be widely practised.

The screen is predominantly accomplished by an adaptation of pure-tone audiometry at specific frequencies, often performed at a fixed level (the sweep test). The pass threshold is generally set at 20 or 25 dB HL, with some districts accepting low-frequency thresholds up to 30 dB HL. One or two tests may be performed, usually during the year of school entry. The school nurse most often performs the test, but some districts use audiometricians, or health visitors (Davis et al., 1997). Testing is generally carried out within the school, where excessive ambient noise may limit specificity. There has been little monitoring or evaluation of the school entry screen. Guidelines for training and testing by non-audiology professionals have, however, been issued (Smith and Evans, 2000).

The yield for bilateral PCHI ≥ 40 dB HL is estimated to be 4 per 10 000 children screened (Davis et al., 1997). Unilateral or mild sensorineural impairments may also be identified, although the clinical implications and benefits of intervention in this group are not established (Haggard and Hughes, 1991). Otitis media with effusion (OME) is highly prevalent at the age of school entry and can affect long-term cognitive development and behaviour and ultimately educational achievement (Chalmers et al., 1989; Bennett and Haggard, 1999; Luotonen et al., 1998). The effectiveness of referral and intervention, however, remains under scrutiny (*Effective Health Care Bulletin No. 4,* NHS Centre for reviews and dissemination) and is currently being addressed in the UK by the TARGET study (*Trial of Alternative Regimens for Glue Ear Treatment*).

The use of screening tympanometry has been considered, but also has low specificity for persisting OME and would not identify sensorineural impairment (Haggard and Hughes, 1991). The value of a single screen for a fluctuating condition such as OME is questionable. Specificity for persisting cases will be low, leading to costly, unnecessary, referrals, and sensitivity may be affected by transient resolution, depending, for example, on seasonal variation. As a consequence, some districts have now discontinued the school entry screen.

Use of a parental questionnaire has been tried as an alternative to screening audiometry. *The Childhood Middle Ear Disease and Hearing Questionnaire* (CMEDHQ) has been developed by the MRC Institute of Hearing Research. Questions relate mainly to a previous or family history of ear symptoms, or current difficulties. A preliminary trial has indicated a high response rate with better specificity, but slightly lower sensitivity than the pure-tone sweep test (Hind et al., 1999). Further trials are anticipated.

There is no evidence to justify further screens after school entry. However, professional vigilance should continue and a hearing test performed on any child experiencing learning or behavioural difficulties or following specific conditions such as meningitis or significant head injury.

Conclusions

The chapter has briefly reviewed the options for early identification of hearing impairment with reference to principles of effective screening. In the first year of life universal neonatal hearing screening has been shown on current evidence to offer the most cost-effective method of detecting PCHI. Although UNHS is relatively new, published reports indicate that it is possible to achieve the screening goals of a high coverage, low referral rate and a high yield. The application of electrophysiological techniques, supported by OAE and tympanometry, allows for initial diagnostic assessment to be rapidly completed. However, a significant minority of PCHI is not present at birth and there is a need for a continuing hearing surveillance programme in infancy and early childhood.

There remain many questions. For example, screening for unilateral and mild hearing impairment is still a subject of debate as, unlike moderate or greater bilateral PCHI, this type of impairment does not fit the screening principles so well. There is little knowledge about the precise degree of loss at which a hearing aid should be fitted and the age at which this should be carried out following detection of a PCHI by a UNHS. The proportion of PCHI present at birth and the onset and time course of acquired hearing losses is not known with precision. To answer these and other questions on screening and surveillance will require major research programmes conducted on large birth populations.

After the first year of life, none of the potential methods for screening are able to meet fully the screening principles set out at the beginning of the chapter. Universal school entry screening is a practical screen and is still implemented in many countries. As UNHS is introduced, further studies are needed to determine whether universal school entry screening is cost effective as part of the overall programme to detect permanent hearing impairment in childhood.

Abbreviations

PCHI: permanent childhood hearing impairment.
UNHS: universal neonatal hearing screening.
TNHS: targeted neonatal hearing screening.
IDT: infant distraction test.
ABR: auditory brainstem response.
AABR: automated auditory brainstem response
ARC: auditory response cradle.
OAE: otoacoustic emissions.
TEOAE: transient evoked otoacoustic emissions.
DPOAE: distortion product evoked otoacoustic emissions.

Definitions

Hearing impairment:
moderate: 40 to 69 dB HL;
severe: 70 to 94 dB HL;
profound: ≥95 dB HL.

Permanent hearing impairment: average (0.5, 1, 2 and 4kHz) hearing levels measured at ≥ 40 dBnHL in the better ear on all occasions.

Congenital hearing impairment: considered to be present at the time of a neonatal screen.

Acquired hearing impairment: considered not to be present at the time of a neonatal screen.

Confirmation of permanent hearing impairment: the date at which tests first indicated permanent hearing impairment with a high degree of accuracy.

Fitting of a hearing aid: the date when the child is first fitted with a hearing aid (not the date when the mould impression was taken).

Screen sensitivity: for those tested, the percentage of cases correctly identified.

Screen specificity: for those tested, the percentage of non-cases correctly identified.

Yield: the number of cases identified by a screening programme.

Chapter 8

Genetics of hearing impairment

AP Read

Introduction

About half of all profound childhood hearing impairment, and a significant but unknown proportion of later onset or milder impairment is caused by mutations at single genetic loci (Morton, 1991). Remarkable progress has been made in the last decade in mapping and identifying the genes involved. The methods that have made this possible will be briefly discussed, then the data summarized for the more significant genes, and finally the implications of all this scientific advance for the working clinician will be considered.

Methods: how the genes are identified

This brief overview describes some of the tools and limitations of current approaches. For more detailed discussion of methods, the reader should consult a suitable textbook, for example Strachan and Read (1999). References are given to the appropriate section of this book.

There is no universal correct way to identify the gene underlying a genetic disease. However, all the many possible methods (summarized in Strachan and Read, 1999, Figure 15.1) converge on testing a *candidate gene* for mutations. One way or another, one gene is chosen from among the 130 000 or so in the human genome. If it is the correct gene, then people with the disease should have mutations in that gene. DNA from patients is analysed to see if the sequence of the gene in the patients differs in any way from the normal sequence. Numerous laboratory techniques are available to answer that question (Strachan and Read, 2000, section 17.1) but problems are still common. None of the techniques is 100% sensitive, and when a deviation from the normal sequence has been found, it may be difficult to know whether the change is pathogenic or just a coincidental rare neutral variant (a 'polymorphism'). For that reason it is desirable to have a panel of unrelated patients available for mutation testing. If a good proportion of the patients has a mutation, and if the mutations include several different sequence variants, none of which is found on testing 100 healthy controls, then it is highly likely that the correct gene has been identified. Further confirmation requires functional studies in a cell-free system, in cultured cells or in genetically engineered mice.

How is the candidate gene chosen? There are many different ways, but almost always the first step is to narrow down the choice by defining the approximate chromosomal location of the gene (mapping it). This is done by studying large families in which the disease is segregating. We need DNA samples from a good number of people (typically 20–30), who could have inherited either the disease gene or its normal allele from their parents, and where we know by clinical examination which possibility in fact happened. We then study DNA markers (common non-pathogenic DNA variants) to try to find one whose transmission through the family tree parallels the transmission of the disease gene. This is called linkage analysis (see Strachan and Read, 1999, section 11.3). If a marker is found that satisfies the statistical test for linkage (measured by the lod score), then the disease gene must be located on the same chromosomal segment as the marker. Given good large families to study, this method typically narrows the candidate region down from 3000 million base pairs of DNA (the size of the whole human genome) to one million to five million base pairs. Such a region might still contain a hundred or so genes. Public databases list the genes in a given chromosomal region and, with the progress of the Human Genome Project, the lists are rapidly becoming more reliable and complete. It then remains to prioritize candidates for mutation testing from among the genes on the list. Clues include the temporal and spatial pattern of expression (presumably the correct gene will be switched on in the inner ear, whether or not it is functional elsewhere as well; genes responsible for developmental defects should be active at the appropriate stage of embryonic development). Genes come in families, and another clue might be a relationship to a gene already known to be implicated in a similar phenotype, in man or model organisms. Knowledge of the biochemical function of the gene may also be relevant, though our ignorance of cell biology means that it is often very difficult to guess the clinical result of mutations in a gene from such knowledge.

From the above, it follows that progress in identifying the genes underlying genetic hearing impairment is crucially dependent on collaboration between clinicians and laboratory workers. However clever the molecular geneticists are, they can achieve nothing unless their clinical colleagues can identify good large families suitable for linkage analysis and collect patients for mutation analysis. A particularly important role of the clinicians is in identifying heterogeneity. Undetected heterogeneity in a collection of families can make linkage analysis almost impossible, whereas identification of subtle distinguishing features can point the way to identifying new disease genes. Finally, alert clinicians picking out patients with chromosomal abnormalities as well as a known Mendelian disease have often provided the vital clue to launch successful gene identification projects. In all these ways, one of the pleasures of working in clinical molecular genetics is the opportunity it provides for fruitful collaboration between insightful clinicians and cutting-edge scientists.

Sources of information

This is a fast-moving area, and for up-to-date information, the reader should consult one of the excellent Internet resources:

- For general information on simply inherited diseases and the underlying genes, OMIM (Online Mendelian Inheritance in Man) is the first choice. Searching this database for a word or phrase will return a series of numbers, each pointing to one entry – for example, Waardenburg syndrome Type 1 is 193500. Clicking on the number brings up a brief clinical description, a more detailed summary of the genetics, lists of references and links to other Internet resources. Online Mendelian Inheritance in Man entries are reliable and generally up to date, but note that new material is usually simply added on to the end of the previous content of a section, so the early parts of an entry for a disease may have been written many years ago.
- Specific information on hereditary hearing impairment is collected on the Hereditary Hearing Loss Homepage, a resource maintained jointly by G Van Camp (Antwerp) and R Smith (Iowa). This lists all the identified and mapped genes and has links to many other Internet resources but is currently a little out of date (www.uia.ac.be/dnalabhhh/).

Progress in identifying the genes: syndromic hearing impairment

Gorlin, Toriello and Cohen (1995) described 427 syndromes in which hearing impairment is a regular or occasional feature. Most are very rare; Table 8.1 summarizes a few of the more frequent syndromes.

Table 8.1. – Examples of syndromic hearing impairment. See text for descriptions of some of the genes. See a human genetics textbook, for example Section 2.5.2 of Strachan and Read (1999) for description of the way chromosomal locations are named.

Condition	Locus	Chromosomal location	Gene (where known)
Alport	*COL4*	Xq22	*COL4A5*
		2q36-q37	*COL4A3, COL4A4*
Branchio-oto-renal	*BOR1*	8q13.3	*EYA1*
	BOR2	1q31	?
Jervell & Lange-Nielsen	*JLN*	11p15	*KCNQ1*
Neurofibromatosis 2	*NF2*	22q	*NF2 (Merlin)*
Pendred	*PDS*	7q21-q34	*PDS*
Treacher Collins	*TCOF1*	5q32	*TCOF1*
Usher Type 1	*USH1A*	14q32	?
	USH1B	11q13.5	*MYO7A*
	USH1C	11p15.1	*Harmonin*
	USH1D	10q	*CDH23*
	USH1E	21q	?
	USH1F	10	?
Usher Type 2	*USH2A*	1q41	*USH2A*
	USH2B	3p23-p24.2	?
	USH2C	5q14.3-21.3	?
Usher Type 3	*USH3*	3q21-q25	?
Waardenburg Type 1	*PAX3*	2q35	*PAX3*
Waardenburg Type 2	*MITF (15%)*	3p14	*MITF*
	Unknown (85%)	?	?
Waardenburg Type 3	*PAX3*	2q35	*PAX3 (+/– or –/–)*
Waardenburg Type 4	*EDNRB, EDN3*	13q22, 20q13,	*EDNRB, EDN3,*
	SOX10	22q	*SOX10*
X-linked + dystonia etc	*DFN1*	Xq22	*DDP*
X-linked with gusher	*DFN3*	Xq13-q21	*POU3F4 (Brain 4)*

Branchio-oto-renal syndrome

The *EYA1* gene is the human homologue of the *eyes absent* gene in the *Drosophila* fruit fly. *EYA1* encodes a transcription factor – that is, a DNA-binding protein that controls the expression of other genes. The results of mutations in man are quite variable, and include the branchio-otic syndrome, previously thought to be genetically distinct from BOR; *EYA1* mutations have also been found in a few humans with eye abnormalities. Only a proportion of BOR patients have detectable *EYA1* mutations; recently a second BOR locus was identified on chromosome 1 (Kumar et al., 2000).

Jervell and Lange-Nielsen syndrome

JLN is one of many examples of hearing impairment caused by defects in ion transport. It is caused by mutations in the voltage-gated potassium channel gene *KCNQ1* (also called *KVLQT1*). People with no functional *KCNQ1* ion channels have JLN; people with 50% of the normal level are clinically normal, whereas people with a level somewhere between 0 and 50% have the heart problem but normal hearing. JLN mutations simply abolish the function of the gene product. Thus homozygotes have JLN but heterozygotes are normal, and JLN is recessive. Some mutations result in production of an altered *KCNQ1* protein that is not only non-functional but partly blocks the function of any normal protein present (a dominant negative effect). People who are heterozygous for such a mutation have the dominant Romano-Ward long QT syndrome, but normal hearing.

Neurofibromatosis 2

All vestibular schwannomas, whether sporadic and unilateral or part of NF2, originate from a cell that has lost both functioning copies of the *NF2* gene. Sporadic VS happens when, by pure chance, an originally normal cell suffers two successive mutations. This is a rare piece of bad luck, hence sporadic VS are unilateral and usually seen in older people (who have had more time to accumulate mutations). People who inherit one mutant *NF2* gene are perfectly normal, because cells can function normally with a single intact copy of this gene. But every cell carries the mutation, and only a single acquired mutation is needed to convert a cell into the precursor of a VS. Given the large number of potential target cells, this is a highly likely occurrence. Hence NF2 affects younger people and often produces bilateral or multifocal tumours. NF2 is a classic example of Knudson's two-hit mechanism of hereditary tumours – see section 18.5 of Strachan and Read (1999).

Pendred syndrome

The *PDS* gene encodes a protein, pendrin, which is involved in transport of chloride and iodide ions. The hearing impairment reflects the general importance of ion transport to cochlear function, and the iodide transport defect explains the goitre. Some PDS mutations cause the non-syndromic *DFNB4* hearing impairment; the reason for this difference is not clear.

Treacher Collins syndrome

The *TCOF1* gene encodes a protein ('treacle') that is probably involved in nucleolar trafficking. Almost all described mutations are predicted to result in premature chain termination during protein synthesis, causing that copy of the gene to produce no functioning protein. How a 50% dosage of treacle protein produces the clinical features of Treacher Collins syndrome is unknown, but the great clinical variability even within families is typical of conditions caused by such dosage sensitivity ('haploinsufficiency'). Branchio-oto-renal and Waardenburg syndromes provide further examples.

Usher syndrome

Usher syndrome has turned out to be remarkably heterogeneous at the molecular level, with so far six different loci implicated in Type 1, and 3 in Type 2 syndrome. Only four have so far been identified. Interestingly, three of the Type 1 loci map to similar locations as non-syndromic loci (Table 8.2), and in the case of *USH1B / DFNB2* the same gene, *MYO7A*, is known to be involved. Unconventional myosins play an important role in the hair cells; mutations in *MYO15* underlie the *DFNB3* hearing impairment, while *MYO6* mutations cause the Snell's waltzer phenotype in mice, and probably will be found in human hearing impairment.

Table 8.2. - Mutations in many different genes can cause non-syndromic hearing loss. Autosomal dominant loci are symbolised DFNA1, DFNA2, etc; recessive loci are DFNB1, DFNB2, etc, while X-linked loci are DFN1, DFN2 etc. See the Hereditary Hearing Loss Homepage, http://www.uia.ac.be/dnalab/hhh/ for more details.

Non-syndromic hearing impairment.

Locus	Chromosomal location	Gene (where known)	Possible overlaps
Autosomal dominant loci (31 described)			
DFNA1	5q31	HDIA1	
DFNA2	1p34	GJB3, KCNQ4	
DFNA3	13q12	GJB2, GJB6	DFNB1
DFNA4	19q13		
DFNA5	7p15	DFNA5	
DFNA6	4p16.3		
DFNA7	1q21-q23		
DFNA9	14q12-q13	COCH	DFNB5?
DFNA10	6q22-q23	EYA4	
DFNA11	11q12.3-q21	MYO7A	DFNB2, USH1B
DFNA12	11q22-q24	TECTA	DFNA8, DFNB21
DFNA13	6p21	COL11A12	
DFNA14	4p16		
DFNA15	5q31	POU4F3	

Table 8.2. (contd)

Autosomal recessive loci (30 described)			
DFNB1	13q12	GJB2	DFNA3
DFNB2	11q13.5	MYO7A	USH1B, DFNA11
DFNB3	17p11.2-q12	MYO15	
DFNB4	7q31	PDS	Pendred
DFNB5	14q12		DFNA9??
DFNB6	3p14-p21		
DFNB7	9q13-q21		DFNB11?
DFNB8	21q22	TMPR553	DFNB10
DFNB9	2p22-p23	OTOF	
DFNB10	21q22.3	TMPRSS3	DFNB8
DFNB11	9q13-q21		DFNB7?
DFNB12	10q21-q22	CDH23	USH1D
DFNB13	7q34-q36		
DFNB14	7q31		
DFNB16	15q21-q22		
DFNB18	11p14-p15.1		
DFNB19	18p11		
DFNB21	11q22-q24	TECTA	DFNA12
USH1C?			
X-linked loci (5 described)			
DFN3	Xq21.1	POU3F4	
DFN4	Xp21.2		
DFN6	Xp22		
Mitochondrial mutations (many described)			
7445insC,		*tRAA^{LEU}*	
A1555G		12S RNA	

Waardenburg syndrome

The label 'Waardenburg syndrome' is applied to a heterogeneous collection of auditory-pigmentary syndromes, all of which have their origin in a dysfunction of melanocytes. See Read and Newton (1997) for a review. Apart from their role in pigmentation, melanocytes also form the pigmented intermediate cells of the stria vascularis, and in their absence there is no hearing. Four types of WS are usually listed.

- Type 1 with dystopia canthorum (outward displacement of the inner canthi of the eyes) is caused by mutations in *PAX3,* which encodes a homeodomain-containing transcription factor expressed in the embryonic neural crest (the tissue of origin of melanocytes). WS1 is dominant, patients are heterozygous, and the pathogenic mechanism is haploinsufficiency.

- Type 2 WS is a melanocyte-specific disturbance, caused in some cases by mutations in the *MITF* transcription factor gene (a master gene controlling differentiation of melanocytes), and in other cases by as yet unidentified gene(s).
- Type 3 WS has the features of Type 1 with additionally limb abnormalities. Most 'WS3' patients have mild muscular hypoplasia of the arms and/or contractures of some joints. This is an occasional variant presentation of WS1, and these patients are heterozygous for *PAX3* mutations similar to those seen in WS1. Very rare patients have a much more severe phenotype with extreme depigmentation, severe dystopia canthorum and amyoplasia of the arms and shoulders. These patients are homozygous for PAX3 mutations, and in at least two cases WS1 was documented in both parents.
- Type 4 WS or Waardenburg-Shah syndrome has the features of WS2 plus Hirschsprung disease. All the affected tissues are derived from the neural crest, and WS4 comprises a heterogeneous set of severe neurocristopathies. Three causative genes have been identified. Mutations in endothelin 3 and its receptor EDNRB usually cause isolated Hirschsprung disease in heterozygotes but WS4 in homozygotes; mutations in the transcription factor SOX10 can cause WS4 in heterozygotes (sometimes with additional neurological problems).

Progress in identifying the genes: non-syndromic hearing impairment

In many families uncomplicated hearing impairment segregates in a pattern consistent with determination at a single genetic locus. Pre-lingual hearing impairment is usually autosomal recessive whereas dominant inheritance is more commonly seen in late-onset hearing impairment. X-linked inheritance is uncommon. There is no simple way to work out how many different genes are involved, although indirect estimates based on population genetics suggested there might be 30 to 100 loci determining autosomal recessive hearing impairment (Morton, 1991). It is also becoming evident that mutations in the mitochondrial genome (inherited exclusively from the mother, though affecting either sex) are a common cause of progressive hearing impairment.

For many years non-syndromic hearing impairment was regarded as genetically intractable. The dominant forms are mostly of late onset and the pattern in families is confused by the frequent co-occurrence of non-genetic age-related hearing impairment (phenocopies). Families with recessive hearing impairment are usually too small for individual linkage analysis, but families cannot be combined for analysis because of the expected extensive genetic heterogeneity. Moreover, frequent deaf–deaf marriages can make it impossible to follow the line of transmission of a deafness gene through a family, and further confusion is introduced by family members who are hearing-impaired for some other reason, despite not inheriting the family gene (phenocopies). For recessive hearing impairment, the solution was to study the large multiply-inbred kindreds that can be found in various societies around the Mediterranean and across the Middle East to the Indian subcontinent. A single kindred can be large enough to give statistically meaningful linkage data, so avoiding the problem of heterogeneity. Dominant hearing impairment of adult onset is amenable to family study where the usual age of onset is relatively early, but little headway has yet been made in identifying genetic susceptibility to presbyacusis or noise-induced hearing impairment.

Ten years of linkage analysis have led to about 30 recessive and 40 dominant loci being mapped (Table 8.2). Progress in cloning the genes is accelerating as the Human Genome Project makes better tools available. Currently the genes responsible for nine recessive and ten dominant forms of non-syndromic hearing impairment have been identified. The gene products are mostly unrelated to each other; they include several membrane proteins (ion channels or connexins), at least two myosin motor proteins and some structural proteins (alpha tectorin and otoferlin). In two cases (*DFNA2, DFNA3*) mutations have been found in two genes at the appropriate chromosomal location in different families, suggesting yet further heterogeneity.

A surprising finding has been that the same gene may be mutated in two or more different types of hearing impairment. Sometimes mutations in the same gene can cause either dominant or recessive non-syndromic hearing impairment – for example, connexin 26 is mutated in recessive *DFNB1* and dominant *DFNA3,* and alpha-tectorin is mutated in dominant *DFNA12* and recessive *DFNB21.* In other cases mutations in the same gene may underlie both a non-syndromic and a syndromic form of hearing impairment. MYO7A is mutated in Usher syndrome 1B, in recessive *DFNB1* and in dominant *DFNA11. PDS* is mutated in Pendred syndrome and in recessive non-syndromic *DFNB4.* The explanation here is likely to centre around the distinction between simple loss of function mutations and dominant negative effects, as described above in connection with Jervell and Lange-Nielsen syndrome. Such dominant negative effects are especially seen when the protein encoded by the gene functions as a multimer. A multimer containing some normal and some abnormal molecules is non-functional, heterozygotes are affected, and so the condition is dominant.

Most loci have been implicated in only one or a few families, but two genes seem to be major causes of non-syndromic genetic hearing impairment, as mentioned below.

Connexin 26

Connexins are proteins that assemble into hexameric units (connexons) in cell membranes and bind to connexons on an adjacent cell to form a gap junction, through which small molecules can pass from one cell to another. Mutations in at least three connexin genes (*GJB2, GJB3* and *GJB6*) have been implicated in non-syndromic hearing impairment. See the Connexin-deafness homepage (References) for further information. By far the major player is connexin 26, encoded by the *GJB2* gene. Mutations in connexin 26 are the cause of *DFNB1* recessive hearing impairment, and also *DFNA3* dominant hearing impairment. *DFNB1* is a major cause of pre-lingual hearing impairment in European populations, accounting for up to half of recessive (unaffected parents, two or more affected children) and 10% to 25% of sporadic pre-lingual hearing impairments in several studies (Estivill et al., 1998a; Denoyelle et al., 1999; Mueller et al., 1999). Moreover a high proportion of all mutations are one particular sequence change, loss of one G from a run of 6 consecutive G nucleotides (30delG, sometimes called 35delG). This has important implications for diagnostic testing, as will be discussed.

Mitochondrial syndromes

Mitochondria have their own small genome, a 16569 base pair circle of DNA containing 37 genes. Mutations in the mitochondrial DNA are the cause of a bewildering variety of disorders, with the hallmark that they are inherited exclusively from the mother. Sperm do not contribute mitochondria to the zygote. Cells contain many mitochondria, and patients with mitochondrial mutations can be homoplasmic (all mitochondria the same) or heteroplasmic (a mixture of mitochondrial types). Heteroplasmy can be transmitted from mother to child, because the egg contains huge numbers of mitochondria.

Mitochondrial DNA is rather variable compared with the nuclear DNA. Thus sequence variants are very common and their significance is often hard to assess. Nevertheless, it is clear that one particular variant, replacement of nucleotide 1555, normally A, by G, is a common cause of hearing impairment. Originally A1555G was identified in patients with aminoglycoside-induced hearing impairment, and it is undoubtedly a major susceptibility factor in this impairment, but additionally it is present in hearing-impaired people with no history of exposure to aminoglycosides. Estivill's group in Spain (Estivill, 1998b) found A1555G in 17/70 consecutive referrals of severe congenital or progressive sensorineural hearing impairment with no other identifiable cause where the proband had at least one other affected relative. Similar results have been found in an independent Spanish series (reported in Torroni et al., 1999) and the detailed DNA analysis suggests that this might be a common mutation throughout European populations. A survey of 480 hearing-impaired students in schools for the deaf in Mongolia (Pandya et al., 1999) found 37 with A1555G. In Estivill's data (1998b) the chance of hearing impairment for a carrier of A1555G with no antibiotic exposure is 40% by age 30, rising to 60% by age 60.

Implications

Identifying the genes causing hearing impairment has several purposes. Biologists hope to gain insight into normal human physiology and development. The genes mutated in non-syndromic impairment presumably encode components of the auditory transduction machinery, while those mutated in syndromic hearing impairment control developmental processes. Identifying the genes should help elucidate the mechanisms of these various processes.

Identifying a disease gene immediately raises the possibility of molecular diagnosis. Whether or not this hope is realistic depends on the precision of the diagnostic question being posed. Consider three possible questions:

1. Does this patient have *any* mutation in *any* gene that will explain her condition?
2. Does this patient have *any* mutation in *this particular gene* that will explain her condition?
3. Does this patient have *one specified* mutation (for example, nucleotide A replaced with G at position 1555) in *this particular gene?*

Question 1 is quite impossible to answer, now or in any likely future. Question 3 on the other hand can be answered cheaply and easily, by a single quick laboratory test. Question 2 is in principle always answerable, but answering it is often too laborious and expensive to contemplate in the context of a routine diagnostic service. Maybe the new technology of gene chips will help here, but even if it does, it will probably be available only for diseases common enough to repay the investment needed to create the right chip.

How practical is it to specify the gene in advance? For syndromic hearing impairment, this is usually possible if the syndrome is identified correctly by clinical examination. Sometimes, as, for example, with Usher syndrome, there may be several suspects, but at least the list is limited. For non-syndromic hearing impairments, clinical examination will give no clue, and the only hope is if experience shows that one particular gene is mutated in a substantial proportion of all patients. In small isolated populations this can be quite a common occurrence; it is less likely in large and open populations.

In general it is not possible to specify the precise DNA sequence change that is sought. For most genetic diseases, unrelated affected people have different mutations and it is necessary to search the whole gene to find a mutation. Genes are long stretches of DNA, thousands or tens of thousands of base pairs long, and this is a major task. However, there are four circumstances in which one can suggest the particular mutation to be tested for:

- If additional family members are being tested for the presence or absence of a mutation that has already been defined in one affected family member.
- If the nature of the disease is such that only one very specific alteration in the gene sequence will produce that effect. An example would be sickle cell disease; in hearing impairment the only possible example that comes to mind is the mitochondrial A1555G mutation in aminoglycoside-induced hearing impairment.
- If the nature of the gene sequence is such that one particular mutational change happens very often, whereas other changes are much less common. An example would be fragile-X syndrome which can be caused by any change that abolishes function of the *FMR1* gene, but in over 99% of cases is caused by one particular change, expansion of a $(CGG)_n$ trinucleotide repeat. Several genes implicated in hearing impairment have mutational hot spots, but so far none has accounted for a high enough proportion of all mutations to be helpful in genetic testing.
- If one particular mutation, inherited from a common ancestor, has by chance spread very widely through a population. The connexin 26 mutation 30delG is the prime example of this (that particular sequence is also a mutational hotspot, which no doubt contributes to its high prevalence).

What molecular diagnostic services are available at present for the clinician? This is an area of rapid change superimposed on great differences between countries and even regions. For most of the important syndromes, mutation testing languishes in the gulf between research and service. Mutation screening of *MYO7A, EYA1, PAX3, MITF, PDS* and other important genes has been offered by the researchers who initially identified these genes, but once they have published a few dozen mutations, they can rarely justify using research funds for further testing. If they are set up to handle invoicing they may be able to continue on a fee-for-service basis. With over 1000 disease genes identified, routine diagnostic laboratories have to restrict themselves to a limited menu of tests. Laboratories are slowly moving towards establishing consortia where in each country (or for rarer diseases, each continent) two laboratories, one primary and one backup, agree to provide a costed service for any particular rare disease. Progress to date has been slow, but hopefully such a service will eventually extend to all the genes involved in hereditary hearing impairment, syndromic and non-syndromic.

Connexin 26 is a special case. The high frequency of the 30delG mutation in many countries clearly justifies routine testing of hearing-impaired children, and technically the test is simple and cheap. The problem is what to do when a hearing-impaired child turns out to have a single copy of the 30delG mutation. This is a common finding: 10/82, 7/47 and 16/96 consecutive children in presumed recessive families in Spain, France and the UK (Estivill et al., 1998a; Denoyelle et al., 1999; Mueller et al., 1999). Does the child have a different mutation in the other copy of the *GJB2* gene, or is the child hearing-impaired for some unrelated reason, but coincidentally a heterozygous carrier of 30delG? Carrier frequencies in many European countries are 1–2%, so the dilemma is a real one. Thus any laboratory offering testing for 30delG must also be able to offer, or at least organize, screening of the whole *GJB2* gene for further mutations, which is expensive and requires specialized skills. The detection rate for ‘second mutations’ is currently often lower than expected, suggesting further work is needed before Cx26 testing can become routine.

Finally, the mitochondrial A1555G mutation may also justify dedicated diagnostic testing. Data from Spain (Estivill et al., 1998b; Torroni et al., 1999) show a remarkably high frequency (51/204 consecutive cases) of A1555G in adult-onset hearing impairment, whether or not there has been exposure to aminoglycosides. If these figures are confirmed, and if they apply to other countries as well, mutation testing would identify the cause of a significant proportion of all adult-onset hearing impairment. Population screening, as always, would be justified only if it resulted in some useful intervention, but a definitive diagnosis is of value in itself to patients and parents who want to know why they or their children are hearing-impaired.

Thus it is clear that the progress of the last 10 years in identifying the specific causes of genetic hearing impairment has greatly extended the scope of diagnostic testing. In the longer term, everybody hopes that the new knowledge will lead to better treatment and maybe prevention or cures. Gene therapy (replacing or removing malfunctioning and defective genes) should eventually produce cures for diseases where the symptoms stem from malfunctioning of the defective gene here and now, and are reversible. It would not help with developmental defects, where the damage was done long ago and is irreversible. Maybe some people are genetically sensitive to particular environmental insults (as with aminoglycosides) and if they could be identified by population screening, they could be singled out for protection. Maybe genetic dissection of the mechanisms of development and function of the auditory system will identify novel targets for drug treatments. These are all developments for the long-term future – but a consistent lesson from the past 20 years of molecular genetics has been that the long-term future often materializes remarkably quickly.

CHAPTER 9

Infectious causes of paediatric hearing impairment

PJ VALLELY, PE KLAPPER AND GM CLEATOR

Introduction

It is estimated that one in every 1000 newborns has significant hearing impairment (Grundfast, 1996). Most of these cases are attributable to heredity or premature birth and the problems associated with neonatal intensive care (Grundfast and Lalwani, 1992; Das, 1996; Roizen, 1999). The etiology of the remainder of the cases of hearing impairment is still largely unknown, but improved methods of diagnosis suggest infection may be a more common cause than previously recognized (Das, 1996; Berrettini et al., 1999). A wide range of infectious agents have been associated with hearing impairment either through direct effects upon organogenesis; direct (cell cytolytic) effects on the organ; or through indirect damage to nerves peripherally or centrally. Childhood immunization programmes in developed countries have considerably reduced the incidence of the diseases caused by many pathogens, but on a world-wide basis infection remains a considerable source of preventable audiological morbidity.

Identification of the cause of childhood hearing impairment can be difficult, but definition of an infectious etiology, where it can be achieved, is of benefit in counselling parents. It may also help anticipate prognosis and allow treatment interventions to prevent further deterioration, and will provide data important to the design and implementation of strategies to control infection within the community.

Infectious causes

The infectious causes of hearing impairment may be divided into the prenatal or congenital and the post-natal or acquired infections (Table 9.1 and

Table 9.2). Definitive data on the prevalence of infective causes of audiological impairment are not available, but a review of 3660 patients attending an otolaryngology clinic suggested that among those with bilateral profound hearing impairment, congenital infection was a predominant cause (Qiu, Yin and Stucker, 1999). The most frequently reported agents of congenital infection are cytomegalovirus, rubella virus, *Toxoplasma gondii* and, in developing countries, *Treponema pallidum* (syphilis). Congenital hearing impairment is sometimes seen as part of a severe syndrome as in the congenital rubella syndrome

Table 9.1. Congenital infectious causes of auditory impairment

Congenital infection	percentage transmission risk and (percentage risk of damage[1])			
	1st trimester	2nd trimester	3rd trimester	Term
Infectious Agent[2]				
Rubella virus	90% (80–90%)	25–70% (17.5–50%)	35%(0%)	100%(0%)
Human cytomegalovirus	40–50% (NK)	40–50% (NK)	40–50% (NK)	100% (probably 0%)
Herpes varicella-zoster	NK (v.low)	NK (0%)	NK (0%)	60% (c.30%)
Herpes simplex virus types 1 & 2	NK (v.low)	NK (0%)	NK (0%)	NK (Moderate to High)
Human immunodeficiency virus	Low (NK)	Low (NK)	Low (NK)	24–50%[3] (c.8%)
Toxoplasma gondii	4–25% (2–10%)	25–54% (2–4%)	65% (0%)	80% (0%)
Treponema pallidum	100% in primary or secondary syphilis (50% risk of premature neonatal death or still birth)[4]			

NK = Not Known

[1]'Damage' represents risk of significant foetal damage when mother experiences infection in pregnancy (e.g. if materno-foetal transmission occurs in 60% of pregnancies and 40% of the foetuses who are congenitally infected are damaged, overall percentage risk of damage is 60/100 × 40 i.e. 24%).

[2]List is only representative, the literature abounds with anecdotal accounts of congenital, peri- and post-natal infections causing auditory impairment in later life.

[3]Without antiviral prophylaxis in 3rd trimester. Variable rate depends upon maternal viral load and presence of other sexually transmitted diseases.

[4]Risk of materno-foetal transmission decreases to 80% in early latent syphilis and to 30% or less in late latent syphilis.

Table 9.2. Acquired infectious causes of auditory impairment

Perinatal and Post-natally Acquired Infection	
	Risk of residual deafness
Bacterial Meningitis	*Streptococcus pneumoniae* - 18-30% *Neisseria meningitidis* - 10% *Haemophilus influenza* - 6% *Mycobacterium tuberculosis* - NK (probably rare) *Borrelia burgdorferi* - Low frequency, hearing loss in 2% of cases
Chronic otitis media	NK (rare)
Fungal Infection	NK (rare, but more common in immunocompromised)
Parasitic Infection	*Treponema pallidum*, *Leishmania donovani*, *Fasciola hepaticum* - NK (rare)
Viral Infection	Measles virus - 1 per 1000 cases of measles Mumps virus - 1 per 10000 cases of mumps Rubella - NK (rare) Herpes simplex viruses - NK (rare) Varicella-zoster - NK (rare, but 48% in cases of Ramsay-Hunt syndrome) Human immunodeficiency virus - NK (rare, but HIV infection may increase risk of auditory morbidity from other infections)

NK = Not Known.

(CRS), but more commonly hearing impairment is the first and/or only manifestation of intrauterine infection. In many cases, impairment is not detected until the child reaches two to four years of age and at this age definition of the causative agent is difficult (see diagnosis below).

Among acquired infections, bacterial infection, particularly where there is leptomeningeal involvement, is often cited as the most common cause of hearing impairment (Bohme, 1985; Newton and Rowson, 1988; Ruben, 1990). However, the common viral infections of childhood, especially mumps and measles and, less often, herpes simplex virus (HSV), herpes varicella-zoster, and parvovirus B-19, are probably more frequent but largely unrecognized, causes of acute or progressive hearing impairment (Keleman, 1958; Rowson, Hinchcliffe and Gamble, 1975; Cotter, Singleton and Corman, 1994).

Congenital infection

Rubella

Epidemiology

Rubella ('German measles') is spread via the respiratory route and is a highly contagious disease. The incubation period is 14 to 21 days and the period of infectivity is from one week before until four days after the onset of a transient erythematous (maculopapular) rash of two or three days' duration. A rash of longer duration and greater severity is seen in older children and adults, sometimes associated with arthritis and arthralgia. Lymphadenopathy involving post-auricular and sub-occipital glands may be seen. In general, illness is self-limiting and complications of infection are rare.

Congenital rubella syndrome (CRS)

Until 1941 rubella was considered as a mild self-limiting disease of childhood. However, following a large epidemic of rubella in 1940 an Australian ophthalmologist (Gregg, 1941) observed a series of 78 babies with similar kinds of congenital cataract, some of whom also had heart disease. In 68 of the cases it was found that maternal rubella had occurred in the first or second month of pregnancy. In subsequent reports deafness and microcephaly were also reported with a preponderance of cases of deafness occurring in infants whose mothers were infected slightly later in pregnancy (mean 2.1 months gestation; reviewed by Hanshaw, Dudgeon and Marshall, 1985). It is now recognized that CRS classically produces a triad of symptoms: cataracts, heart defects, and sensorineural hearing impairment. However virtually every organ may be involved and severely affected infants will also show intrauterine growth retardation, central nervous system defects, hepatosplenomegaly, thrombocytopenia, petechia, purpura, and thyroid disorders (Cooper, Prelud and Alford, 1995). The only deficits that commonly occur alone are perceptive hearing impairment and pigmentary retinopathy following infection after the first eight weeks of pregnancy (Miller, Cradock-Watson and Pollack, 1982). Prior to control of maternal rubella through vaccination, it is estimated that 10% of all pregnant women became infected and that 30% of the foetuses from these mothers were affected (Green et al., 1965).

Pathogenesis

Foetal infection with rubella results from a primary maternal infection, the timing of which is crucial for the development of CRS. The earlier in pregnancy that the virus is contracted, the poorer the prognosis for the foetus. The overall rate of transmission of infection to the foetus is 90% during the first trimester, but there is gradation of transmission rates from 100% in the first month of gestation reducing to 80% in the third month. During the second and third trimesters the risk falls to 70% and 25–35% respectively. The reduction in rates of transmission possibly reflects the maturation of the placenta after the first trimester allowing it to limit transfer of the virus, or it may be due to the increased resistance to rubella virus infection of differentiated foetal cells (Cooper et al., 1995). When infection does occur the risk of damage to the foetus is 80% to 90% (principally heart, eye and hearing deficits) during the first trimester. This reduces to 5–17.5% (principally hearing deficits) in the second trimester, and is effectively zero if maternal infection occurs during the last trimester (Klapper and Morris, 1990).

Auditory impairment is the most common manifestation of congenital rubella infection occurring in 65% to 80% of those infected (Peckham, 1972; Cooper et al., 1995; Wolinsky, 1996). The hearing impairment may not be evident at birth but may develop progressively or be delayed into later childhood or even early adulthood. Similarly, 20% of children with CRS develop insulin dependent diabetes mellitus by the time they reach adulthood (Menser, Forrest and Bransby, 1978) and about 5% develop thyroid dysfunction (Hanid, 1976). A 20-year follow up study of infants born with CRS found long-term progressive damage to the central nervous system affecting eyesight, hearing and intellectual and motor functioning (Givens et al., 1993).

Control of infection

To date, no effective antiviral drugs have been developed to treat rubella virus infection. Administration of hyperimmune immunoglobulin has been claimed to reduce maternal viraemia and thereby reduce the rate of transmission of infection. However, early identification of infection may be problematic and no clinical trials of efficacy of this therapy have been reported (Best and Banatvala, 2000). The mainstay for control of rubella virus is prevention, and the success of this strategy may be gauged by the current rarity of CRS in developed countries.

Rubella vaccine is unusual in that it is not given to protect the individual to whom it is administered, but rather to protect the unborn child with whom that individual may have later contact. Universal childhood immunization of both sexes is designed to eradicate or at least prevent the epidemic spread of virus in the population. The alternative strategy of selective pre-pubertal vaccination provides protection to the pregnant woman and thus to the foetus but does not prevent or reduce virus circulation in the community. Universal childhood immunization was introduced in the US in 1969. However between 1985–96, 122 cases of CRS were reported in the US (Schluter et al., 1998), 44% of whom were born to Hispanic non-immunized mothers. High immigration levels and continued circulation of rubella in the community because of childhood vaccine uptake rates of <90% have meant that CRS continues to occur in the US. In 1970, the UK introduced a programme of selective immunization of pre-pubertal females. This led to large reduction in CRS (Figure 9.1) but did not eliminate it, and cases continued to be reported because of epidemics of rubella occurring in non-immunized children. Universal vaccination was thus introduced in 1988 and has been effective in eliminating epidemic spread. However, worldwide, CRS continues to be a problem. The WHO report that a universal childhood immunization programme now exists in 92% of developed countries, contrasting with only 36% of countries with transient economies, and 28% of developing countries (Robertson et al., 1997). On a global scale a high burden of CRS (0.6–2.2 per 1000 live births) still exists (Cutts et al., 1997).

Cytomegalovirus

Epidemiology

Human cytomegalovirus (HCMV; human herpes virus 5) is one of the eight herpes viruses capable of causing human infection (Van Loon, Cleator and

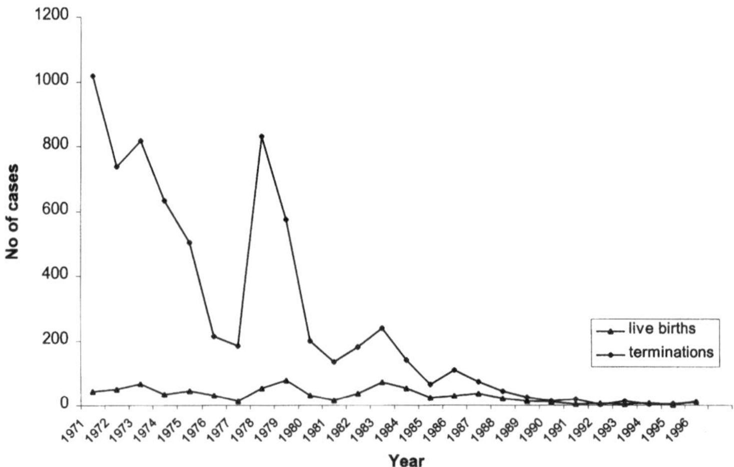

Figure 9.1. Registered congenital rubella births (in England, Scotland and Wales) and terminations (England and Wales only) for rubella contact or rubella disease (excludes those associated with inadvertent rubella vaccination in pregnancy) 1971–1996. Data kindly provided by Dr Pat Tookey.

Klapper, 1999) and has been shown to be endemic in every human population surveyed (Gold and Nankervis, 1982). Herpes viruses are relatively fragile and transmit most easily by direct contact between warm and moist mucosal surfaces. HCMV is transmitted predominantly by oropharyngeal secretions, but may be transmitted by urine, blood, cervical and vaginal secretions, semen, tears, faeces and in breast milk (Stagno et al., 1980). In common with all herpes viruses, HCMV establishes latency in its host following primary infection. Periodic reactivation occurs and virus is intermittently shed in saliva, urine and other secretions from healthy, asymptomatic carriers (Britt and Alford, 1996). This continued excretion ensures the successful circulation of the virus within the population. Antibody seroprevalence generally increases with age, but age of first acquisition varies widely among populations. Seroprevalence is higher and occurs at a younger age in developing countries and in lower socioeconomic groups (Gold and Nankervis, 1982; Britt and Alford, 1996). In higher socio-economic groupings, infection may be delayed and peaks of infection are seen in early adulthood.

Infection occurring in infancy is usually asymptomatic. Infection in adolescence or adulthood may be asymptomatic or may produce an infectious mononucleosis-like syndrome clinically indistinguishable from the more commonly described Epstein–Barr virus mediated infectious mononucleosis or glandular fever. However, HCMV can cause more significant disease in two groups: the immunocompromised, including recipients of organ transplants and individuals with acquired immune deficiency syndrome (AIDS) in whom CMV mediated pneumonitis, retinitis, gastrointestinal disease and encephalitis are often seen (Cinque et al., 1998); and secondly, in the congenitally infected neonate.

Cytomegalic inclusion disease (CID)

Human cytomegalovirus is now recognized as the most frequent cause of congenital infection in humans and is the leading non-hereditary cause of congenital sensorineural hearing impairment (Peckham et al., 1987; Hicks et al.,1993; Schildroth, 1994).

Congenital CMV infection occurs in approximately 1% of all newborns (Alford et al., 1990; Dobbins, Stewart and Demmler, 1992). Of these infected children 10% are symptomatic at birth, with half exhibiting the severe symptoms characteristic of CID. Unlike rubell avirus, HCMV is only weakly teratogenic and malformations associated with congenital disease arise from tissue destruction rather than interference with organogenesis. Cytomegalic inclusion disease involves multiple organs and causes prematurity and intrauterine growth retardation, petechiae, jaundice, hepatosplenomegaly, purpura, and microcephaly. Mortality among severely affected neonates may be as high as 30% (Stagno et al., 1983) with death typically occurring as a result of liver dysfunction, blood disorders or secondary bacterial infection. Permanent central nervous system sequelae are also common, including sensorineural hearing impairment, mental retardation, cerebral palsy, seizures, blindness and other visual defects. Hearing impairment is the most common neurological abnormality associated with congenital CMV infection and ranges from mild to profound (Britt and Alford, 1996). Although difficult to obtain precise figures, it is estimated that 60% of infants born with symptomatic CMV infection will suffer hearing impairment (Bopanna et al., 1992). A further 10%–15% of those asymptomatically infected at birth will also develop progressive hearing impairment or deterioration as a direct result of the congenital infection (Fowler et al., 1997).

Pathogenesis

In some geographic areas seropositivity rates of 90% to 100% have been recorded in women of child-bearing age. In Europe and the US, however, rates of between 50% and 80% are more usual (Stagno, 1995). Consequently, in the latter countries, significant numbers of women of childbearing age are susceptible to primary infection with HCMV. Although vertical transmission can occur during both primary and recurrent disease the consequences for the foetus are generally much more severe following primary maternal infection (Stagno et al., 1982).

Infection of the mother during pregnancy may occur via the oral or sexual route. Initially, a small amount of viral replication occurs in local epithelial cells. Human cytomegalovirus then enters the blood and it is during this viraemic phase that virus is probably passed transplacentally to the foetus. Reactivation of latent virus in the cervix is believed to be the source of foetal infection when CID occurs as a result of recurrent maternal infection. In addition to *in utero* infection HCMV can also be acquired perinatally during passage through the birth canal or post-natally as a result of virus shedding in breast milk and direct maternal contact.

Control of infection

In contrast to rubella, where it is possible to predict outcome in relation to timing of maternal infection, HCMV transmission may occur at all stages of pregnancy (Stagno et al., 1982). The risk of severe congenital damage is probably higher in the first half of gestation (Stagno, 1995). However, termination of all pregnancies complicated by primary CMV infection cannot be recommended. Neither identification of primary maternal infection nor direct evidence of foetal infection is predictive of outcome and only one in 30 pregnancies complicated by primary HCMV infection will result in the birth of a HCMV-damaged baby (Klapper and Morris, 1990).

A number of antiviral drugs have been developed for the treatment of HCMV infections (Cinque et al., 1998) and several novel compounds are under investigation (Martinez et al., 1999). Currently three antiviral drugs are available for the therapy of life-threatening HCMV infection; Ganciclovir, Famciclovir and Cidofovir. Unfortunately none is licensed for use in pregnant women or neonates because all are associated with significant side effects. The most widely available compound Ganciclovir is foetotoxic, toxic to bone marrow and may cause permanent infertility in women. This narrow therapeutic to toxic dose ratio precludes its use when most babies of infected mothers develop normally. The development of a vaccine to protect seronegative women from primary infection is desirable and a number of candidate vaccines have been proposed (Griffiths, 2000). However, as yet no effective immunization strategy is available and the situation is complicated by the occasional occurrence of CID in association with recurrent maternal infection (Figure 9.2). Eradication of congenital infection through immunization, a reasonable prospect for rubella, may not be achievable for CMV.

Toxoplasmosis

Epidemiology and pathogenesis

A less common cause of delayed hearing impairment arises from congenital infection with the protozoan parasite *Toxoplasma gondii*. Infection is usually asymptomatic and resolves spontaneously but may be associated

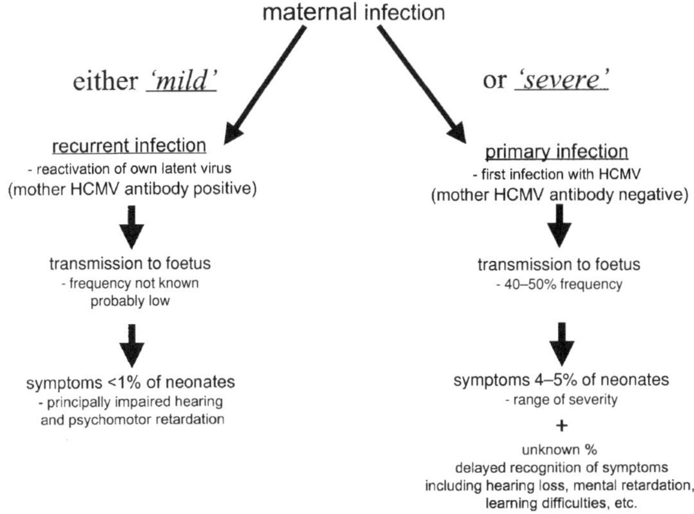

Figure 9.2. Risks and outcome of HCMV infection in pregnancy.

with a mild mononucleosis-like illness or 'flu-like' symptoms. However, as with HCMV, infection with *Toxoplasma gondii* can cause disease in the immunocompromised and severe congenital infection.

The parasite infects a wide range of both wild and domestic animals and appears to be transmitted to man via two main routes: consumption of undercooked meat from animals previously infected with *Toxoplasma gondii* or through direct or indirect contact with cat faeces (Figure 9.3).

Congenital toxoplasmosis

Congenital toxoplasmosis occurs when the mother acquires a primary infection during pregnancy. Estimates for the incidence of congenital toxoplasmosis range from 0.1 to 10 cases per 1000 live births (Roberts, Boyer and McLeod, 1998). Maternal infection in the first trimester of pregnancy carries a low risk of transmission to the foetus (4% to 25%) but a high risk of severe damage (40%) evidenced at birth (Desmontes and Couvreur, 1974; Daffos et al., 1988). As pregnancy progresses, the rate of transmission to the foetus increases (to 65% in the last trimester) but the risk of severe damage conversely reduces to effectively zero in the last trimester (Desmontes and Couvreur, 1974; Daffos et al., 1988). Severe cases of congenital toxoplasmosis are thus rare but show all or some of the tetrad of symptoms described by Sabin (1941) – chorioretinitis, cerebral calcification, hydrocephalus and mental subnormality. However, mild

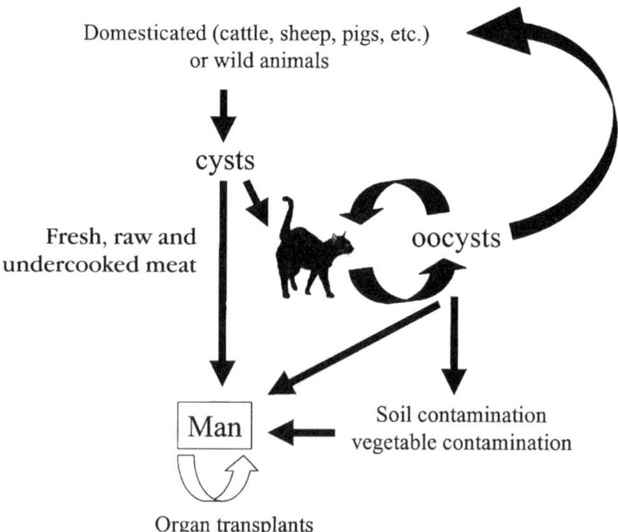

Figure 9.3. *Toxoplasma gondii* lifecycle and routes of human infection.

infection with *Toxoplasma gondii* may be underdiagnosed. As with HCMV, the majority of infected infants may be born symptom free but develop late sequelae. Retinal disease is the most common of these but late development of hearing impairment and some degree of mental retardation also occur, sometimes up to two decades later.

Control of infection

The principal method for the control of congenital toxoplasmosis is a strategy of primary prevention through health education. This involves educating mothers as to how toxoplasmosis is acquired and how infection may be prevented. A strategy of secondary prevention, which involves serological screening for infection throughout pregnancy has been adopted in some countries where seroprevalence of toxoplasmosis is high and the cost-benefit studies have indicated the need for such a programme (Conyn-Van Spaendonck and Van Knapen, 1992). Such strategies have reduced animal–human transmission and contributed to the general lowering of toxoplasma seroprevalence observed in developed countries since 1969 (Klapper and Morris, 1990).

Detection of specific toxoplasma antibody (IgA and IgM) in foetal blood, *in vitro* culture and detection of the parasite DNA in foetal blood and amniotic fluid can achieve identification of foetal infection (Couvreur, 1999; Robert-Gangneux et al., 1999). Where foetal infection is confirmed in the first trimester and detailed ultrasound study reveals abnormal morphological signs, termination of pregnancy is an option. Because the outcome of infection can be difficult to predict, specific treatment is an alternative when termination is not elected. Therapy with pyrimethamine, sulphadiazine and a folinic acid supplement for three weeks followed by three weeks of therapy with the antibiotic spiramycin is advised. This schedule is repeated throughout the pregnancy. When *in utero* infection is only identified at birth, the alternating three weeks of therapy is given to the infant over a period of one year. Treatment is important to prevent progressive post-natal morbidity including hearing impairment.

Treponema pallidum (syphilis)

Epidemiology

The development of the long-acting penicillins in the 1950s and the introduction of serological screening programmes for syphilis in pregnant women brought about a dramatic reduction in cases of both sexually and congenitally transmitted syphilis. However, the World Health Organization estimates that 12 million new cases of infectious syphilis still occur each year (CDSC, 1996) with highest rates in sub-Saharan Africa and South and

Southeast Asia (Linglof, 1995). The incidence of syphilis in the US increased in the late 1980s, partly due to a change in the reporting guidelines which expanded the definition of the syndrome, but also due to an increase in the actual numbers of cases of syphilis. By the early 1990s this had again declined and the 1998 data, which suggests an overall incidence rate of 20 cases of infectious syphilis per 100 000 population, with three cases of congenital syphilis per 100 000 live births, is the lowest rate yet recorded in the US (MMWR, 1999). In the UK the incidence of syphilis has declined to 0.47 per 100 000 (PHLS, 1999). However, the resurgence of the disease in Russia and the Baltic States (Linglof, 1995) is having an impact across Europe and there have been recent outbreaks in the UK (Deayton and French, 1997), Finland (Hiltunen-Back et al., 1996) and Italy (Smacchia et al., 1998) linked to contact with this region. Thus, even in countries where syphilis is well controlled the threat from imported syphilis is constant.

Congenital syphilis

Although many infants born to mothers with primary or secondary syphilis will be premature, stillborn or die during the neonatal period, the majority born with congenital syphilis are asymptomatic at birth. Symptoms may appear at any time within the first two years of life, when they are termed 'early' manifestations, or if they occur after this they are considered as 'late' manifestations.

Active, disseminated foetal infection and the subsequent inflammatory response produce very early manifestations (three to seven weeks after birth). Hepatosplenomegaly, lesions on the skin, rhinitis, inflammation of the long bones, anaemia and thrombocytopenia together with low birth weight and failure to thrive are seen. Where deafness is a complication of congenital syphilis it appears as a late manifestation, typically when the child is eight to ten years of age, although occasionally it may be delayed until adulthood. Onset is sudden and usually occurs as part of 'Hutchinson's triad' (Fiumara and Lessell, 1970), which includes notched incisor teeth, interstitial keratitis and eighth cranial nerve deafness. Damage to the cranial nerve is thought to result from a persistent and ongoing inflammatory response to the infection. Impairment of hearing may be unilateral or bilateral and initially involves higher frequencies, with normal conversational tones affected later. Facial abnormalities – a 'saddle' nose, protuberant mandible, central nervous system (CNS) abnormality (mental retardation, optic nerve atrophy) and bone or joint involvement (frontal bossing of the skull, 'saber' shins, hypertrophy of the sternoclavicular joints) – may also be present and point to a diagnosis of congenital syphilis.

Pathogenesis

Congenital infection occurs by transplacental transfer of the organism from the infected mother, and can occur at any stage of pregnancy. However, the prognosis for the foetus is considerably worse if infection occurs during the first or second trimester.

Both primary maternal syphilis and untreated secondary syphilis threaten the foetus. Primary maternal syphilis will result in prematurity, stillbirth or death in the first year of life in 35% of cases, with a further 40% developing symptoms of congenital disease. In secondary syphilis 10% develop symptoms of congenital disease and 10% may be stillborn. Pregnancy during the first year of an untreated early syphilis infection has an 80% to 90% risk of transmission to the foetus. This risk declines over time and by the fourth year of infection transmission to the foetus is rare.

Control of infection

The development of ante-natal maternal screening programmes is the key to prevention of congenital syphilis. When infection is identified, penicillin is the treatment of choice and although antibiotic therapy during pregnancy can be problematic (Rolfs, 1995), effective therapy is essential if a favourable outcome to the pregnancy is to be achieved. Congenital syphilis, and particularly late congenital syphilis, is extremely rare in developed countries. However, the recent resurgence in primary and secondary syphilis among young women suggests that constant vigilance is required and late congenital syphilis must continue to be considered as a cause of childhood hearing impairment.

Other congenital infections resulting in hearing impairment

Herpes simplex virus

Congenital deafness has been attributed to infection with herpes simplex virus (HSV) (Veltri et al., 1981). Most cases of infection appearing in the neonatal period are a result of perinatal or post-natal acquisition of virus. Baldwin and Whitley (1989) considered that only 5% of all babies born with neonatal HSV had been infected *in utero*. This was based on the criteria that such infection would result in symptoms (skin vesicles or scarring, chorioretinitis, and/or hydranencephaly) within the first 24 to 48 hours of life. The reported incidence of neonatal herpes varies from extremes of one case in 2500 live births (Whitley, 1993) to 1.65 per 100 000 live births reported in a UK survey (Tookey and Peckham, 1996). Thus, *in utero* infection with HSV is most probably a rare occurrence but the mortality rate is high and most children who survive have neurological sequelae including hearing impairment.

Herpes varicella-zoster virus

Primary infection with herpes varicella-zoster virus (VZV) during the first trimester and early part of the second trimester can, rarely, result in transmission of the virus to the foetus. At birth, infants have cutaneous scars and exhibit a range of congenital damage including eye abnormalities, limb deformation, cortical atrophy, mental retardation and hearing impairment. It is possible that milder cases occur with residual auditory morbidity only apparent in later life.

Other infections

A number of other organisms associated with congenital infection have, occasionally and anecdotally, been cited as a cause of audiological morbidity. These include Epstein–Barr virus, Human herpes viruses 6, 7 and 8, measles virus, mumps virus, parvovirus B-19, enteroviruses, and lymphocytic choriomeningitis virus, *Borrellia burgdorferi* (Lyme disease), and Mycoplasmas. A major problem of proving an association between congenital damage and maternal infection with these agents is the rarity with which maternal infection during pregnancy is proven. This is compounded by the often long interval between birth and observations of hearing impairment in an infant.

Acquired infections

Principal causes of acquired infections leading to hearing impairment

Mumps virus

Mumps is a distinctive childhood illness characterized by swelling of one or both parotid glands. In areas where vaccination is administered routinely the infection is now rare. However, mumps remains endemic in many areas of the world. The typical salivary gland swelling usually occurs within 24 hours, progresses for two or three days and subsides within one week. The most common complications are orchitis, pancreatitis and aseptic meningitis (5% to 25% of cases – Gershon, 1995).

Hearing impairment is a rare but serious complication, occurring in five of every 10 000 cases of mumps. The onset of hearing impairment is sudden and usually unilateral (80% of cases). It occurs as part of the acute infection, usually in association with aseptic meningitis and is often accompanied by vertigo, tinnitus, ataxia and vomiting. The overall severity of the infection does not determine whether hearing impairment will be a feature. Mumps hearing impairment tends to be profound and permanent, preferentially affecting the higher frequencies although it may remain unnoticed for a time, especially if the child is very young at infection (Kayan, 1990). Asymptomatic mumps virus infection has recently been demonstrated to be a cause of sudden and total bilateral deafness (Unal et al., 1998). It has been suggested that such asymptomatic infection may be responsible for some cases of unexplained, mild, sudden hearing impairment (Okamoto et al., 1994).

Although mumps sequelae such as hearing impairment are rare, the consequences when they do occur are severe. For this reason mumps immunization, given as part of the mumps, measles and rubella (MMR) vaccine is now routine in most developed countries.

Measles virus

Measles virus infection (rubeola), is the most contagious of all the childhood diseases. The characterizing features of the infection are the appearance of the pathognomonic enanthem, Koplik's spots, on the buccal mucous membranes, followed within one or two days by a generalized maculopapular rash. Infectious virus continues to be shed until approximately four days after the appearance of the rash, contributing to the epidemic spread. Although the disease is usually self-limiting, occasionally complications are seen. The most common sites of involvement of measles complications are the respiratory tract (pneumonia), the CNS (acute encephalomyelitis or, later, sub-acute sclerosing pan encephalitis (SSPE)) and the ear (otitis media and virus-induced sensorineural hearing impairment).

Permanent hearing impairment following measles virus infection occurs in up to 1 in 1 000 cases. The loss is usually sudden and bilateral, and occurs at the same time as the appearance of the measles rash. Prior to the introduction of measles vaccine, the virus was the cause of 3% to 10% of all acquired hearing impairment in children (Lindsay, 1973).

Complications resulting from childhood measles infection remain a problem, particularly in developing countries. However, measles vaccine, either presented alone or given as a combined measles, mumps and rubella (MMR) vaccination has been demonstrated to be safe and effective. The WHO-implemented global strategy has the ultimate goal of eradicating the infection (CDC, 1997).

Bacterial meningitis

Epidemiology

In contrast to the more common viral ('aseptic') meningitis that is usually mild and self-limiting, bacterial meningitis is associated with high mortality and high levels of residual morbidity. At least 50 different species of bacteria can cause meningitis (Table 9.3). The main types involved are Meningococcus species, Pneumococcus species, Group B Streptococcus, *Escherichia coli, Listeria monocytogenes, Haemophilus influenza B* and *Mycobacterium tuberculosis.* In premature babies and neonatal cases *Escherichia coli* (*E.coli*), Group B Streptococcus, and *Listeria monocytogenes* predominate (Dawson, Emerson and Burns, 1999) while *Haemophilus influenza, Streptococcous pneumoniae,* and *Neisseria meningitidis* are common in childhood. Overall, sensorineural hearing impairment occurs in approximately 10% of all cases of bacterial meningitis (Baraff, Lee and Schriger, 1993). However pneumococcal meningitis is particularly associated with auditory complications with an incidence of sensorineural hearing impairment of 18% to 30% (Rasmussen, Johnson and Bohr, 1991).

Pathogenesis

Infection of the central nervous system usually follows septicaemia after the organism has first colonized a mucosal surface. Perinatal acquisition may result from contact with infected maternal mucosal secretions (Peter and Nelson, 1978), whereas in an older child infection is most likely to be acquired following colonization of the nasopharynx. Bacteria replicate in the blood stream, and gain access to the brain most frequently via the choroid plexus. However, it is possible for an organism to gain direct entry into the CNS via a middle-ear infection or from a paranasal sinus. Occasionally severe head trauma can allow bacterial invasion of the meninges.

Damage to hearing is thought to occur early in the infection, probably within the first 24 to 48 hours (Brookhouser, Auslander and Meskan, 1988). As this is typically around the time of admission to hospital, hearing impairment is usually apparent within six hours of first assessment (Richardson et al., 1997). Both clinical studies and animal models have

Table 9.3. Causes of bacterial meningitis

Neonates	Gram negative bacilli (e.g. *Escherichia coli*, Group B streptococci, *Listeria monocytogenes*
Infants	*Haemophilus influenzae*, *Neisseria meningitidis*, *Streptococcus pneumoniae*, *Mycobacterium tuberculosis*
Older children	*Neisseria meningitidis*, *Streptococcus pneumoniae*, *Listeria monocytogenes*, *Mycobacterium tuberculosis*, *Staphylococcus aureus* (in skull fracture)

shown that duration of infection before antibiotic treatment begins is strongly linked to development of auditory impairment, and early administration of therapy is essential to prevent permanent impairment (Bhatt et al., 1995; Richardson et al., 1997; Winter et al., 1998). In some cases the hearing impairment is temporary, with improvement noted over a two-week recovery period. No improvement in recovery of hearing beyond the initial two-week period has been observed (Kaplan et al., 1984; Vienny et al., 1984). Conversely, no reports of 'late' onset hearing impairment have been described, although hearing impairment in a neonate occurring in the course of the meningitis may not be apparent until the child is older. The pattern of hearing impairment varies, but usually it is bilateral, severe and permanent involving both high and low frequencies (Nadol, 1978; Dodge et al., 1984; Kaplan et al., 1984; Vienny et al., 1984; Baldwin, Sweitzer and Friend, 1985).

Control of infection

Bacterial meningitis is always a medical emergency necessitating prompt and aggressive antimicrobial therapy. However, there is increasing evidence (see 'pathology of hearing impairment') that deafness due to meningitis is partly or wholly due to an inappropriate host inflammatory response to the bacteria or its products. For this reason, administration of steroid therapy, such as dexamethasone, together with the antibiotics has been suggested (Kaplan et al., 1984; Odio et al., 1991). However, this adjunct therapy remains controversial with other studies showing no reduction in hearing impairment when dexamethasone is given (Wald et al., 1995; Richardson et al., 1997).

As with most infections, prevention of bacterial meningitis is preferable to, and more successful than, treatment. Perinatal infection may be controlled by prospective study of the mother. Common genitourinary infections including bacterial vaginosis, trichomoniasis, chlamydia, and gonorrhoeae result in large numbers of babies being born prematurely. These babies suffer complications frequently requiring neonatal intensive care and the long-term consequences of these infections are cerebral palsy, mental retardation, blindness and hearing impairment (McGregor and French, 1997). Controlled trials suggest that many premature births could be prevented by identification and treatment of bacterial vaginosis in pregnancy (Hillier et al., 1995). Undoubtedly, improved surveillance and identification of 'at-risk' pregnancies may prevent many cases of neonatal infection. The vaccine against *Haemophilus influenzae* type B is now widely administered in childhood. Meningococcal vaccines effective against serogroup strains A and C are available and vaccine for serogroup B is under active development.

Other causes of acquired infection causing hearing impairment

Mycobacterium tuberculosis

Cases of *Mycobacterium tuberculosis* infection have increased in recent years and drug resistant forms of the bacterium threaten existing control of the disease. Tuberculosis involving the middle ear can be a first indication of the infection. Chronic otorrhoea and perforations of the tympanic membrane are seen and without prompt anti-tuberculous therapy complications of infection including the development of tuberculoma may result in permanent hearing impairment (Skolnik, Nadol and Baker, 1986).

Borrelia burgdorferi (Lyme disease)

Lyme disease, caused by infection with the tick-borne spirochaete *Borrellia burgdorferi,* results in frequent neurological complications and permanent sensorineural hearing impairment (Logigian, Kaplan and Steere, 1990). In common with other spirochaete infections, the manifestations of Lyme disease are varied and may be characterized as early, intermediate or late stages of the disease. Neurological symptoms, including hearing impairment are a part of the late manifestation of the disease. The exact mechanism of hearing impairment is unknown, but it is possibly due to direct damage to the auditory centre, the eighth cranial nerve, or labyrinthitis.

Fungal infections

Fungal infections resulting in hearing impairment are rare but meningitis caused by *Candida albicans* has been noted, particularly in babies of low birth weight. In addition *Cryptococcus neoformans,* Aspergillus species, and *Pneumocycstis carinii* may all cause meningitis with residual auditory impairment in immunocompromised patients.

Visceral leishmaniasis

A number of protozoal infections are capable of producing CNS infections that may include hearing impairment among their residual morbidity. For example, visceral leishmaniasis caused by *Leishmania donovani* can cause retrocochlear hearing impairment. Nerve conduction studies suggest demyelination as a principle cause of hearing impairment that resolves after successful treatment of the infection (Hashim et al., 1995).

Rubella

Post-natal rubella rarely affects hearing. Where it has been reported, it affects adults rather than children and presents as unilateral sensorineural hearing impairment (Kobayashi, Suzuki and Nomura, 1994), contrasting with the profound bilateral hearing impairment seen following congenital rubella infection.

Human immunodeficiency virus (HIV)

Most HIV infection in children results from perinatal transmission. Although the infections encountered by the HIV-positive child are those common in childhood, impaired immunity may render them severe, chronic, and more frequently recurrent. Thus the child is potentially susceptible to all of the infectious causes of hearing impairment described previously. In addition, HIV itself has been suggested to be an ototoxic virus, since hearing impairment is seen in HIV-infected patients who do not have evidence of significant immunosuppression (Marra et al., 1996). Overall the prevalence of hearing impairment in HIV-infected children is unknown, but studies suggest that up to 49% of individuals with HIV show some degree of audiological abnormality (Lalwani and Sooy, 1992; Madriz and Herrera, 1995).

Herpes simplex and herpes varicella-zoster viruses

Neonatal HSV infection is rare but can have severe manifestations. It usually occurs in neonates without protective maternal HSV antibody and infection with HSV-2 is typically more severe than that caused by HSV-1. If untreated, mortality exceeds 50% and children with disseminated infection have the worst prognosis. Even with prompt administration of specific antiviral chemotherapy, survivors may have various degrees of psychomotor retardation and hearing impairment is common among these.

An analogous disease, severe neonatal chickenpox (varicella) may occur when maternal varicella presents within five days of delivery. Neonatal VZV infection is fatal in approximately 30% of cases and, as with neonatal HSV infection, survivors often exhibit some degree of hearing impairment.

Other infections

It is likely that many cases of sudden hearing impairment are attributable to infection and the causes will undoubtedly emerge as diagnostic methodology continues to improve. In addition to congenital infection both perinatal and post-natally acquired *Treponema pallidum* infection can result in loss of hearing. Clinical symptoms are of unilateral or bilateral hearing impairment but may also present as Ménière's syndrome (Hendershot, 1978; Rothenberg, 1979). Many viral infections of the central nervous system can produce residual auditory impairment as a result of central or peripheral nerve damage. Epidemics of CNS infection may have, as late sequelae, increased occurrence of auditory impairment such as observed in tick-borne encephalitis in children (Cizman et al., 1999). Damage incurred through such infection is unpredictable and in many cases an aberrant immune response triggered by a severe virus infection is a more plausible explanation of audiological deterioration than direct viral involvement. Microbial associated toxicity (as for example in pneumococcal infection) or toxicity indirectly caused as a result of infection (for example, in fulminant viral hepatitis where excessive bilirubinaemia has been suggested as a cause of cochlear damage) presents a further source for infection associated hearing impairment.

The pathology of hearing impairment associated with infection

Hearing impairment following infection may result from direct cytolytic effects of the pathogen within the inner ear, from immune mediated damage due to the inflammatory response to the organism, or as a consequence of damage to the auditory nerves following CNS infection.

A number of early studies examined the temporal bones taken post-mortem from infants congenitally infected with rubella or CMV, or who died after measles or mumps infection (Lindsay and Hemenway, 1954a, 1954b; Lindsay, Davey and Ward, 1960; Myers and Stool, 1968; Davis, 1969; Bordley and Kapur, 1977). These studies described common histopathological features, principally of endolymphatic labyrinthitis, with pathological changes limited almost entirely to the membranous labyrinth; in particular, the cochlear duct, saccule and utricle. However, although the common pathology indicates a common mechanism of damage to the specific audiological structures, it is evident from the detail of the reports that the significant lesions may be mediated differently depending on the individual pathogen involved.

Lindsay and Hemingway (1954b) reported the case of an infant who had died after measles complications. The structures in the cochlea showed degeneration that was greater at the basal coil and diminished towards the apex so that, in the basal coil, only slight remnants of stria remained and Corti's organ was absent. Only a small fraction of the normal number of nerve fibres remained and the ganglia were greatly reduced. In the middle and apical coils more of the stria and organ of Corti was present and the nerve cells were approximately normal in number, but there were areas in the remaining stria vascularis of the apical coil where a localized inflammatory reaction around actively proliferating foci of infection was evident. They suggested that the viral infection of the inner ear occurred via the stria vascularis, beginning at the basal coil. Release of virus and inflammatory cells into the endolymph caused infection further into the coils of the cochlea, with resultant destruction of the nerve cells secondary to the initial infection. The stria vascularis in the cochlea is a site rich in capillaries, and therefore a likely portal of entry for the blood borne virus.

In 1968, Lindsay et al. (1960) described the temporal bone pathology in a case of mumps deafness. Similar to the measles case described above, they found that the pathologic changes were confined primarily to the cochlear duct and consisted of degeneration of the stria vascularis, the organ of Corti and the tectorial membrane in the basal coil of the cochlea, with damage diminishing progressively towards the apex. However, the case described was unusual for mumps deafness in that it was bilateral. Earlier work (Evenberg, 1957) suggested that hearing impairment resulting from mumps infection more usually occurred because of viral invasion of the meninges. Encroachment of the localized meningeal lesion on the acoustic nerve would produce a pathology more likely to lead to unilateral hearing impairment.

Congenital rubella is now thought to be unique in that its principal effect is that of a teratogen interfering with the genesis of normal organs. Inner ear malformation manifests as a lack of development of hair cells and supporting cells especially in the apical coil of the cochlea. The tectorial membrane is found rolled up against the limbus in contact with Reissner's membrane and is enclosed in a sheath of flattened cells. The saccular membrane may be hypertrophic and adherent to a degenerated macula, or collapsed and the stria vascularis may be partly or totally absent (Lindsay and Hemenway, 1954a). It is likely that rubella acts on the epithelial cells of the developing labyrinth resulting in the cochleosaccular degeneration described (Strauss and Davis, 1973).

Myers and Stool (1968) were first to examine the inner ear pathology in a fatal neonatal case of cytomegalic inclusion disease. In contrast to the changes noted in some other viral inner ear infections no obvious involvement of the organ of Corti or curling of the tectorial membrane was noted in this or later studies (Davis, 1969; Strauss, 1990). For most viral infections, demonstration of the actual virus within the ear has not been achieved, presumably because the temporal bones are examined at too late a stage in the infection. In the case of CMV however, characteristic cytomegalic nuclear inclusions have been described, located in the epithelial cells of the cochlea, saccule, utricle and semicircular canals and demonstrating the susceptibility of the entire ear to this virus.

Indeed, evidence for more extensive distribution of virus than the areas of manifest cellular damage has been provided by the use of CMV specific immunofluorescent antibodies, which demonstrated the presence of viral antigen in the organ of Corti, and in neuromas of the eighth cranial nerve (Stagno, et al., 1977). In 1979, Davis et al. isolated CMV from the perilymph of an infant who died from congenital CMV. In a further study, the same group (Davis et al., 1981) reported a congenitally CMV-infected infant who showed no evidence of CMV-induced hearing impairment and no histopathologic changes to the inner ear. The child died of encephalitis of undetermined etiology, but which was presumed to be due to HSV. Post mortem, CMV was isolated from the inner ear fluid, but not from the adjacent brain tissue. The infant was five months old and the authors suggested that CMV is capable of persisting in the ear for prolonged periods without causing destruction to the cochlea. They speculated that the delayed and progressive hearing impairment following congenital infection may have been due to the virus either slowly causing direct damage to the critical inner ear cells, or to a delayed host immune response causing immunopathologic damage.

The presence of an inflammatory cell response in most cases that have been investigated has raised the possibility that the damage to the inner ear is partly due to an immunopathological response as well as direct viral cytopathology. In support of this hypothesis, Harris, Fan and Keithley (1990) described an animal model for CMV labyrinthitis wherein a positive relationship between the degree and extent of inflammatory reaction in the cochlea and hearing impairment was found. No such correlation existed between CMV antigen level and hearing impairment. The authors suggested that the inflammatory response may be of more importance in causing inner ear damage than is the direct effect of the virus. More recently, a case was reported which described the temporal bone histopathology in a child who died at 14 years of age from the sequelae of congenital CMV infection (Rarey and Davis, 1993). No virus could be isolated from the inner ear (or from any other tissues) but the damage to the ear structures was more extensive than that previously reported from the infant cases. Atrophy of the stria vascularis and loss of cochlear hair cells was noted along the entire length of the basilar membrane. There was evidence of damage to vestibular as well as cochlear structures and the overall finding was of chronic immunopathologic damage.

Collectively, the histopathology of the CMV-infected inner ears suggests that hearing impairment in the acute stage of the disease is caused by viral cytolysis. Whereas the delayed or progressive hearing impairment often associated with congenital infection may result from damage caused by the immunological response to the infection.

It has been suggested that the hearing impairment associated with bacterial meningitis may result from bacterial or inflammation-induced damage to the auditory nerve, or from lesions in the brainstem or higher centres. However, although there are few recent reports describing the pathology of the inner ear in cases of hearing impairment following meningitis in humans, earlier studies and data derived from animal models, provide evidence that the principal cause is a cochlear lesion (Igarishi and Schucknecht, 1962; Wiedermann et al., 1986; Kaplan et al., 1989; Bhatt, Halpin and Hsu, 1991; Kay, 1991; Bhatt et al., 1993). It is known from human studies that bacteria accumulating in the subarachnoid space can invade the cochlea via the cochlear aqueduct (Igarishi and Schucknecht, 1962) and that the resulting labyrinthitis causes damage to the inner ear.

Experimental data show that introduction of antigen into the inner ear of an animal previously sensitized systemically, produces an immune response in the ear against the antigen. The resulting cellular infiltration and inflammation, release of cytokines and triggering of the complement cascade are all likely to damage the delicate cochlear tissue. However, it is not evident why this immune-mediated pathology should cause damage to the auditory processes more frequently than to other neurological structures, nor why the pneumococcal organism causes hearing impairment more often than do other etiological agents of meningitis. Although there is little doubt that inflammatory mediated damage plays an important role in hearing impairment resulting from infection, further data suggest that in some infections, the bacterial products themselves are directly ototoxic. In particular the pneumococcal toxin, pneumolysin, has been found to induce severe damage to the inner ear in experimental meningitis. When the toxin was introduced directly into the scala tympani, lesions appeared on the hair cells within a few minutes suggesting that the toxin is able to cross the basilar membrane, and that its effect is caused by a direct, rather than an indirect action (Comis et al., 1993). A similar experiment using the *E.coli* endotoxin produced lesions also but the effect was much less severe and occurred more slowly. It is possible that the potency of pneumolysin may account for the increased ototoxicity of pneumococcal meningitis.

Whether directly or indirectly mediated, pathological damage to the various cell types in the cochlea will result in loss of hearing. As transduction of sound pressure into electrical impulses is dependent on intact stereocilia, damage to the hair cells would inevitably disrupt this process. Similarly, damage to the nerve endings at the base of the hair cell would interfere with the generation of nerve impulses along the auditory nerve (Osborne et al., 1995). As auditory hair cells are not thought to be capable of regeneration in mammals, including humans, damage to the hair cells would lead to permanent hearing impairment. Damage to nerve endings, on the other hand, is more likely to be temporary. Stereocilia have been shown to be highly susceptible to pneumolysin (Winter et al., 1998) which might explain the higher incidence of permanent hearing impairment following pneumococcal meningitis.

In summary, hearing impairment resulting from infection, although not completely understood, is likely to be mediated by a number of mechanisms that are dependent on the organism involved, the stage of disease, and the immune response mounted against the pathogen. Rubella appears to be the only organism that causes deafness by interfering with foetal inner ear development. Where central nervous system infection occurs, damage to the acoustic nerves is possible. Alternatively, the organism may invade the inner ear from the meninges or from the blood system and cause direct cytopathic damage, in particular to the delicate cochlear structures. This damage may be compounded by the indirect, immunopathologic, effects of the immune response mounted against the pathogen. In some cases, particularly perhaps following congenital CMV infection, the virus persists in the inner ear and a delayed immune response occurring several years later may be responsible for late onset hearing impairment.

Laboratory diagnosis and treatment

The identification of an infectious cause of hearing impairment is often problematic. In many instances intra-uterine or perinatal infections are not apparent or symptoms are mild and non-specific. Associated hearing impairment may not be apparent for months or even years after the initial infection. In such circumstances conventional diagnostic procedures designed to culture the pathogen or identify some component (for example, antigen or nucleic acid) of the causative organism will fail. Often serological investigation will be the only viable route to establish a diagnosis and because of the length of time elapsing between infection and observation of hearing impairment, such evidence may at best be circumstantial.

Initial valuable information may be gained by obtaining a detailed clinical and family history, including where possible, immunization records for the child, details of foreign travel and times of exposure to likely causal agents. The physical and audiological examination should include neurological and ocular tests as these can often guide laboratory investigation. Relevant information should then be communicated to the diagnostic microbiology and virology services to enable appropriate laboratory investigations to be carried out.

Congenital infection

Identification in the immediate post-natal period

Identification of the causative agent is most easily achieved in the period immediately following birth. However, as many of the congenital infections that may result in later hearing impairment are asymptomatic at birth, it is usually only the minority of cases exhibiting severe symptoms that will be investigated at this time.

Culture of virus and detection of virus antigen in cells from the urine, or detection of virus DNA by the nucleic acid amplification technique; the polymerase chain reaction (PCR), represent reliable methods for the detection of HCMV excretion (Revello et al., 1994; Oda et al., 1995). It is probable that virus isolation from saliva is also a good marker of infection (Balcarek et al., 1993). Symptomatic neonates with congenital cytomegalovirus infection shed virus in urine for periods of two or more years post-partum. The congenitally infected foetus appears to develop immunological 'tolerance' to the pathogen and an appropriate immunological response is delayed. Prolonged excretion of virus thus provides clear evidence of congenital infection, and failure to identify an immune response to the virus in the neonate does not preclude intra-uterine infection.

In contrast to HCMV congenital infection, infections with rubella virus, *Treponema pallidum* and *Toxoplasma gondii* usually result in production of specific IgM antibody in the neonate. Toxoplasmosis may also be identified by culture of the parasite (intra-cerebral inoculation of suckling mice) and/or identification of *Toxoplasma gondii* DNA by PCR. In the case of syphilis, if papules or mucosal ulcers are available for examination, *Treponema pallidum* may be observed in these samples using dark-field microsocopy.

The diagnosis of congenital infection with HSV or VZV may be achieved by virus culture, detection of viral DNA and by electron microscopic examination of vesicle fluids. Maternal serology will usually reveal the presence of virus specific IgM in initial samples, followed by IgG in later sera. The neonate may initially be seronegative with the appearance of IgM antibody delayed for six months or more. Negative neonatal serology does not therefore preclude a diagnosis of HSV or VZV infection.

Investigation of possible maternal infection is as important and urgent as investigation of the neonate. The maternal antenatal serological specimen should be retrieved wherever possible to allow comparative pre- and post-natal serology. Diagnosis of congenital infection is best established by comparison of the results obtained in the maternal and the neonatal specimens (Table 9.4).

Table 9.4. Investigation of congenital infection and infection evident in the neonatal period: diagnostic specimens and appropriate tests

Infant

	PCR	**Culture**	**Serology (IgG & IgM)****
Urine	(+)	+	–
Throat swab	(+)	+	–
CSF	(+)	+	+
Blood	(+)	+	+
Vesicles or other lesions	(+)	+	–

In newborn infants investigation of both mother and baby is essential

(+) Test may be appropriate in certain circumstances

** Determination of IgG avidity is a valuable adjunct to IgM detection in defining recent infection. In recent infection low avidity IgG antibody will be detected while in old or recurrent infection high avidity IgG antibody will be present.

Mother

Serological investigation for recent infection with:

Herpes simplex virus
Herpes varicella-zoster virus
Human cytomegalovirus
Human immunodeficiency viruses 1 and 2
Hepatitis B
Rubella virus
Toxoplasma gondii
Treponema pallidum

Where possible examine routine ante-natal blood specimen in parallel with post-natal blood specimen.

Identification after the neonatal period

During the first six to nine months of life caution must be exercised in interpretation of serological test results because the detection of antibody may merely reflect passively transferred maternal antibody rather than infection (Table 9.5). Serological investigation of a child that reveals *Treponema pallidum* or *Toxoplasma gondii* infection after six to nine

Table 9.5. Acquired infection: diagnostic specimens and appropriate tests

	PCR	Culture	Serology (IgG & IgM)**
Urine[1]	–	+	–
Blood	(+)	+	+

[1]Important specimen for detection of HCMV congenital infection. Virus excretion can occur for 2 or more years post-natally.

Serological diagnosis is likely to be the mainstay of diagnosis in the asymptomatic child or in a child being investigated at a late stage. Serological investigation should include investigation of both child and mother and, if appropriate, siblings or other immediate family members. Where possible, examine mother's routine ante-natal blood specimen in parallel with post-natal blood specimen.

Select appropriate laboratory tests in relation to maternal, family and geographical history.

months of age provides supportive evidence for congenital or early infection with these agents because these are rare infections of childhood. At 12 to 15 months of age, detection of antibody to rubella may or may not reflect congenital infection since immunization against rubella is given at this time. Similarly the detection of HCMV, HSV or HVZV antibody cannot provide clear evidence of congenital infection since most primary infections with these viruses occur in childhood (Van Loon et al., 1999).

Post-natal infection

Bacterial meningitis, particularly when presenting with bacterial septicaemia is a major medical emergency. While meningitis is usually secondary to a bacteraemia, infection can also result from spread from a focus of infection in the ear, sinuses or from a skull fracture. A variety of rapid diagnostic procedures including antigen detection, nucleic acid hybridization and PCR techniques have been developed to supplement conventional blood and CSF culture procedures. However, not all cases are amenable to diagnosis. Prompt administration of antibacterial agents, although essential for patient management, may preclude identification of the causal agent, whilst cryptic sites of infection may limit the availability of organism in conventional diagnostic specimens (blood and CSF). A wide variety of organisms may cause such infection and the type of organism involved will vary with age (Table 9.3).

Acute stage viral infections in children may be diagnosed by virus culture, identification of specific viral antigens using ELISA-based techniques or by detection of specific nucleic acids using molecular assays such as PCR. It must be remembered however, that it is a feature of most virus infections that, by the time symptoms are evident, the peak of viral replication is over and thus, if a virus is to be identified, early collection of appropriate specimens is essential. Serological investigation of infection can be achieved later, either via detection of virus specific IgM or by detection of a rising level of virus specific IgG antibody in suitably spaced specimens.

Summary

Infection is a significant cause of paediatric hearing impairment. Except in the case of CMV, hearing impairment is rarely the only, or principal, feature of the infection. However, the delayed onset of deafness attributed to some infections, particularly congenital ones, makes it likely that the role of infectious organisms in the epidemiology of hearing impairment is presently underestimated. A number of viruses, only briefly considered here, have been occasionally associated with loss of hearing in children or young adults and it is likely that, as diagnostic methods improve, further associations will be made. The decline in hearing impairment attributed to rubella, measles and mumps viruses, and to some forms of bacterial meningitis, demonstrates the success of an effective immunization programme. Future improvements in both the diagnosis of paediatric infection and vaccine development promise continued decline in the incidence of preventable childhood hearing impairment.

CHAPTER 10

Adverse perinatal factors associated with hearing impairment

VE NEWTON

Introduction

Animal experiments and clinical investigations have implicated a number of perinatal factors as causative of sensorineural hearing impairment. These include low gestation and low birthweight, hypoxia, hypoxic-ischaemia, hyperbilirubinaemia, sepsis and the use of aminoglycosides. Determining whether any or all of these potential causative factors have actually given rise to the hearing impairment of any one particular infant is more problematic. The hearing impairment may have been caused by events that occurred earlier in the pregnancy and the perinatal problems may have been a result of these factors. Traumatic events around the time of birth may occur in families with a history of genetic hearing impairment, in instances of congenital intrauterine infection or other congenital conditions. Whereas it was once believed that birth trauma caused cerebral palsy, Nelson and Ellenberg (1986) were able to show that in many cases the cause predated the time of birth. Retrospective allocation of a perinatal etiology is therefore not straightforward for the clinician.

For the reasons given above the investigation of a sensorineural hearing impairment is important in spite of a history of perinatal problems, to see if any pre-natal cause can be identified. These investigations should be carried out as soon as possible after the hearing impairment has been identified. A careful history would include time of onset of the hearing impairment, its course and whether or not it was associated with balance problems. A family history should be taken and should include both a history of hearing impairment and a list of features in family members that could indicate a syndrome. Autosomal dominant conditions can be highly variable in expressivity and only specific questions would indicate the presence of a syndrome. A history of syncopal episodes in a family member or early death could indicate a recessively inherited syndrome with a manageable cardiac conduction defect.

Examination of the child is important to detect craniofacial abnormalities that may indicate a particular syndrome and it is necessary to see other members of the immediate family. Seeing other close relatives who have a hearing impairment from birth or early childhood could also be helpful. Laboratory investigations should include serology to identify the TORCH infections and other tests should include an ECG, serum creatinine and urinalysis. A magnetic resonance scan or CT scan should be performed as this investigation may reveal a cochlear or neural defect indicating that the cause of the hearing impairment was early in intrauterine development. Ophthalmological examination is important as children with a hearing impairment have a greater likelihood of visual defects, but also because examination of the fundi may help to indicate that a congenital infection has occurred. Increasingly, it will become possible to test for specific gene mutations as part of the investigation protocol.

Prevalence of sensorineural hearing loss

The proportion of sensorineural hearing loss attributed to perinatal causation is shown in Table 10.1 Comparison between studies is made difficult by the different criteria used to define the hearing-impaired population under investigation and the different criteria used to allocate cases as being of perinatal origin (Davidson et al., 1988). In some instances the criteria are not specified.

Table 10.1. Proportion of sensorineural hearing impairment attributable to perinatal causes

Author	Year	Hearing loss criteria (dB HL, BE)	Frequency Range (kHz)	Type of study	% Perinatal causes
Parving	1984	>35	0.5–4	Population	14
Newton	1985	>25	0.5–4	Population	13.5
Parving	1988	>35	0.5–4	Population	10.1
Das	1991	>25	0.5–4	Population	12.7
Van Rijn and Cremers	1991	>35	0.25–8	School-based	14.9
Fortnum and Davis	1997	>35	0.5–4	Population	6.1
Sutton and Rowe	1997	>25	0.5–4	Population	6.8

BE – better ear.

Perinatal risk factors for hearing impairment

Davis (1993b) found that an increased risk of hearing impairment was associated with birth asphyxia where the Apgar score was <5 at five minutes and where there was a history of fits and ototoxic drugs. The Joint Committee on Infant Hearing, US, issued a position statement in 1994, which gave the following perinatal indicators for sensorineural hearing loss in neonates: birthweight <1.5 grams, hyperbilirubinaemia requiring exchange transfusion, Apgar scores of 0–4 at one minute or 0–6 at five minutes and mechanical ventilation lasting five days or more, ototoxic drugs, including aminoglycosides but not limited to these, given in multiple courses or in conjunction with loop diuretics (ASHA 1994) (see Figure 4.3). Risk factors identified by various investigations are shown in Table 10.2 (page 223).

Low gestation and low birthweight

The prevalence of sensorineural hearing impairment in babies of low gestation is higher than in term infants and more than one adverse perinatal factor may be operative at the same time. As a result of improvements in perinatal care more babies of low birthweight (<2500 g) are surviving than in previous years. Extremely low birthweight babies (<800 g) with gestation ages as low as 23 and 24 weeks now survive as a result of the introduction of assisted ventilation, surfactant therapy and possibly antenatal steroids (Hack and Fanaroff, 1999). The prevalence of sensorineural hearing impairment in this population varies from 0–4% in reported studies (Marlow, Hunt and Harlow, 2000).

Babies born with gestational ages <32 weeks or birthweight <1500 g were investigated by Veen et al. (1993) in a cohort of 1338 infants. At the age of five years they were able to obtain audiograms from 890 out of 966 survivors and it was found that 1.5% had a sensorineural hearing impairment and 13.8% a conductive or unspecified hearing loss. Intracranial haemorrhage, sepsis and assisted ventilation were significantly related to sensorineural hearing impairment.

Infants born at 24 to 26 weeks' gestation were followed up until the age of five years in an Australian study described by Doyle (1995). Of the 95 children examined only two had a sensorineural hearing impairment requiring the use of hearing aids. In Canada, a follow up of 646 infants weighing 500 g to 1249 g at the age of two to three years revealed hearing loss in 1.3%. Darlow et al. (1997) conducted a prospective study of 413 very low birthweight (VLBW) infants and 286 children were alive and traceable at the age of seven years. Four (1.3%) of the children were found to have a hearing impairment of sufficient degree to warrant hearing aids, half the number with a severe visual impairment.

Naarden and Decoufle's (1999) investigation into the association of sensorineural hearing impairment and birthweight used data from a population-based surveillance programme in the Atlanta, Georgia area of the US. Birth weight categories were >4000 g, 3000 g to 3999 g, 2500 g to 2999 g, 1500 g to 2499 g and (VLBW) < 1500 g. Hearing impairment was defined as an average loss of at least 40 dB in the better ear over the range 500 Hz, 1 and 2 kHz. They found that prevalence rates (PR) and relative risks (RR) of presumed congenital sensorineural hearing impairment amongst the 169 children identified were inversely proportional to their birthweight categories. Prevalence rates for hearing impairment were 4.1/10 000 for those in the >4 000 g group, 3.7/10 000 for those weighing 3000 g to 3 999 g, 6.6/10 000 among those weighing 2500 g to 2999 g, 12.5/10 000 for those weighing 1 500 g to 2 499 g and, in the group of VLBW infants, PR was 51/10 000 and the RR was 13.9. Children in all birthweight categories were at higher risk for hearing impairment if they had additional developmental defects but particularly so if VLBW. There was no significant difference in the risks for moderate, severe or profound hearing impairment between different birthweight groups.

A birthweight <1 500 g and gestation <32 weeks were not found to significantly raise the risk of neonatal hearing impairment in the study reported by Meyer et al. (1999). It was suggested that these findings were different from those of previous investigations as a result of improvements in perinatal care and a reduction in the complications associated with prematurity.

Babies of low gestation may be exposed to all the aforementioned factors but still not develop a sensorineural hearing impairment. When they do develop a hearing defect then it may not be possible to determine which of the factors was causative as a result of the various interactions that exist.

Hypoxia/hypoxic-ischaemia

Infants may suffer hypoxaemia as a result of a number of events including birth asphyxia, recurrent apnoea, respiratory distress syndrome, meconium aspiration and pneumonia. Infants suffering hypoxic-ischaemia or hypoxia have been found in some instances to develop a sensorineural hearing impairment whereas others apparently undergoing equivalent hypoxic events are found subsequently to have normal hearing. There may, however, be minimal residual damage not detected by standard audiometric test protocols. Razi and Das (1994) investigated high-frequency hearing in children who had a history of hypoxia and compared their thresholds at 8–18 kHz with those of a control group with no adverse perinatal history. Both groups had normal audiograms within the range 250 Hz–8 kHz. They found that there were significant mean threshold differences between the study and control groups at thresholds of 12 kHz and above with thresholds worse in the group that had experienced perinatal problems.

D'Souza et al. (1981) reported the outcome for 26 children who experienced severe perinatal problems and only one infant was found to have a sensorineural hearing impairment. This infant was born at full term weighing 2.8 kg. A heartbeat was not detectable until five minutes after birth and it took more than 30 minutes to establish spontaneous respiration. The audiogram showed normal hearing at 250 Hz and 500 Hz and a steeply sloping sensorineural hearing impairment affecting higher frequencies.

In 1991, Anand, Gupta and Raj examined a group of 24 newborn infants with a history of asphyxia and hypoxic-ischaemic encephalopathy (HIE) and a group of 20 newborn infants without evidence of neurological abnormality. All of the babies were tested using an auditory brainstem response test (ABR). Twenty-two % of the infants with HIE had ABR abnormalities and these were found more frequently in babies with Stage 11 HIE. They concluded that birth asphyxia complicated by HIE was a significant risk factor for hearing impairment.

Jiang (1995) investigated the long-term effects of perinatal and post-natal asphyxia on developing auditory brainstem responses (ABR) of three groups of infants. Groups A and B had experienced perinatal asphyxia and Group C post-natal asphyxia. Group A (n = 48) gestational age 34–42 weeks, with no evidence of neurological abnormality; Group B (n = 41) gestational age 34–41 weeks, with neurodevelopmental defects; Group C (n = 14) gestational age 38–41 weeks. The ABR was performed six months after the asphyxial episode. Ten of the children in the perinatal asphyxia groups had threshold elevation and none in the post-natal group.

The conclusion reached by Jiang was that residual neurodevelopmental defects such as a sensorineural hearing loss were most likely to follow a prolonged period of hypoxic-ischaemia, probably as a result of cardiovascular collapse and cerebral-ischaemia. In the study there was no correlation between hearing impairment and the presence of neurodevelopmental defects. Most of the children who had residual neurodevelopmental deficits had normal hearing, whereas some of the children with a hearing impairment had no neurodevelopment defects. The poor correlation between peripheral hearing outcomes and those for neurodevelopment was thought to be explained by the variation in individual susceptibility to the effects of hypoxic damage. In the discussion of his findings Jiang referred to the known differential susceptibility of tissues to hypoxic damage and the possibility that the susceptibility to selectively damage either the peripheral auditory system or the central nervous system, could vary amongst individuals.

Jiang suggested that there was a critical period during the period of development of the peripheral auditory system when there was a particular sensitivity to the effects of hypoxia. This period was thought to possibly extend from some time pre-natally until shortly after birth, possibly the third post-natal month.

In an investigation involving 355 infants treated with ECMO (extracorporeal membrane oxygenation), Graziano et al. (1997) observed that the risk for hearing loss was significantly greater in neonates with a $PaCO_2$ below 14 mm Hg and those experiencing delay in ECMO treatment.

Most reports of hearing impairment after hypoxic insult have involved low gestation infants but term babies have also been found to have a hearing loss after hypoxic damage. Das (1991) reported five term/post-term infants with a history of severe birth asphyxia who were subsequently found to have a profound sensorineural hearing impairment.

A survey of published studies over the preceding 15–20 years was carried out by Borg (1997) who observed that in the majority birth asphyxia was not correlated with complicated deliveries. He noted that prolonged artificial ventilation and persistent pulmonary hypertension seemed to be important antecedents of hearing impairment. Borg concluded that pre-natal, perinatal and post-natal hypoxic-ischaemia was more likely to be associated with subsequent hearing impairment than pure hypoxia and that perinatal hypoxia was more likely to be associated with a temporary hearing loss than a permanent one. A prolonged stay in a neonatal intensive care unit and the duration of artificial ventilation were found to be the best predictors of hearing impairment of perinatal origin.

Hyperbilirubinaemia

Serum bilirubin levels represent a balance between the production of bilirubin and its elimination from the body. Hyperbilirubinaemia is more prevalent in low-birthweight infants than term infants for several reasons. Production of haemoglobin is greater and the process of elimination is less efficient. At birth 70% to 90% of haemoglobin is of the fetal type but over the first two or three months after birth it is replaced by adult haemoglobin. Fetal haemoglobin is more fragile and the life span of the red cells is of shorter duration than in term infants. Fetal haemoglobin has a greater affinity for oxygen than adult haemoglobin but it is less readily released into the tissues. The immature liver is less able to conjugate the bilirubin than the liver of the term infant and so is less able to eliminate an excess of bilirubin.

Acidosis, protein binding, hypoxia and intracranial haemorrhage facilitate bilirubin toxicity (Gustafson and Boyle, 1995). Bilirubin toxicity occurs when the amount of free bilirubin exceeds the binding capacity of the infant's plasma proteins or when there is severe acidosis. In acidosis unconjugated bilrubin is displaced from albumen and there is an increase in free bilirubin levels. The serum level at which bilirubin becomes toxic is dependent upon the gestational age of the baby with term infants being more resistant to toxic damage than babies of low gestation. Deposition of bilirubin may occur in the cochlear nuclei and in the basal ganglia and give rise to kernicterus. Toxicity is related to interruption in the respiratory chain in the mitochondria (Singer, 1991).

Experiments with Gunn rats have shown that neither asphyxia or jaundice alone led to hearing impairment but a combination of high plasma bilirubin levels and asphyxia in 10-day-old rats produced a progressive hearing impairment (Silver, Kapitulnik and Sohmer, 1995).

The type of hearing impairment associated with hyperbilirubinaemia was described by Fisch and Osborne (1955) in a group of 27 children with haemolytic disease of the newborn. The hearing loss affected the high frequencies and, in the group investigated, the degree of hearing loss was moderate or severe. Most also had cerebral palsy of the chorio-athetoid type.

Van de Bor et al. (1992) reported the five-year outcome of hyperbilirubinaemia in low birthweight infants at the age of five years. The babies were part of a National Collaborative Study of 1338 pre-term and small-for-gestational-age infants born in the Netherlands. They found that there was no significant relationship between mean maximum serum total bilirubin concentration and the risk of an adverse outcome. In children with an intracranial haemorrhage during the neonatal period it was discovered that the risk of a handicap increased significantly for each 50 μmol/L increase in bilirubin but no dose relationship was observed in the absence of an intracranial haemorrhage. Six children in the study had a significant sensorineural hearing impairment.

The hearing loss resulting from hyperbilirubinaemia is retrocochlear rather than cochlear in origin. Reversible changes in auditory brainstem evoked potentials have been shown in infants with hyperbilirubinaemia treated with exchange transfusions (Rhee et al., 1999). Care has to be taken in interpreting the results of hearing tests on neonates with a history of hyperbilirubinaemia. The high-serum bilirubin levels may result in a click-evoked auditory brainstem response test exhibiting abnormal or absent waveforms that, on reduction of these levels to normal, results in restoration of normal waveform morphology. Infants with a history of hyperbilirubinaemia should be given an otoacoustic emission test as well as an auditory brainstem response test when referred for audiological assessment. Where otoacoustic emissions are present normally but the auditory brainstem evoked response test is abnormal this would indicate a potentially reversible auditory neuropathy.

In recent years treatment with phototherapy, exchange transfusion and the use of anti-D immunoglobulin has reduced the incidence of toxic effects as a result of hyperbilirubinaemia.

Sepsis

Sepsis is particularly prevalent in low-birthweight babies. It is a major cause of morbidity in infants weighing <750 g with between 30% and 50% having one or more bouts of septicaemia during the period they are in hospital (Hack and Fanaroff, 1999).

Neonatal meningitis is a potential cause of permanent hearing impairment and affected infants should be referred for audiological assessment before being discharged from hospital. The most common organisms involved are *Escherichia coli,* Group B Streptococcus and *Listeria monocytogenes* (Dawson et al., 1999). The infection is thought to reach the ear via the cochlear aqueduct and cause a labyrinthitis.

Sensorineural hearing impairment occurs early in the illness and may be reversible during the first 48 hours (Richardson et al., 1997). It is usually bilateral and symmetrical but may be asymmetrical and there may be vestibular as well as cochlear damage. Adjunctive dexamethasone therapy reduces the incidence of severe hearing impairment as a result of *Haemophilus influenzae* type b and for pneumococcal meningitis when given with or before parenteral antibiotics (McIntyre et al.,1997).

In the process of healing there may be ossification of the lumen of the cochleae. Infants with a profound hearing impairment as a result of meningitis need to be monitored using an MR scan so that if a cochlear implant is needed this can be inserted prior to the degree of ossification of the cochlea precluding the introduction of the optimal array of electrodes.

Ototoxicity

Aminoglycosides and loop diuretics are used frequently in the management of the sick neonate and are potential causes of sensorineural hearing impairment.

Aminoglycosides

Aminoglycosides are bacteriocidal antibiotics and are particularly active against aerobic gram negative bacteria. Their principal adverse effects are ototoxicity, nephrotoxicity and neuromuscular blockage. Individual aminoglycosides vary in the degree to which their ototoxic effects are targeted upon particular organs. It has been suggested that the acute effects of aminoglycoside toxicity are distinctly separate from the effects of chronic toxicity. Acute ototoxicity is associated with high dosage and is believed to result from blockade of calcium currents in outer hair cells and this is reversible. Chronic ototoxicity is more common, may be irreversible, and depends upon the balance between production of the toxin and its detoxification (Schacht, 1993). It may relate to the area under the concentration time curve and the total dose administration (Barclay, Kirkpatrick and Begg, 1999). Ototoxicity is closely related to prolonged administration and higher total dose (Borradori et al., 1997).

The risk of ototoxicity as a result of aminoglycosides therapy is related to the duration of treatment and clearance of gentamycin from the body is slow. The effects of gentamycin are potentiated by concurrent treatment with loop diuretics such as frusemide. As gentamycin is excreted via the kidney, patients with renal impairment are at greater risk of ototoxicity than those with normal renal function.

Schacht (1993) postulated that enzymatic transformation of gentamycin to a metabolite or an 'activated' molecule was part of the ototoxic mechanism. There is evidence that free radical mechanisms are involved in the activation process (Crann and Schacht, 1996). Experiments on guinea pigs support the involvement of iron and free radicals play a critical role in the toxic effects of aminoglycoside antibiotics.

Transplacental ototoxicity has been demonstrated in animals. Postnatally, rats given gentamycin have suffered greater effects upon the auditory brainstem response when the antibiotic is given during the period of development of the auditory system than in the adult rat. A sensitive period for aminoglycoside ototoxicity has also been described in human neonates indicating that the premature baby is more susceptible than adults (Henley and Rybak, 1995).

Gentamycin is the aminoglycoside that is most commonly used and is both cochleotoxic and vestibulotoxic. The effect upon the vestibular system is greater than upon the cochlea. The frequency of cochlear toxicity averaged 8.3% for gentamycin in one large survey of patients given on average daily dosage of 3.9 mg/kg (Kahlmeter and Dahlager, 1984).

Previously aminoglycosides were administered in divided doses. Serum levels were determined to avoid peak concentrations >10 mg/l and troughs >2 mg/1. Multiple administration of aminoglycosides has more recently been replaced by once daily dosage. Transitory high concentrations of aminoglycosides do not result in a high uptake of the drug by cochlear tissues because of the saturation of cell binding sites (Langhendries et al., 1998).

Bailey, Kirkpatrick and Begg (1999) reviewed nine meta-analyses of the use of aminoglycosides and concluded that there was no significant increase in ototoxicity with once-daily dosage. A prospective controlled randomized study was carried out on 50 children aged six months to 18 years. Peak, four-hour, eight-hour and trough gentamycin concentrations were measured and hearing tested. There was no evidence of ototoxicity and the researchers concluded that once-daily dosage enhances the bactericidal effects as a result of peak concentrations and avoids toxicity.

Monitoring of concentration levels is still required with once daily dosage and methods using mid-dosage interval concentrations to gauge drug exposure are recommended (Barclay et al., 1999).

Barclay et al. (1999) described the damage as a result of gentamycin ototoxicity. This begins in the outer hair cells of the basal turn of the cochlea and results in a high-frequency hearing impairment. Subsequently the damage extends towards the apex of the cochlea resulting in middle and lower frequency hearing becoming affected. Tinnitus may be the initial symptom. Vestibular damage may also occur resulting in ataxia, positional vertigo and oscillopsia. Animal experiments have indicated that gentamycin reduces or abolishes the suppression effects of the medial efferent system (Henley and Rybak, 1995).

Hearing impairment as a result of gentamycin ototoxicity may be unilateral or bilateral, reversible or permanent (Winkel et al., 1978). Damage to the auditory system may not be apparent immediately but may appear after some delay and be progressive. In an investigation of the prevalence of hearing impairment in an at-risk neonatal intensive care unit, 137 (1.4%) of the 835 infants studied were found to have a hearing impairment >30 dB. All children had received aminoglycosides but only one had no other risk factors (Hess et al., 1998).

In recent years there have been several reports of a mitochondrial mutation that renders affected individuals susceptible to developing hearing impairment when treated with aminoglycosides in therapeutic doses (Hu et al., 1991; Prezant et al., 1993). A point mutation 1555 A-G in the ribosomal RNA has been found in various countries in families with hearing impairment following aminoglycoside administration (Fischel-Ghodson, 1996). This offers the possibility of prevention of hearing impairment by using alternative antibiotics where possible when those susceptibility to develop hearing damage are identified.

Loop diuretics

There have been a number of experimental studies that have investigated the ototoxicity of loop diuretics. Aniko and Sobin (1987) examined the effects of ethacrynic acid in mice and discovered hair cell damage in the organ of Corti with involvement of the supporting cells at higher drug concentrations. Ryback et al. (1991) administered frusemide to young rats and showed that those that were nine to 28 days old had a greater reduction of endocochlear potential than those aged more than 30 days. They also had oedema and histological changes in the stria vascularis whereas the older rats did not. This indicated the existence of a critical period during which the animals are susceptible to loop diuretics. Low birthweight babies could be particularly susceptible to the effects of frusemide as the half life is prolonged in these infants (Henley and Rybak, 1995).

In 1991, Brown, Watcho and Sabo gave an account of a case-controlled study of 35 neonates with a sensorineural hearing impairment and a group of age-matched controls. Multivariate analysis of potential causative factors was carried out and frusemide was identified as the only significant factor. More recently Marlow et al. (2000), investigating antecedents of sensorineural hearing loss in infants <33 weeks gestation, found that frusemide use in the presence of serum creatinine levels >60 mmol/l was associated with an increased risk of sensorineural hearing loss.

Incubator noise

Exposure to excessive noise is known to cause a sensorineural hearing impairment in adults and experiments performed by Douek (1976) indicated that young guinea pigs suffered noise damage when exposed to loud noise averaging 80 dB for seven days. In the NICU the environmental sound levels range from 45 dB to 135 dB and they may be exposed to high levels of noise for prolonged periods (Zahr and de Traversay, 1995). The noise levels found in NICUs exceed the recommendation of the American Academy of Pediatrics that noise levels in NICUs should not exceed 58 dB (American Academy of Pediatrics, 1994). Zahr and Traversay (1995) put earmuffs on infants, which attenuated noise levels by 7 dB to 12 dB and observed that these babies had significantly higher mean oxygen saturation levels and less fluctuation in oxygen saturation than a control group. The infants wearing earmuffs also had fewer behavioural state changes and slept more. Testing the babies' hearing was not part of the investigation.

Children who were in incubators as babies do not show a notch in the audiogram at 4 kHz and this has been thought to indicate that there was no noise damage. The intensity levels to which babies are exposed in incubators vary according to the type of incubator. In most instances the noise level is below 85 dB HL. It is possible that the immature auditory system and the mature system respond differently to damaging levels of noise and a different pattern of hearing loss would be produced.

Noise exposure and the use of aminoglycosides are synergistic in producing auditory damage. Pye and Collins (1991) observed that aminoglycosides given to guinea pigs in a non-damaging dose could potentiate the effects of noise at just damaging levels when both are present at the same time. The neonate being treated with therapeutic doses of aminoglycosides and exposed to noise in an incubator could be at particular risk for hearing impairment.

More research is needed to determine whether or not there is more than a theoretical risk of infants developing a hearing loss as a result of exposure to noise in incubators in combination with other potentially damaging agents.

Degree of hearing impairment

The degree of hearing impairment reported in studies has varied and most reports have indicated that where the hearing impairment is severe or profound there are usually associated neurological abnormalities.

Newton (1985), in a population study of 111 children with a bilateral sensorineural hearing impairment, identified 15 (13.5%) of the children as having a hearing impairment of perinatal origin. Of these, seven had a loss over the frequency range 0.5 kHz to 4kHz of <80 dB HL and eight >80 dB HL. The proportions in each degree category did not differ significantly. Das (1988) reported that 20 out of the 24 children with a hearing loss attributable to perinatal causation had hearing impairments >80 dB HL over the same frequency range. In a later study, published in 1991, Das noted that out of 22 children whose hearing impairment was attributed to perinatal events, 20 had hearing impairments averaging >80 dB HL over the frequency range 0.5 kHz to 4 kHz. Five were term or post-term infants who had experienced birth asphyxia. In contrast, Sutton and Rowe (1997) noted that there were more mild and moderate hearing impairments amongst the group thought to have a perinatal etiology than in other investigations.

Additional disabilities

Newton (1985) found disabilities were significantly higher in those children with a hearing impairment as a result of perinatal disorders than in other etiological groups with the exception of those resulting from intrauterine infections. Amongst a group of 145 children with mild to severe neonatal encephalopathy followed up at the age of eight years by Robertson et al. (1989), 16% had a major impairment such as cerebral palsy, blindness, cognitive delay, convulsive disorder, and severe hearing impairment.

In the 22 children with perinatally acquired hearing impairment described by Das (1991) two-thirds had a major disability. These included severe visual defects, developmental delay and neurological disabilities.

Amongst a group of 145 children with mild to severe neonatal encephalopathy followed up at the age of eight years by Robertson, Finer and Grace (1989), 16% had a major impairment such as cerebral palsy, blindness, cognitive delay, convulsive disorder and severe hearing impairment.

The frequent association of other deficits together with sensorineural hearing impairment has implications for management. These children will need the input of a multidisciplinary team to enable them to maximize their potential (see Chapter 16).

Conclusion

Adverse conditions around the time of birth are potential causes of sensorineural hearing impairment particularly for the lower birthweight neonate. Some babies seem to be more prone than others to sustain damaging effects and genetic factors could be involved in their greater susceptibility. To what extent perinatal factors are coincidental or causative of a hearing impairment in individual infants is often difficult to determine and arrival at a conclusion too often relies upon the weight of probability rather than the results of specific tests. A better understanding is needed of the pathophysiology surrounding the birth process, particularly as it impinges upon the auditory system, and of the extent to which genes have a role in determining the outcome for the neonate. More specialized monitoring of events preceding and during birth need to be developed to enable a prospective rather than a retrospective approach to the question of causation of a subsequent hearing impairment.

Table 10.2: Perinatal risk factors for hearing impairment

Authors	Year	No. of infants	Population description	Gestation (wks)	Birth weight (g)	No. with SN hearing loss + perinatal factors	Risk factors for hearing loss identified
Abramovitch et al.	1979	111	intensive care survivors	26–35	<1500	10	apnoeic episodes; indirect SB≥ 170μmol/l has an additive effect
Thiringer et al.	1984	146 HI	HI children born in two hospitals	26–43	1150–3470	17	hypoxic lung disease (apnoea + respiratory distress) needing ventilation
Bergman et al.	1985	72	36 HI NICU survivors + 36 NH survivors	=<36	=<1500	36	prolonged respirator care; hyperbilirubinemia; hyponatremia; hyperbilirubinemia
Duara et al.	1986	278	intensive care + well baby nurseries	36±4.2	<1500	4	low birthweight; perinatal asphyxia; prolonged hospital stay
Swigonski et al.	1987	137	NICU survivors		<1250	4	IVH/PVH, apnoea, major craniofacial abnormalities; possibly SB↑and congenital infections
Halpern et al.	1987	820	ICN survivors	<38	+<1500	50	time in intensive care; gestational age; craniofacial abnormalities
Salamy et al.	1989	24	intensive care survivors	<34	<1500	12	frusemide dose + duration ± aminoglycosides; acidosis pO_2<50mmHg; high total SB
Veen et al.	1993	890	Pre-term + small-for-gestational-age infants	<32	<1500	13	IPPV and/or CPAP; intracranial haemorrhage; sepsis
Eavey et al.	1995	40	NICU survivors	28–42	1360–3950	23	ventilation
Ertl et al.	2001	164	NICU survivors	30.4±3.7	1410±280		hypernatremia; amnioglycosides

CPAP = continuous positive airways pressure; HI = hearing impaired; ICN = intensive care nursery; IPPV = intermittent positive pressure ventilation; IVH = intraventricular haemorrhage; NH = normal hearing; PVH = periventricular haemorrhage; NICU = neonatal intensive care; SB = serum bilirubin.

CHAPTER 11

Craniofacial syndromes and hearing impairment with special reference to syndromes with external ear anomalies

CWRJ CREMERS

Introduction

Since the middle of the nineteenth century, genetic syndromes with hearing impairment as a main feature have been recognized, like Usher syndrome (Von Graefe, 1858; Liebreich, 1861), branchio-oto-renal syndrome (Paget, 1877, 1878), Treacher Collins syndrome (Berry, 1899) and osteogenesis imperfecta (Dent, 1897; Van der Hoeve and De Kleyn, 1917). At this moment over 450 syndromes with hereditary hearing impairment have been described and this number is still increasing (Gorlin et al., 1995). Recently, gene identification and mutation analysis have provided a molecular basis for most of the more common genetic deafness syndromes. This has led more frequently to splitting than to lumping of previously reported clinical syndromes. Some excellent books and catalogues are available to assist in reaching syndromal diagnoses in individual cases (Gorlin et al., 1995; Tewfik and der Kaloustian, 1997).

This chapter will focus only on a few groups of somewhat analogous syndromes to provide some ideas about genetic deafness syndromes and their delineation.

External ear anomalies and genetic hearing impairment

Unilateral or bilateral aural atresia

Aural atresia includes an anotia or microtia of the auricle. In almost all cases it is combined with a bony atresia of the external ear canal. An atretic bony plate will be there instead of a tympanic membrane. A 40 dB to 60 dB conductive hearing impairment will exist in the affected ear. The sensorineural component of the hearing impairment will mostly be within the range of 0 dB to 20 dB.

Aural atresia can be part of a series of syndromes like hemifacial microsomia, Treacher Collins syndrome, branchio-oto-renal syndrome, craniosynostosis syndromes, del (18q) syndrome caused by a deletion of long arm of chromosome 18, thalidomide embryopathy, branchio-oculofacial syndrome, MRKH-syndrome and some 20 occasional syndromes (Gorlin et al., 1995).

The etiology of isolated unilateral or bilateral atresia of the ear canal is only in about 10% genetic. An autosomal dominant and autosomal recessive pattern of inheritance has been reported, the first one being the most frequent (Cremers, 1985; Gorlin et al., 1995). The etiology of the remaining 90% remains mostly unknown. A multifactorial etiology remains an option.

Hemifacial microsomia (Goldenhar syndrome, oculo-auriculo-vertebral spectrum)

This condition is a predominantly unilateral malformation of craniofacial structures that develop from the first and second branchial arches. The many terms used for this complex indicate the wide spectrum of anomalies described and emphasized by various authors (Gorlin et al., 1995). About 10% of the patients have a bilateral involvement.

In most cases of unilateral aural atresia there is a slight but unnoticed unilateral hemifacial microsomia. This can be made visible by placing a wooden spatula between the upper and under jaw. This spatula will turn upwards to the affected side, which shows the underdevelopment of that side of the face. Malocclusion is frequent. The presence of an epibulbar dermoid is common. Blepharoptosis or narrowing of the palpebral fissures occurs also on the affected side. Lower facial weakness on the affected side can occur.

Severe cranial and cerebral involvement occur in the so-called extended hemifacial microsomia. Cervical spine and cranial base anomalies, cervical vertebral fusions, spina bifida, scoliosis, abnormal ribs, heart anomalies, renal anomalies including also renal agenesis and vaginal atresia (extended MRKH-syndrome) (Strübbe et al., 1994) are reported. In rare families an autosomal dominant pattern of inheritance has been shown. It is essential to be careful in this diagnosis and to exclude other first and second branchial arch syndromes. In most cases the etiology of this affection remains unknown. A multifactorial etiology remains an important option, including a genetic background.

Treacher Collins syndrome (Mandibulo-facial dysostosis; Franceschetti-Zwahlen-Klein syndrome)

Berry (1889) and Treacher Collins (1900) were ophthalmologists for isolated cases (Berry, 1899) and a mother and daughter (Treacher Collins, 1900), and reported the unusual facies with malar hypoplasia, the downslanting palpebral fissures and the coloboma of the inferior eyelid. They illustrated their clinical reports with excellent portrait drawings.

The portraits of the mother and daughter (Treacher Collins, 1900) show the anomalous auricles. The initial firm report of this syndrome was by Zwahlen in his thesis (Franceschetti and Zwahlen, 1944). Franceschetti later on extended his work by providing overwhelming evidence about the presence of this autosomal dominant inherited syndrome. Most patients have normal intelligence but microcephaly and some mental retardation can occur.

The anti-mongoloid slanting and the lower lid colobomas are very striking. The facies is characteristic. There is hypoplasia of the mid-face with a retrognathia blind fistula between the auricle and angle of the mouth. Choanal atresia and pharyngeal hypoplasia are occasional abnormalities (Sphrintzen et al., 1979).

Incomplete penetrance is more common than reported in the textbooks (Marres et al., 1995a). Hypoplasia of the zygoma arch to be shown by X-ray (Water's projection) is the most sensible/sensitive feature when the other characteristic features are lacking. Non-penetrance has also been overlooked for a long time (Marres et al., 1995a). Mutations of the TCOFI-gene are causative for this syndrome. Cases of non-penetrance or doubtful incomplete penetrance can be diagnosed by mutation analysis of the TCOFI-gene (Dixon et al., 1996).

The hearing impairment is purely conductive but is not a necessary feature. In severe cases there is bony atresia of the external ear canal with or without microtia or anotia. In those cases the bone-anchored hearing aid is the best method for hearing rehabilitation (Mylanus et al., 1998). There can be a conductive hearing impairment as result of malformation of the ossicular chain. Surgical intervention to restore hearing can be considered (Marres et al., 1995a). Middle-ear anomalies in Treacher Collins syndromes are partially quite specific and knowledge about this is helpful (Marres et al., 1995a).

Nager acrofacial dysostosis syndrome (preaxial acrofacial dysostosis)

Nager acrofacial dysostosis (Nager and DeReynier, 1948) is a mandibulo-facial-dysostosis associated with radial defects. Almost 100 cases have been

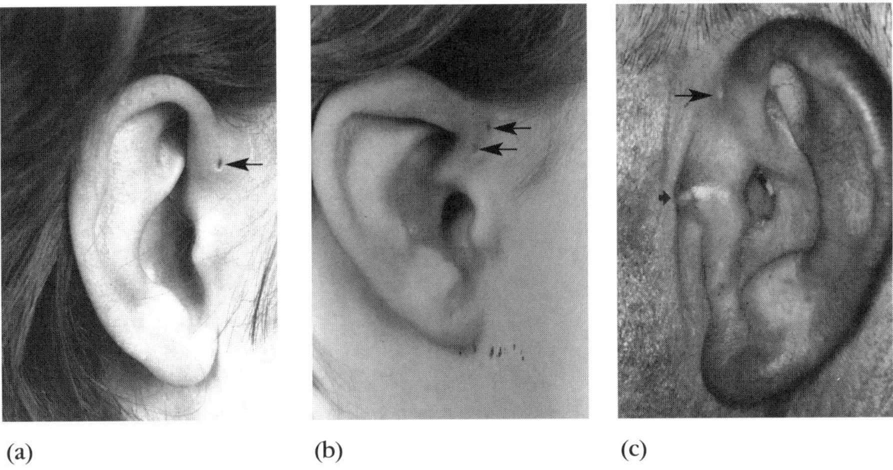

(a) (b) (c)

Figure 11.1. Three auricles from 3 different patients with Branchio-oto-renal syndrome showing a pre-auricular sinus (thin black arrow) and a dysmorphic superior helix in each. A pre-auricular appendage (thick black arrow) is present in one of them.

reported. Radial ray abnormalities are a common feature. Thumb hypoplasia or aplasia, triphalangeal thumb, symphalangism, double thumb and syndactaly are common features (Gorlin et al., 1995). Most cases are sporadic. Autosomal dominant and autosomal recessive inheritance is considered. Non-penetrance could be possible, hiding an autosomal dominant pattern of inheritance. A chromosome 9q32 translocation was found (Zori et al., 1993).

Branchio-oto-renal syndrome (ear-pit hearing loss syndrome, Branchio-oto syndrome)

The Branchio-oto-renal (BOR) syndrome (McK No. 601653) (McKusick, 1988) has an autosomal dominant pattern of inheritance. Main features are slight malformation of the auricles, pre-auricular sinuses, hearing impairment, branchiogenic cervical fistulas of the second branchial arch and renal dysplasia. Penetrance of the disease is almost totally complete, but expression of the symptoms varies. In particular the severity of the hearing impairment and renal abnormalities varies (Melnick et al., 1976; Fraser et al., 1978; Cremers et al., 1980, 1981; Widdershoven et al., 1983; Gimsing and Dyrmorse, 1986; McKusick, 1988; Chen et al., 1995).

Hearing impairment can be of the conductive, mixed or sensorineural type. Hypoplasia of the cochlea has been demonstrated histologically and radiologically (Fitch et al., 1976; Cremers and Fikkers van-Noord, 1980). A widened vestibular aqueduct has been described after histological examination and after radiological examination (Dagillas et al., 1992; Chen et al., 1995). A review of the literature showed progression of the sensorineural component of the hearing impairment in a few cases (Fourman and Fourman, 1955; Shenoi, 1972; Brusis, 1974; Fraser et al., 1978; Bourguet et al., 1996).

Reconstructive surgery for the congenital conductive component is possible, but it is generally difficult to achieve satisfactory results (Kluyskens et al., 1966; Cremers et al. 1981; Cremers et al., 1993).

Prevalence of the BOR syndrome is estimated to be 1:40 000. The BOR gene is EYA1, which lies on 8q13.3 (Abdelhak et al., 1997; Vincent et al., 1997; Kumar et al. 1998a). The BOR syndrome is genetically and clinically different from a very similar branchiogenic syndrome. This syndrome is not linked to the EYA1-locus (Marres et al., 1994; Kumar et al., 1998b).

Recently, detailed CT and MRI studies of BOR-syndrome have been published. These showed, in almost all patients, hypoplasia of the cochlea and in some patients an incomplete intrascalar separation, a dysplastic vestibule, a hypoplastic lateral semicircular canal, an enlarged vestibular aqueduct and an enlarged endolymphatic duct and sac (Ceruti et al., 2001). The question has arisen of whether or not the enlarged vestibular aqueduct and/or an enlarged endolymphatic duct and sac are related to a progressive hearing impairment (Kemperman et al., 2001; Stinckens et al., 2001). Long-term audiometric data in BOR syndrome are scarce (Kemperman et al., 2001).

From the group of branchiogenic syndromes a new syndrome has been recognized that is almost similar to the branchiogenic syndrome. Its features are hearing impairment, pre-auricular sinus, external ear anomalies and commissural lip pits (Marres and Cremers, 1991; Marres et al., 1994). It has been linked to chromosome 1 (Kumar et al., 1999).

Again a new syndrome has been reported showing dysmorphic auricles, lip pits and conductive hearing impairment in one family. The pattern of inheritance is autosomal dominant. Gene-linkage excluded linkage to the EYA-1 locus (BOR-syndrome) and to the Marres-Cremers syndrome on chromosome 1.

In one case an exploratory tympanotomy showed a congenital anomaly of the ossicular chain including a dysmorphic incus and a stapes ankylosis. Hearing was improved successfully by interposing a piston from the malleus to the vestibule (Koch et al., 2000).

Lacrimo-auriculo-dento-digital syndrome (Levy-Hollister syndrome)

Features of this autosomal dominant inherited disorder include nasolacrimal duct obstruction with chronic dacrocystitis, absent lacrimal

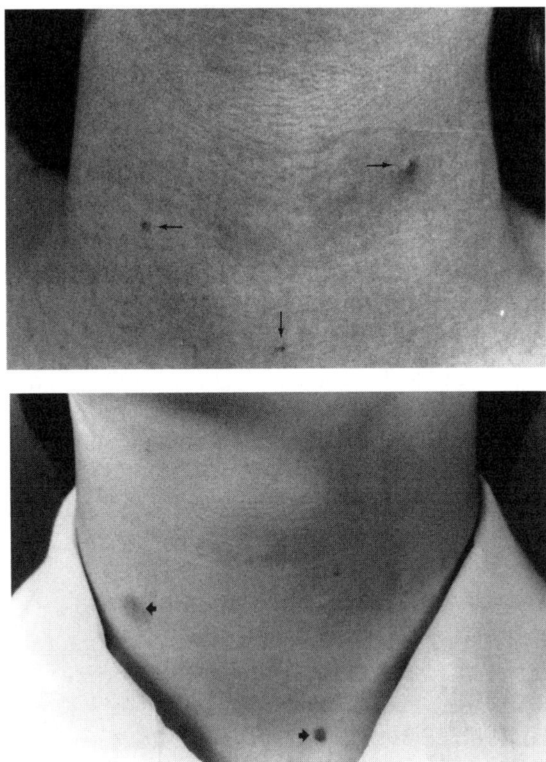

Figure 11.2. Second branchial arch fistulas in two teenagers (black arrow). Their openings can be found halfway or lower along the sternocleidoid muscle. Their openings are sometimes in a pigmented area. A midline fistula is most unusual.

puncta, cup-shaped ears, peg-shaped teeth with enamel hypoplasia, various preaxial digital anomalies and congenital, mostly sensorineural, hearing impairment. The most remarkable features are congenital unilateral or bilateral hearing impairment, the cup-shaped auricles and the preaxial digital anomalies including shortening of the radius, triphalangeal thumbs, thenar muscle hypoplasia and other digital anomalies. The congenital conductive hearing impairment has been operated successfully.

CHARGE association

The term CHARGE association was introduced in 1981 by Pagon et al. (1981) and refers to a combination of congenital malformations. The mnemonic CHARGE designates the most frequently occurring anomalies in the constellation. 'C' indicates coloboma of the retina, 'H' heart defects, 'A' choanal atresia, 'R' genital hypoplasia, and 'E' ear anomalies, including a typical hypoplasia of the auricle and/or deafness. No hereditary pattern has been found. Translocations involving chromosome 6 and 8 have been reported. A locus for a gene causing CHARGE association may reside in the region of 14q22-q24.3 (North et al., 1995).

The inner-ear anomaly consists of a specific form of labyrinthine dysplasia that includes a hypoplasia of the cochlea and the saccule and complete absence of the utricle and the semicircular canals. The temporal bone anomalies represent a specific form of labyrinthine dysplasia. Normal otolith vestibulo-ocular responses to the off-vertical axis rotation test was found in seven out of seven CHARGE patients having no semicircular canals in the CT scan and no canal vestibulo-ocular responses to earth-vertical axis rotation (Gyuot and Vibert, 1999; Wiener-Vacher et al., 1999). The delay of the development of walking is considered to be due to severe sensorineural, visual and vestibular deficits.

Hearing impairment is conductive or sensorineural and often asymmetrical (Brown and Israel, 1991; Hurst, Meinecke and Baraitser, 1991). The auricle is mostly low-set and posteriorly angulated, asymmetric and cup-shaped. A pronounced ridge of the vertical part of the superior helix can be remarkable. Other otolaryngological manifestations are retrognathia, facial asymmetry, feeding difficulties, trachea-oesophageal fistula, oesophageal atresia, cleft lip/palate and upper airway abnormalities.

CHARGE association should be considered in all cases with ocular colobomas, mental retardation, vertebral anomalies and cleft palate/lip.

Klippel-Feil anomaly

The only characteristic of this syndrome is fusion of the cervical vertebrae. Associated anomalies are scoliosis, kyphosis, spina bifida occulta, urinary tract anomalies, hypospadia, cryptochismus, short webbed neck and low posterior hairline, sensorineural and conductive hearing impairment have been reported (Stewart and O'Reilly, 1989). The etiology of this anomaly is unknown. It will probably have a heterogeneous background. One of the genes responsible may be located at 5q11.2 or 17q23 (Fukushima et al., 1995).

Other syndromes that include Klippel-Feil anomaly are Wildervanck syndrome, Duane anomaly, MURCS-association, Noonan syndrome and Turner syndrome. The major clinical features are fused cervical vertebrae, abducens palsy with retracted globe and sensorineural and/or conductive hearing impairment.

Wildervanck syndrome

This syndrome is characterized by inner-ear deafness, with Klippel-Feil and Duane anomalies. This may be unilateral or bilateral. The Duane anomaly includes abducens paralysis and globe retraction with narrowing of the palpable fissures on attempted adduction. The hearing impairment may be sensorineural, conductive or mixed, and unilateral or bilateral. Severe inner-ear anomalies on CT scans and conventional polytomography are a classical feature (Windle-Taylor et al., 1981; Keeney, Gebarski and Brunberg, 1992). The etiology of this syndrome is unclear.

Gorlin et al. (1995) considers the Klippel-Feil anomaly, the Duane anomaly and Wildervanck syndrome as a heterogeneous group of anomalies that have much in common in their presentation.

Craniosynostosis syndromes

Crouzon syndrome, Saethre-Chotzen syndrome, Apert syndrome and Pfeiffer syndrome are the most common craniosynostosis syndromes having hearing impairment (50%) as a feature. Even atresia of the bony air canal can occur (10%). The hearing impairment is conductive and the result of fixation of the ossicular chain by stapes ankylosis and/or fixation of the malleus and incus in the epitympanum. The mastoid and the middle ear are smaller in size by the hypoplastic development of the temporal bone. Only occasionally surgical results have been reported to improve hearing mainly by stapes surgery (Boedts, 1967; Cremers, 1981).

Crouzon syndrome is characterized by craniosynostosis, maxillary hypoplasia, shallow orbits and ocular proptosis, mild ocular hypertelorism, midfacial hypoplasia, malocclusion and relative mandibular prognathism. Variability in expression is well-known in Crouzon's syndrome, which has an autosomal dominant pattern of inheritance with variable expression.

Pfeiffer syndrome is characterized by craniosynostosis, broad thumbs, broad great toes and occasionally partial soft tissue syndactyly of the hands. The pattern of inheritance is autosomal dominant. Most cases are sporadic.

Saethre-Chotzen syndrome is characterized by craniosynostosis in combination with a broad and variable pattern of malformations like facial asymmetry, ptosis of eyelids, low-set frontal hairline and brachydactyly. The pattern of inheritance is autosomal dominant. Most cases are sporadic.

Apert syndrome is characterized by craniosynostosis, mid-facial malformations and syndactyly of the hands and minimally involving digits 2, 3 and 4. The hearing impairment is conductive. Serous otitis media and its sequelae were common. Congenital stapes ankylosis has been reported (Bergstrom et al., 1972; Philips and Miyamoto, 1986). Associated anomalies of the airway like tracheal stenosis, obstructive sleep apnoea and cor pulmonale resulting in early death have been reported. The pattern of inheritance in Apert syndrome is autosomal dominant. Most cases are sporadic.

CHAPTER 12

Otitis media: diagnosis and management

MD GRAHAM, TG DELAP AND M GOLDSMITH

Introduction

Since it was first described by Hippocrates in 450 BC otitis media has continued to be one of the most commonly diagnosed conditions in infancy and childhood. In England otitis media with effusion remains the most common cause of hearing impairment and indication for surgical intervention in children (Freemantle et al., 1992). The literature reports that 70% of children will have had one or more episodes of otitis media by their third birthday (Stein et al., 1983).

While the paediatric population are most commonly affected, adults also may suffer from any of the different forms of otitis media. While both sexes are equally affected, there appears to be a racial predominance, and Native Americans, Eskimo groups and Australian aboriginal children appear to have a higher prevalence. Apart from a genetic predisposition in the above groups, other epidemiological factors have been identified, many of which may be related to socioeconomic status. Breast feeding appears to confer protective factors, reducing the number of episodes of otitis media in children and delaying the age of onset (Anianson et al., 1994). This data has been corroborated by other groups (Sassen, Brand and Grote, 1977; Duffy et al., 1997). Unquestionably breast milk contains a protective factor which remains to be identified. The previously held concept that the protective benefit was due to the position or method of feeding appears to have been rejected (Paradise et al., 1994).

Anatomical abnormalities such as cleft palate and immune deficiency states predispose to an increased incidence of otitis media. There are a number of studies that have shown that children in day care, particularly during the first two years of life (Wald, Guerra and Bayers, 1991), are at a greater risk of the condition. This is likely to be due to cross-infection of micro-organisms from different households. The number of children within the day care group appears to directly correlate with the frequency of infection. Pre-natal factors such as low vitamin C intake and high alcohol consumption during pregnancy may also increase the incidence (Stenström and Ingvarsson, 1997). Secondary smoke in the home environment remains unproven as a risk factor but the weight of evidence appears to suggest that this is the case and physicians should continue to advise appropriately.

Classification

The recently described classification by Harkness and Topham (1998) is a valuable working one. Otitis media *per se* represents an inflammatory condition of the middle-ear space cleft, without reference to etiology or pathogenesis. The definition of 'chronic', namely duration greater than eight weeks, was agreed at the Second and Third International Symposia on Recent Advances in Otitis Media with Effusion (Paparella et al., 1985). A working classification is necessary for accurate clinical diagnosis, and hence the planning of further management. It is also essential for communication between professionals.

Pathophysiology

The seasonal variation in the incidence of OME is well documented. This relationship to respiratory infection is still under scientific evaluation. It may simply be the case that both recurrent acute otitis media and otitis media with effusion are common conditions in childhood. Workers who support a bacterial origin for OME will argue that bacteria have been cultured from effusions (up to 40% in some studies) and that this may be an underestimate given the practical difficulties of obtaining a culture. *Haemophilus influenza, moraxella catarrhalis* and streptococcus are the most frequently cultured micro-organisms. Furthermore, the hypothesis that adenoidal hypertrophy resulting from chronic infection acts as a source of micro-organisms is widely held. Whether adenoidectomy is beneficial in the management of OME as a consequence of correction of an obstructed Eustachian tube or because of the removal of a source of infection, remains unclear.

Diagnosis

To establish a diagnosis a full otological history must be obtained. Typically, acute otitis media presents with otalgia, fever and irritability, and vomiting and diarrhoea may be present in association. The presence of pain may be suddenly alleviated by the onset of otorrhea, an event typically associated with perforation of the tympanic membrane. Vertigo and facial palsy should also be investigated. Hearing impairment will also be present. Indeed, in its chronic form hearing impairment may be the only symptom, and owing to the insidious nature of the condition the patient may have gradually become accustomed to this attendant morbidity. Examination entails a thorough assessment of the head and neck to ascertain the presence of predisposing conditions, namely adenoid hypertrophy, cleft palate or accompanying rhinosinusitis. A careful nasopharyngeal examination should be performed to exclude the possibility of pathology at that site.

Clinical diagnosis of otitis media may be hampered by the lack of co-operation with the examination by the patient, particularly in the paediatric age group. A history in pre-lingual patients is, by definition, collateral and cases of Munchausen syndrome by proxy have been described in the literature. A screening programme for hearing impairment in high-risk children exists in many developed countries, but may unfortunately still be lacking in developing countries.

Otoscopy

Otoscopy remains the most important part of the physical examination to establish a diagnosis of otitis media. Prior to visualization of the tympanic membrane it is essential to meticulously clean the external auditory meatus to obtain a full view of the tympanic membrane. Use of the binocular microscope will afford a magnified view, which will facilitate cleaning and minimize the risk of iatrogenic trauma. In addition, a magnified view of the detail of the tympanic membrane is obtained.

Otoscopy must be performed methodically, or subtle pathological findings may be missed. The external auditory meatus must be examined for foreign bodies and skin diseases including tumours and defects. In examining the tympanic membrane the handle of malleus should be identified initially, followed by the division between the pars flaccida and pars tensa, namely the anterior and posterior malleolar folds. The long process of the incus and stapedius tendon may be seen in some cases. Perforations of the tympanic membrane should be noted and classified according to type, namely marginal or central, position, namely anterior, inferior or posterior, and size (Figure 12.1). Large central perforations may be classified as subtotal, whereas large marginal perforations may be classified as total (Figure 12.2).

Colour is a somewhat subjective finding, but should be considered. Thickening of the tympanic membrane may reduce the degree of transparency. Tympanosclerotic plaques, indicative of previous disease or surgical intervention, may be noted. The presence of middle-ear effusion may be confirmed by a dull hue. Where a definite air-fluid level or bubbles are seen the diagnosis can be made with greater confidence (Figure 12.3).

Retraction of the tympanic membrane may be present, as manifested by apparent shortening of the handle of the malleus. In severely retracted cases the long process of the incus or the head of the stapes may be draped by the tympanic membrane (Figure 12.4). It may be difficult to differentiate adhesions or indeed perforations from retracted tympanic membranes.

Pneumatic otoscopy is essential in order to form a judgement as to the mobility of the tympanic membrane. A good seal must be obtained, while variable pressures are exerted on the external ear. Bi-directional brisk tympanic membrane movement is the normal finding. Mobility will be absent or reduced when middle-ear effusion is present. Combinations of different tympanic membrane findings (colour, position and mobility) are considered to be the most reliable indicators of the presence or absence of otitis media with effusion (Karma et al., 1993). Acoustic emittance measurements will confirm the findings of pneumatic otoscopy, providing objective information on tympanic membrane and ossicular chain mobility. These instruments are capable of recording tympanograms, measuring stapedial reflexes.

Mobility may also be assessed clinically using Valsalva or Toynbee manoeuvres. In a Valsalva manoeuvre the patient endeavours to expire against a closed nose and lips, thus forcing air into the Eustachian tube. Overperformance of forceful insufflation must be avoid as lethal intracranial complications have been reported (Finsnes, 1973).

In patients complaining of vertigo it is imperative to exclude the presence of a positive fistula sign. A positive sign is present if the patient complains of dizziness or demonstrates deviation of the eyes away from the examined side or indeed a jerk nystagmus towards the examined side, following elevation of the external ear pressure using a Siegle speculum or tragal pressure. False positive results may occur following a perilymph leak. A false negative result may occur because of poor technique or in the presence of vestibular failure.

Repeat evaluations, or indeed even examination under general anaesthesia, may be required before a proper assessment of the ear can be made. Laboratory cultures and further courses of topical or systemic medications may be needed in individual cases, and co-existent nasopharyngeal conditions may require medical or surgical attention.

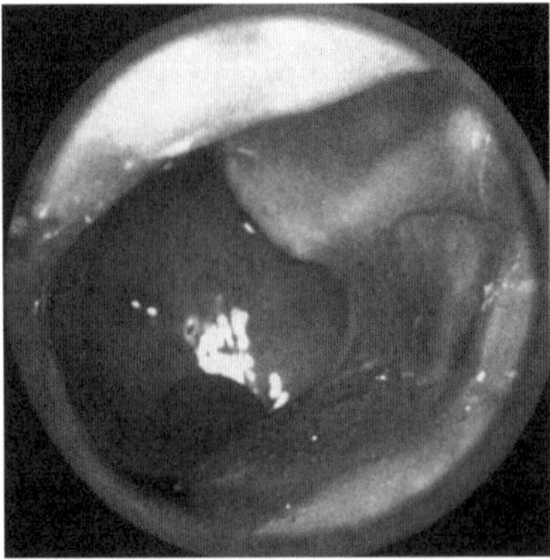

Figure 12.1. Chronic non-suppurative otitis media. Tubotympanic disease.

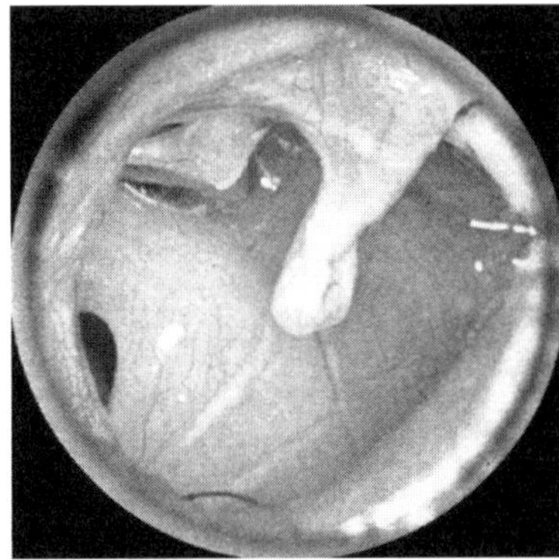

Figure 12.2. Right subtotal perforation.

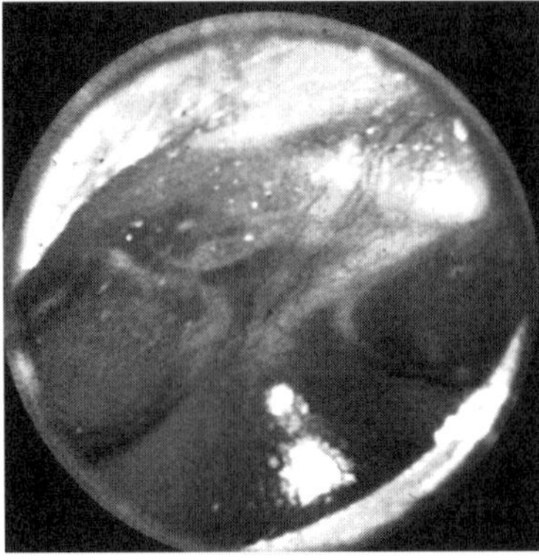

Figure 12.3. Fluid level right tympanic membrane.

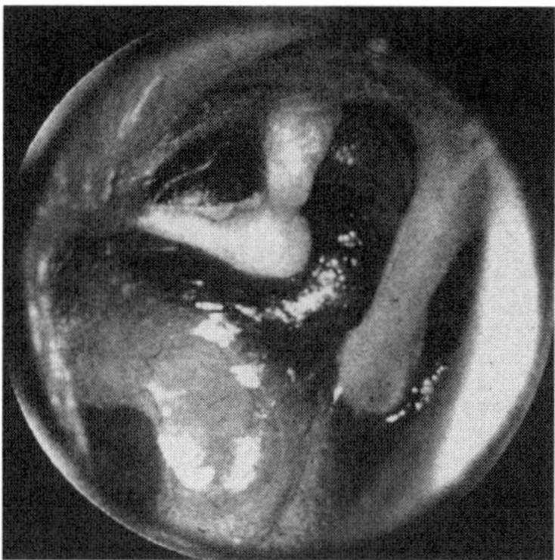

Figure 12.4. Severely retracted tympanic membrane, right ear. Incudo-stapedial joint and round window niche are clearly visible.

Audiological testing

Prior to embarking on sophisticated audiological testing, a clinical evaluation should be performed by the physician. Gross speech tests, although crude, may be helpful in identifying malingering or simply the presence of a hearing impairment. Tuning fork tests are essential, and the Weber test and Rinne test should be performed in all cases. Tuning forks of 256, 512, 1024 and 2048 Hz should be used. A quiet room is essential, and the tines of the fork should be held parallel to the external meatus at a distance of 1 cm from the entrance to the meatus. The Rinne test is considered positive if the perceived sound by air conduction is louder than that audible by bone conduction. A positive result is obtained in normal cases, and in most patients with a unilateral sensorineural hearing loss. A negative result will occur in patients with a conductive hearing loss greater than 15 to 20 dB HL. A false Rinne negative result will occur where a severe sensorineural hearing loss occurs in the test ear, and results in transmission of the auditory stimulus across the skull to the non-test cochlea. It is important to use a Bárány noisemaker to exclude such an occurrence. The Bárány noisemaker is used to emit white noise into the non-test ear to exclude the possibility of cross-over hearing to that side.

The Weber test is performed by applying the tuning fork to the midline and testing for laterality. In symmetrical hearing impairment or normal hearing the patient will experience the auditory stimulus in the midline. The stimulus will lateralize to the better-hearing ear in cases of unilateral sensorineural hearing impairment, and will lateralize to the affected ear in cases of unilateral conductive hearing loss.

Other tuning fork tests, such as the Bing test, the Gellé test and the Lewis test, are rarely used in clinical practice.

Tympanometry

Tympanometry is a reliable non-invasive simple test of short duration that is valuable in the assessment of patients with a variety of middle-ear pathologies. Five main types are described, namely Type A, normal middle-ear function, which are sub-classified into a shallow and a deep type. A scarred or thickened tympanic membrane may give a similar picture. The shallow type A tympanogram is produced by ossicular fixation, whereas the deep high compliance tympanogram is suggestive of ossicular discontinuity. The Type B tympanogram indicates poor middle-ear compliance, and is present in cases of middle-ear fluid, otitis media or cholesteatoma. A Type C tympanogram, indicative of abnormal negative middle-ear pressure, may also be present with the latter three entities, or indeed in the presence of a scarred or thickened tympanic membrane. Tympanometry is valuable when combined with otoscopy for confirmation of the diagnosis, or as an aid to diagnosis where otoscopy is equivocal. It is also valuable as a screening test of ear disease. When performing audiometry, it is important to bear in mind that a mixed hearing impairment may be mistaken for a conductive hearing loss, if careful masking is not performed.

Medical management

In clinical practice, antibiotics are indicated in cases of acute suppurative otitis media. Amoxycillin or ampicillin are usually appropriate as first-line antibiotics in community-acquired infection. A drug with beta-lactamase activity may be required in refractory cases.

In acute non-suppurative otitis media, antibiotics are not indicated, and simple analgesia is generally adequate. If, however, symptoms persist for more than 48 hours or the child develops a fever, the child should be reassessed and antibiotics recommended. The role of systemic decongestants and antihistamines remains unproven, but they are anecdotally beneficial to certain patients.

In cases where middle-ear effusions have persisted for more than three months, the effusion is considered chronic. As the primary handicap in this situation is prolonged hearing impairment, some physicians argue that the provision of hearing aids will avoid the need for surgery and restore full cognitive and language development. This has cost implications, however, and may be disconcerting for some children. Myringotomy and ventilation tube insertion is the preferred treatment in the authors' view, as discussed below.

Pre-operative treatment

Chronic otitis media may be a result of systemic illness, including diabetes, agammaglobulinemia, adrenal cortical insufficiency, chronic leukemia, hepatic or renal disease or dietary insufficiency. An allergic tendency appears to increase the risk of otitis media with effusion. A full overall physical assessment, supplemented if necessary by appropriate clinical investigation, will elucidate these factors. The patient should be comprehensively assessed from an anaesthetic point of view and counselled with respect to the potential complications that may arise during surgical treatment. In cases of chronic suppurative otitis media, efforts are made to provide an optimal surgical field prior to operation. Middle-ear toilette using the binocular microscope is essential. Systemic antibiotics are rarely required. In cases of mucoid discharge insufflation of boric acid powder may be helpful. Anti-fungal and antibiotic ear drops may be used where indicated.

Surgical treatment

The broad indications for surgery are:

- tympanic membrane perforation;
- chronic ear infection;
- ossicular discontinuity.

Surgery should be performed urgently in the presence of persistent vertigo, facial paralysis and impending or recognized intracranial complications.

Myringotomy

Myringotomy and ventilation tube insertion remains the commonest surgical procedure performed in the UK. Mandell et al. showed that children with chronic otitis media with effusion had significantly less time with effusion following tube insertion than when compared with either myringotomy alone or no surgery (Mandell et al., 1992). Maw and Bawden (1994) found in their study that the placement of a unilateral tube was equivalent in efficacy to an adenoidectomy, but the combination was more effective in reducing the overall duration of otitis media with effusion. Post-tube insertion tympanosclerosis appears to be related to the presence of the tube rather than the incidence of acute otitis media episodes (Stengstrom et al., 1996).

A number of different tube types have been used. These may be broadly categorized into long-stay tubes and short-stay tubes. A follow up series of long-stay tubes reported a 33% rate of persistent tympanic membrane perforation, and a 48% rate of patients with one or more tube-related complications (Mangat, Morrison and Daniwalla, 1993). It was noted that all these complications increased in incidence if the tube remained *in situ* for longer than 36 months. The lesser mass of the mini-shah tube has been associated with less tympanosclerosis (Dingle et al., 1993). Earlier extrusion rates were noted by the same authors in a different publication in a further study (Hampal, Flood and Kumar, 1991). Takasaka et al. (1996) showed that tubes could be removed without risk of otitis media with effusion recurrence if tubes had functioned for at least 18 months, if tympanometric equivalent ear volume was at least 3 ml, Eustachian tube function was normal, and there was no nasal airway disease or well-controlled nasal airway disease. Tonsillectomy confers no additional benefit to adenoidectomy in improving 12-year outcomes in severe chronic secretory otitis media with effusion (Maw and Bawden, 1993).

Consideration must be given to the function of aeration and drainage of the middle ear via the Eustachian tube. The patency of the Eustachian tube lumen may be assessed by having the patient perform auto-inflation, by Politzerization, or by special manometric study. A randomized clinical trial of auto-inflation compared with observation in Danish children with chronic otitis media with effusion showed a two-week positive effect of approximately 50% based on tympanometry (Stengerup, Sederberg-Olssen and Balle, 1992).

Myringoplasty is a term used to describe the procedure used to repair a perforated tympanic membrane. The middle ear is inspected during the procedure to exclude the presence of middle-ear disease. The procedure may be performed via a permeatal, post-auricular, or endaural approach. Most commonly, connective tissue grafts are used and temporalis fascia or tragal perichondrium is usually chosen. Homograft materials are no longer favoured in view of the risk of slow virus transmission. The connective tissue graft chosen functions as a scaffold over which the squamous and mucosal layers regenerate. Approximately four weeks' healing time is required for neovascularization to occur.

Tympanoplasty without mastoidectomy

This term, coined by Wuhlstein in 1953, is used to describe surgical reconstructions of the middle-ear hearing mechanism following disease processes. A myringoplasty is generally performed as one of the steps in the procedure. This procedure is performed in most cases of simple chronic otitis media, chronic adhesive otitis and tympanosclerosis. Removing a portion of the outer attic wall can augment middle-ear exposure. A full evaluation can then be made and the need for a formal mastoid exploration established. Pathologic middle-ear processes such as the presence of squamous epithelium, infection, osteitis or tympanosclerosis may then be assessed. Special attention must be directed at areas that are difficult to access, such as the sinus tympani. Care must be taken to eliminate all foci of infection in both the bony and soft tissues.

Wuhlstein has described five types of tympanoplasty. In a *type 1* tympanoplasty restoration of the normal middle-ear hearing mechanism is achieved. This may simply require division of adhesions in conjunction with a myringoplasty. In a *type 2* reconstruction of the defective ossicular chain is achieved by restoring continuity between the tympanic membrane and a partially destroyed ossicular chain. In a *type 3* direct transmission of sound waves occurs by a columellar effect using a surgically performed *myringostapediopexy*. In a *type 4* a mobile footplate is left exposed in the absence of an ossicular chain. Sound transmission is directly to the oval window, and protection from a Baffle effect is afforded by protecting the round window. In a *type 5* the oval window is completely closed by bony fixation, and a fenestra is performed in the horizontal semicircular canal and covered by a skin graft. Type 4 and type 5 procedures have largely been abandoned for the interposition of an artificial columella or the interposition of a bony, cartilaginous or synthetic prosthesis to the footplate.

Artificial materials such as Teflon, hydroxyapatite or stainless steel, and the autograft bone, usually ossicular bone, are most commonly used for ossicular chain reconstruction. Artificial materials are preferred in instances where autograft bone is unavailable or infiltrated with disease process. Hydroxyapatite appears to fulfil many of the criteria for an ideal prosthesis.

Surgery on a better or only-hearing ear is contraindicated unless useful hearing may be attained with the use of a hearing aid on the contralateral side. Tympanoplasty is contraindicated in the presence of a non-functional cochlea, malignant neoplasms of the outer or middle ear, and *Pseudomonas* infections in diabetics. Relative contraindications include poor Eustachian tube function and extensive middle-ear fibrosis.

Tympanoplasty with mastoidectomy

In ears where the pathological process extends into the mastoid air cell system, surgical exploration is necessary (Figure 12.5). Complete eradication of disease is the primary aim of surgical intervention. Surgery may be carried out via an endaural or a post-aural incision.

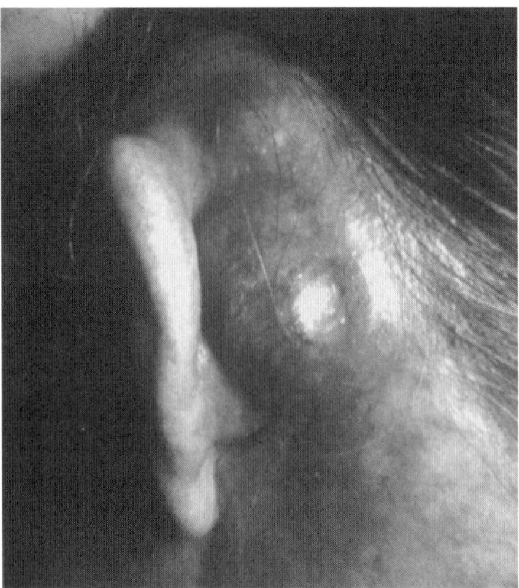

Figure 12.5. Left subperiosteal abscess.

Cholesteatoma of the middle ear and mastoid is generally an acquired disorder in which keratinizing squamous epithelium has become displaced into the middle ear or mastoid and results in an accumulation of keratin debris. In its congenital form, which is uncommon, there is no obvious connection between the external meatus or tympanic membrane. Acquired cholesteatoma generally presents as a keratin-filled retraction pocket or is mistaken for a simple perforation. Most commonly it affects the pars flaccida. The true cause of cholesteatoma remains speculative, but a number of theories exist as to its pathogenesis. A number of otologists believe that non-keratinizing epithelium of the middle ear and mastoid undergoes metaplasia. Others contend that epithelial emigration occurs across the margin of the tympanic membrane into the middle ear. It may be the case that epithelial migration across a perforated tympanic membrane occurs along surfaces denuded by previous trauma, stimulated by a loss of contact inhibition. This finding can be repeated experimentally in the animal model. A further theory is that epithelial cells from the keratinizing epithelium of the pars flaccida migrate in isolation and proliferate. Perhaps the theory that is most widely accepted is that tympanic membrane retraction occurs secondary to negative middle-ear pressure or infection. Once the retraction pocket becomes sufficiently large, keratin is unable to migrate laterally. It thus accumulates and expansion of the cholesteatoma results in destruction of tissue locally. This destruction may be due to simple pressure, the result of enzymatic action or a combination of both.

Classic radical mastoidectomy is performed only rarely today, and involves removal of all middle-ear structures, including the tympanic membrane, malleus and incus, tensor tympani muscle and mucosa. In addition, the orifice of the Eustachian tube is blocked and healing occurs by secondary intention. *Modified radical mastoidectomy* as proposed by Bondi endeavoured to preserve the middle-ear space and exteriorize the pathological process. Periodic ear cleaning is required to remove excessive debris and wax accumulation within the mastoid bowl post-operatively. A large meatoplasty is performed at the time of the initial procedure in order to facilitate self-cleansing and ease surgical toilette. An overly large meatoplasty can result in cosmetic dissatisfaction and temperature sensitivity (Naclerio, Nealy and Alford, 1981). The procedure may be performed working posteriorly through a canal wall backwards. Tumarkin revived an approach initially described by Stake in which the cholesteatoma sac is initially exteriorized in the posterior mesotympanum or epitympanum and followed posteriorly with removal of only the amount of bone that is necessary for its complete exteriorization. Less normal mastoid bone is thus removed and the resultant mastoid cavity is in general smaller. Further advantages include the easy assessment of depth with respect to the tympanic ring, and the early identification of ossicles and facial nerve. The medial osseous canal wall may primarily be repaired where indicated, furthermore. Shorter operating times are also noted (Naclerio et al., 1981).

Closed tympanomastoidectomy

House and Sheehy (1980) modified the combined anterior and posterior tympanotomy approach advocated by Jansen, to include drilling out of the facial recess and staging the ossicular reconstruction. The aim of retaining the posterior canal wall to retain as normal an anatomical configuration as possible offered advantages over canal wall down techniques, in that more rapid healing occurred, and the need for frequent ear cleanings was obviated. The need to keep the ear meticulously dry was also avoided, and fittings of hearing aids were facilitated. Closed tympanomastoidectomy requires greater surgical skill and increases operative time. A second look procedure needs to be performed within 18 months to two years as residual or recurrent cholesteatoma needs to be excluded. The otoendoscope may be of value when performing this type of surgery. Closed techniques may be the preferred treatment in children to avoid the need for life-long mastoid cavity care, which may be considered quite distressing in the office setting. Average recidivism rates in children have been quoted at approximately 30% with results from different series varying from 7% to 57% (Dodson et al., 1998). Poor Eustachian tube function and the presence of good pneumatization of temporal bones in children, as well as the effect of growth factors elaborated in childhood have all been proposed as reasons for cholesteatoma being clinically noted to be a more aggressive disease in childhood.

Intact bridge tympanomastoidectomy

The intact bridge tympanomastoidectomy developed by Paparella and Jung (1984) is a one-stage procedure that combines features of both the open and closed techniques. A flexible approach is adopted as dictated by the pathological findings perioperatively.

All forms of mastoid surgery share the same primary objective, namely total eradication of disease with a dry, safe ear. An additional but secondary objective is the retention of functional hearing and restoration with tympanoplastic techniques. In unilateral cases where no useful hearing remains and distressing persistent discharge is present, consideration may be given to performing a mastoid obliteration procedure.

Complications of suppurative otitis media

Otological complications tend to result more from chronic middle-ear disease rather than acute disease in current clinical practice. The likelihood of the development of complications depends upon both patient and bacterial factors. Host resistance, advanced age, intercurrent chronic disease and previous history of recurrent otitis media will predispose to the possibility of complications occurring. Poorly pneumatized temporal bones are at more risk than well-pneumatized ones.

The type and virulence of the infecting organisms and the level of susceptibility to chemotherapeutic agents are also obviously important. Inadequate treatment may result in spread of disease.

Infection may extend via a number of potential routes. The oval and round windows, the cochlear and vestibular aqueducts, the dihiscences in bony coverings may constitute potential pathways despite the presence of normal anatomy. Infection may also spread via bony defects resulting from neoplastic erosion, previous surgery, or accident. Most commonly this type of pathway is the mechanism of disease extension following acute infections and tends to occur early. Infection may spread through the small veins through bone and dura. The vascular system within intact bone may be similarly affected. These complications frequently arise in the early post-operative period. In chronic ear disease the usual method of infective spread is by means of bony erosion and this tends to manifest later. Surgical removal of the source of infection is required.

Complications of suppurative otitis media may be extracranial or intracranial. The *extracranial* complications include:

- subperiosteal abscess;
- facial paralysis;
- labyrinthitis;
- petrousitis.

The *intracranial* complications encountered are:

- meningitis;
- brain abscess;
- lateral sinus thrombophlebitis;
- otitic hydrocephalus.

Conclusion

Otitis media remains a challenging clinical entity as we enter the 21st century. Screening programmes and modern diagnostic methods have led to earlier recognition of the condition, but the available treatment modalities remain unsupported by strong scientific evidence. An increasing prevalence, the emergence of drug-resistant organisms, higher patient expectation and the financial issues raised by surveillance and treatment, will undoubtedly remain subjects of debate in the future. The widespread use of ventilation tubes is likely to remain unchanged until an effective medical treatment becomes available and accepted. Hope beckons in the field of immunotherapy, where viral vaccines are being evaluated for efficacy and safety, in the belief that upper respiratory pathogens may be the initiating factor in otitis media with effusion, and that this condition in turn may be a germinal event in all middle-ear disease. Molecular genetics may also unfold some valuable knowledge in the future with regards to the underlying etiologies. Improvements in technology such as otoendoscopic equipment may reduce the morbidity from surgical intervention. In the interim, we must continue to work with rational management plans based on our existing knowledge and experience.

CHAPTER 13

Central auditory processing disorders

RW KEITH

Introduction

Purposes of the chapter

Central auditory processing disorder (CAPD) is an area of expanding professional interest among audiologists and others who work with individuals who have problems of auditory reception, expressive and receptive language, reading and attention. There is increasing information in the literature with regard to the identification and management of children and adults who have CAPDs. More efficient and effective test batteries are being developed, as are strategies for management or remediation of persons with CAPD. There remain many questions about assessment and remediation of persons with CAPD but much is currently known. The purposes of this chapter are to provide information on the broad construct of central auditory processing disorders (CAPDs), to discuss the diagnostic approach to individuals who are thought to be at risk for CAPD, and to briefly review some remediation approaches to individuals diagnosed as having CAPD. Hopefully the information provided here will encourage audiologists to further investigate this interesting problem, and to expand their personal scope of practice to include central auditory testing and remediation.

Definition of CAPD

For many years professionals and parents concerned about auditory processing were constrained by lack of agreement on basic definitions of central auditory processing disorders. Individual authors were inclined to offer their own definitions, and there was great disparity among those opinions. In 1995 an American Speech Language Hearing Association

(ASHA, 1996) task force on central auditory processing consensus development met to define central auditory processing and its disorders. A second purpose was to define how the disorders can be identified and ameliorated through intervention.

According to the task force, central auditory processes are the auditory system mechanisms and processes responsible for the following behavioural phenomena:

- sound localization and lateralization;
- auditory discrimination;
- auditory pattern recognition;
- temporal aspects of audition, including;
  - temporal resolution;
  - temporal masking;
  - temporal integration;
  - temporal ordering;
- auditory performance decrements with competing acoustic signals;
- auditory performance decrements with degraded acoustic signals.

The ASHA statement specifies that these mechanisms and processes are presumed to apply to non-verbal as well as verbal signals and to affect many areas of function, including speech and language. They have neurophysiological as well as behavioural correlates. Further, many neurocognitive mechanisms and processes are engaged in recognition and discrimination tasks. Some are specifically dedicated to acoustic signals, whereas others (for example, attentional processes, long-term language representations) are not. With respect to these non-dedicated mechanisms and processes, the term *central auditory processes* refers particularly to their deployment in the service of acoustic signal processing.

The ASHA consensus statement defines a central auditory processing disorder (CAPD) as an observed deficiency in one or more of the behaviours listed above. For some, CAPD is presumed to result from the dysfunction of processes and mechanisms dedicated to audition; for others, CAPD may stem from some more general dysfunction, such as an attention deficit or neural timing deficit, which affects performance across modalities. It is also possible for CAPD to reflect coexisting dysfunction of both types.

The ASHA statement leaves open many questions about specifics of test administration but it serves as an important landmark in the arena of auditory processing. For the first time, a nationally recognized organization agreed on a definition that served to formally systemize thinking about CAPD.

In the UK the term *obscure auditory dysfunction* (OAD) is sometimes used to describe persons between 15 and 55 years with 'convincing self report of auditory disability accompanied by normal pure-tone thresholds' (Saunders et al., 1992). The auditory test battery used to identify persons with OAD include:

- history;
- pure-tone thresholds;
- speech thresholds and discrimination in noise;
- pure-tone threshold in white and narrow band noise;
- masking level difference;
- gap detection of temporal resolution;
- otoacoustic emissions;
- dichotic listening tests.

Obscure auditory dysfunction appears to be similar to what is known in the US as central auditory processing disorder, and the test battery contains elements that are similar to that identified by the ASHA panel.

Whatever definition of CAPD is eventually agreed by participating professionals, the diagnosis and remediation of central auditory processing disorders in children and adults is complex because of the wide range of intellectual, behavioural, educational, psychological, medical and social issues associated with CAPD. The complexity of this disorder (or perhaps these disorders) requires transdisciplinary involvement in the assessment and remediation of affected persons and that audiologists involved in this area be widely read in a variety of subjects.

Characteristic behaviour

Children with CAPD are known to exhibit a wide range of behaviours and experience a number of language and learning problems, they often exhibit some of the following characteristics (Keith, 2000):

- normal pure-tone hearing thresholds – some have a significant history of chronic otitis media that has been treated and/or resolved;
- may respond inconsistently to auditory stimuli – children often respond inappropriately but at other times they seem unable to follow auditory instructions;
- may have difficulty with auditory localization skills – this might include an inability to tell how close or distant the source of the sound, and an inability to differentiate soft and loud sounds. There are also frequent clinical reports that these children become frightened and upset when they are exposed to loud noise, and often hold their hands over their ears to stop the sound;

- may have difficulty with auditory discrimination;
- may have deficiencies in remembering phonemes and manipulating them (for example, in tasks such as reading, spelling and phonics, as well as phonemic synthesis or analysis – Katz et al., 1992: p. 84);
- may have difficulty understanding speech in the presence of background noise.
- may have difficulty with auditory memory, either span or sequence, and poor ability to remember auditory information or follow multiple instructions;
- may have poor listening skills characterized by decreased attention for auditory information, distractibility or restlessness in listening situations;
- may have difficulty understanding rapid speech or persons with an unfamiliar dialect;
- may frequently request that information be repeated – for example, one teacher described these children as saying 'huh?' and 'what?' frequently.

The profiles of these children often include significant reading problems, poor spelling, and poor handwriting. They may have articulation or language disorders. In the classroom, they may act out frustrations that result from their perceptual deficits, or they may be shy and withdrawn because of the poor self-concept that results from multiple failures. Children who exhibit these behaviours are candidates for central auditory testing (Keith, 2000).

These examples are only a few of the characteristics of persons with CAPD. Not every child with an auditory processing problem will exhibit all of the characteristics mentioned here. The number of problems experienced by a given child will be an expression of the severity of the CAPD, with symptoms ranging from mild to severe.

Central auditory processing disorder versus attention deficit hyperactivity disorder

One of the special challenges of central auditory testing is the frequent history of decreased attention, distractibility, or restlessness in listening situations, a history that is similar to children with attention deficit hyperactivity disorder (ADHD). When that history exists, it is necessary to determine whether an individual is experiencing a primary CAPD or ADHD. Controversy has existed whether CAPD and ADHD represent the same or separate developmental disorders (Burd and Fisher, 1986; Gascon et al., 1986; Keller, 1992). However, Chermak et al. (1998)

compared professionals' rankings of behavioural symptoms of ADHD and CAPD in order to examine the degree to which professionals responsible for diagnosis of these disorders ranked them in a mutually exclusive manner. They concluded that audiologists and paediatricians listed a number of behaviours that differentiated CAPD and ADHD. They are shown in Table 13.1 in rank order.

Table 13.1. Behavioural signs in ADHD and CAPD

ADHD	CAPD
Inattentive	Difficulty hearing in background noise
Distracted	Difficulty following oral instructions
Hyperactive	Poor listening skills
Fidgety or restless	Academic difficulties
Hasty or impulsive	Poor auditory association skills
Interrupts or intrudes	Distracted
	Inattentive

Check lists

Another approach for the identification of children who should be tested for the possible presence of CAPD includes the use of various checklists of auditory performance (Fisher, 1976; Sanger et al., 1985; Smoski et al., 1992). Among these the Children's Auditory Processing Performance Scale (CHAPPS) developed by Smoski et al. (1992) is used to systematically collect and quantify the observed listening behaviours of children. This is a questionnaire consisting of 36 items concerning listening behaviour in a variety of listening conditions and functions. According to the authors the clinical applications of this scale are to identify children who should be referred for a CAP evaluation, and to prescribe and measure the effects of therapeutic intervention.

History

The assessment should begin with careful observation of the child, with particular attention to the auditory behaviour patterns described previously in this chapter. Care should be taken to identify strengths as well as weaknesses, and to note performance in other modalities including vision, motor coordination, tactile response, speech and language.

When possible, an in-depth history from the child's caregiver should be taken. Rosenberg (1978) called the case history 'the first test' because of the value of the information obtained. He pointed out that a carefully taken history can be extremely useful in differentiating among various problems, can supplement results from auditory tests, and can help in making decisions about the child's educational management.

The case history should be taken systematically to avoid missing important information. The person taking the history should provide an opportunity for caregivers to state their concerns about the child, to describe the child's behaviours, and to express any other related concerns. Specific information that should be requested includes information about:

- auditory processing, language and learning problems that exist in the family;
- the mother's pregnancy;
- conditions at birth, the child's growth and development, health and illnesses;
- general behaviour and social-emotional development;
- speech and language development;
- hearing and auditory behaviour; and
- educational progress.

The specific questions asked of parents will depend on the setting in which the testing is being done, and the purpose of the examination. Areas to be investigated in the history when a CAPD is suspected are listed in Table 13.2 (pp. 252–3).

Auditory neuropathy

An auditory problem that is related to, but apparently different from a typical central auditory processing disorder is auditory neuropathy. The basis of this disorder appears to be some combination of problems between the axon terminal of the inner hair cell and dendrite of the spiral ganglion neurons or the axons of the spiral ganglion neuron with the auditory nerve in their course to the brain stem (Stein et al., 1996). Starr et al. (1996) provided further information to suggest that auditory neuropathy is an auditory nerve disorder. According to Sininger et al. (1995) and Hood (1998) the symptoms seen in auditory neuropathy include:

- mild to moderate elevation of auditory thresholds to pure tones by air and bone conduction;
- present otoacoustic emissions (OAEs);
- absent acoustic reflexes to ipsilateral and contralateral tones;

Table 13.2. Model for taking a case history (Keith, 1995)

Area	Information needed
Family history	History of any family member's difficulty in school achievement The language spoken in the home
Pregnancy and birth	Unusual problems during pregnancy or delivery Abnormalities present in the child at birth
Health and illness	Childhood illnesses, neurological problems, history of seizure, psychological trauma, head trauma or injury, middle-ear disease, allergies Drugs or medications prescribed by the physician
General behaviour and social –emotional development	Age-appropriate play behaviour, social isolation, impulsiveness, withdrawal, aggression, tact, sensitivity to others, self-discipline
Speech and language development	Evidence of articulation or receptive/ expressive language disorder Ability to communicate ideas verbally Ability to formulate sentences correctly Appropriateness of verbal expression to subject or situation
Hearing and auditory behaviour	Ability to localize sounds auditorily Ability to identify the sound with its source Reaction to sudden, unexpected sound Ability to ignore environmental sounds Tolerance to loud sounds Consistency of response to sound Need to have spoken information repeated Ability to: follow verbal instructions listen for appropriate length of time remember things heard pay attention to what is said comprehend words and their meaning understand multiple meanings of words understand abstract ideas

Table 13.2. (contd)

Area	**Information needed**
	Discrepancies between auditory and visual behaviour
Non-auditory behaviour	Motor coordination: gross, fine, eye-hand Hand dominance Visual perception Spatial orientation Any unusual reaction to touch
Educational history and progress	History of progress in school Reading, math, musical and art ability

- absent to severely abnormal ABRs in response to high level stimuli and inability to suppress OAEs;
- word recognition ability poorer than expected for pure-tone hearing loss configuration;
- absent masking level differences (MLD).

The problems of auditory neuropathy are beyond the scope of this chapter but readers should be aware of its existence. Sininger states that auditory neuropathy and CAPD are different entities because 'CAPD is characterized by normal hearing while auditory neuropathy involves the peripheral auditory system and hearing loss.' According to Starr et al. (1996) auditory neuropathy 'could be one etiology for some cases with the disorder known as central auditory processing disorder', especially those in whom pure-tone thresholds were elevated. Whether they are different, or whether auditory neuropathy is a subset of central auditory processing disorders, is still to be determined.

Auditory tests and interpretation

Statistical qualities of central auditory tests

One challenge in the UK is the need to develop a battery of central auditory tests that are standardized to provide results with sufficient reliability and validity to have confidence in the findings. For example, central auditory tests must emphasize assessment of auditory perceptual abilities while de-emphasizing auditory processing strategies that include cognitive and memory aspects of audition. Central auditory tests must also avoid the confusion of interpreting results created by cross-modality picture-pointing tasks. Central auditory tests must be produced to precise technical specifications under state-of-the-art conditions. They must be normed on an adequate sample of individuals of the appropriate age for whom testing is intended. Finally, they must be presented in the language of the individuals to be tested. Results of previous research (Gat and Keith, 1978; Keith et al., 1987) indicate that linguistic background has a significant impact on the individual's ability to perform on sensitized speech tests, such as those used in central auditory tests. In the UK there are many children and adults who are not native speakers of English, and so results of tests presented in the English language may be contaminated by linguistic background. The linguistic factor carries over to the hazards of using well-standardized tests using American-accented English, such as SCAN-C (Keith, 1999) and SCAN-A (Keith, 1994). For those tests, the normative data obtained with American children will not be valid for children of the UK because of the possible contamination of accent. For all those reasons, it is necessary to develop tests that use non-linguistic signals, or to develop a battery of speech measures using 'received pronunciation' with standard British accent, such as that formerly used by newsreaders of the British Broadcasting Corporation (BBC).

Test reliability is described by Anastasi (1982: p. 102) as the 'consistency of scores obtained by the same persons when re-examined with the same test on different occasions, or with different sets of equivalent items, or under other variable examining conditions.' If a test is well designed and if the trait being measured is stable, then the relative standing of a subject from one testing to another testing should not change substantially and the correlation between scores obtained on two separate occasions should be moderate to high in magnitude. Unfortunately there are few studies that document the reliability of central auditory tests currently in use, and reliability data are seldom provided in test manuals.

Regarding the validity of central auditory tests, there are different kinds of validity, and understanding the various definitions is necessary. Briefly, a test is considered valid if it measures what it is designed to measure. Unlike reliability, estimates of validity cannot come from one large administration of a single test. Instead, an entire body of information on validity must be obtained over a time. Establishing the validity of a test is a complex task because validity must be studied in relation to particular uses of the test.

There are at least two ways of determining test validity. One is to test persons with proven lesions involving the CANS (Musiek et al., 1994). Test validity can also be shown with patients who do not have a known lesion but have long-standing demonstrable problems of auditory reception. These are persons with normal hearing, no known lesion of the brain, excellent language and intelligence, who, by every indication from their history, cannot process auditory information efficiently. Abnormal central auditory test findings on these persons show another way of validating these measures. Examples of research supporting validity of testing based on individuals with normal hearing and listening problems include Middelweed (1990), Rodriguez et al. (1990), Chermak et al. (1989) and Jerger et al. (1989).

Assessment of peripheral hearing prior to central auditory testing

Before any attempt is made to diagnose a child as having CAPD it is necessary to rule out the presence of a conductive or sensorineural hearing problem. Therefore comprehensive audiometry, including pure-tone air and bone conduction threshold tests, tympanometry, and speech audiometry must be administered prior to the central auditory tests. The recent addition of otoacoustic emissions provides additional opportunity to verify normal cochlear hair cell function prior to CAP testing.

In general, central auditory testing is done when hearing is within normal limits, defined as thresholds between 0 and 15 dB HL for the frequencies 500 through 4000 Hz and within 5 dB for adjacent octave frequencies. When a unilateral hearing impairment is present only monaural sensitized speech tests can be administered. When there is a sloping hearing loss present, it may be necessary to identify central auditory tests using pure-tone stimuli that can be administered at frequencies of 'normal' hearing. When children have a history of otitis media and fluctuating hearing impairment it is unwise to administer central auditory tests based on a previous hearing test, and auditory thresholds should be obtained just prior to the test. Because of the residual effects of early hearing impairment on central auditory processing, children with histories of frequent colds or chronic middle-ear disease should be carefully watched for signs of central auditory processing disorder (Menyuk, 1992; Gravel and Ellis, 1995).

Behavioural tests of central auditory function

Some basic principles apply to central auditory assessment. It is known that most conditions affecting central hearing pathways produce no loss in threshold sensitivity. Therefore, pure-tone tests do not generally identify CAPDs. In addition, undistorted speech audiometry is not sufficiently challenging to the central auditory nervous system to identify the presence of a central auditory lesion/disorder. It is generally true that only tests of reduced acoustic redundancy (distorted speech materials called sensitized speech tests by Teatini, 1970) are sufficiently challenging to the auditory nervous system to identify a central auditory lesion/disorder.

Sensitized speech tests use various means of distortion of the speech stimuli to reduce the intelligibility of the message. Distortion can be accomplished in many ways including high- or low-pass filtering that reduces the range of frequencies (filtered speech testing). Another technique is to reduce the intensity level of speech above a simultaneously presented background noise (auditory figure ground testing). Speech is distorted in the time domain by interrupting the speech at different rates, and by increasing the rate of presentation (time-compressed speech). The basic principle of sensitized speech testing is that persons with normal auditory sensitivity and central auditory pathways can understand a distorted speech message. However, when a central auditory disorder is present, speech intelligibility is poor. The construct of sensitized speech testing is extremely powerful and forms the basis of all behavioural speech tests of central auditory function.

Tests of temporal processing

The first group of central auditory tests listed by the ASHA panel includes tests of temporal process. According to a number of investigators the ability to process basic acoustic parameters such as frequency and duration may predict speech intelligibility (Phillips and Farmer, 1990; Thompson and Abel, 1992; Tallal et al., 1993; Merzenich et al., 1996; Tallal et al., 1996). Specifically, auditory discrimination is dependent on the ability to hear formant frequency transitions of speech. Thus, deficits in ability to 'hear' small differences in timing aspects of ongoing speech create speech discrimination errors, even though hearing thresholds may be normal.

The general range of temporal discriminations that must be made during running speech is as follows. The distinction between the duration of the voice onset time (VOT) of consonants such as /p/ versus /b/ is approximately 20 ms (Eimas, 1975a) but the duration of the silent interval itself may vary across a range from 65 ms to 125 ms. Any circumstance that interferes with the perception of these intervals – either internally or externally – will affect the learner adversely. For example, excessive room reverberation can mask these intervals and reduce speech intelligibility (McCroskey et al., 1981).

A number of techniques for assessing different temporal aspects of acoustic signals are available. They include assessment of thresholds for brief tones, testing for temporal ordering and sequencing of tonal or click stimuli, and discrimination of time-compressed speech. All of these techniques find that disturbances in the temporal aspects of audition are related to cortical lesions. These findings are summarized in several references (Pinheiro and Musiek, 1985; Baran and Musiek, 1991; Olsen, 1991;

Thompson and Abel, 1992). Two specific examples of tests of temporal processing include the Duration Patterns Test (Musiek et al., 1990) and the Auditory Fusion Test – Revised (McCroskey and Keith, 1996).

The Duration Patterns Test (Musiek et al., 1990) is a sequence of three consecutive 1 000 Hz tones with one differing by being either longer (L) (500 ms), or shorter (S) 200 (ms), in duration than the other two tones in the sequence. The tones have a rise/fall time of 10 ms and an interstimulus interval of 300 ms. Six different sequences, LLS, LSL, LSS, SLS, SLL, and SSL are used in the test. A total of 30 to 50 three-tone sequences are presented monaurally or binaurally at 50 dB re: spondee threshold (ST). Prior to testing, five to 10 practice items are provided to each subject to ensure their understanding of the task (Hurley and Museik, 1997). Subjects respond to each stimulus presentation with a verbal description of the sequence heard, pointing response and/or humming. A percentage correct score is computed with performance below 70% considered abnormal by some investigators although normative data are limited (especially for children) at the time of this writing (Hall and Mueller, 1997: p. 535). According to Musiek and his co-authors, the duration patterns test is sensitive to cerebral lesions while remaining unaffected by peripheral hearing impairment. The test is also free of effects of linguistic background.

The Auditory Fusion Test – Revised (AFT-R) (McCroskey and Keith, 1996) is designed to measure one aspect of audition, namely temporal resolution that is sometimes called 'gap detection'. The method of evaluating temporal resolution in the AFT-R is through determination of the auditory fusion threshold. The auditory fusion threshold is measured in milliseconds (ms) and is obtained by having a listener attend to a series of pure tones presented in pairs. The silent time interval (the interpulse interval) between each pair of tones increases and decreases in duration. As the silent interval changes, the listener reports whether the stimulus pairs are heard as one tone or two tones. The auditory fusion threshold is the average of the points at which the two tones, for the ascending and descending interpulse interval (IPI) series, are perceptually fused and heard as one.

The Auditory Fusion Test – Revised can be used to identify a temporal processing disorder that may account for language learning problems. The AFT-R is viewed as a test of temporal integrity at the level of the cortex. Even though it is a cortical measure the test has a low linguistic and cognitive load – for example, the listener must simply respond by indicating whether one or two tone pulses were heard. As with the duration patterns test, the AFT-R is unaffected by peripheral hearing impairment or linguistic background.

Monaural degraded speech tests

One of the most common complaints among children with auditory processing disorders is their inability to communicate when background noise is present. Therefore speech-in-noise testing may be indicated to identify when the child's ability to communicate in the presence of noise is substantially below what is expected for a child's age level. For that reason, it may be beneficial to use different competing signals (for example, a single speaker versus multi-talker speech babble background) at different signal-to-noise ratios (for instance +8, +4, and 0 dB S/N). Research finds that linguistic materials (such as multi-talker speech babble background noise) are more effective maskers than speech-spectrum noise (SSN), even though the SSN has the same long-term spectrum and amplitude as the meaningful multi-talker competing message (Sperry et al., 1997). Other research finds that white noise and narrow band noise are also less effective than speech babble for masking speech. For many years it has been known that there is a great deal of variability among normal subjects in their ability to discriminate speech in a noise background (Keith and Tallis, 1970). As a consequence, when speech-in-noise testing is done to identify central auditory processing disorders, it is important to know the cut-off of normal performance for the S/N ratio and type of noise used in the test.

Low pass filtered-word tests are a category of tests in which speech is degraded by removing part of the frequency spectrum. Some authors consider this a test of auditory closure that is defined as the ability to understand the whole word or message when part is missing. Early research (Willeford, 1976) showed reduced performance on filtered word testing in children who are poor listeners who have central auditory dysfunction. Willeford's early studies have been subsequently verified by other authors (Costello, 1977; Keith and Farrer, 1981; Deitrich et al., 1992). Presumably the child with CAPD is unable to resist acoustic distortions of speech, resulting in poor listening abilities in acoustic environments that are less than optimal.

Filtered word tests are available with different cut-off frequencies and filter slopes (Keith, 1986, 1994; Bornstein et al., 1994). Filtered word test results are particularly vulnerable to high frequency hearing impairment, so it is important to rule out peripheral hearing impairment prior to testing. In addition, as with all central auditory testing, it is important to know the mean and range of scores obtained on normal subjects for the filter conditions used.

Some tests of low redundancy monaural speech include:

- Pediatric Speech Intelligibility (PSI) test (Jerger, 1987);

- Auditory Figure Ground and Filtered Words subtests of SCAN, SCAN-C, and SCAN-A (Keith, 1986, 1994, 2000);
- Time Compressed Speech (VA CD, 1992).

Binaural tests of separation or integration

Dichotic speech testing is typically administered to determine hemispheric dominance for language shown by asymmetrical ear responses and to assess neuromaturational development of the auditory system. Dichotic listening tests involve the simultaneous presentation of different acoustic stimuli to the two ears. Commonly used stimuli include digits, consonant-vowel (CV) nonsense syllables incorporating the six stop consonants (p, t, k, b, d, g) paired with the vowel /a/, words, spondees, and sentences. With the exception of the Staggered Spondee Word Test (SSW), the dichotic signals are recorded with simultaneous alignment of onset and off times.

Dichotic tests are generally administered at comfortable listening levels under earphones. The listener is required to repeat or write what is heard. There are two types of listening instructions given to subjects, free recall or directed-ear testing. Free recall allows the subject to respond to whatever was heard in either ear. Directed-ear testing requires the subject to report what was heard in the right or the left ear first. Tests vary whether they require reporting of what was heard in one or both ears. When instructions require the subject to respond to both stimuli, the first ear reported will show better scores and higher reliability than the second ear reported (Millay et al., 1977). The right-ear performance is typically better in young subjects, reflecting the ear-to-dominant-hemisphere relationship, so children will usually report what is heard in the right ear first under free recall conditions. Directed-ear listening therefore provides better estimates of the true ear score difference and reliability of test scores in the left ear. Directed-ear listening provides additional diagnostic information. For example, Obrzut et al. (1981) found that children with learning disabilities exhibited a marked switch in ear advantage on directed right and directed left-ear-first responses. That is, they yielded a right ear advantage when directed to respond from the right ear first, and a left ear advantage when directed to respond from the left ear first.

In general, for normal subjects, all dichotic test results show a right-ear advantage under free recall and directed-ear testing. A right-ear advantage is typically present whether the child is right or left handed. For one thing, handedness does not necessarily indicate hemispheric dominance for language (Knox and Roeser, 1980). Further, Satz (1976) reported that a strong REA is an extremely probable predictor of left hemispheric specialization for speech and language function. However, Satz found that a left-ear advantage predicts right hemispheric function for language only rarely. The greater the linguistic content of the signal (from consonant vowels to words, spondees, and sentences) the larger the right-ear advantage (the larger the difference between the right- and left-ear scores). As the central auditory nervous system matures, the left-ear scores improve and the right-ear advantage becomes progressively smaller. At age 11 or 12 years the auditory system is adult like in terms of performance on dichotic testing.

Abnormal dichotic speech test results typically fall in one of the following categories:

- poor overall performance;
- enhanced right-ear advantage in the directed-right condition and enhanced left-ear advantage in the directed-left condition;
- a marked left-ear advantage for both directed-right and directed-left ear conditions.

Abnormal performance on dichotic tests indicates delays in auditory maturation, underlying neurological disorganization or damage to auditory pathways. Left-ear advantages for all test conditions indicate the possibility of damage to the auditory reception areas of the left hemisphere, or failure to develop left-hemisphere dominance for language. These abnormalities are related to a wide range of specific learning disabilities including central auditory processing disorders, language, learning and reading. Longitudinal testing will help the audiologist discern whether maturation is occurring. If repeat testing after an appropriate interval (for example, after a year) shows little change or no change in dichotic test scores it is likely that the central auditory system is damaged or disordered. The greater the disorder, the more likely that residual deficits will remain in later years.

Some dichotic tests include:

- Dichotic Digits (Musiek et al., 1991, VA CD, 1992)
- Dichotic Words (SCAN and SCAN-A, Keith, 1986, 1994)
- Dichotic Spondees (SSW, Katz, 1962)
- Dichotic Sentences (SCAN-C , Keith 2000 and SCAN-A, Keith 1994)
- Dichotic Syllables, Digits, Sentences (VA CD, 1992)

Binaural interaction procedures

Masking level differences (MLD)

The masking level difference (MLD) refers to the difference between thresholds obtained under two binaural masking paradigms termed homophasic and antiphasic. According to Wilson, Zizz and Sperry (1994) a homophasic condition is one in which the signals in two channels are in phase with one another and the noises in two channels are in phase with one another (S_0N_0). An antiphasic condition is one in which either the signals or noises in the two channels are 180 degrees out of phase (S_0N_π or S_π N_0). Masking level differences have been used for many years in psychoacoustic research and in the clinical evaluation of brainstem function. MLDs are obtained by obtaining binaural masked thresholds for either pure tones or speech under homophasic and antiphasic conditions. The thresholds for the homophasic (for example, noise in phase at the two ears and signal in phase at the two ears; S_0N_0) minus the antiphasic conditions (for example, noise in phase at the two ears and signal out of phase at the two ears; S_π N_0) is the MLD. This effect is sometimes called the binaural release from masking. The MLD can be 10 to 15 dB for pure tones and is frequency dependent with the largest effects in the lower frequencies (300 Hz to 600 Hz). The MLD for speech is smaller than for pure tones (Wilson et al., 1994). Subjects must have normal hearing to maximize the MLD, because peripheral hearing impairment has a substantial effect on reducing the size of the MLD. Brainstem lesions can reduce or eliminate the MLD (Olsen and Noffsinger, 1976). Early research by Sweetow and Reddell (1978) found reduced MLDs in children with suspected auditory perceptual problems. They found that tonal MLDs were effective in discriminating children with auditory perceptual dysfunction from normal children, but speech MLDs were not. Current interest in the MLD is directed at the fact that it is a non-linguistic task that may identify dysfunction in the processing of auditory information at brainstem levels.

Electrophysiological tests of auditory function

For many years clinicians have used electrophysiological measures to assess the central auditory nervous system. There are several measures available for these purposes including auditory brainstem responses (ABR), middle-latency responses (MLR), long-latency auditory evoked potentials (LAEP), event-related potentials called P-300, and mismatch negativity (MMN). McPherson (1996) describes the long-latency auditory evoked potentials as consisting of perceptual and cognitive processes. Called exogenous and endogenous potentials, the components from 90 to 200 ms are generally related to the acoustic features of the stimulus, while the P-300, contingent negative variation (CNV) and later components are related to cognition where the subject consciously recognizes the presence of a change in the acoustic stimuli. Electrophysiological responses add an additional dimension to the central auditory test battery and may help to understand the neurophysiological substrata of CAPD.

Auditory brainstem responses (ABR)

The ABR is a series of neurological responses that are assumed to reflect the sequence of activity of the auditory nerve and nerve tracts and nuclei of the ascending auditory pathway (Moller, 1985). These compound action potentials result from an acoustic stimulus of fast rise time (a click) and occur within the first 10 ms following the stimulus. Because the ABR reflects pontine-mesencephalic transmission of neural activity, it is a measure of central auditory processing at the brainstem level. Investigators have reported abnormalities in the ABR in children with central auditory processing and language-learning disorders (Worthington, 1980; Jerger and Jerger, 1985). Stein and Kraus (1988) report various studies showing ABR abnormalities in patients with confirmed hydrocephalus, autism and Down's syndrome. Lynn et al. (1983) reported ABR abnormalities in patients with olivopontocerebellar degeneration, and Keith and Jacobson (1994) report ABR abnormalities commonly observed in patients with multiple sclerosis. These and other studies indicate the sensitivity of ABR measurements to the presence of brainstem abnormalities.

Middle-latency responses (MLR)

The middle-latency components of the auditory evoked response occur within the first 100 ms following the presentation of an effective auditory stimulus (Kileny, 1985). The specific generator of the MLR is unknown but is felt to represent a diffuse response of the auditory cortex (Kraus et al., 1982). Infant and adult MLRs have different morphologies and the infant requires a lower high-pass filter, for example, 10 Hz, compared to adults for whom the MLR can be obtained using a 30 Hz high-pass filter. Kraus et al. (1985) reported that detectability of the MLR increased significantly as a function of age. Detection of MLR Na components increased from 75% to 90% as subject age increased from zero to 20 years while detection of the Pa component increased from 40% to 90% during the same time frame. There continues to be question whether attention, including sleep states and effects of barbiturate anaesthesia, has an affect on the MLR. Research published by Osterhammel, Shallop and Terkilson (1985) found substantial changes in morphology and latencies of the MLR during sleep. Kraus et al. (1989) found that wave Pa was consistently present during wakefulness, alpha stage 1 and REM sleep. They interpret their data as indicating that the MLR in children is not haphazard and that it can be reliably obtained during certain states of arousal. Nevertheless, caution should be taken in obtaining MRL data under conditions of sleep, and subjects should be awake and alert for optimal data collection.

Several reports in the literature indicate that MLR is a useful technique for assessment of individuals with CAPD (Ozdamar and Kraus, 1983; Jerger et al., 1988; Fifer and Sierra-Irizarry, 1988). Chermak and Museik (1997: p. 136) recommend measurement of the MLR from both cerebral hemispheres using a C3, C4, and Cz electrode array. They state that the electrode on the hemisphere near a lesion will have reduced amplitude, with reduction of 50% considered diagnostically important. While there is substantial MLR data on patients with central auditory lesions, less has been published on subjects with CAPD. Therefore, as Chermak and Musiek (1997) indicate, sensitivity and specificity data on MLR in subjects with CAPD is not currently known.

P-300 and mismatched negativity (MMN)

The P-300 is an endogenous cognitive evoked potential event with diffuse bilateral cortical distribution that is triggered by cognitive activity. This response is consistently elicited by target stimuli as long as the subject is attending to them, and as long as the subject performs adequately. The P-300 requires an 'oddball' paradigm in which rarely occurring stimuli are randomly presented within a succession of frequently occurring stimuli. Subjects are required to attend to the rare stimuli while ignoring the frequent stimuli. The response includes the N1 and P2 exogenous components to the frequent stimuli and a P-300 response to the rare stimulus, indicating perception of the contrast between the two stimuli (Kileny et al., 1997). The P-300 is strongly influenced by attention, alerting, arousal and subject psychological state. The response has been used in many ways to study information processing, and as such is used for the study of language, central auditory processing, and attention deficit disorders (Kraus et al., 1995; McPherson, 1996).

By contrast the mismatch negativity (MMN) response is an automatic response that requires no attention to the task. It can be elicited by a small acoustic difference in stimuli and is therefore suitable for the assessment of speech perception (Kraus et al., 1995; Sandridge and Boothroyd, 1996). The MMN occurs approximately 100 ms to 300 ms after the stimulus onset. Sandridge and Boothroyd, (1996) summarize previous research of MMN as indicating that it is elicited by changes in frequency, duration and intensity. It can be elicited with complex stimuli such as speech and can be elicited when differences between stimuli are near psychophysical thresholds. As such, the MMN is another tool for the study of central auditory processing and its disorders. A caveat for audiologists who plan to use MMN in clinical assessment of individual subjects was published by Dalebout and Stach (1999). Their research found that MMN was not present in one-third of listeners in their sample of normal young adults, suggesting the possibility of false positive outcomes in a clinical situation.

Central auditory testing in the UK

In the UK, the problem of test choice is seen in a wider context, and the relatively low volume of routine diagnostic tests for CAPD has meant few studies of batteries of tests. In dyslexia, British research has been directed towards basic rather than applied questions – particularly the neurological underpinning of the disorder – and there is similar emerging research in CAPD. In this way the national research agenda can be driven by priority issues in determining the allocation of resources to the identification and assessment of children within a limited cash system. For example, there exists a variety of perceptions on the prevalence of CAPD and the impact on the child, parent and teacher in terms of quality of life. However, for none of these is there an unbiased quantitative estimate.

To guide the national research agenda Berrie and Haggard (personal communication, 1999) conducted a questionnaire survey of the relevant UK clinicians. Four groups of audiologists were targeted: members of the British Association of Audiological Physicians, members of the British Association of Community Doctors in Audiology, educational audiologists and all heads of audiology clinics in the UK. Opinions about the nature of CAPD varied but there were distinct majority views on three points. They were that children with CAPD also have general dysfunctions, the issue of overlap with other disorders remains to be resolved, and the main consequence of the disorder is difficulty hearing speech-in-noise.

Few respondents (5%) used specifically developed tests of central auditory processing as a method of assessment, and only 11% used a speech-in-noise test. The usual form of assessment (31% of respondents) was standard speech discrimination tests administered in a face-to-face test situation or through speech audiometry. Although the practitioners were aware of the limited specific value of such tests, the emerging importance of Health Technology Assessment in the UK means that advancement on this relatively limited clinical picture will require additional evaluative information on the benefits to the patient from more sophisticated diagnosis and management.

Language testing

Language tests are designed to assess areas of strength and weakness for all aspects of language including discrimination, phonology, receptive language, expressive language, prosody and pragmatics. Non-standardized language sampling and standardized language measures are both used by speech language pathologists for assessment. That information is used in the development of remediation programmes for children with central auditory processing and language disorders. The ASHA (1996) consensus statement on CAPD points out that clinicians should be cautious in attributing language/learning difficulties to CAPD in any simple fashion. Clinicians should not infer the existence of CAPD solely from evidence of learning disability or language impairment or vice versa.

Management and remediation

There is beginning to be agreement about therapy approaches to take following assessment of auditory processing and the identification of an auditory processing disorder. Two terms are commonly used in discussing follow up of a CAPD diagnosis, including management and remediation. Some authors believe that these two terms have distinct meanings and implications for the CAPD. Remediation is an actual altering of the central auditory nervous system function while management involves modifying behaviour, performance or environment with compensatory or cognitive techniques. The following is a brief overview of strategies for management and remediation of auditory processing disorders (Keith and Fallis, 1998).

Basic intervention strategies

The basic intervention strategies are:

- medical;
- perceptual training;
- compensatory;
- cognitive;
- management of environment.

Medical therapy is the use of drugs or surgery in the treatment of an auditory processing disorder. An example of a medical therapy strategy is the prescription of a stimulant medication for the treatment of ADHD.

Perceptual training addresses the temporal aspects of audition. The strongest evidence of the benefits of this type of therapy come from studies completed by Merzenich et al. (1996) and Tallal et al. (1996). These authors describe the positive effects of computer-based games that train or modify temporal deficits in children. Merzenich et al. used a perceptual identification task to assess auditory sequencing. A correct response in the exercise was a faithful reproduction of the order of two-stimuli sound sequences. Performance functions indicated that all children showed substantial and progressive gains in their abilities to sequence these fast, brief stimuli. In a companion study, Tallal et al. reported on perceptual training, again using computer games, of children with temporal processing deficits. The duration of the modified speech signal used was prolonged by 50% while preserving spectral content and natural quality. The authors claim that training results in dramatic improvements in recognition of rapid speech and non-speech stimuli as well as improvements in speech discrimination and language comprehension abilities.

Compensatory techniques (auditory skills development) are used to strengthen perceptual processes and teach specific academic skills. There are many different approaches to teaching auditory skills that assist the central auditory processing disordered child in academic, social and emotional worlds. A brief description of various auditory skills follows. References related to these auditory skills are added for the reader to further pursue a specific method. This list does not include all of the compensatory techniques available to the teacher, parent or therapist of a CAPD child:

- speech sound discrimination (auditory discrimination) – (Sloan, 1986);
- auditory analysis;
- phonemic synthesis (auditory synthesis) – (Katz, 1983);
- auditory memory – (Butler, 1981);
- auditory figure-ground – (Gillet, 1993);
- prosody training;
- temporal processing deficit – (McCroskey, 1986; Merzenich et al., 1996; Tallal et al., 1996).

An excellent resource regarding the management or remediation of auditory skills may be found in Kelly (1995).

Cognitive training involves teaching the child to actively monitor and self-regulate their message comprehension skills and develop new problem-solving skills. Cognitive therapy may include language training (linguistic or metalinguistic), vocabulary development, and the teaching of organizational skills (Chermak and Musiek, 1992).

Butler (1981) reported on the teaching of mnemonic strategies to assist the CAPD child. She suggests using rehearsal, paragraphing, imagery, networking (building bridges to store new concepts), analysis of new ideas, and using key ideas to think systematically. According to Butler, these and other techniques improve memory ability in children.

Cognitive therapy may also include the teaching of organizational skills. These skills include teaching the child:

- how to follow directions;
- how to use written notes;
- self-monitoring strategies;
- to know what they know;
- to learn to listen and anticipate;
- to ask relevant questions;
- to know how to answer questions.

Finally, *management of the environment* includes such things as preferential seating in the classroom to enhance the signal-to-noise (S/N) ratio, increase visual communication between teacher and student, and allow the teacher to monitor the student's activities more effectively. Other environmental strategies include use of classroom amplification or personal assistive listening devices to enhance the S/N ratio. Carpeting of classrooms and use of drapes or other soft fabrics on the walls and windows absorbs sound and reduces reverberation in a room.

Jerger and Allen (1998) point out that the lack of specificity of central auditory test batteries 'can complicate the remediation and management of children diagnosed as having CAPD on the basis of such measures.' Their philosophical position is that 'our goals should be reoriented toward determining the normalcy/abnormalcy of the component processes involved in spoken word recognition.' In practical terms that philosophy translates into determining subtypes of central auditory processing disorders in children. Some efforts are being made in that regard at the time of this writing, although more is required. For example, based on the Staggered Spondaic Word Test results, Katz and his colleagues (Katz et al., 1992: p. 81) developed a model that can be used for understanding the CAPD and developing a remediation programme. Their model includes four categories: Phonemic Decoding, Tolerance-Fading Memory, Integration and Organization. Bellis (1996: p. 193) describes four categories of disorders including: Auditory Decoding Deficit, Integration Deficit, Association Deficit and Output-Organization Deficit. Both Katz and Bellis recommend management suggestions based on the CAPD category to which the child is assigned. Similarly, Fallis-Cunningham and Keith (1998) proposed that decisions for remediation should be based on results of central auditory tests. Table 13.3 provides examples of this model.

These models for categorizing subgroups are simplistic, and often without clear definition or agreement of what tests or test findings place a child in a certain category. Nevertheless, they represent early efforts to systematize the assessment and remediation of CAPD.

Table 13.3. Remediation algorithm based on results of central auditory tests (Fallis-Cunningham and Keith, 1998).

Disorder	Remediation
Disorder of temporal processing	Perceptual training (modify speaker rate), auditory discrimination, phoneme training, computer assisted remediation (e.g. FastForward, Earobics)
Disorder of auditory figure ground or other monaural degraded speech test	Reduce noise in environment Classroom management including preferential seating Use of FM system or other assistive listening device
Disorders of binaural separation /maturation	Receptive and expressive language remediation usually provided by a speech-language pathologist.

CHAPTER 14

Progressive hearing loss

D LUCAS

Introduction

After the initial shock of the confirmation of their child's hearing loss, parents tend to ask three questions: the first is 'when will he talk?' the second 'why me?' and the third 'will it get worse?' This latter question is almost impossible to answer unless the diagnosis (etiology) has been accurately identified; even then, there are many occasions when professionals are as shocked as parents to discover that the hearing loss is progressing. It is clearly wrong to assume that the impairment will not change but confirmation, or even suspicion, of change presents both parties with significant problems.

For families, the resolution of grief following the confirmation of the hearing loss may become impossible. They dread each visit to the audiology department, anticipating further bad news. They must constantly adjust to the changes in their child's ability to communicate and to use his or her residual hearing, to the type of hearing aids provided, to the school he or she will attend, to his or her eventual future in society. They may have to contemplate a decision about cochlear implant. They are in a state of constant uncertainty, enhanced by a sense of powerlessness, which may fuel their anger towards the professionals responsible for their child's care or to other family members or previous professionals whom they may seek to blame. Young children are remarkably stoical about changes in their disease or disorder; older children, however, may become extremely distressed, tearful and depressed as they struggle to cope with the change in their circumstances and ability to participate.

Although recognizing the needs of the child and family to be paramount, thought must be given to the dilemmas facing professionals. Gauging how much information to give, when to give it and how to break the news is professionally challenging. The late identification of permanent childhood hearing impairment is vexing and raises both doubts and assumptions about the onset or natural history of the hearing loss. Frequently, professionals will question the validity of their previous findings and must therefore deal with their own uncertainties, especially if the diagnosis is not obvious and only retrospectively is there thought to have been the possibility of active and potentially successful intervention.

Presentation

Deterioration of hearing may present in a variety of ways. The child, a parent or teacher may remark upon poorer responses to sound or instructions. Older children may complain of reduced speech perception, a complaint that must be taken seriously, even in the presence of an unchanged pure tone audiogram. Deterioration in behaviour is a frequent complaint, the child becoming naughty or disruptive, persistently tired or aggressive, increasingly demanding or withdrawn, refusing even to use sign language. Hearing aids may be rejected, despite previously established use. Older children may become reluctant to attend school or socialize or have apparently irrational fears, for example, of shopping or the dark. Frequently, the presenting complaint will be about the poor performance of the hearing aids. Tinnitus, vertigo, headache or noise intolerance may be directly or indirectly related to the progression. Savastano, Savini and Andreoli (1993) suggested that most children had symptoms of cochlear recruitment. The clarity of speech may deteriorate; conversely, speech may be better than anticipated in a child who presents with severe to profound loss in early childhood. Only rarely is there a clear history of a precipitating event.

Prevalence

Accurate information on what proportion of children have progressive (and/or fluctuating hearing loss) is difficult to obtain and relates almost entirely to sensorineural hearing loss (SNHL). Progressive SNHL is thought to occur in 2% to 32% of children depending on the criteria used (10, 15 or 20 dB HL) and the population studied. Various researchers have surveyed general or selected populations, seeking to link progression to etiology, age and audiometric configuration but, with the identification of hearing loss remaining at over 18 months of age in most children, early information about hearing thresholds will be missing and conclusions speculative: the mean age at first assessment was 33 months in one retrospective study (Berrettini et al., 1999).

Brookhouser et al. (1994) identified 6% of 365 ears to progress by 10 dB or more, a further 57% having fluctuating losses with gradual progression. Walch et al. (2000) also used a 10 dB change and found 32% of children to have progressive losses in their group of 106 children, the progression most commonly occurring between one and two years of age. Berrettini et al. (1999) identified 6.2% of 178 children in whom the hearing loss was progressive based on a recorded change of 20 dB at two or more frequencies but Newton and Rowson (1988) perceptively thought that their 9% of 177 children might be an underestimate. They used a 15 dB change as their parameter as did Parving (1988) who suggested 2% to 4% of a cohort of 138 children but as many as 16% based on a 10 dB difference. This group included post-meningitic children. Levi et al. (1993) studied 92 children retrospectively over 15 years, finding that 22.8% of them demonstrated progression, all of whom had more than a mild hearing loss when first identified.

Progression is thought to be faster in those under five or six years of age (Newton and Rowson, 1988; Savastano et al., 1993) when accurate behavioural thresholds may be more difficult to obtain. Deterioration is described across all frequencies although high frequencies may deteriorate first. Experience suggests that further loss of hearing is likely to occur where there is an island of much better hearing remaining: indeed, Newton and Rowson (1988) found that deterioration was always greatest in the better-hearing ear in asymmetrical hearing loss and Berrettini et al. (1999) commented that the least affected frequencies tended to deteriorate the most. Progression tends to be gradual rather than sudden, although a combination of progressive and fluctuating is possibly more common (Brookhouser et al., 1994). There does not seem to be any sex difference.

Confounding issues

Otitis media with effusion is as common in the child with permanent hearing impairment as in the general population: glue ear may add up to 40 dB to the hearing threshold. Anxious children may add another variable, that of a spurious (non-organic) overlay. Behavioural and electrophysiological tests are not directly comparable and tests in very young children can be fraught with hazard in interpretation with variable reproducibility (Parving, 1988). Even auditory brainstem (ABR) testing can be misleading and requires careful knowledge and experience. Poorer performance may be due to malfunction of the hearing aids. More powerful hearing aids are needed to deliver the same gain as the ear grows and canal resonance changes. Increased demands on language will be confused with deterioration of hearing.

With the increase in targeted neonatal screening, reports are emerging of infants who have passed the screen but who have subsequently been found to have a progressive SNHL (Nield et al., 1986; Konkle and Knightley, 1993; Borradori et al., 1997). Ototoxic drugs (such as furosamide), which are frequently used in the sick neonate, have been linked to progression, but reports have also highlighted the possible implication of extra-corporeal membrane oxygenation (ECMO), a technique used only in very sick infants with severe cardiorespiratory failure (Cheung et al., 1996; Graziani et al., 1997). Parker (personal communication) found that intermittent positive pressure ventilation (IPPV) of more than five days duration and the administration of ototoxic antibiotics were positively correlated with subsequent progressive SNHL in infants from neonatal intensive care units (NICU) who had passed the neonatal screen. The lack of a family history may be misleading: some of these children may yet be found to carry the A1555G mitochondrial mutation. Others will turn out to have acquired their hearing loss through later events, but an association of onset with subsequent illness must be treated cautiously: illness, like times of festival, may merely act as a temporal marker, an aide memoire. With the advent of universal neonatal screening, it will be vital to establish a dedicated targeted further 'screen' during the first year of life for those infants considered to be most at risk for historical or clinical reasons.

Assessment

The late identification of congenital SNHL means that progression may have been missed by professionals who have a tendency to describe as 'congenital' all severe to profound sensory hearing losses in those under two years of age. This underlines the importance of a careful history and the necessity of believing parents who are generally correct in their observations of their child's responses to sound and perplexed by the changes that they have observed, only to be dismissed by professionals at a time that is already very distressing for them. Where possible, a detailed history should be taken first from the child, using a sign language interpreter where necessary. Children will give a very clear description of their symptoms, uncontaminated by the fear and worry that frequently clouds the comments of their parents. It is not unknown for them to have omitted to tell their parents about changes in their hearing acuity until after the clinic has identified the further loss.

Clinical examination is mandatory. It is interesting to reflect on how often children with significant SNHL have their hearing accurately measured but no steps are taken to identify whether or not there are other clinically relevant signs: examination of the ears, nose and throat is frequently all that is considered necessary. Subtle dysmorphisms including external ear anomalies (pre-auricular pits, sinuses and epidermoids), eye manifestations (colour, setting, shape, cataracts, colobomata, retinal signs), palatal and dental abnormalities, and neck signs (branchial pits and sinuses, goitre, webbing, head tilt) should be sought. The skin should be examined for excess lentigines, cafe au lait spots, freckling in the axillae, haemangiomata. The heart should be examined, the blood pressure taken. The hands and feet must be inspected for the signs of additional digits, webbing, unusual morphology of the fingers and creases. The hair must be carefully inspected for signs of unusual pigmentation as this does not always occur as the classical white forelock and may also extend into the eyebrows. Is there synophrys? Where is the nasal root? Careful neuro-otological examination, including eye movements and observation of gait, may identify previously unsuspected vestibular or neuromuscular dysfunction. Examination of first-degree relatives may elicit the features of dominantly inherited conditions.

Investigations

Further investigation will be dictated by the findings on anamnesis and examination. Imaging of the petrous temporal bones is probably the single most useful investigation using high resolution axial CT scan for suspected bony anomalies, although the new generation of MRI scanner is the choice for definition of nerves and soft tissues and will, hopefully, supercede CT in the near future. Cuts of 1.2 mm on CT are essential if the widened vestibular aqueduct is to be demonstrated. Densitometry will clarify the extent of otosclerosis or cochlear otospongiosis.

As up to 64% of children with SNHL have some sort of eye or visual defect (Siatkowski et al., 1994; Guest, personal communication, 1999), all children should be examined by an ophthalmologist who is familiar with the visual and ophthalmic implications of permanent childhood hearing impairment.

Blood tests should look for abnormalities of renal function and of thyroid function in those with a goitre and must include syphilis serology. Anaemia has been linked with progressive hearing loss (Savastano et al., 1993) as have the haemoglobinopathies. In very young infants, identified before immunization or exposure, a search must be made for rubella and cytomegalovirus (CMV) antibodies. Other blood tests will be determined by clinical findings or the age at presentation. They may include ESR, autoantibodies and anti-cardiolipins.

Urinary metabolic screen is of debatable value but the progressive loss of Refsum syndrome may be identifiable in this way. A search for cells, protein and blood in the urine is mandatory. The presence of renal anomalies is simply demonstrated by renal ultrasound.

There is no excuse for not undertaking an ECG. The hearing loss has been described as progressive in Jervell and Lange -Nielsen syndrome.

Pure-tone audiometry of first degree relatives is mandatory.

Etiology

Most progressive hearing loss is ascribed to genetic causes: late-onset progressive SNHL is a feature of dominant inheritance and early onset of recessive inheritance. Barr and Wedenberg (1965) found progression in 50% of presumed familial hearing loss, at least two of these children having had normal measured responses in infancy. Although Brookhouser et al. (1994) suggested that only 14% were genetic, another 7% had a positive family history. Levi et al. (1993) did not find progression to be linked with any specific etiology. Newton and Rowson (1988) echoed earlier authors in pointing out the frequent finding of progression in association with intrauterine infection with CMV and rubella. Berrettini et al. (1999) excluded all recognized syndromal hearing losses from their retrospective group, finding that 5/11 patients had an inherited hearing loss, one was due to CMV, one to an anatomical abnormality (widened vestibular aqueducts, which may actually be genetically determined) and four were of unknown etiology. Savastano et al. (1993) excluded all known causes of hearing loss to give an idiopathic group, the only possible correlate being with a mild iron deficiency anaemia in those less than six years old: this is reported to occur in 6% to 27% of this age group anyway (Childs et al., 1997; Oti-Boateng et al., 1998; Wilson et al., 1999; Requejo et al., 1999). There have also been reports of cochlear abnormalities, including a widened vestibular aqueduct, in children with confirmed congenital CMV (Baumann et al., 1994). See Table 14.1.

Genetic non-syndromal progressive hearing loss

Autosomal dominant sensorineural

Up to 25% of congenital profound hearing loss may be dominantly inherited. The majority of these cases are non-syndromal and, therefore, without any warning signs or specific features, hence the importance of carefully reviewing children at risk based on an accurate history of the onset of the hearing loss in the adult members of the family. It would be wrong to omit consideration of those losses that are only described in adults; the stigma of deafness and the relative paucity of facilities for identification may have prevented earlier identification in older family members. Variability of expressivity is characteristic of dominantly inherited disorders so it is unsurprising to find that, although the shape of the

Table 14.1. Commonest ages of onset of progressive hearing loss in children.

Age band	Etiology
0–5 years	Autosomal recessive X-linked Jervell and Lange-Nielsen syndrome Perinatal events Congenital cytomegalovirus Congenital rubella Mucopolysaccharidoses
5–10 years	Autosomal dominant Osteogenesis imperfecta Alport syndrome Alström syndrome Marshall syndrome Noonan syndrome
10–20 years	Otosclerosis Usher Type 3 Mitochondrial Down's syndrome Turner syndrome Norrie syndrome Congenital syphilis Autoimmune Noise
Any age	Bacterial meningitis Ototoxic drugs Widened vestibular aqueducts Tumours Trauma

audiogram may be similar between family members, the level of hearing loss and the speed of change can be quite variable.

Although most dominantly inherited progressive losses are said to commence in the high frequencies, almost every configuration of audiometric pattern has been described: first or second decade onset SNHL above 2 kHz progressing to severe in mid and high frequencies in later life (Khetarpal et al., 1991; Lalwani et al., 1997; Van Camp et al., 1997); early childhood onset high-frequency loss progressing diagonally across the audiogram from high frequencies to low; mid-frequency saucer-shaped loss with high frequency progression (Paparella, Sugiura and Hoshino, 1969); low frequency SNHL starting in the first decade and progressing to profound across all frequencies in adult life (Leon et al., 1981); pre-lingual onset severe to profound.

Discrimination between these hearing losses was made primarily by the pattern of progression and time of onset. Nowadays, however, it is the identification of different gene loci that is enabling a more accurate classification. A number of different linkages have been demonstrated on a variety of chromosomes (Leon et al, 1993; Brown et al, 1997; Van Camp et al., 1997). See Table 14.2.

The sensorineural loss in the best known dominantly inherited syndrome, Waardenburg Type 2, may be progressive in some families (Hildesheimer et al., 1989).

Table 14.2. Identified chromosome linkages in autosomal dominant progressive sensorineural hearing loss.

Linkage	Chromosome	Onset	Progression	Reference
DFNA1	5q31	Low frequency 1st decade	Profound 4th decade (Monge's deafness)	Leon et al (1981)
DFNA2	1p32	High frequency Early loss ? congenital	Mid and high frequency 3rd – 5th decade 1dB per octave per year	Van Camp et al (1997) Marres et al (1997)
DFNA3	13q12	Pre-lingual Mod/severe	Severe/ profound	Chaib et al (1994)
DFNA4	19q13	2nd decade	Profound by 5th decade	Chen et al (1995)
DFNA5	7p15	High frequency Early childhood	To include low frequency 4th – 5th decade	Van Laer et al (1997)
DFNA6	4p16.3	Low frequency 2nd decade		Lesperance et al (1995)
DFNA9	14q12 – q13	Progessive and Vestibular disturbance		De Kok et al (1999)
DFNA11	11q			Tamagawa et al (1996)
DFNA13	6p	Progressive 2–4th decades		Brown et al (1997)

Otosclerosis and otospongiosis

These have long been recognized as characterized by dominantly inherited conductive hearing loss with an onset typically in the middle years of life, often hastened by pregnancy. Onset in childhood is said to be rare but may occur more commonly than is recognized, the disease being reported in five year olds. Some children, with a family history of otosclerosis, present with a sensorineural or mixed hearing loss, CT scan demonstrating the typical picture of cochlear otospongiosis. There is debate, however, as to whether cochlear otospongiosis and the progressive stapes fixation of otosclerosis are the same condition. As well as the condition itself being progressive, there are risks attached to surgical intervention, although results are encouraging with 90% maintaining an air-bone gap of less than 20 dB over several years (Millman et al., 1996; Lippy et al., 1998). Success with stapedectomy may correlate with less severe footplate fixation in the younger patient (Robinson, 1983). Some children, however, will become profoundly deaf.

Autosomal recessive sensorineural

There are a number of non-syndromal sensorineural hearing losses described, but ascertainment is poor due to the very wide clinical heterogeneity in these families. There do seem to be two patterns: one of early onset with progression to profound by five years of age (Mustapha et al., 1998), the other being predominantly high frequency.

Genetic syndromal progressive hearing loss

Disorders of bone and progressive hearing loss

Osteogenesis imperfecta

There are a number of craniotubular dysplasias, inherited variably in a dominant or recessive manner, which affect the temporal bone. Progressive mixed hearing loss during childhood is an almost universal feature. A particular example of this mix of inner and middle-ear pathology is to be found in the bone disorder Camurati-Engelmann disease (Huygen et al., 1996). Progressive mixed loss is also reported in association with chondrodysplasias.

Families with type 1 autosomal dominantly inherited osteogenesis imperfecta show the typical triad of multiple fractures, blue sclerae and hearing loss, the latter said to commence most commonly at the end of the first decade. The hearing loss was always thought to be conductive, due to stapes fixation, fracture or anomalous ossicular articulation. It is now realized that, despite the variable expressivity of the gene, a sensory component is the rule rather than the exception, being progressive in up to 50%, starting at under 30 years of age as a mild high-frequency loss and continuing to include the low frequencies (Shapiro et al., 1982; Pederson, 1984). The hearing loss does not seem to be related to either the severity or the frequency of the fractures. More severe degrees of sensory loss are often accompanied by vestibular symptoms.

Eye problems and progressive hearing loss

Pigmentary disorders of the retina are the best recognized of the variety of eye disorders that can be associated with childhood progression of genetic hearing loss. Other syndromes include corneal dystrophy (autosomal recessive), cataracts (autosomal dominant), ophthalmoplegias, optic atrophies, high myopia and retinal aplasia leading to detachment (Norrie syndrome). Onset of the progression ranges from early childhood to the second decade and from slow progression in the high frequencies only to severe to profound within 10 years. It is important to remember that retinal pigment ('salt and pepper retinopathy') and cataracts form part of the typical findings in congenital rubella.

Usher syndrome Type 3

Linked to chromosome 3q, this is the least common of the heterogeneic group of Usher syndrome, in which retinitis pigmentosa develops at the end of the second decade resulting in night-blindness and visual field defects. It is thought to represent from 1% to 4% of patients with Usher syndrome and is characterized by progression of the initially mild hearing loss, which is not usually congenital. There seems to be a far higher prevalence in Finland (Pakarinen et al., 1995), perhaps as much as 40%. There have been some reports of progression in other types of Usher syndrome, but these may represent incorrect classification.

Alström syndrome

Alström syndrome is a complex recessively inherited condition in which pigmentary retinal degeneration is usually the presenting feature, progressive SNHL, truncal obesity, acanthosis nigrans and abnormalities of lipid and glucose metabolism being apparent later. Non-insulin-dependent diabetes mellitus and growth retardation occur in adolescence (Sebag, Albert and Craft, 1984; Marshall et al., 1997). Edward syndrome is very similar but it is accompanied by significant learning difficulties.

Marshall Stickler syndrome

Progressive mixed loss is described in Marshall syndrome, which is most likely to be dominantly inherited with other features including severe myopia, cataracts and saddle nose. It is uncertain as to whether this syndrome is distinct from Stickler syndrome where the main features are high myopia leading to retinal detachment, cleft palate and spondyloepiphyseal dysplasia with progressive SNHL in 80% (Zlotogora et al., 1992).

Mucopolysaccharidoses (MPS)

The mucopolysaccharidoses are a complex collection of specific lyzosomal enzyme deficiency disorders, usually presenting within the first two to three years of life with deterioration in developmental progress, coarsening of the facial features and a variety of other system manifestations depending on the enzyme involved. All are autosomal recessively inherited with the exception of Hunter syndrome, which is X-linked. The progressive deterioration in physical, neurological and mental function in most of these conditions supercedes concerns about hearing.

At least five types are known to be associated with conductive hearing losses but progressive SNHL is less well recognized (Hayes et al., 1980). The pathology is complex involving both the middle ear and semicircular canals. The progressive conductive hearing loss of Hurler syndrome (MPS 1-H) is now known to be associated in many children with a progressive SNHL. About 25% of those with Maroteaux-Lamy syndrome (MPS Vl) have a progressive conductive hearing loss as do 25% to 50% of those with Hunter syndrome (MPS ll) (Lyons Jones, 1997). Morquio syndrome (MPS lV) is generally milder than the other MPS but virtually all patients with type A develop a progressive SNHL by the second decade (Kasman-Kellaret et al., 1999).

Renal problems and hearing loss

A number of nephritides have progressive SNHL amongst their features; in Epstein syndrome, hearing loss and macrothrombocytopenia develop before the age of 10 years with renal symptoms developing later (Epstein et al., 1972). The SNHL of Charcot-Marie-Tooth disease (nephritis with sensory and motor neuropathy) is slowly progressive from childhood (Raglan et al., 1987). Other types begin in adolescence and progress to profound loss with renal failure. Brown et al. (1993) reported on two types of renal tubular acidosis of infantile and juvenile onset: the more severe infantile version presents typically with failure to thrive in the first year of life with a severe and possibly progressive SNHL.

Alport syndrome

This is a syndrome of specific glomerulonephritis and SNHL with axial myopia, anterior lenticonus (progressing to cataracts) and macular or perimacular flecks. As in most of the nephritides associated with progressive hearing loss, the patient usually presents with haematuria. Males are more severely affected and the picture is of progressive renal dysfunction leading to failure. Typically, the hearing loss commences in the midfrequencies, progressing to the high frequencies and further as renal function deteriorates, at the end of the first decade of life, although Sirimanna and Stephens (1997) have pointed out that the hearing loss often starts before 10 years of age. The pattern of disease progression tends to be individual to the family, nearly all cases involving distinct mutations because of poor male fitness (Barker et al., 1997). The commonest variety is X-linked (85%) with the remainder being predominantly autosomal recessive (Brunner, 1996).

Widened vestibular aqueducts

Much excitement has been generated over the past 15 years by the radiological identification of the widened vestibular aqueduct (WVA) and the link with progressive SNHL (Valvassori and Clemis, 1978; Levenson et al., 1989). Carlo Mondini gave the original description of this anomaly in 1791 in association with the abnormal basal turn and distal sac, which we now recognize as the Mondini cochlea. The two do not necessarily coexist, however, and do not form a syndrome in their own right. The symptoms are characteristic: a progressive or fluctuating, mixed or SNHL, change often being precipitated by a minor blow to the head or pressure change, such as air travel. Episodes of hearing loss usually result in a permanent raising of hearing thresholds although there may be some return towards the original levels. Occasionally, the hearing loss is total and sudden. Many patients also complain of vestibular symptoms and tinnitus. The presenting hearing loss ranges from high frequency (often late in identification) to profound and even conductive. Over 70% are bilateral (Valvassori and Clemis, 1978; Arcand et al., 1991).

The confirmation of the presence of WVA is dependent upon careful CT scan although axial and sagittal MRI may demonstrate an enlarged endolymphatic duct and sac when the CT findings are equivocal (Dahlen et al., 1997; Phelps et al., 1997). There is no robust evidence that the rate of progression, ultimate hearing level or pattern of loss is related to the size of the aqueduct (Zalzal et al., 1995). The puzzle is in elucidating the relevance of the bony anomalies in those patients without enlarged endolymphatic sacs or without progression of the hearing loss.

The association between the Mondini cochlea and the autosomal recessively inherited Pendred syndrome (profound SNHL with goitre) has long been recognized, but WVA are now being found in around 80% of those with Pendred (Cremers et al., 1998). Although examination of the neck for a goitre should be undertaken regularly in deaf children, caution is appropriate. Some deaf children with goitre will turn out to have Hashimoto's thyroiditis rather than Pendred (O Mahoney et al., 1996), and goitre frequently does not develop until adult life (if at all) and is often difficult to detect in those under five years old. Perchlorate discharge may be misleading (Reardon et al., 1997) and genetic investigation into a large Pendrin gene (chromosome 7q) does not always come up with a definitive result.

Chen et al. (1995) identified 11 out of 24 ears to have WVA in patients with branchio-oto-renal syndrome. A history of dominant inheritance and the discovery of pre-auricular pits/sinuses, lacrimal sinuses, branchial cysts and sinuses or renal anomalies should enable clinical differentiation.

A surgical approach to stabilizing the hearing loss or restoring the hearing in patients with WVA has been tried but without conferring any sustained benefit (Jackler and De La Cruz, 1989; Wilson et al., 1997; Welling et al., 1998). It is likely that previously described benefit in some patients may be related to the natural history of fluctuation; some patients will lose all their residual hearing following surgery.

Miscellaneous

There are a number of other associations described with progressive SNHL, such as gonadal dysgenesis (Perrault syndrome), progressive pontobulbar palsy with progressive vestibular dysfunction (Brucher et al., 1981) and Chiari malformation (Johnson et al., 1994). There are anecdotal reports of progressive high-frequency SNHL associated with hydrocephalus, although it is most likely that this is associated with the events giving rise to the hydrocephalus. It is uncommon to find progressive SNHL with a large jugular fossa and bulb (Good et al., 1995). Progressive high-frequency loss to about 65 dB has been found in the dominantly inherited otodental syndrome (Gorlin et al., 1995).

X-linked deafness

A number of X-linked non-syndromic hearing losses have been described, the most widely recognized association being that of progressive mixed hearing loss with perilymphatic gusher. The hearing loss becomes evident in the first year of life and is accompanied by vestibular dysfunction. A CT scan may show the typical findings of a bulbous internal acoustic meatus with a deficiency in the bone between the lateral end of the meatus and the basal turn of the cochlea.

Other X-linked syndromes with progressive hearing loss are linked to a variety of neurological deficits or optic atrophy. In Norrie syndrome (bilateral congenital blindness due to maldevelopment of the retina and a variety of other ocular features), some 30% of patients develop a progressive SNHL in adult life. Onset may be detected in childhood, although this may be masked by a progressive worsening of cognitive function. Zachmann, Fuchs and Prader (1992) described X-linked adrenal hypoplasia with progressive loss in the second decade of life progressing rapidly to profound deafness within seven years.

Mitochondrially determined progressive hearing loss

Mitochondrial DNA encodes the mRNA necessary for effective cell metabolism. There are a variety of complex disorders now recognized to be associated with mitochondrial inheritance, transmitted entirely by the mother. These may be syndromic or non-syndromic.

The progressive high-frequency hearing loss of Kearns-Sayre syndrome (progressive ophthalmoplegia and retinitis pigmentosa) usually starts under the age of 20 years: four children have been described as presenting with hypoparathyroidism and progressive deafness (Wilichowski et al., 1997). In both Kearns-Sayre and MERRF (myoclonic epilepsy, ragged red fibres, ataxia, dementia, optic atrophy, A8344G and A8356G) hearing loss is reported to occur in 50% of cases, sometimes as the sole manifestation of the disease (Reardon and Harding, 1995). MELAS (myopathy, encephalopathy, lactic acidosis and stroke-like episodes, A3243G) is of gradual onset in adult life: SNHL often commences in the high frequencies during the second decade, occurs in about 30%, and is often the presenting feature with or without vestibular symptoms (Ensink, Camp and Cremers, 1998). Gold and Rapin (1994) reviewed the literature to determine whether SNHL could be a marker for particular phenotypes but progressive loss seems to occur in all ages in a variety of types of mitochondrial disease.

Although mitochondrial disease is predominantly described in adults, it may present in childhood with a moderate to severe hearing loss. Unfortunately, this will be at that vulnerable age when hearing loss is thought to be spurious (non-organic): diagnosis is therefore delayed, especially if the condition has not been recognized in the mother.

It is now thought that the susceptibility to SNHL with aminoglycosides is dependent on A1555G mitochondrial inheritance (Estivill et al., 1998b). An initially mild high-frequency progressive SNHL is also reported in susceptible family members who are not known to have been exposed to aminoglycosides (Usami et al., 1998) so it seems that many, if not all, of those with the mutation will become deaf anyway, just that the age of onset is earlier in those who have received the antibiotics. The real worry is that gentamycin is offered free to health clinics by the government of at least one country (Newton, personal communication) and is easily purchased across the counter in others where injectable drugs are regarded as being more efficacious: this presents significant opportunities for good evidence-based public health work.

Chromosomal syndromes

Down's syndrome (trisomy 21)

The commonest hearing deficit in children with Down's syndrome is that related to otitis media with effusion and its complications. A progressive high-frequency SNHL commences in the teenage years in as many as one-third (Davies, 1988; Roizen et al., 1993). Evenhuis et al. (1992) found that 56 of 59 ears in middle-aged patients with Down's syndrome had SNHL. Buchanan (1990) suggested that this might be early onset presbyacusis, a term that itself is falling increasingly into disrepute as the hearing loss of older age is recognized to be multifactorial and often related to both genetic and environmental factors.

Turner syndrome (XO and mosaics)

Turner syndrome is variable in both genotype and phenotype so the characteristic XO configuration with short stature, ovarian agenesis, short webbed neck and increased carrying angle with a shield chest is not always found. Chronic ear infections occur in 60% to 80% of patients in early childhood, 40% to 70% having a conductive hearing loss and 40% to 60% a progressive mid-frequency sensory dip (Watkin, 1989; Sculerati et al., 1990; Stenberg et al., 1998). Although typically described as occurring in the teenage years, the sensory loss has been identified in at least one reported six-year-old. Hultcrantz, Sylven and Borg (1994) found that all 45XO and 45XO/46Xi(Xq) mosaics had a mid-frequency dip, whereas only 31% of 45XO/46XX did; Hultcrantz and Sylven (1997) suggested that if no dip was found by early adult life, future problems with hearing would not occur.

Noonan syndrome

Progressive high-frequency hearing loss, present in perhaps 50% (Qiu, Yin and Stucker, 1998) may be the presenting feature in this relatively common dominantly inherited syndrome of short stature, congenital cardiac anomalies, webbed neck and mild learning difficulties.

Perilymph fistulae

The significance of perilymph fistulae in progressive SNHL remains debatable. Most protagonists firmly believe that early identification followed by surgical intervention will stabilize hearing (Myer et al., 1989; Kohut et al., 1996). Parnes and McCabe (1987) found six children out of 16 with proven fistulae were less than two years old when their symptoms commenced; 56% of their patients were also intermittently dizzy. The association of fistulae with minor head trauma (before the recognition of WVA) (Myer et al., 1989), with WVA and with radiological abnormalities (Belenky et al., 1993) has prompted the suggestion that all children with relevant symptoms should undergo CT scan (Weissman et al., 1994). Patients with residual hearing following transverse fracture of the temporal bone may have a perilymph fistula and surgery may preserve residual hearing (Lyos et al., 1995).

Intrauterine infection

Cytomegalovirus (CMV)

It has long been recognized that congenital CMV can be associated with SNHL. The estimated prevalence of congenital CMV is 0.3% to 0.4% of live births in the UK, although it may be as high as 2.2% in other countries. Boppana et al. (1992) noted decreased hearing in 56% of those infants with symptomatic infection in whom the hearing was assessed. Unfortunately, only some 10% of infants with congenital CMV are symptomatic at birth and therefore likely to be screened for hearing impairment. Of asymptomatic infants, about 5% will later manifest symptoms of the disease, SNHL being the most common (Peckham, 1989).

Several authors have commented on the unexpected deterioration of hearing thresholds in children with congenital CMV: Dahle et al. (1979) found four out of 12 children to have progressive losses and Williamson et al. (1992) five out of eight. A further child in Williamson et al.'s study developed a unilateral SNHL in the first year of life with subsequent deterioration. Hickson and Alcock (1991) noted deterioration in the first four years of life in five children referred for audiological assessment. In a large study of 307 children with asymptomatic congenital CMV, Fowler et al. (1997) found that 7.25% had SNHL, of whom 50% deteriorated between the ages of two and 70 months. Fluctuation was a significant finding in 22.7% of those with proven SNHL. Further, some 18.2% of children did not appear deaf when first screened but became deaf at 25 to 62 months. The latency and reactivation of herpes viruses is well recognized and it is possible that this represents a reactivation response to an unknown stimulus. Some of these children may also have vestibular symptoms (Huygen and Admiraal, 1996) leading to the suggestion that congenital CMV should come into the differential diagnosis of delayed endolymphatic hydrops. Cytomegalovirus inclusion bearing cells have been found in both the cochlea and the vestibular labyrinth, but reports of virus in the organ of Corti and spiral ganglia are conflicting (Strauss, 1990). Abnormal radiological findings (such as intracranial calcification and periventricular radiolucencies) are strongly linked to SNHL, although not necessarily to progression.

There is no safe immunization against CMV, so active disease may occur in more than one pregnancy (Williamson et al., 1992). As neonatal hearing screening programmes targeting at-risk infants will only identify about 14% of the asymptomatic deaf children (Hicks et al., 1993), deafness due to congenital CMV infection may be misdiagnosed as a recessively inherited hearing loss and any progression similarly falsely ascribed.

Congenital rubella

Progression of the hearing loss (Sheridan, 1964; Newton and Rowson, 1988) is thought to occur early in life and has been reported as being accompanied by significant cochlear recruitment. Wild et al. (1989) reported only one of 68 children with congenital rubella to have a documented progressive loss. In this study, however, only eight children had been tested before the age of six months, and diagnostic tests were frequently not undertaken until after the first birthday. In contrast, Das (1996) found evidence of progression in four out of 18 children, based on a change of 20 dB.

Congenital syphilis

The classical early findings of congenital syphilis (snuffles, rash, anaemia, jaundice and osteochondritis) are easily overlooked. The distinctive features of saddle nose, Hutchinson's teeth and mulberry molars will not be apparent until later. The most consistent finding to raise suspicion of the diagnosis is interstitial keratitis, present in 73% of 15 patients in Steckelberg and McDonald's (1984) retrospective study. Although congenital syphilis is traditionally associated with a progressive SNHL commencing at the beginning of the second decade, the time of onset can vary from early childhood to middle age. The hearing loss may be unilateral, bilateral, asymmetrical, of gradual onset over several years or occur with devastating rapidity as a sudden profound loss. Patients may also complain of tinnitus or vertigo, leading Karmody and Schuknecht (1966) to suggest that symptoms were all related to a hydropic picture. Spirochaetes may linger in the labyrinthine fluids for some time and osteitis and middle-ear thickening are also described. Active disease should be treated with penicillin and steroids.

Syphilis remains the great imitator in the pantheon of disease. Its incidence is increasing with the spread of HIV-positive people. It must always be considered in progressive and sudden SNHL.

Bacterial meningitis

Progression following bacterial meningitis is variable and unpredictable. In a retrospective study, Woolley et al. (1999) found 22% of 59 children had a fluctuating or progressive loss, which stabilized between three months and four years after the initial illness. They did not discover any predictive variables for progression in the initial illness. Fluctuations may be attributable to secondary endolymphatic hydrops (Rosenhall and Kankunnen, 1981). Labyrinthitis ossificans is thought to account for many of the cases of progression but this is not always demonstrable on CT scan: MRI is therefore mandatory, if cochlear implant is to be considered for these children, as the window of opportunity may be very narrow.

Autoimmune inner-ear disease

Of adult patients with rapidly progressive SNHL, one-third to a half had antibodies to 68kd inner-ear antigen (Moscicki et al., 1994; Gottschlich et al., 1995). Atlas, Chai and Boscato (1998) in 36 patients with classical Ménière's disease found 'strong evidence' of antibodies to inner-ear proteins. Berrettini et al. (1998) noted that progressive hearing loss is rare in the systemic vasculitides but may be amenable to treatment with steroids and cyclophosphamide or, eventually, with methotrexate and plasma exchange. Autoimmune disorders are rare in children, but Hisashi et al. (1993) reported a 15-year-old who presented with sudden SNHL and vertigo which partly responded to steroids. Systemic lupus erythematosis was subsequently diagnosed.

Anticardiolipin antibodies have been implicated in adults with sudden onset and progressive SNHL (Toubi et al., 1997). The youngest patient reported was 20 years old. Brodie et al. (1992) have described macrothrombocytopenia with progressive SNHL. The onset appeared to be before the third decade but the platelet disorder may start in early childhood.

The increasing prevalence of HIV has prompted consideration of a paediatric immunodeficiency syndrome (Madriz and Herrera, 1995). It is recognized that AIDS results in increased susceptibility to a variety of viral and bacterial disorders, often presenting in uncommon ways, and associated with progressive sensorineural hearing loss.

Ménière's disease

The classical triad of tinnitus, episodic vertigo and fluctuating low tone SNHL is rare in children (Meyerhoff, Paparella and Shea, 1978), although it is suggested that a secondary endolymphatic hydrops may be more common than is realized (Rodgers and Telischi, 1997). Temporal bone studies of infants and children showed bulging in Reissner's membrane in the cochlear duct in 16.9%, more commonly in those with congenital anomalies (Bachor and Karmody, 1995).

Acoustic neuroma

It is uncommon to find vestibular schwannomas presenting in childhood (Ishikawa et al., 1997). Almost exclusively, they will occur in children with neurofibromatosis Type ll (NF2), probably first described by Wishart in 1820. Most cases present with unilateral symptoms of the neuroma, including tinnitus, progressive hearing loss and, occasionally, dysequilibrium: some present with other types of schwannoma or intracranial or spinal tumours. Childhood cataracts may occur in 20% and this, together with a family history, may alert the clinician. Café au lait spots are uncommon but a search should be made for them in the axillae.

In a literature review, however, Chen et al. (1992) found only 16 cases reported before the age of 15 years; by 1999, this number had grown to 18. Management will be related to tumour size, growth and symptoms: surgical removal is commonly necessary and efforts are being made with new techniques to preserve hearing. Unfortunately, most of these patients end up with bilateral profound losses. The provision of a brainstem implant to give some access to sound may be considered for these young patients in the future.

Ototoxicity and progressive hearing loss

Drugs

A range of drugs has been identified over the years to be associated with the development of sensorineural hearing loss. These include aminoglycoside antibiotics, salicylates, loop diuretics and chemotherapeutic agents.

Research continues into the genetic predisposition to ototoxicity: evidence is emerging of additive effects between chemical ototoxicity and noise. It remains to be seen whether or not other chemotherapeutic agents only have an otoxic effect if there is a genetic predispostion.

Cisplatinum induces a dose-related progressive sensory loss, enhanced by previous irradiation. Littman et al. (1998) used distortion product otoacoustic emissions to try to predict who would be affected. At least one case of sudden total hearing loss has been reported following a single course of Cisplatin (Domenech et al., 1988) and others have warned of the risk of further progression even when treatment has ceased (Sweetow and Will, 1993).

Noise

Exposure to sustained or sudden loud noise has long been recognized to be a potent inducer of SNHL in adults. With the advent of personal stereo systems and the school disco, the increasing popularity of pop concerts (where the success of the evening is partly measured by the temporary threshold shift of the avid fan) and the increasing prevalence of the ubiquitous mobile phone and its toy equivalent, attention is being paid to noise as a potential hazard for young people.

Squeaky toys for babies, often used by parents as an indicator of good hearing, may emit sounds from 78 dBA to 108 dBA. Toy pistols and other weapons can emit levels as high as 150 dB (Luxon, 1998). There are anecdotal reports of noise levels as high as 90 dB in incubators although measurements nowadays suggest that 60 dB to 70 dB is more likely. The effect of noise may be enhanced by ototoxic drugs in these vulnerable children: we do not, however, have a clear idea of the effects of noise on the young ear.

Mansfield, Baghurst and Newton (1999) suggested that, in young adults, outer hair cell damage occurs firstly in the region of 2 kHz as measured by transient evoked otoacoustic emissions. Ising et al. (1997) looked at 569 pupils aged 10 years to 17 years and estimated that 40% might have significant hearing loss after 10 years if the same exposure continued. This study showed a somewhat higher relative risk in the less educated pupil. Alberti (1995) has suggested that noise-induced hearing loss is rare before the age of 10 years and states 'If ringing persists more than 30 minutes after listening to intense sound or if fullness of hearing persists for more than a very few hours, the young person almost certainly has hypersensitive ears and is at risk of hearing loss from levels of sound which are generally not damaging.'

Hearing aids

Given the clear recognition that noise can cause SNHL, it was natural to implicate the powerful hearing aids provided to young children in the progression of their loss. Although a number of authors have addressed the question in both retrospective and prospective studies, evidence is lacking (Reilly et al., 1981; Azema et al., 1994; Walch et al., 2000). Streppel et al. (1997) commented on the increasing numbers of children being identified as having progressive SNHL but, in a prospective study of 16 children, could find no evidence that this was linked with hearing aid provision.

Middle-ear disease

It is suggested that chronic middle-ear disease may lead to SNHL in as many as 50% of patients (Muchner, 1981; Paparella et al., 1984). Some children with chronic or recurrent acute otitis media have impaired hearing in the very high frequency range (12 kHz to 20 kHz) with normal hearing across the recognized speech frequencies (Margolis et al., 1993). There is no substantial evidence to confirm that middle-ear disease causes significant SNHL affecting general communicative ability in children (Walby et al., 1983; Kaplan et al., 1996).

Fageeh et al. (1999) found that the speech reception thresholds of 13% of children (total 173) operated on for cholesteatoma, both acquired and congenital, became worse post-operatively. A sensorineural hearing loss occurred in one child (0.5%) who had a congenital cholesteatoma extending over the lateral semicircular canal and round window niche. Congenital cholesteatoma is also reported in association with branchio-oto-renal syndrome where progressive hearing loss in association with WVA has also been described (Rajput et al., 1999; Worley et al., 1999).

Treatment

A variety of treatment regimens have been proposed over the years with little in the way of evidence to support them. The suspicion is that physicians are treating their own natural anxiety and that of the parents, rather than expecting to find any change. Thus betahistine (Soucek et al., 1985), ubiquitin (extract of calf thymuses) (Reron, Turowski and Olszewski, 1995), glycerol, calcium antagonists and some cerebral vasodilators have all been tried but without notable or sustained success; the use of many of these substances might be frowned upon in children. Carbogen was thought to have had some success when adults with sudden hearing loss were re-evaluated one year after treatment (Fisch, 1983). The use of high-dose oral steroids, hyperbaric oxygen and bed rest (during any identified acute phase of deterioration) remain a staple protocol for some clinicians but there is no real evidence of success and confining an otherwise well young child to bed is a challenging proposition.

There are some specific remedies for particular conditions, such as etidonrate sodium for otosclerosis (Kennedy, Hoffer and Holliday, 1993) but this only showed a trend towards stabilization in adults. Fluoride has been tried but side effects outweigh benefit. Patients with moderate-to-severe hearing loss who were positive for inner-ear protein antibodies responded better to steroids (Moscicki et al., 1994). Co-enzyme Q10 may prevent progression of the loss in some mitochondrial disorders (Seki et al., 1997; Suzuki et al., 1998). Children with symptoms suggestive of endolymphatic hydrops may benefit from restriction of salt and caffeine intake and the judicious use of diuretics.

Surgical approaches have now mostly been discounted except where there is a clear history of perilymph fistula, where ventilation of the middle ears in intercurrent glue ear is necessary for health reasons, in some cases of otosclerosis, and where there is a risk of meningitis in severe Cock's deformity of the inner ear in combination with progression of the hearing loss.

Management

The aim of management must be to maintain the child's confidence and rate of progress in development and learning. The mainstay of management, therefore, must be continuous rehabilitation and support. Addressing the child's needs as well as the parents', introducing psychological support, reviewing hearing aid provision, communication mode and educational environment must all be undertaken promptly and sensitively. Parents may cling onto the child's earlier potential with more hearing and be reluctant to adapt to different needs, especially if this involves a change of school or the introduction of signing. Feelings of guilt may supervene, especially where the loss is recognized to be genetically determined or due to some potentially avoidable cause.

The child and family will be under a number of increased stresses at this time. They must deal with the increasing impairment in the child and the impact that this has on the child's ability to function and the reaction, if any, of those around them. They may have to address other major health or ability problems. More frequent visits to the audiology centre result in time away from school, reduced academic achievement and reduced confidence; teasing may occur both because of poor achievement and because of increased hearing difficulty. From research on children with chronic illness, much depends on how the child's mother reacts, whether there is a large network of friends and family to support them, or whether support is distant and fragmented (Eiser, 1990). Siblings may perceive the extra attention as 'unfair'.

Children cope with bad news in a variety of ways, depending on their age. They need more than just the facts about their increased hearing loss – they need tactics and strategies to maintain their self-esteem, to be able to explain their situation to others and to resolve the conflict that may arise with their social and personal lifestyle. The unpredictable nature of progression makes it difficult for the child and family to adjust. Their sense of belonging to a common community may be disturbed. Many older children ask to talk to other children who have had the same experience, as do their parents.

Much of the burden of additional emotional and practical support in the pre-school child will fall on the visiting teacher of the deaf, who is often already a family confidant; finding support is much more difficult for the families of children who are already attending school and have less contact with their child's peers and teachers.

Experience shows that it is often difficult to encourage services to respond quickly to a change in a child's circumstances and all too often the school-age child is left floundering in mainstream provision long after he or she has actually requested additional support or a change to special education. Specialist speech and language therapists for the deaf are in short supply but their help is invaluable in evaluating speech and language acquisition and supporting its development.

Clinical psychologists with knowledge and experience of deaf children are thin on the ground but invaluable in encouraging resolution of the grief in parents, children and siblings, in advising on behaviour and in addressing specific issues such as tinnitus. There may be a social worker for the deaf available to offer wider experience or a counsellor with specific training. Explanation to the child's peers and siblings may moderate the social effects of the greater loss.

Programmable hearing aids with a flexible gain may enable the child with a progressive loss to function more effectively in different situations. Digital hearing aids may offer some additional benefit in due course, although their application to the profoundly deaf is presently limited. The provision of assistive listening devices should not be overlooked. The frustration and grief of independent children will only increase if they find that they are now totally dependent on family or peers for everyday activities such as getting up in the morning.

Appropriate investigation and genetic counselling must always be offered to the child and family. Where the etiology of the loss is in doubt, careful medical review is essential, as is regular review of the hearing of siblings who may develop a progressive loss at a different age from the recognized child (Madell and Sculerati, 1991) and go undetected for significant periods, especially if they have previously been determined to have normal hearing.

Little is written on what happens to a progressive hearing loss. It is clear that not all continue to profound levels but it is not known what determines the level that is reached; it is likely that this will turn out to be a combination of factors. Where the loss seems to be progressing to profound it is appropriate to discuss cochlear implant with the child and family. The decision as to when to commence this discussion is difficult; some families regard the suggestion with horror as it underlines the unthinkable and removes all possibility of recovery. Children, in particular, are already struggling to adjust to their worsening hearing and often have stormily mixed feelings about a procedure that will change things again. Other families grasp the thought of an implant as a lifeline to the restoration of hearing and may have quite unrealistic expectations of the procedure and benefit of implant. Referral should be made as early as discussions with the child and family will allow, so that close coordination between the implant team and the local services can be developed and the procedure actively considered before the child is really struggling. Many of these children, even if congenitally deaf, will make good use of the electrical signal (Bellman, 1987).

Conclusions

The identification and management of progressive hearing loss in children remains one of the most difficult aspects of audiological practice. It requires a high index of suspicion, robust audiometric and clinical facilities and professional honesty with both families and children. Fortunately, the integrated working of the multidisciplinary team of professionals in paediatric audiology departments facilitates an effective and supportive approach to these difficulties, underpinned by careful liaison with local professionals and charitable support networks.

There is a quietly voiced suspicion that progression of hearing loss is more common than previously, but this may be a false premise, related to earlier age of identification, more carefully structured review and more reliable audiometry.

There are a multitude of syndromes identifiable in association with progressive hearing loss, many of which will present to paediatricians in other fields, so clinical collaboration, research, publication and dissemination remain of vital importance if the needs of the child and family are to be addressed promptly and empathetically.

The unravelling of the human genome with the continuing increase of interest in hearing impairment amongst geneticists is contributing to the identification of those disorders that may yet be amenable to pre-symptomatic identification, prevention or direct treatment. The recognition that genetic predisposition may be necessary for the adverse effects of some environmental factors underlines the importance of careful further research, public health information and preventive work.

Acknowledgement

With thanks to Dr. Katherine Harrop-Griffiths for invaluable help in the literature search.

CHAPTER 15

Children with a unilateral sensorineural hearing impairment

FH BESS, AM ROTHPLETZ AND J DODD-MURPHY

Introduction and background

A long-standing premise among hearing healthcare providers has been that children with unilateral sensorineural hearing impairment experience few, if any, communicative or psychoeducational problems. The time-honoured management strategy for this population was to identify the hearing impairment, inform the parents that the hearing impairment exists, but assure them that there was no problem, always recommend classroom seating preference and, occasionally, experiment with the use of a hearing aid. Since the 1980s, however, we have come to realize that children with unilateral hearing impairment can be at risk for a number of complications including communicative deficits, social-emotional problems and academic failure (Bess, 1982; Bess and Tharpe, 1984; Bess, Tharpe and Gibler, 1986; Culbertson and Gilbert, 1986; Bovo et al., 1988; Oyler and Matkin, 1988; Brookhouser et al., 1991; Tharpe and Bess, 1991; Bess, Murohy and Parker, 1998).

This chapter offers an overview on children with unilateral sensorineural hearing impairment. To this end, the chapter focuses first on background information pertinent to unilateral hearing impairment and includes such topics as binaural versus monaural listening, speech understanding in adverse listening situations, and learning and educational issues. Second, a review of the current status of this population and recommendations for identification and management is provided.

Binaural versus monaural listening

Some of the problems experienced by children with unilateral hearing impairment can be explained, in part, by their lack of binaural processing mechanisms. That is, two ears provide a distinct listening advantage over one ear alone. Factors that contribute to a binaural listening advantage include: binaural summation (Scharf, 1968), localization (Humes, Allen and Bess, 1980; Konkle and Schwartz, 1981; Newton, 1983), head-shadow effects (Tillman, Kastin and Horner, 1963); and binaural release from masking (Norland and Fritzell, 1963).

Binaural summation

When a sound is presented simultaneously to two ears it is perceived louder than if the same sound is presented monaurally. Research has demonstrated that binaural thresholds for pure-tone and speech stimuli are better than monaural thresholds by approximately 3 dB. That is, when two ears are equated for hearing sensitivity, individuals with normal hearing receive binaural gains for both tonal and speech stimuli. This binaural advantage is even greater at suprathreshold levels. For example, a stimulus presented at a level of 30 dB SL to one ear has about the same loudness as a 24 dB SL stimulus presented simultaneously to both ears – a 6 dB effect. Binaural gains can be as large as 10 dB for stimuli presented at 90 dB SL (Fletcher and Munson, 1933; Hirsh and Pollack, 1948; Scharf, 1968). Depending on the severity of their hearing impairment, individuals with unilateral hearing impairment may not experience binaural summation – a phenomenon that is also thought to contribute to the ease of listening.

Although a 3 dB binaural threshold advantage may seem unimportant, it has considerable effects on speech understanding. A 3 dB increase can result in an 18% improvement in monosyllabic word recognition scores and a 30% improvement for sentential materials (Konkle and Schwartz, 1981).

Localization

Another binaural phenomenon is the ability to localize a sound source in the horizontal plane. Predictably, individuals with a unilateral hearing impairment exhibit considerable difficulty with localization tasks. Interaural differences in time (ITD) and intensity (IID) provide a physical basis for the localization of sound in the horizontal plane. Sounds are localized on the side that receives the more intense signal level or earlier stimulation. The cue (ITD or IID) that predominates in sound localization depends on the frequency of the sound stimuli. Specifically, the ITD is the predominant cue for low-frequency sounds and the IID is the predom-inant cue for high-frequency sounds. In summary, the localization of sounds is largely dependent upon a listener's ability to process between-ear differences in the time of arrival or the intensity of the auditory stimulus.

Individuals with a unilateral hearing impairment have limited access to IID or ITD cues. Without such cues, one must depend on less reliable cues (loudness, pinna effects, head movements) to localize sounds in the horizontal plane.

Head-shadow effect

The 'head-shadow effect' occurs when the head serves to attenuate sounds propagating to the ear farther from the sound source. It is most salient when a sound is directed at a 45° angle towards the listener. This 'head shadow' causes a reduction in the intensity of the signal at the far ear. Specifically, for a sound source at 45°, the 'head shadow' can attenuate speech (complex) signals 6 dB to 12 dB in the far ear relative to its level in the near ear.

For a normal-hearing listener, the head-shadow effect does not generally affect speech recognition. Regardless of where a primary and competing source originate from, the normal listener can attend at will to the ear having the better S/N ratio.

The impact of the head-shadow effect for individuals with unilateral sensorineural hearing impairment depends upon the orientation of the listener. The effect is most profound when the primary signal comes from one source and a competing message or noise comes from a different source. If the primary signal originates from the side of the impaired ear and the noise originates from the listener's good ear, the resulting listening condition is most adverse for individuals with a unilateral sensorineural hearing impairment.

The 'head-shadow effect' can create problems in speech understanding for individuals with a unilateral hearing impairment. The effect is greatest for high-frequency sounds. Because high-frequency consonants carry 60% of speech intelligibility, individuals with a unilateral hearing impairment experience significant speech recognition difficulty when the signal source is initiated on the side of the impaired ear.

Binaural release from masking

Consider the situation in which a noise masker and a signal are presented binaurally to a normal hearing listener over headphones. If different interaural manipulations are imposed on the masker from those imposed on the signal, the signal becomes more detectable than if the same manipulations are imposed on both masker and signal or if the masker and signal are presented to only one ear (Grantham, 1995). When masking noise is presented identically to both ears while speech signals are presented interaurally phase-reversed, the release from masking is approximately 3 dB to 8 dB (Licklider, 1948). This binaural release from masking is believed to result from the auditory system's ability to compare the stimuli to the two ears and effectively reduce or cancel the masking noise, thereby yielding a better S/N ratio than occurs in either ear alone (Stern, 1995).

Binaural release from masking is one factor underlying the real-world phenomenon known as the 'cocktail-party effect'. The 'cocktail-party effect' refers to the ability of an individual to tune into one conversation in a room of competing conversations. Under these circumstances, the auditory system is able to take advantage of the fact that the primary conversation has a different ITD from that of the competing conversations due to their different spatial locations (Yost, 1997). Clearly, a person with a unilateral hearing impairment would be unable to take advantage of this difference.

Several studies have demonstrated the positive effects of binaural release from masking on speech recognition in adverse listening situations (Nordlund and Fritzell, 1963; Carhart, 1965; Harris, 1965; Moncur and Dirks, 1967; MacKeith and Coles, 1971). For normal-hearing subjects, speech recognition improves for binaural stimulation over monaural stimulation, even if in the monaural case the ear is in a favourable position for the primary signals. Binaural speech recognition is also superior to monaural recognition in reverberant conditions – a 3 dB signal-to-noise (S/N) ratio advantage exists for binaural listening over monaural listening.

In summary, binaural hearing offers a number of important listening advantages over monaural hearing. These advantages have clear implications for understanding speech under routine daily living activities. The benefits of binaural hearing are particularly apparent in communicative situations where background noise and/or reverberation exist.

Speech understanding in adverse listening situations

As with normal hearers, individuals with a unilateral hearing impairment are often confronted with the task of listening in a variety of adverse listening situations – situations that can interfere with the ease of listening. These difficult listening situations can presumably impose a deleterious effect on classroom learning.

A child's ability to hear the teacher and make fine-grained auditory discriminations is highly dependent on the acoustical conditions of the classroom, particularly the S/N ratio. S/N ratio is the relationship between the primary speech or signal of interest (such as the teacher's voice) and background sounds (for example other talkers, hallway noise, air-conditioner noise, and classroom clatter). A poor S/N ratio and reverberant conditions not only degrade speech perception ability but also negatively affect behaviour, concentration, attention, reading/spelling ability, and academic outcomes (Finitzo-Hieber and Tillman, 1978; Blair, 1985; Bess and Tharpe, 1986; Ross, 1990; Leavitt and Flexer, 1991; Crandell, 1993; Crandell, Smaldino and Flexer, 1995a).

Unfortunately, the classroom is not an ideal listening environment for normal-hearing students, much less for students with unilateral sensorineural hearing impairment. Finitzo-Hieber and Tillman (1978) reported that, based on the monosyllabic word discrimination performance of normal-hearing children, an adequate classroom listening environment would have a S/N ratio of at least +6 dB (preferably +15 dB) and reverberation time of less than 0.04 s. Gengel et al. (1971) reported that children with hearing impairment require a S/N ratio of +20 to 30 dB for maximum speech understanding. Saunders (1965), however, found that the S/N ratio in a typical classroom ranged from +5 to +1 with a reverberation time of 0.6 to 1.2 s. Other studies have reported S/N ratios of +5 to -7 dB HL (for example, Saunders, 1965; Blair, 1985; Ross, 1990; Crandell, 1993; Crandell, Smaldino and Flexer, 1995). These findings suggest that a S/N ratio and reverberation time commonly found in classrooms is unacceptable even for children without educational disabilities.

It is possible that the listening conditions of classroom environments interfere with the communication and learning of many children with a unilateral hearing impairment. In fact, normal-hearing children yield significantly more errors in speech discrimination when classroom noise is present than in quiet conditions. The noise and reverberation levels, typical of many classroom settings, can mask many of the important cues needed for speech understanding. Therefore, children who already miss some of the salient acoustic cues for speech because of their unilateral hearing impairment will experience even greater difficulties under acoustic conditions often encountered in schools.

Several studies have demonstrated the undermining effects of noise and reverberation on the speech understanding of both normal-hearing children and children with hearing impairment – including those with unilateral hearing impairment. These studies have demonstrated that children with hearing impairment experience greater debasement in word recognition as noise and reverberation increase (Ross and Giolas, 1971; Nober and Nober, 1975; Finitzo-Hieber and Tilman, 1978; Boney and Bess, 1984; Crandell, 1993). In addition, children with even minimal degrees of hearing impairment experience more difficulty than their normal hearing peers. Finally, the more adverse the listening situation, the greater the disparity in speech perception performance of normal-hearing children and children with hearing impairment (Crandell, 1993).

Learning and educational issues

When one considers the probable adverse effects of noise on the speech understanding of persons with unilateral sensorineural hearing impairment, it is not surprising that many of these children experience academic problems as well. Evidence suggests that fine-grain speech-perception skills are critical to language development and learning. Elliot, Hammer and Scholl (1989) found that measures of fine-grained auditory discrimination classified nearly 80% of children age six-to-eight years as possessing normally or demonstrating language learning difficulties. Others (Goetzinger et al., 1962; Clark and Richards, 1966) report that weaknesses in the auditory discrimination of speech sounds is one of the most frequent causes of poor reading skills. Such findings suggest that academic achievement is highly dependent on the student's ability to perceive and discern word-sound differences.

It seems probable that the speech understanding difficulties many children with unilateral sensorineural hearing impairment experience in noisy conditions contribute to academic problems. Downs and Crum (1978) reported that processing demands during auditory learning are significantly greater under competition than under quiet conditions. Classroom noise may produce deleterious effects on learning performance of children, particularly children with hearing impairment. Increased effort is required to attend selectively to an auditory signal when the acoustical environment is adverse. If this energy is not expended there is a concomitant decrease in learning performance. That is, optimal learning may be compromised if the processing demands of a task are increased. It is possible that unilateral hearing impairment accompanied by noise and reverberant conditions typical of most classrooms makes learning a highly demanding task, resulting in reduced academic performance of many children with a unilateral sensorineural hearing impairment.

Children with unilateral sensorineural hearing impairment

Given the discussion presented above concerning the advantages of binaural hearing, the problems children have understanding speech in noise, and learning and educational issues, it is not surprising to note that some children with a unilateral hearing impairment experience a variety of communicative, psychoeducational and psychosocial problems. This section will address our current knowledge on unilateral hearing impairment in the areas of epidemiological considerations, auditory performance, educational performance, language, cognitive skills and functional health status.

Epidemiological considerations

The epidemiology of unilateral sensorineural hearing impairment is an important consideration when examining the nature of the problem, determining methods for identification and planning strategies for intervention. Epidemiological issues pertinent to unilateral sensorineural hearing impairment include: prevalence, age of identification and etiology.

Prevalence

Findings from studies examining the prevalence of unilateral sensorineural hearing impairment in children have been variable depending upon the criteria used to define a hearing impairment. Using a criterion of >45 dB HL in the affected ear, Berg (1972) reported the prevalence of unilateral sensorineural hearing impairment in school-age children to be three per 1000, increasing to 13 per 1 000 if a stricter criterion (26 dB HL or worse) is used. Bess et al. (1998) reported a prevalence of 3 per 1000 among school-age children using an average threshold criterion of 20 dB or worse. Individuals with a unilateral hearing impairment are more likely to be male (62%) than female (37.7%) and are slightly more likely to have left-ear impairment (52%) (Evenburg, 1960). Currently, no prevalence data exist for children under the age of three years.

Age of identification

Unilateral sensorineural hearing impairments have traditionally been identified much later in life than bilateral hearing impairments. Because unilateral hearing impairment does not appear to have a pronounced affect on early language development, the impairment often goes unnoticed until it is discovered in a routine school screening (Bess, 1986). Hence, the average age of identification of children with unilateral hearing impairment is 5.6 years. With advancement in hearing screening technology and the recent trend toward universal newborn hearing screening, it is probable that many more children with unilateral hearing impairments will be identified at younger ages.

Etiology

The cause of unilateral hearing impairment is idiopathic in about 35% to 66% of cases (Kinney; 1953; Evenberg, 1960; Tarkkanen and Aho, 1966; Brookhouser et al., 1991). It is suspected that congenital factors are associated with unilateral hearing impairment in 75% of the cases, with heredity being the most common etiology. In past decades, the mumps virus was a common contributor to unilateral hearing impairment, however, most developed countries have experienced a 90% to 95% decrease in the incidence of mumps due to immunization efforts (Brookhouser et al., 1991). Another possible cause for unilateral sensorineural hearing impairment is middle-ear disease with effusion. Hunter and co-workers (1996) reported that young children with an early history of ear disease can experience hearing impairment in the high frequencies, especially if a history of multiple intubations exist. It is theorized that bacterial products are transmitted through the round window causing damage to the basal end of the cochlea. The findings of Hunter and colleagues were reaffirmed in a follow-up publication (Margolis, Saly and Hunter, 2000). Other factors associated with acquired unilateral hearing impairment are meningitis, head trauma and noise trauma.

Auditory performance

Localization

Children with unilateral sensorineural hearing impairment experience significant problems localizing sound on the horizontal plane. Bess et al. (1986) reported on the localization scores of a group of children with unilateral hearing impairment (N = 25) and contrasted these data to a matched group of children with normal hearing. Localization scores for the unilaterally hearing-impaired children were significantly poorer than the scores of normal-hearing children at the two frequencies tested (500 Hz and 3000 Hz). Predictably, localization scores were positively correlated with the degree of hearing impairment. That is, as hearing impairment in the impaired ear worsened, localization errors also increased.

Speech recognition

Studies concerned with speech-recognition abilities of children with unilateral sensorineural hearing impairment are sparse. Bess et al. (1986), examined the speech-recognition skills of children with unilateral sensorineural hearing impairment and a matched group of normal listeners (N = 25) at different S/N ratios using nonsense syllables. Children with unilateral hearing impairment exhibited significantly greater difficulty understanding speech than did their normal hearing counterparts under all listening conditions. A summary of the data reported by Bess and co-workers is shown in Figure 15.1.

This figure illustrates the mean nonsense syllable recognition scores (percentage correct) across several S/N ratios for a group of normal-hearing children and children with unilateral sensorineural hearing impairment. The hearing-impaired children were assessed in the monaural direct and monaural indirect conditions, whereas the normal hearers were tested in the monaural direct condition only. Interestingly, it is seen that the unilaterally hearing-impaired children performed poorer than the normal hearers across all monaural direct conditions. When the primary signal is directed to the good ear with noise striking the poor ear at full impact, unilaterally hearing-impaired children did not perform as well as their normal peers. Moreover, the more adverse the listening situation, the greater the discrepancy between the unilateral subjects and their normal-hearing counterparts. In the monaural indirect condition, the children with unilateral hearing impairment show a marked breakdown in speech recognition even under the most favourable S/N ratios. The ability to understand speech varied based on the degree of hearing impairment; children with the more severe impairments performed poorer than children with the milder hearing impairments. Clearly, children with unilateral sensorineural hearing impairments experience far greater difficulty understanding speech in the background of noise than children with normal hearing, especially in the monaural indirect condition.

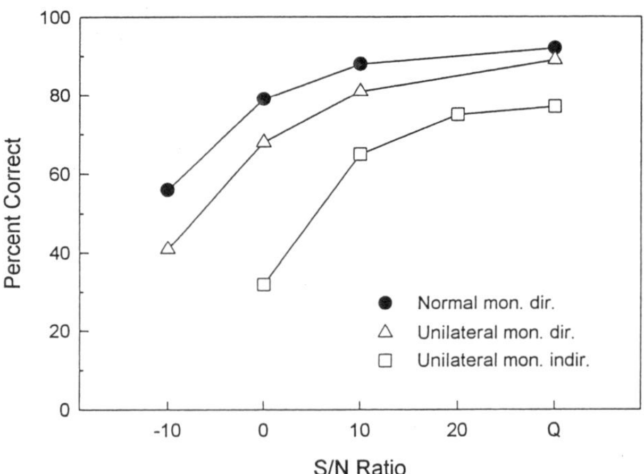

Figure 15.1. Mean sound field composite scores (in per cent) on the nonsense syllable test across several S/N ratios for normal children and children with unilateral hearing impairment. The hearing-impaired children were assessed in the monaural direct and monaural indirect conditions, whereas the normal-hearing children were tested in the monaural direct condition only. (Redrawn with permission from Bess FH (1986), Children with unilateral sensorineural hearing loss. *Ear and Hearing* 7:(1)2–54.)

Bess and co-workers (1986) also examined the speech-recognition abilities of children with unilateral hearing impairment as a function of those who had failed a grade and those who had not failed a grade, and as a function of right-ear impairment versus left-ear impairment. The findings from this analysis are shown in Figures 15.2 and 15.3. The speech recognition performance scores for children who had failed a grade versus those who did not fail are shown in Figure 15.2. There is a tendency for children who experience difficulty in school to perform more poorly in the monaural direct position than children who perform satisfactorily in school. Note, for example, that children who have failed a grade perform poorer than normal listeners and children who have not failed a grade across all listening conditions.

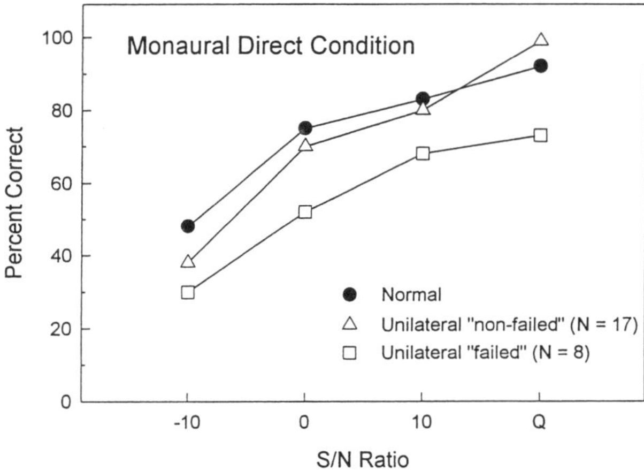

Figure 15.2. Mean sound field composite scores (in per cent) on the nonsense syllable test across several S/N ratios for children with unilateral sensorineural hearing impairment as a function of those who had failed a grade and those who have not failed a grade. The children were assessed in the monaural direct condition only. (Redrawn with permission from Bess FH (1986) Children with unilateral sensorineural hearing loss. *Ear and Hearing* 7:(1)2–54.)

The data obtained for ear effects are shown in Figure 15.3. A definite trend exists for right-ear-impaired subjects to perform more poorly than left-ear-impaired subjects across all listening conditions. Right-ear-impaired subjects performed poorer than normal-hearing children and poorer than left-ear impaired subjects.

The data on ear effects were confirmed by Jensen and co-workers (1989b) who examined the speech recognition skills of 30 children with

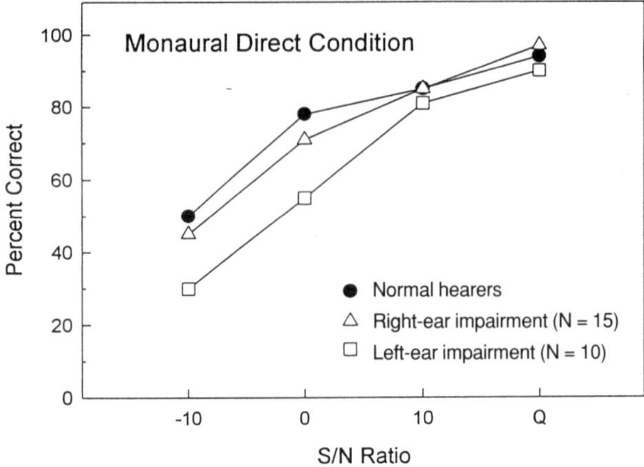

Figure 15.3. Mean sound field composite scores (in per cent) on the nonsense syllable test across several S/N ratios for children with unilateral sensorineural hearing impairment as a function of right-ear impairment versus left-ear impairment. The hearing-impaired children were assessed in the monaural direct condition only. (Redrawn with permission from Bess FH (1986) Children with unilateral sensorineural hearing loss. *Ear and Hearing* 7:(1)2–54).

unilateral hearing impairments that were matched to a control group of normal listeners. Using interrupted speech in a background of noise, they found that right-ear impaired subjects performed significantly poorer than left-ear impaired subjects.

Educational performance

Children with unilateral hearing impairment experience far greater difficulty in school than children with normal hearing. In fact, children with unilateral sensorineural hearing impairment are ten times greater at risk for academic failure than their normal-hearing counterparts. A breakdown of the grades typically failed by children with unilateral hearing impairment is shown in Figure 15.4.

Note that the largest number of children failed in the first grade; however, many children failed grades two through seven. Boyd (1974) was one of the very first to examine the effects of unilateral hearing impairment on educational performance. Boyd reported that 38% of their children with unilateral impairments exhibited reading problems, 31% exhibited spelling problems, and 23% had problems in arithmetic. Bess and colleagues (1986) reviewed case history data from 60 school-age children with unilateral hearing impairment and found that 35% failed at least one grade – these data rank in comparison to an overall failure rate of 3.5% for the school district norm. Overall, 48.3% of the sample of unilaterally hearing-impaired children experienced significant academic problems that required either resource assistance or grade repetition. These data have been validated from a number of other studies in the US and Europe (Bovo et al., 1988; Jensen and Jensen, 1989a and b; Oyler and Matkin, 1991). It appears that right-ear-impaired subjects are at greater risk for academic failure than left-ear-impaired subjects (Bess, 1986; Oyler and Matkin, 1991). In fact, according to Oyler and Matkin (1991), unilaterally hearing-impaired children with right-ear impairment are five times more at risk for academic failure than children with left-ear impairment.

Even children with mild unilateral hearing impairments (20 dB HL to 45 dB HL) can be at risk for academic failure. Bess et al. (1998) examined the educational status of children with minimal sensorineural hearing impairments. More than half of their population exhibited unilateral hearing impairment. Of this group, 40% had failed at least one grade.

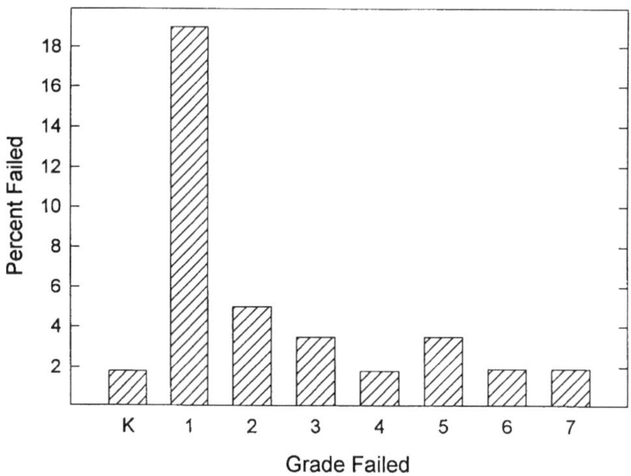

Figure 15.4. Percentage distribution showing the grades failed by 60 children with unilateral sensorineural hearing impairment. (Redrawn with permission from Bess, F.H. (1986), Children With Unilateral Sensorineural Hearing Loss, *Ear and Hearing*, 7:(1)2–54.)

Language and cognitive skills

Children with unilateral sensorineural hearing impairment appear to exhibit good language skills – a fact that makes it difficult to identify these children early. A comparison of performance scores on the WISC-Revised for unilateral hearing-impaired children (N = 25) and a matched group of normal-hearing children is summarized in Figure 15.5.

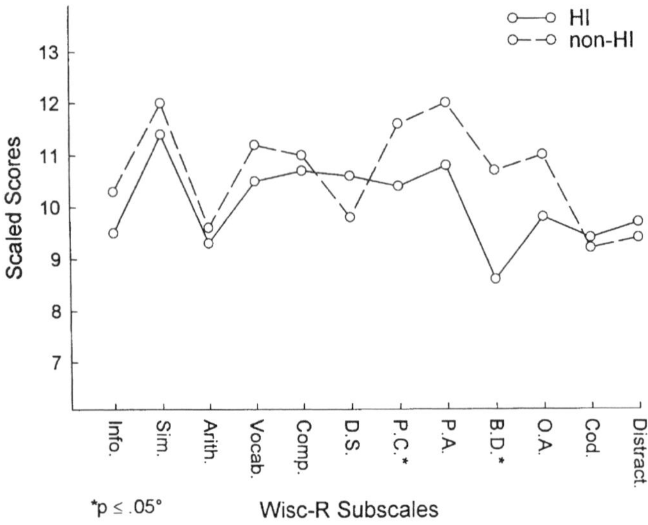

Figure 15.5. Performance scores on the subtests of the WISC-R for children with unilateral hearing impairment (HI) and a matched control group of children with normal hearing (non-HI). (Redrawn with permission from Bess FH (1986) Children With Unilateral Sensorineural Hearing Loss. *Ear and Hearing* 7:(1)2–54.)

It is seen that few differences exist between the two groups; significant differences are noted only for the subscales picture completion and the block design. However, an analysis within the group with unilateral hearing impairments revealed that:

- children with severe to profound hearing impairments exhibited significantly lower full-scale IQs than children with milder hearing impairments; and
- children with unilateral sensorineural hearing impairment who failed a grade in school exhibited verbal IQs significantly lower than unilaterally hearing impaired children who had not failed a grade.

The academic performance of the unilaterally hearing-impaired children and their matched controls on the Wide Range Achievement Test (WRAT) revealed that the hearing-impaired children showed significantly greater problems than the normal-hearing children on word recognition (decoding) and on spelling. No differences were found between the two groups, however, on arithmetic – a non-verbal task (see Table 15.1).

Table 15.1. – Comparison of unilaterally hearing impaired children (N=25) and a matched group of normal listeners on individual achievement measures.

	Wide Range Achievement Test (Standard Scores)		
	Word recognition	Spelling	Arithmetic
Unilateral group	100.4	97.5	99.2
Normal Group	109.3	107.5	96.3
Significance	p = 0.03	p =0.01	NS*

*Not significant.

Functional health status

Finally, children with unilateral sensorineural hearing impairment also exhibit functional difficulties. Bess and co-workers (1986) noted that unilaterally hearing-impaired children experienced difficulties in such general areas as dependence/independence, attention to task, emotional ability, and peer relation/social confidence. Some unilaterally hearing-impaired children misbehave to gain attention and often appear frustrated or anxious. In the peer relation/social confidence category, hearing-impaired children were more often rated as aggressive toward peers and not initiating interaction with their peers. Overall, when teachers were asked to rate whether the children were average, above average, or below average academically, there were marked differences between the unilateral hearing-impaired children and normal-hearing children. Only 39% of the hearing-impaired group versus 53% of the normal-hearing children were rated as average. Twenty-two percent of the hearing-impaired children versus 42% of the normal-hearing children were rated as above average. In direct contrast, 39% of the hearing-impaired versus 5% of the normal-hearing children were rated as below average. In another study, Bess et al. (1998) examined the functional status of school-age children with minimal sensorineural hearing impairment – many of these children had unilateral impairments. Children with minimal sensorineural hearing impairment exhibited greater dysfunction than normal-hearing children on such psychosocial domains as behaviour, energy, stress, social support and self-esteem.

Identification and management of children with unilateral sensorineural hearing impairment

Strategies to identify and manage children with unilateral sensorineural hearing impairment have been limited because unilateral hearing impairment was traditionally considered inconsequential. As noted earlier, conventional management has been to provide the child with unilateral hearing impairment preferential seating in the classroom. However, in view of current data, it is evident that a more aggressive approach to identification and intervention is needed. The long-standing approach of simply recommending classroom seating preference and a possible hearing aid will not be sufficient for many children with a unilateral sensorineural hearing impairment.

Early identification of unilateral sensorineural hearing impairment in children and appropriate intervention may serve to minimize any disparaging effects on academic and social-emotional development. In addition, if we could target children with unilateral sensorineural hearing impairment who appear to be at greater academic/functional risk and in need for early intervention, educational resources may be more prudently distributed. Three disciplines of professionals are likely to encounter children with unilateral sensorineural hearing impairment – audiology, speech-language pathology and psychology. The following review represents some identification and management considerations for each of these disciplines.

Audiological considerations

Early intervention efforts depend upon early identification of unilateral sensorineural hearing impairment. As previously noted, unilateral sensorineural hearing impairments have traditionally been identified much later in life than bilateral hearing impairment due to the inconspicuous nature of the disability. If there is congenital causation, the hearing impairment should ideally be identified before the child enters school, preferably by two years of age – early identification can then lead to early intervention. Behavioural assessment procedures conducted in sound field settings are not sufficiently sensitive to identify unilateral impairment, and should, therefore, be supplemented with behavioural assessment under earphones and/or electrophysiological measures, such as immittance otoacoustic emissions and auditory evoked responses.

When a child is identified with a unilateral hearing impairment, otological follow-up is recommended. In addition, it is essential that the child is followed audiologically to monitor hearing in both the normal and the impaired ear. Furthermore, middle-ear status should be closely regulated, especially in the early years. A conductive overlay, secondary to otitis media with effusion, can cause significant problems for children with unilateral sensorineural hearing impairment, particularly if the good ear is affected. This is especially critical for younger children who are most prone to experience recurrent bouts of otitis media, and are typically transitioning through a time of rapid speech and language learning.

Decisions regarding audiological management of unilateral sensorineural hearing impairment should be made upon a case-by-case basis, depending upon the individual needs of the child. Therefore, deliberate audiological, speech-language, and educational monitoring of the child's progression is essential. If a child is performing well in school and seems to be adjusting well to the impairment, then preferential seating in the classroom and routine monitoring of his or her progress may be sufficient. For many children with monaural hearing impairment, however, more aggressive intervention is warranted.

Effective management of children with unilateral hearing impairment may depend on a communicative link between the audiologist and the child's parents, teachers, physicians, and other professionals who come in contact with the child. Each of these individuals gains important information about the child, and their expertise is essential to maximize the child's education and intervention. Audiologists have expertise in the specific nature of the child's hearing impairment and are, therefore, in a good position to provide practical information and recommendations to parents and teachers. Furthermore, they can serve as advocates for the child by attending IEP meetings and making specific suggestions regarding classroom seating, amplification, the acoustical environment, and the possible needs of speech-language assessments.

Conversely, the child's teachers and other professionals (such as child-care providers or speech-language pathologists) have an abundance of knowledge about a given child that may not be readily available to the audiologist, such as the child's academic progress and social skills. In addition, because they observe the child on a daily basis, they may be the first to recognize a change in performance that may indicate a change in hearing status or the need for more aggressive management. Finally, parents may be the most instrumental experts on their child. Children interact with their parents off and on many hours of each day; therefore, parents are sources of a plethora of information on their child and typically have the most vested in their success. Parents should not be treated as onlookers but should be encouraged to become actively involved with their child's audiological and educational management. To a large extent, the child's success in school will depend upon the co-operation, understanding and support given by parents.

Many children with unilateral hearing impairment may reap significant educational benefits from the use of amplification in the classroom. In the past, contralateral routing of signal (CROS) hearing aids were the only amplification system recommended for individuals with a unilateral hearing impairment. However, the use of CROS hearing aids with children has been met by only limited success. As previously discussed, children with unilateral hearing impairments are likely to have the greatest difficulty listening in adverse listening conditions, but have little difficulty in quiet conditions. Intervention should therefore address listening conditions with high levels of background noise (such as the classroom) in which these children experience the most difficulty. Unfortunately, CROS hearing aids do nothing to rectify a poor S/N ratio or reverberation; these devices merely amplify all sound in the environment. Frequency modulated (FM) technology is the preferable choice for children with unilateral sensorineural hearing impairment.

The purpose of FM systems is to improve the S/N ratio reaching the child's ear. This goal is achieved by placing a microphone on the person speaking and transmitting his or her voice via FM signals to a headset. This system maintains an optimal S/N ratio by allowing the child to receive the teacher's voice from any location in the room at an intensity that is stronger than the ambient noise (Ross, 1990). If fitted properly, a personal FM system can improve the S/N ratio by 20 dB to 30 dB (Hawkins, 1984). The situation is comparable to the teacher speaking within six inches of the child's ear, no matter where the teacher or the child is located in the classroom (Flexer, 1996). FM systems significantly enhance the speech recognition abilities of children with unilateral hearing impairment in classroom-like listening conditions (Kenworthy, Klee and Tharpe, 1990; Updike, 1994). In order to minimize the risk of over-amplification, it is important that an audiologist is involved with the fitting and maintaining of these devices. It is recommended that the FM system be coupled with an open earmould and that the high-frequency gain is set at 12 dB to 15 dB at one-half the volume rotation, with an SSPL-90 not to exceed 105 dB to 100 dB. Of course, the use of sound field amplification is another effective way in which to overcome the problem of poor acoustical conditions.

Speech and language considerations

Although unilateral hearing impairment does not often produce obvious effects on speech and language acquisition, children with monaural hearing impairment should be closely monitored for subtle speech and language problems. Customary protocols for speech-language evaluations for children include both screening and full-scale assessments. The purpose of screening is not to diagnose a speech or language problem or to make specific recommendations, but to identify children for whom more comprehensive testing is warranted. Screening can take the form of standardized screening tests, parent referrals or professional referrals. It is important to note that formal screening tests may not be sensitive to some of the subtle language problems that children with unilateral sensori-neural hearing impairment may exhibit. Though slight, these problems may have detrimental effects in how well the child copes with the demands of the classroom where verbal skills such as reading, writing and oral discussion are emphasized. It is recommended that information from parents and teachers regarding the child's progress supplement formal screening tests.

A full-scale speech-language evaluation is indicated if a child fails a screening test or if there is concern from the child's parents, teacher, audiologist, or physician regarding speech or language development. Comprehensive speech-language tests serve to ascertain the child's current level of speech and language functioning, to diagnose a speech or language disability, and to determine appropriate intervention strategies. Full-scale speech and language tests should assess language production (for example, spontaneous language sample, or formal articulation/ expressive language tests), receptive vocabulary, syntactical understanding, language comprehension, and if necessary, non-verbal cognitive functioning.

Like standardized screening tests, comprehensive language batteries can also be insensitive to the subtle speech-language deficits that children with sensorineural hearing impairment may experience. For this reason, it is recommended that specific information from parents and teachers regarding the child's speech and language development be obtained to complement formal test batteries.

Speech-language deficits in many children with unilateral sensorineural hearing impairment are not the result of the hearing impairment, per se, but secondary to the causal agent of the hearing impairment. For example, research has indicated that, in a significant percentage of children with unilateral hearing impairment who exhibit speech-language or educational deficits, the suspected etiology of the hearing impairment was bacterial meningitis, viral infection, or other casual factor associated with neurological damage (Bess and Tharpe, 1986). These etiologies may also have considerable behavioural effects on the child. The importance of a thorough case history, therefore, cannot be overstated in assessing the child's current state of functioning and risk for developing speech-language, academic or social-behavioural problems. These factors should also be considered when constructing intervention strategies for the child.

Educational and social considerations

As previously discussed, many children with unilateral sensorineural hearing impairment will encounter significant academic and/or psychosocial problems requiring comprehensive assessment and resource services. As with audiological and speech-language management, a thorough case history should be the foundation of the assessment. The case history should tap into medical information from the pre-natal period, past illnesses that might have some effect upon the child's learning or behaviour, social/family data, records of school performance and descriptive social/behavioural information. The case history may suggest some aspect of the child's development that may be related to the current problems and may provide some information regarding the specific nature of the child's difficulties.

There exists no universal assessment battery for children with unilateral hearing impairment; therefore, the assessment should be based on an hypothesis-testing approach. That is, the battery of assessments should be based upon the presenting symptoms of the child, and should be intended to evaluate a specific hypothesis regarding the child's strengths and deficits. In addition, the battery of assessment should be completed with the end goal of obtaining a profile of documented strengths and weaknesses for each child that can form the basis for future educational planning.

Once diagnostic information on the specific nature of the child's deficits has been obtained, educational programming becomes the key to successful intervention. Since the passage of Public Law 94-142 in the US – now the Individuals with Disabilities Education Act (IDEA) – public schools have been required to provide a variety of special education services, tailored to the individual needs of the child. These services may include self-contained classroom placement, resource training for part of the day combined with a regular classroom placement for the remainder of the day, or itinerate services from a resource teacher who provides consultation to the child's regular classroom teacher regarding appropriate educational modifications. Of paramount importance to the success of educational intervention is the involvement of the child's family. Under IDEA, parents have the right, through the Individualized Education Plan (IEP), to actively participate in the planning of the goals and types of services their child receives. Audiologists should inform parents of their rights and should empower them to become advocates for their child.

Afterword

In summary, although not every child with unilateral hearing impairment will exhibit communication or academic problems, research has indicated that many children with unilateral hearing impairment will experience significant problems. A recurring profile for unilaterally hearing-impaired children who are at-risk for communicative and psychoeducational problems include:

- early age of onset,
- perinatal or post natal complications,
- severe to profound hearing impairment, and
- right-ear impairment.

For these children, preferred seating is not sufficient to effectively manage their educational needs. Children with unilateral sensorineural hearing impairment compose a heterogeneous group with variable needs, and therefore, require individualized assessment and intervention strategies. Planning of appropriate education strategies depends on detailed evaluation and input from professionals of multiple disciplines. Intervention efforts should be based on the specific strengths and weaknesses of the child and should be modified according to the child's progress. Finally, the involvement of parents is an essential component to the successful intervention of any child with a unilateral hearing impairment.

Acknowledgements

Preparation of this chapter was supported, in part, by the Robert Wood Johnson Foundation.

CHAPTER 16

Management of the hearing-impaired child

S SNASHALL AND J WITANA

Prevention

Dealing day by day with children in whom hearing impairment has not been prevented it is easy to forget that immunization against rubella, monitoring of ototoxic drugs and control of middle-ear disease can reduce the prevalence of hearing impairment in children, and prevention of deafness should always be our priority (De la Mata and De Wals, 1988; Hinman, Hersh and de Quadros, 1998).

Management aims

The ultimate goal of all those involved in the management of the child with hearing impairment is for the child to grow up into a socially well-adjusted, integrated, competent adult, with good communication skills, good employment prospects, and above all, one who is happy (Arnold, 1982; Hindley et al., 1994; Bellman, 1998; Hindley and Parkes, 1999).

In order to achieve this, the professionals involved in the care of the child should aim at a number of targets, such as early identification, effective amplification, and language competency appropriate to the child's maturity. With optimal educational facilities children can then access the curriculum, and make friends and be integrated within their peer group.

Standards of care

Quality standards of managed care have been set by consensus (for example NDCS, 1996) as each child deserves the highest standard of care regardless of geography and degree of deafness. Although inequity due to geography cannot usually be addressed by the providers of audiological care, they can ensure that all children within their care receive the same attention. Cochlear implant programmes have set standards of care, which are applicable to all children with hearing impairment, and the targets to which they aspire can be adapted to children who are not candidates for implantation (Ling and Nienhuys, 1983). For example, the results of implantation are known to be best in those treated early, with much less advantage after the age of seven years (Bellman, 1988). This means that detection and early management of congenital deafness needs to be such that habilitation can be well established, and response scientifically evaluated before the age of two years (Yoshinaga-Itano et al., 1998). There is therefore no scope for complacency or pragmatism in the management of children with *any* degree of hearing impairment and each aspect must be addressed meticulously.

Key elements of management

The management of a hearing-impaired child is a continuing process that begins at screening and diagnosis and only ends when care is transferred to adult services at school leaving. Although each stage will present unique challenges to the team, there are some aspects that will apply in one form or another throughout the process. At every contact each of these key elements will be considered, even if one is taking precedent over another at that particular visit. Key elements include:

- *accurate hearing assessment* at all ages, using objective tests if required and including loudness tolerance measures;
- *language evaluation,* including pre-treatment baseline assessment, regular monitoring and recommendations regarding communication by a specialist speech and language therapist;
- *effective amplification* scientifically based on real ear measurements as well as subjective testing, which should include open set speech discrimination;
- *educational provision* by advisory teachers for the hearing-impaired, monitoring of attainment, identification of special needs;
- *etiological investigation,* including detection of other impairments, planned in stages as the child matures;
- *detection of imbalance, vertigo and tinnitus* and their management;
- *medical and surgical treatment* for middle-ear disease or perilymph fistula, control of otitis externa, steroids or vasodilators for inner-ear events, detection of associated medical conditions of eyes, kidneys, heart, thyroid and so forth;

- *social and emotional care* of both the child and family, including identification of a key worker, such as a paediatric nurse, and provision of deaf role models;
- *provision of information* that is unbiased, relevant and accessible, including introduction to voluntary bodies;
- *child-centred decision making,* by parents initially, but progressively by the child with regard to amplification, communication and educational strategy in a way that promotes subsequent choice and integration;
- *shared care of special children* such as those with craniofacial disorders, severe medical conditions, or other handicaps;
- *tailored care* for immigrants, homes where the language is different from the language used for education and healthcare, and those children from homes where the main carer is unable to spend sufficient focused time with the child;
- *ensuring appointments* are planned in such a way that sufficient information is collected to monitor outcome and good care delivered by the many professionals involved, without the child and family being overburdened by too many visits.

The management team

A wide variety of people become involved at different stages of the child's life. The most important members of the team are of course the child, the parents and the family, with a *key worker* linking the family with other members of the team (Bysshe, 1995; NDCS, 1996). Successful teamwork depends upon a common policy with interdisciplinary respect and flexibility, decisions being taken collectively around the child. Often these children will be under the care of more than one team and here there is need for respect between the teams and good communication systems. Child-held records are useful in this respect.

The professional team includes doctors, audiologists (scientific and technical), hearing aid professionals, speech and language therapists, advisory teachers, psychologists, counsellors and social workers. Voluntary organizations such as deaf children's societies are advocates of children and their families in a variety of ways.

Once the child is identified as having special educational needs, the education service plans how to provide for those needs. Social services maintain a register of hearing-impaired and other disabled children. Many hearing-impaired children will have additional handicaps. For these children, the team may include advisory teachers for the visually impaired, physiotherapists, occupational therapists and others.

Roles within the team

All team members have core skills and are aware of the special expertise of other members. The team needs to be composed of professionals drawn from the full spectrum of health skills, including speech and language therapy, and also requires active input from the education service regardless of the age of the child. Although a given professional may have expertise and responsibility in a particular area, other team members can influence decision making in that area as the child has to be treated as a whole, not a sum of parts.

Areas of responsibility include:

- *advisory teacher* – day-to-day advice on developing awareness of sound language development and educational policy;
- *audiological technician/scientist* – undertaking and interpreting tests, selection, fitting and maintenance of hearing aids;
- *doctor* – investigating, diagnosing, treating the whole child and the family, being an advocate of the child;
- *nurse* – health visitor or other key worker support for the family;
- *parent* – chief observer and worker with the child;
- *psychologist/counsellor/ family-liaison officer* – providing psychological support to parents and child;
- *speech and language therapist* – monitoring language and communication development and providing advice and therapy;

Management at diagnosis

Care of the hearing-impaired child actually begins with the screening process and the first screening failure must be handled with sensitivity if unnecessary anxiety is to be avoided and an atmosphere of trust created. At this stage the only intervention is referral for diagnostic testing, but this will inevitably create a need for information and support; it is the moment of diagnosis that is the most critical point in the life of the hearing-impaired child and his or her family.

Paediatric audiology is full of pitfalls and it is sound practice to seek a second opinion if there is any doubt about diagnosis or management. Easy access to a second opinion is also helpful to parents struggling to come to terms with bad news. From the outset an open mind and an ability to listen to the concerns and preferences of both parents and others is essential for successful management. In some countries, there is a statutory obligation upon the doctor to inform the education service as soon as hearing impairment is diagnosed, and at the same time to put the parents in touch with the relevant voluntary organization. Individual targets for management at diagnosis regardless of age are given in Table 16.1.

Table 16.1. Management targets at diagnosis

- determination of level of hearing
- explanation and supportive counselling for the parents
- written information about deafness, voluntary organizations, timescale of assessments and interventions and roles of team members
- baseline assessment of communication
- investigation and explanation of cause
- identification of other handicaps
- collection of family audiograms
- assessment of amplification needs (using tone pip auditory brainstem responses if required)
- provision of appropriate amplification
- notification to Education Services
- genetic counselling
- introduction to a deaf role model

Diagnosis at age one to four months

If the hearing impairment has been detected by neonatal screening, the infant may be as young as two weeks of age at diagnosis and in some instances, especially with universal screening, the situation may be totally unexpected. The parents may already be coping with the consequences of extremely premature or complicated birth and not able to deal with an additional handicap. Professionals are faced with the dilemma of detecting hearing impairment early in order to ensure rapid habilitation of the child, whilst not interfering with parent-child bonding (MacRae, 1979). Overall, the benefits of early amplification outweigh the disadvantages (Kittrell and Arjmand, 1997; Lenars, 1997; Waltzman et al., 1998) and management before the age of six months is known to facilitate normal language acquisition (Yoshinaga-Itano et. al., 1998) but habilitation should proceed with sensitivity and caution.

Lack of adequate information regarding both hearing status and the presence of other impairments presents problems when attempting early habilitation. Challenges to diagnosis also include the effect of neurological damage upon the startle response and the auditory brainstem evoked response; otoacoustic emissions at times being normal in the presence of neural deafness; and middle-ear dysfunction masquerading as, or masking, sensorineural hearing impairment. Alternatively, test results may be normal, and falsely reassuring in the presence of a progressive hearing impairment such as that due to metabolic acidosis, rubella or some types of genetic hearing impairment. Parents and professional alike have to recognize the limits of the information and take decisions on management accordingly. The true picture will gradually become clear as the infant matures and regular assessments will therefore be needed.

Another hurdle to be overcome in effective management is the extremely small and soft ear canal and a pinna that is not firm enough to support a hearing aid. Sometimes body-worn hearing aids are the only solution to acoustic feedback until the ear has grown and the child is able to sit up. As the ears are growing, impressions for earmoulds will be required at least monthly. The hearing aids are likely to need changing at least once during this period and by six months transfer to behind-the-ear hearing aids is usually possible.

Speech and language therapy is concerned with developing interactive skills, attention-getting devices, and child-directed speech ('motherese'), all of which are a positive encouragement to bonding. Communication patterns will emerge, and it is useful for the speech and language therapist to be involved from the outset, as other factors might influence the infant's ability to communicate and policy will need to evolve with time.

Diagnosis at five to 12 months

Management at five to 12 months presents fewer practical problems than either earlier or later diagnosis, whilst remaining within the timeframe of 'early' diagnosis. Information about true hearing status increases as the child responds behaviourally to sound, but has not yet become a 'difficult-to-test' toddler. Both the distraction test and visual reinforcement audiometry give reliable information. The benefit from amplification can also be assessed behaviourally. The ears are large enough to support hearing aids and head control allows post-aural hearing aids to be worn. At this age sedation may be required for objective tests of hearing, but the nervous system has matured and more reliance may be placed upon the brainstem evoked responses. Middle-ear function may be a confounding factor from this age onwards and tympanometry is required.

The speech and language therapist and the advisory teacher can now assess voice and communication skills and the approach to language acquisition can be discussed and planned. Questions regarding prognosis can begin to be answered, and referral for an opthalmological opinion can be made.

Late diagnosis from 12 to 60 months

Diagnosis after the age of 12 months fails to comply with quality standards (NDCS, 1994) and can cause various problems. The later the diagnosis, the more likely the parents are to experience anger as a prime component of their bereavement reaction, and this aspect will need to be addressed in the initial supportive counselling. However, by now, additional handicaps will be easier to recognize, or may already be known.

Visual reinforcement audiometry is very useful at this age (Bamford and McSporran, 1993) and insert earphones allow each ear to be tested separately (Gravel and Traquina, 1992). In spite of this technique, hearing assessment can be extremely difficult in both toddlers and in children with communication disorders, and some of these children will require confirmation of diagnosis with brainstem evoked responses under sedation. From the age of nine months children are very aware of the distress of their parents and it is advantageous to separate breaking the bad news of the diagnosis from the taking of the aural impression. Alternatively impressions can be undertaken at the same time as brainstem auditory evoked responses.

The older a child is at the time of diagnosis, the more urgent is the establishment of effective management and communication strategy. This is because the critical period of language acquisition dictates that both choice of amplification (hearing aid/cochlear implant) and communication medium should be decided well before the age of four years, and where possible, before the age of two years. Identification and management of co-existing middle-ear disease must happen in parallel with management of the deafness if delays to diagnosis are to be avoided at this stage. Speech and language therapists and advisory teachers for the hearing impaired will be involved in the child's habilitation from the outset.

Ongoing management in the pre-school period

The emotional needs of the parents will continue to affect management after diagnosis, although time invested at diagnosis will lessen this need subsequently. There is a recurring need to measure hearing accurately, monitor any changes and establish loudness tolerance. During this period, the hearing aid prescription will be under continuous review as more information becomes available and the ears become large and firm enough to sustain more powerful, and relatively larger, instruments. Benefit from amplification can be measured behaviourally, or amplified hearing responses can be measured objectively with real ear measurements or brainstem evoked responses under sedation. Middle-ear disease is likely to require active treatment in this period.

Regular, consistent input from the advisory teacher for the hearing-impaired child is vital, and speech and language assessment should be undertaken at least annually, with regular therapy as required. The success or otherwise of management will be reflected in the development of language. From the age of two years, the need for special education will be evaluated.

Etiological investigation, detection of other impairment, care of the emotional needs of the child and family, and choice of communication strategy are described in more detail in the next section, but they apply as much to the pre-schooler as to the schoolchild. Table 16.2 sets out the ongoing management targets in both the school and pre-school child.

Ongoing management of the schoolchild

The year-on-year management of the schoolchild revolves around determination of cause of hearing impairment, provision of amplification, speech and language therapy, meeting special educational needs, and the support of the child and family. At each review appointment new concerns and issues will be addressed. In particular the presence of *tinnitus, imbalance* and *vertigo* needs to be elicited and managed appropriately. Hearing, retinal, renal and thyroid function require monitoring. Otitis externa can cause difficulties at this stage and may require specific treatment or the use of hypoallergenic earmoulds.

As the child enters school, decisions will have been taken on whether education should be in a mainstream setting, a special unit or a special school, taking communication strategy into account. Educational progress will then be monitored and contribution made to the annual educational

Table 16.2. Management targets in the school and pre-school child:

- establish true threshold of hearing in sound field
- undertake pure-tone audiometry with earphones
- monitor any change in hearing
- measure loudness discomfort levels
- identify other handicaps
- detect and treat middle-ear disease; identify and treat otitis externa
- monitor language development
- set communication strategy
- provide speech and language therapy as required
- provide optimum hearing aids at all times; develop care of hearing aid
- monitor benefit from amplification
- ensure child is receiving support and advice from teacher for the hearing-impaired
- detect any emotional problems in child or family
- refer for cochlear implant if required
- undertake etiological investigation, including ECG
- provide easy access for medical advice as required
- consider other educational needs in addition to hearing

review. Hearing aid prescriptions may need to be changed, a child in an aural environment may require sign language or total communication, or a child in a total communication environment may be able to drop sign language and transfer to an aural school/unit, for example, after cochlear implantation. Decisions will also be made regarding classroom support and any additional aids to amplification such as radio or FM systems. Many of these decisions will involve the team as a whole and some will be entirely the province of the education authority. Difficulties arise when team decisions have resource implications for one service rather than another.

At each pivotal change in the child's life the parents and the child will undergo a further bereavement reaction, which requires recognition and support. Throughout the child's school life a high degree of awareness should be maintained for bullying or abuse. As the child matures, his or her opinion is sought regarding management and he or she gradually empowered to become independent.

Unilateral hearing impairment is often detected by school screening audiometry, having been previously unsuspected and investigation of cause and associated symptoms is as important as with bilateral impairment. The effect upon language, education and wellbeing is less obvious and can easily be overlooked, so that they still need the involvement of advisory teachers and may need FM systems in the classroom. Audiological monitoring is required as these children may develop vertigo, tinnitus or deafness in the better ear, which can present as an emergency.

Investigation strategy

Throughout the management of the hearing-impaired child, the question 'why?' influences the approach of all concerned, but especially the parents. Knowledge of the cause of deafness is helpful in enabling the parents, and later the child, to come to terms with the disability and also for genetic counselling. The process of exhaustive investigations spread over time may be costly both in emotional terms to the family and financially, and may still leave unanswered questions (Marlin et al., 1998). The aim of investigation is to establish the cause of the hearing impairment and to find any other related conditions, which may require intervention. Identification of cause may be urgent if the parents are in the process of planning the next pregnancy as the birth of a second deaf child in the family can be devastating if unexpected. Table 16.3 lists the investigations undertaken in stages by the time they leave school.

The timing of these investigations will vary from child to child. For example, in most cases CT of the petrous temporal bones would not be done until the child is old enough to lie still, but if cochlear implantation is being considered it will be done much earlier. Some investigations such as ophthalmological assessment have to be repeated at intervals. What follows is an attempt to indicate where the timing of investigations fits into the overall management of the hearing-impaired child.

Investigations undertaken as soon as possible after birth

Detailed family history and physical examination are the starting points for diagnosis of etiology, but further items of family history are likely to emerge over the years. Blood tests at this stage include metabolic and endocrine screen, chromosome analysis, examination for sickle cells, antibody screens for toxoplasma, rubella, CMV, herpes and HIV. Infections in pregnancy cannot be ascertained if these antibody tests are carried out after the child has had the opportunity for acquired infection. If dysmorphism, such as ear pits, is present then renal ultrasound is undertaken in the neonatal period. Vestibular responses to rotation by rotating the child in the examiner's arms are investigated in the first six weeks of life.

Investigations undertaken in the first year

If diagnosis has been delayed, the investigations undertaken in the newborn period are still required. The most important next step is visual and retinal examination by an ophthalmologist both for etiological diagnosis and detection of additional impairment. A full developmental assessment is required as other handicaps must be detected early for

Table 16.3. Investigations to be undertaken

- past medical history
- family history
- family audiograms
- whole child examination for dysmorphism
- motor and general development
- speech and language assessment
- chromosomes, sickle cells
- urinalysis, renal function
- renal ultrasound
- thyroid function and perchlorate test
- viral antibodies, autoantibodies
- vestibular function
- ophthalmology
- ECG
- CT and MRI

appropriate management to begin. Vestibular assessment may be undertaken at this age using propping and righting reflexes and the vestibular-ocular reflex in response to rotation with the child sitting on a parent's lap. Family audiograms are also collected.

Investigations in the pre-school period

There is ongoing monitoring of communication, motor and general development. If there is any deterioration in hearing, or lack of response to habilitation, CT or MRI imaging may be required, although this is best left until later if possible so that sedation can be avoided. Electrocardiography (ECG) will detect the long QT syndrome (Mosavy and Shafegh, 1976) and this is useful as fits and 'funny turns', including benign paroxysmal vertigo of childhood, can present at this time.

Investigations undertaken between the ages of six and 18 years.

Full vestibular assessment is now possible and should be undertaken. Both CT and MRI studies can be undertaken without sedation. At this stage, a series of urine analyses begins as Alport's syndrome may present with haematuria from the age of six years. The urine should be examined at six, 12 and 18 years. Ophthalmological examination should also be repeated at these ages as clinical signs of Usher syndrome may develop. As more information becomes available, the proportion of children in whom no cause for the deafness can be found decreases, but the cause may never be found in up to 30% of children with congenital deafness (Feinmesser et al., 1986).

Investigating acquired/progressive hearing impairment

Although the commonest causes of acquired hearing impairment are meningitis and trauma, inexplicable hearing impairment can arise at any time and, for these children, a full medical and investigative strategy is required as rare disorders such as sarcoidosis or leukaemia can present in this way. At least 20% of children born with hearing impairment have deteriorating hearing thresholds, and this is usually genetic, although hearing impairment due to meningitis can also change with age. These children should already have had full investigation of etiology but results may need to be reviewed and additional tests undertaken.

Management of emotional need

The emotional distress of the parents is obvious at diagnosis and the way in which this is managed will influence the reactions of the child and family for years to come (Meadow-Orlans, 1995). Later to emerge is the emotional deprivation and frustration of deaf children, and then their own grieving for their handicap. Rejection of the deafness, by either parent or child, can be expressed as desire for 'invisible' hearing aids, or repeated damage to, or loss of, the device. Much, if not most, of the ongoing emotional support of the child and family will come from other family members and friends and these unseen individuals also suffer an emotional impact that requires recognition and care, although not necessarily from the team involved with the child. Voluntary bodies also give emotional support. Once at school communication difficulties may restrict the development of close friendships just at the time that it is most needed (Mindel and Vernon, 1971). Teenagers can be encouraged to involve their closest friends in their management as this can be a way of overcoming the barriers that can seem insuperable at this age.

Another major source of encouragement and strength to child and family alike is meeting a suitable role model (Watkin et al., 1998) and this should be a standard component of the initial management. Deaf adults and their families can cut through many of the concerns of the parents/carers, can provide communication models, and can give the child a positive goal and a break from the struggle of communicating with hearing people. Deaf families themselves have different emotional needs as they search for the best way to help their children to succeed in a hearing world. The support required is different but no less important to management as, for example, the team can be instrumental in facilitating integration between the deaf and hearing communities. The psychological needs of the deaf child and his or her family, and how to manage them, are described in more detail elsewhere in this book.

Amplification strategy

The aim of amplification is to compensate for the hearing impairment and thus make speech accessible. Much of the effort in the early years will be related to amplification as professionals and parents alike struggle to ensure consistent use of hearing aids that provide sufficient gain without feedback, whilst constantly being aware of the possibility of overamplification. Measurement of gain will be both behavioural and objective, but open set speech discrimination is required to measure benefit from amplification, and this should be attempted as soon as possible, using specially designed material if necessary (Bellman, 1998). As the children grow up, they express their own preferences, initially in terms of appearance but rapidly in terms of quality of sound. One of the first things they learn is to take responsibility for their own instruments. This is not usually a problem if there is good benefit, but hearing aids of little or no benefit are rejected sooner or later.

Amplification and outer-ear disease

Hearing aids inserted into the ear (especially small ears) can impede the epithelial migration in the external auditory canal and trap cerumen, blocking the ear and facilitating the development of chronic otitis externa, thus creating difficulties in the use of conventional hearing aids. Allergic reactions to earmoulds can also be a major problem and should be prevented by hypoallergenic material and topical steroids where necessary. Regular aural toilet may be required in collaboration with otolaryngology. In severe cases of external ear disease or deformity, bone-anchored hearing aids may be needed.

Amplification and middle-ear disease

Although a dry perforation does not pose a problem, an aural discharge does. Aural discharge may arise from a cholesteatoma or from recurrent infections of middle-ear mucosa by pathogens entering directly through the perforation. Although the infection is treatable, microsuction in children can be difficult and may be impossible without anaesthetic. If the infection cannot be controlled medically, surgery in the form of myringoplasty or mastoidectomy may achieve a dry ear, otherwise a bone-anchored hearing aid may offer a solution. Close collaboration with otolaryngology is required and team decisions should be taken in dealing with these complex children, many of whom will also have craniofacial abnormalities involving other surgical specialties.

Why, when and where to refer for cochlear implant

Delay in hearing spoken language permanently impoverishes linguistic skills (Miller,1997) so referral must not be delayed, certainly beyond the age of four years, but preferably before the age of two years. Profound deafness is rare enough for services to require centralization in order that adequate experience is developed for high-quality care. Cochlear implant centres deal exclusively with children whose disability is great enough to require a more radical approach to amplification than that of conventional hearing aids. Children are referred when the hearing levels, wearing the best available hearing aids, are inadequate or the child simply does not seem able to access the sound received at the eardrum. Children are assessed holistically to see not only whether the child is suitable for the implant but whether the implant is suitable for the child. This holistic approach is equally relevant to any potential hearing aid user. Many parents who have been unable to accept the severity of the hearing impairment can do so once they know their child has been fully assessed at such a centre, even if an implant is not recommended. Post-meningitic severe/profoundly hearing-impaired children are referred immediately and are fast-tracked throughout the whole process because of the danger of cochlear ossification.

Communication strategy

Unfortunately, this has been a controversial area for at least two centuries. Initially, it was felt that sign language resulted in linguistic impoverishment, but there is now evidence to suggest that a child's linguistic expression can be as wide in either language (Knell and Klonoff, 1983). There was also concern that, as sign language was easier to learn, it would prevent the deaf child from acquiring spoken language whereas, in fact, early exposure to sign enhances spoken language (Dee, Rapin and Ruben, 1982; Notoya, Susuki and Furukawa, 1994). Gesture evolves as a spontaneous language in deaf children and progresses easily into formalized sign language (Goldin-Meadow and Mylander, 1984). There are thus ethical, and possibly legal, implications if these natural means of communication are denied at the normal age for language development (Siger, 1978). Children with additional speech and language disorders may not access spoken language despite hearing the sound components of speech and may eventually need to transfer to a signing medium. Although language development will be most successful if the optimum communication system is delivered within the time frame of normal language acquisition, the correct communication system cannot always be predicted from the information available in the first two years of life.

One solution to these difficulties, which is of proven effectiveness, is to teach language by total communication (communication by all means, sign, gesture, speech, lip reading, hearing and expression). This also allows the child to be bilingual and integrated within both deaf and hearing society (McLeod and Bentley, 1996).

Communication strategy is reconsidered at every review appointment when outcome is assessed in terms of communication and language development. Further details of alternative methods of communication are given elsewhere in this book.

Special educational needs

An education authority may not have a statutory duty to children under the age of two years and only a limited duty in the pre-school years. It is, however, obvious to all concerned that the children need teachers involved in their management from diagnosis, even if that is at the age of two weeks. Advisory teachers for the hearing impaired provide unique, frequent, input from diagnosis throughout the pre-school period. As diagnostic techniques have improved the age of first intervention has fallen and approximately 30% of hearing-impaired children may now be found in the neonatal period.

Any educational placement has resource implications in terms of manpower, equipment and environment, and each education authority will develop its own policy based on need and available resources. Although boarding placements inevitably lead to some isolation from the family, placement in mainstream school can be more isolating, and therefore associated with more distress, than an environment with other hearing-impaired children (Hindley et al., 1994). The support needs to be intensive for some children if they are to succeed academically (Musselman, Wilson and Lindsay, 1989). Placements may need to change over time (Farrugia and Austin, 1980; Musselman et al., 1989). It is within the remit of the team to contribute to the identification of special educational needs but these needs may not be met within local resources. The parents/guardian and the child make the final decision on what they want and must have ownership of the educational and management strategy if it is to succeed. Ultimately for the child to be happy in his or her environment the system has to fit the child, not the child be made to fit in with the existing system (Hindley et al., 1994).

Management of transition of care at school leaving

As the child matures the responsibility for decisions on management issues should be transferred to the child. This transfer of responsibility should be gradual and dependent on the parent/child interactions as it is easy for parents to be overprotective. At this stage the child has been fully investigated and should have a good understanding of the cause of his or her deafness and genetic counselling is offered. Children should have a copy of, and understand, their audiograms. Any emotional needs should have been recognized and met. Care is transferred to the adult medical and hearing aid clinics, which the young adult should be able to access independently, using a sign-language interpreter if required. Any reason for poor compliance with hearing aids should have been identified and a solution provided. The child's further education plans should be discussed and, if a geographical move is contemplated, a summary report provided. Contact should have been established with social services and they should be aware of their rights as disabled employees/students. Table 16.4 summarizes the targets for management at this stage.

Outcome and effectiveness

Commissioners of services for hearing-impaired children need to know whether the intervention is cost effective and whether it is effective in terms of attaining the aims and objectives set both for the individual child

Table 16.4. Target of management at transition

- identify progressive loss
- establish cause
- make sure hearing aid prescription is optimal for new education placement
- refer for genetic counselling if required
- establish independent access to health care
- provide summary report of audiology throughout childhood
- review emotional needs and address as required
- cater for social needs, e.g. Deaf Clubs to minimize social isolation in school leaving

and for the service. Real outcome measures may be applied prospectively or retrospectively and used to predict future outcome and thereby help in planning early strategy. There are three aspects of outcome in the short term that should be measured on at least an annual basis.

Communication

Communication includes language development and perception of sound using amplification. The best measure of aided hearing is open set speech discrimination (Makhdoum, Snik and Van den Broek, 1997; Waltzman et al., 1997). Tonal thresholds may be used in the absence of any open set discrimination.

Language development is the core short-term outcome measure using standardized tests such as the Reynell Developmental Language Scales to assess year-on-year gain. The value of these tests was demonstrated by Robbins, Svirsky and Kirk (1997) when they used this outcome to show that deaf children make half the language gains of their normal-hearing peers, but attain the same gain as hearing children after cochlear implantation. Speech and language skills can be assessed on a five-point category rating scale for sign ability, overall communication, speech reception and speech intelligibility (Geffner et al., 1978).

Education

National standards for the curriculum are available against which the achievements of the child can be measured. Commonly used outcome measures for the hearing-impaired population are reading ability (Notoya, Suzuki and Furukawa, 1996) and educational placement (Allen and Dyer, 1997).

Social and emotional development

This is a difficult area to quantify and includes the development of age-appropriate behaviours, family dynamics and the quality of life for the child and family, the psychological wellbeing of the child and other family members, the quality of relationships with peers and family, and normalization of child rearing (Dee et al., 1982; NDCS, 1996; Lane and Bahan, 1998). Children need to develop confidence in themselves and acceptance of their deafness (Ridgeway, 1998).

Long-term outcome measures

For these we must observe the young adult. There is some information on psychiatric problems at this time (Hindley et al., 1994; Ridgeway, 1998) but very little in terms of employment profiles and personal fulfilment.

Conclusion

Does our current management strategy produce hearing-impaired adults who are fulfilled and happy? Despite all our effort we do not really know/want to accept the answer to this question. The greatest need for the future is the development of specific, quantifiable outcome measures of both short-term and long-term effectiveness, and for these to be rigorously applied and honestly evaluated. We might then be able to comply with Bellman's plea to become more child-centred and make the environment fit the child (Bellman, 1998).

Acknowledgment

Much of the philosophy of this chapter reflects the content of the Seventh David Edward Hughes Lecture 'The Effect of Cochlear Implantation upon Paediatric Audiology' given by Dr Sue Bellman, consultant at the Great Ormond Street Cochlear Implant Programme, on 29 May 1998, six months before her death.

Chapter 17

Selecting amplification for children

D Toe

Introduction

Henry Ford offered his consumers a wide choice of colours for their Model-T Ford. He said they could have 'any color – so long as it's black.' Similarly, limited hearing aid choices were available to hearing-impaired listeners in the past. Choices may still be severely limited by financial constraints in countries that have just begun to address the hearing needs of their children. Despite some misconceptions, it has never been the case in the provision of amplification that any hearing aid is better than none. There is great potential to do harm with an aid that overamplifies or underamplifies sound for a child. In the former scenario, the child's residual hearing may be damaged. In the latter, wearing aids with too little gain may quickly convince children that hearing aids are of little use to them. This chapter will outline critical aspects in the theory and practice of fitting hearing aids to children.

Basic components of a hearing aid

All hearing aids operate upon similar principles. A simple block diagram is shown in Figure 17.1. A microphone converts mechanical acoustic energy into electrical current. The amplifier in the hearing aid increases the amplitude of the electrical current, which corresponds to an increase in the intensity of the sound energy. The receiver or earphone converts the amplified electrical signal into acoustic energy and delivers it to the ear via an earmould (air conduction) or a bone vibrator (bone conduction). Hearing aids may be worn on the body, whereby the microphone and amplifier are worn on the chest and a separate receiver is worn at ear level, or at ear level. Ear-level aids can be behind-the-ear (BTE), in-the-ear (ITE) or in-the-canal (ITC). The most practical and commonly worn aid for small growing ears is the BTE aid worn with a custom earmould.

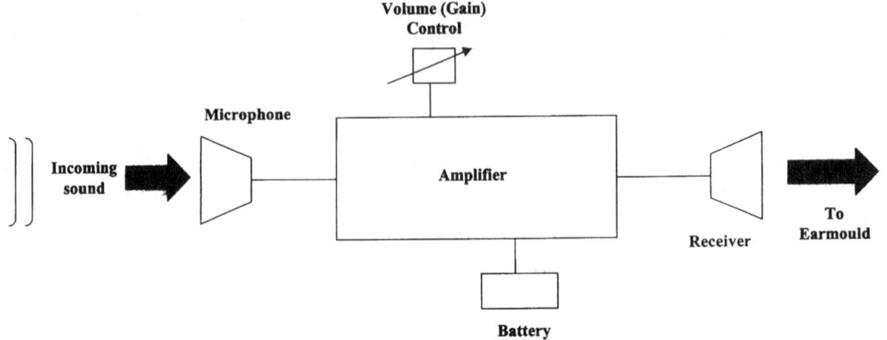

Figure 17.1. Block diagram for a simple hearing aid.

Principles and aims of amplification

The main purpose of a hearing aid is to amplify speech so that it is audible and comfortable to listen to. Audibility is critical – speech that cannot be heard cannot be understood – but it is not everything. Audibility is not perfectly correlated with intelligibility. There is little point amplifying sound to the point of discomfort because it will inevitably lead to aid rejection or a reduced volume setting. Byrne and Ching (1997) point out that as hearing impairment increases the contribution made by a given amount of audibility decreases. Increasing high-frequency audibility in the high frequencies may even result in reduced speech recognition (Murray and Byrne, 1986). What appears to be critical is the balance between low-frequency and high-frequency amplification and the contribution of each to the overall loudness and comfort associated with aided listening.

Defining hearing aid performance

Fitting hearing aids to children involves a careful process of selecting and adapting a particular hearing aid to an individual child. A first step in understanding this process involves defining hearing aid performance; that is, establishing how much amplification a hearing aid provides. The characteristics of hearing aids are described using the terms *gain, frequency response, saturation sound pressure level (SSPL)* and *distortion.* A brief description of each of these electroacoustic hearing aid characteristics is presented in Table 17.1.

Table 17.1. Terminology for the electroacoustic characteristics of hearing aids

Terminology	Electroacoustic characteristics of hearing aids
Gain	Gain is the difference in decibels between the input signal and the output signal. In a hearing aid test box, the gain of an aid is measured by presenting a signal of 50 or 60 dB to the hearing aid microphone and measuring the output of the hearing aid in a 2cc coupler. By subtracting the input from the output gain can be calculated at individual frequencies. Gain can be assessed with the aid on full volume (full on gain) or on a child's user volume (user gain).
Frequency Response	Hearing aid frequency response is determined by measuring hearing aid gain across a wide range of frequencies (eg. 125 Hz to 10000 Hz using a constant input level). All sound systems are limited in the range of frequencies that they can amplify and typically hearing aids amplify across the range of 200 to 6000 Hz.
Saturation Sound Pressure Level	The saturation sound pressure level, also known as the Maximum Power Output and the SSPL90, is the greatest sound pressure that can be produced by a hearing aid. It is measured with the aid on full volume using an input signal of 90 dB SPL.
Distortion	Distortion occurs in a hearing aid when the sound leaving the hearing aid varies from the sound entering the hearing aid. The addition of distortion to the amplified sound may reduce speech intelligibility for the hearing-impaired listener. Harmonic distortion occurs when new frequencies are generated in the amplifier that are whole number multiples of the fundamental frequency of the input signal. Harmonic distortion increases with increases in volume setting making it undesirable to fit children with an aid that is to be worn near maximum

Measuring hearing aid performance

Hearing aid measurement in the 2cc coupler

The electroacoustic characteristics of an individual hearing aid can be measured by attaching the hearing aid to a 2cc coupler to simulate some of the properties of an average adult ear. The 2cc coupler is placed in a soundproof test chamber. A tone of a specified input level is generated in the test box and the specified level is maintained at the hearing aid microphone. The output of the hearing aid is measured in the 2cc coupler. *Gain* is calculated by subtracting the input from the output. The gain of the hearing aid will vary across the frequencies tested, hence the *frequency response* of the aid is measured in the test box to establish the amount of gain in the hearing aid at each frequency. *Saturation sound pressure level* can also be measured in the hearing aid test box by using a high input level of 90 dB that aims to fully saturate the hearing aid. The aid is turned to full volume. Saturation sound pressure level is tested across the frequency range. The graphs in Figure 17.2 show gain, frequency response and SSPL for a hearing aid on full volume. Distortion can also be measured in the hearing aid test box.

The 2cc coupler measures serve several useful purposes. They are critical for quality control to ensure that individual hearing aids match up to manufacturers' specifications. In 1977, a set of standards was established by ANSI (American National Standards Institute) that required the hearing aid industry to undertake a set of 2cc coupler measures and express hearing aid performance according to a standardized set of rules. The manufacturer specifications provide an important guide to hearing aid performance. However, each individual aid can vary by up to 12 dB from the specification sheet and still be within acceptable tolerances (Northern, 1992). It is therefore important to measure each aid in the hearing aid test box prior to commencing the selection process.

The 2cc coupler measures provide a valuable starting point for hearing aid selection. They allow the audiologist to select an appropriate hearing aid to try with a hearing-impaired child. However, 2cc coupler measurements will not accurately predict hearing aid gain or SSPL in the real ear, particularly in a small child's ear. Consequently, further real-ear measurements of the hearing aid characteristics are required.

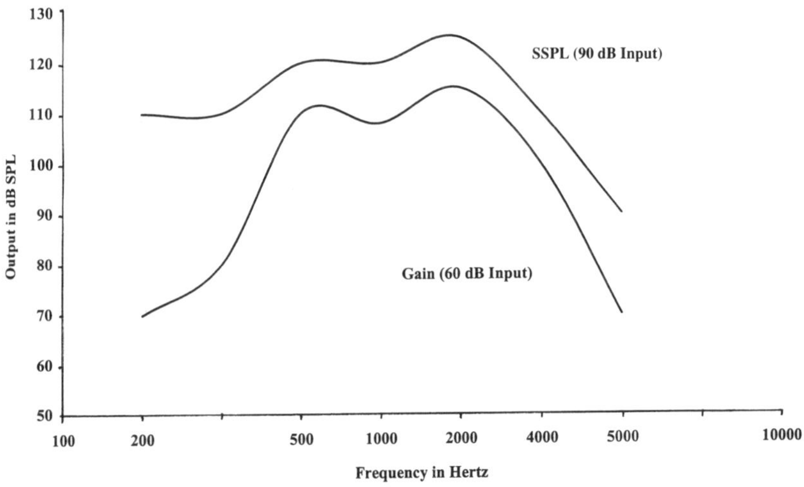

Figure 17.2. Gain and frequency response (60 dB input) and SSPL (90 dB input) characteristics of a BTE hearing aid measured with a 2cc coupler in a hearing aid test chamber.

Real-ear probe microphone measurements

The development of equipment to measure hearing aid performance via a microphone placed near the tympanic membrane represents a small revolution in hearing aid fitting. Using this equipment, the audiologist is able to measure the real-ear gain, output, SSPL and harmonic distortion of a hearing aid while it is worn by a hearing-impaired child or adult. The procedure is quick, objective, accurate and reasonably non-invasive.

A small rubber probe tube attached to a measurement microphone is placed into the unaided and unoccluded ear canal. The child is seated beside or in front of a loudspeaker. The loudspeaker generates a test signal, such as a frequency sweep of warble tones or a speech weighted broadband signal, and the output is measured in the ear canal. By comparing the SPL in the ear canal to the SPL at a reference microphone placed near the pinna, the real-ear unaided response (REUR) can be established.

Keeping the probe microphone in place, the hearing aid is then placed on the child's ear, set on user volume and the procedure is repeated, this time measuring the SPL at the eardrum when the hearing aid is worn. By comparing the SPL in the ear canal to the SPL at the reference microphone the real-ear aided response of the aid can be established, showing how much amplification the aid provides at each frequency in the real ear. Alternatively, the REAR can be compared to the REUR to generate a measure of insertion gain. Insertion gain is the amount of gain delivered to a child or adult wearing a hearing aid that he or she did not have prior to the hearing aid fitting. It is the net effect of placing an earmould into the child's ear and amplifying the sound with a hearing aid. Table 17.2 contains a summary of the terminology for probe tube real-ear measurement.

Hearing aids behave quite differently in the real ear than in the 2cc coupler. Real-ear probe microphone measurement offers a very reliable tool for verifying hearing aid performance in the real ear but real-ear measures are not hearing tests. They measure how the hearing aid amplifies sound in an individual ear, thus reflecting the acoustic characteristics of that ear.

Sound field thresholds and functional gain

A third means of measuring hearing aid gain involves obtaining a child's unaided thresholds in the sound field and then comparing these with the child's aided thresholds measured with his or her hearing aids on the selected user volume.

The formula for calculating functional gain is:

Functional gain = unaided thresholds – aided thresholds

Table 17.2. Terminology used for real-ear measurement of hearing aid performance

Terminology	Description of real-ear measurement
Real-ear Unaided Response REUR	The SPL as a function of frequency in the unoccluded, unaided ear canal with the probe tube at a specified point in the ear canal and in a specified sound field.
Real ear Unaided Gain REUG	The difference in decibels between the SPL in the ear canal and the SPL at the field reference point (reference microphone) in the unaided, unoccluded, ear with the probe tube at a specified point in the ear canal and in a specified sound field.
Real-ear Aided Response REAR	The SPL, as a function of frequency, with the hearing aid in place and turned on and the probe tube at a specified point in the ear canal and in a specified sound field.
Real-ear Aided Gain REAG	The difference in decibels, as a function of frequency, between the SPL in the ear canal and at the field reference point (reference microphone) with the hearing aid in place and turned on and the probe tube at a specified point and in a specified sound field.
Real-ear Insertion Gain REIG	The difference in decibels between the REAR and the REUG, made at the same measurement point and in the same sound field.
Real-ear Saturation Response RESR	The SPL, as a function of frequency, with the hearing aid in place, and as close as possible to full volume, at a specified point in the ear canal with a specified sound field and at a stimulus level sufficiently intense to operate the hearing aid at SSPL
Real-ear to Coupler Difference RECD	The difference in decibels, as a function of frequency between the output of the hearing aid in the real ear and the output of the hearing aid in the 2cc coupler, taken with the same input signal and hearing aid volume setting

Adapted from Mueller HG and Hall JW Audiologists' Desk Reference Volume II: Audiologic Management, Rehabilitation and Terminology. San Diego, CA: Singular Publishing Group (1999)

Where unaided thresholds have been measured in HL under headphones they can be converted to SPL in the free field using the figures in Table 17.3.

In the past, sound field thresholds have enjoyed great popularity as a means of verifying hearing aid performance in the real ear. However they have a number of significant disadvantages. Test-retest reliability for aided thresholds has been established with adults by Hawkins et al. (1987) as

±15 dB. Unaided thresholds have similar test-retest confidence limits. Consequently, a measure of functional gain may vary from one day to another by as much as 30 dB with no real change in the amplification provided by the hearing aid. Test-retest reliability is likely to be even larger for young children (Stuart, Durieux-Smith and Stenstrom, 1990). Obtaining a full set of aided thresholds can be time consuming. Moreover, testing only at octave frequencies often masks the presence of peaks and troughs in the hearing aid frequency response.

With the development of real-ear probe microphone measurement there is no need to rely upon sound field threshold testing. In most cases, hearing aid performance can be verified using probe tube measures with even very young children. However, under some circumstances, sound-field threshold testing remains of value:

- Where queries remain regarding the unaided thresholds. Aided sound field thresholds can assist in confirmation of the accuracy of unaided thresholds when consistent with the coupler gain in a child's hearing aid.
- Where a child has a profound corner audiogram and the presence of true hearing is in question. A child with vibrotactile thresholds may appear to be well aided when tested using real-ear probe tube measures but obtains very little benefit from amplification if the responses are vibrotactile.
- When a child will not co-operate for probe microphone measurement. Young children may need considerable support and orientation to the probe tube before they will accept it in their ear. Active children in the two-to-three-year-old age group can make challenging candidates. Good tips for obtaining results with this age group, or any reluctant child, include watching a video with no sound, using a sticker reward system and allowing the child to watch the process using a small mirror.
- When there is soft wax present, this may block the probe tube.

Table 17.3. Minimum audible field (MAF) figures for transforming dB HL to dB SPL

250	500	750	1000	1500	2000	3000	4000
13	6	4	3	2	0	–3	–4

Source: ISO Draft International Standard 389-7 (December, 1993) corrected for monaural listening and semi-diffuse field.
Note. To convert HL to SPL: HL + MAF = SPL.

Fitting amplification to children: special considerations

Amplifying sound for small ears

The residual volume of air between the tip of the earmould and the eardrum is significantly reduced in a child as compared to an adult. Consequently, the output of a hearing aid worn in a small ear is likely to be higher than in the ear of an adult. Feigin et al. (1989) demonstrated that real-ear to coupler differences were larger in children and the magnitude of that difference varied with age, with larger real ear to coupler differences found in younger children. As a consequence, 2cc coupler measures may significantly underestimate the SPL in the real ear. This highlights the importance of probe microphone measures to assess both gain and SSPL. While some attempts have been made to verify real-ear performance using sound field testing in the past, assessment of real-ear SSPL has been particularly neglected. This hearing aid characteristic has frequently only been assessed in the 2cc coupler. It seems likely that there have been young children fitted with unnecessarily high real-ear SSPL, possibly resulting in further deterioration of their hearing impairments.

Amplification and auditory development

Normally hearing infants can make very fine speech discriminations early in infancy. Pioneering work by Eimas (1974, 1975b) using the high amplitude sucking procedure showed that one- and four-month-old babies could discriminate between syllables from different phonetic categories. Many more studies have since extended the body of knowledge regarding infants' considerable capacity to make fine speech discriminations. Nozza's work in this area has particular relevance to the fitting of hearing aids to young children.

Nozza et al., (1990) showed that infants were capable of discriminating speech in noise but they required a signal-to-noise ratio of 6–12 dB more than adults for the same task. Nozza and his colleagues also studied speech perception in infants while simulating a hearing impairment using a reduced signal intensity (Nozza, Rossman and Bond, 1991) or by filtering the speech signal (Nozza, 1998). They showed that infants required an additional 8-10 sensation level to discriminate speech sounds level as compared to adults. At a recent conference on early amplification for children, Nozza (1998) concluded that infants require greater signal intensity and a better S/N ratio than adults to perceive speech optimally. One untested conclusion that could be drawn from these studies is that a young child requires more gain and better listening conditions for speech perception than an adult with the same degree of hearing impairment.

Amplifying speech for young language learners

Adventitiously deafened adults are usually competent users of spoken language with a great capacity to compensate for their gradual loss of sensory input. In comparison, congenitally deaf and hearing-impaired children are faced with the dual task of learning to listen with amplification and learning language simultaneously. In this situation, every piece of sensory input becomes critical.

Approaches to the selection and verification of amplification for children

The modern hearing aid market seems full of much-vaunted new technology: programmable aids, signal processing aids, digital hearing aids, and wide range dynamic compression. However, the wonders of new technology are of little use to a hearing-impaired child, if an appropriate procedure is not used to match the hearing aid selected to the characteristics of the child and their hearing impairment. Having decided that a child is a hearing aid candidate, the first and most essential step in the process is the selection of the hearing aid characteristics for the child. Two approaches to this task are the traditional approach (also known as the empirical or experimental approach) and the theoretical approach (or prescriptive approach). The first step for both approaches involves obtaining a reliable and reasonably accurate picture of the child's hearing impairment either via behavioural assessment or by using objective electrophysiological assessment. Beyond this, the two approaches differ significantly in their conceptualization and execution.

Traditional approaches

Superficially, the traditional or empirical approach to hearing aid selection has considerable face validity. It is based firmly in the belief that it will be possible to clearly demonstrate that one hearing is better than another in the audiology clinic. The traditional approach follows the procedure outlined in Table 17.4.

The face validity and sense of comfort associated with this traditional approach is somewhat outweighed by some of the approach's disadvantages. Many of them centre upon the reliability and sensitivity of the tools commonly used to evaluate the aids selected, sound field aided thresholds and speech perception and reception measures.

Basing hearing aid selection upon repeated sound field threshold measures with a range of aids presumes a certain level of sensitivity in the assessment tool used. As already discussed, sound field thresholds have limited test-retest reliability and the limited attention span of small children dictates that only a few frequencies can be tested in any single test session. Testing at main octave frequencies often masks the inter-octave peaks and troughs in the hearing aid's frequency response. Sound field aided threshold assessment is also sensitive to environmental background noise and the internal noise of the hearing aid, which may mask true thresholds at low intensity levels. Macrae's (1982) investigation of the impact of ambient noise and internal noise levels upon aided threshold results concluded that it was not possible to obtain valid aided thresholds for hearing impairments less than 30 dB HL.

Comparing a set of aided thresholds to the 70 dB average speech spectrum was first proposed by Gengel, Pascoe and Shore (1971) as a way of making judgements about a child's aided access to speech sounds. Although a popular procedure it also has limitations and does not qualify as a valid procedure for hearing aid selection (Jordt et al., 1997). Aided thresholds can clearly show detection thresholds across the frequency range but they do not show the impact of the output limit of the hearing aid upon the speech spectrum at suprathreshold levels, thus providing potentially misleading information about the sensation level at which the speech spectrum may be heard. This may help to explain why some children do not meet the expectations set by the aided audiogram.

Schwartz and Larson (1977) compared the hearing aid performance of 10 hearing-impaired children using three different procedures, aided sound field thresholds, speech sensation levels and a procedure that estimated the child's aided dynamic range for speech. All three procedures indicated similar results for those with mild and moderate hearing impairments but showed that for severe to profound hearing impairments, aided thresholds overestimated the audibility of conversational speech. Seewald, Ross and Stelmachowicz (1987) and Stelmachowicz and Lewis (1988) posited an explanation for this. Their studies examined the interaction between hearing-aid gain, the output limiting characteristics of the hearing aid and the effects of input signals higher than 70 dB RMS. They concluded that the interaction between the output limits of the hearing aid and higher input levels were not accurately represented by sound field aided thresholds.

Using speech reception thresholds or perception scores to select a hearing aid is also problematic. Finding a sufficiently sensitive test that is appropriate for the child's developmental level is extremely hazardous. The recent developments with cochlear implants have resulted in considerable refinement of speech perception tests but there are few appropriate for children under five. Even when assessing older children the sensitivity of the test remains an issue. Thornton and Raffin (1978) have demonstrated that, depending upon the number of items in the test, quite large differences in speech perception scores are required before one score is significantly different from another score.

Repeated aided threshold or speech perception testing can be a very slow process. Children become easily fatigued and distracted. Without their cooperation it is impossible to apply this approach to aid selection. In addition, there remains the dilemma of pre-selecting the most appropriate aids. Can clinicians really be sure that they have compared the most suitable aids for the child? Although clinical experience is highly valuable, without some theoretical model for ascertaining what is an optimum hearing aid fitting it will always be difficult to be absolutely confident in the aids pre-selected for trial.

Although traditional approaches have been popular in the past (Hedley-Williams, Tharpe and Bess, 1996), their general appeal appears to be in decline (Seewald, 1998). Perhaps audiologists have finally begun to grasp some of the significant disadvantages of this approach and look to methods more firmly grounded in theoretical models and modern methods of audiological assessment.

Table 17.4. Guide to hearing aid fitting using a traditional approach

Step-by-Step Guide to a Traditional Approach to Hearing Aid Fitting for Children
1. Assess the child's hearing thresholds
2. Pre-select hearing aids based upon clinical experience and the range of aids available
3. Manufacture custom-made earmould
4. Child returns to clinic for hearing aid fitting
5. Evaluate and compare pre-selected hearing aids with child based on
(a) soundfield aided thresholds
(b) speech reception thresholds
(c) speech perception test score
1. Aid yielding the 'best' results is selected and fitted to the child
2. Gather feedback from parents, child and teachers to fine tune the hearing aid fitting

Theoretical approaches to hearing aid selection

Theoretical approaches use a model or theoretical rationale that aims to optimize the audibility of speech according to the degree and configuration of hearing impairment. A set of figures is derived from this model. These permit the audiologist to precisely select the electroacoustic characteristics of a hearing aid based upon the child's unaided hearing thresholds. These may be expressed as 2cc coupler figures, sound field aided thresholds, or as real-ear gain. Theoretical approaches are often referred to as prescriptive approaches because hearing aid characteristics are specified or prescribed according to the theoretical model. A guide to hearing aid selection using a theoretical approach is shown in Table 17.5.

There are several advantages associated with choosing to use a theoretical or prescriptive approach to select a hearing aid for a child. First, the theory or model for optimizing the child's reception of speech is clearly stated and open to scrutiny. Second, it is a systematic procedure that clearly specifies criteria for pre-selection of hearing aid and verification following fitting. Third, it can be implemented with some confidence by both experienced and inexperienced audiologists. It does not rely upon clinical experience for hearing aid selection. Fourth, it is time efficient, usually one hearing aid is pre-selected for the child on the basis of 2cc coupler measures and then modified to fit the targets of the prescriptive procedure during the real-ear verification process. Prescriptive procedures that rely upon real-ear measurement for aid verification have eliminated most of the problems of reliability and fatigue associated with sound field and speech perception testing.

Several well-documented prescriptive approaches have been developed over the past 20 years. Some of the better known include POGO II (Schwartz, Lyregaard and Lundh, 1988), DSL (Seewald, 1992; Seewald et al., 1993) and the National Acoustic Laboratories' revised procedure (NAL-RP) (Byrne and Dillon, 1986; Byrne, Parkinson and Newall, 1990). Selection of a specific procedure is important because each procedure will prescribe a different amount of gain and power for the hearing-impaired individual. Deciding which prescriptive procedure is best depends upon the target population, the clinician's personal philosophy and some careful evaluation of the theoretical models that underpin each procedure.

Table 17.5. A guide to hearing aid fitting using a theoretical or prescriptive approach

A Step-by-Step Guide to a Theoretical Approach to Hearing Aid Fitting for Children
1. Assess unaided hearing
2. Manufacture custom-made earmould
3. Pre-select hearing aid in 2cc coupler based upon theoretical set of criteria ie., set of prescriptive targets
4. Fit aid to child and verify aid fitting with a measure of real-ear gain. Adjust hearing aid to fit performance criteria/targets (e.g., sound field thresholds, insertion gain, real-ear aided response)
5. Evaluation of hearing aid fitting and fine tuning of aid fitting based upon feedback from parents and teachers

Two theoretical selection procedures frequently used with children will be briefly reviewed here: the Desired Sensation Level (DSL) approach and the National Acoustics Laboratories (NAL-RP) approach.

The Desired Sensation Level approach to hearing aid selection for children

The earliest versions of this approach appeared during the 1980s. Its stated goals are to provide children with amplified speech that is audible, comfortable and undistorted across the broadest relevant frequency range possible (Seewald et al., 1987). This approach has been specifically developed for children and is cognizant of the arguments regarding the importance of adequate amplification during the early language learning years and the differences between young children's and adults' speech-perception skills.

Gain and frequency response selection in the DSL approach originates from a set of desired sensation levels (DSL) across the frequency range for the long-term speech spectrum. These desired sensation levels are dependent upon frequency and degree of hearing impairment. From these desired sensation levels, targets for real-ear aided gain, real-ear insertion gain, and sound field thresholds have been generated. In addition, the approach specifies targets for real-ear saturation response based upon theoretical work by Pascoe (1988).

The DSL approach has incorporated the use of probe microphone measurements so that all measurements are specified in the ear canal. Hence, there are no conversions or corrections and a child's resulting hearing aid fitting can be clearly presented as his or her dynamic range for speech showing unaided thresholds, the amplified speech spectrum and the real-ear saturation response of the aid, all as if measured in the ear canal.

A very significant, innovation in the DSL approach has been the use of the 'real-ear to coupler difference' procedure, whereby the only real-ear measurement performed with the child is to establish their individual real ear to coupler difference (Seewald, Sinclair and Moodie, 1994). This single real-ear measurement may only take a few seconds. The audiologist can apply this information to 2cc coupler measures to accurately predict the real-ear aided response and real-ear saturation response. Several aid settings or aids can be trialed to select the one that best meets the real-ear validation targets without having to undertake further tests with the child.

Targets for selection of gain and frequency response and SSPL setting can be calculated by hand or generated efficiently using the DSL method software. The most recent version of this software (DSL 4.1 for Windows) allows the audiologist to fit hearing instruments with wide range dynamic compression.

The National Acoustic Laboratories (NAL) approach to hearing aid fitting

The first version of the NAL procedure was introduced in Australia in 1976. This approach aims to amplify the long-term speech spectrum so that it is comfortable and equally loud across the frequency range. Byrne and Tonnison (1976) based their estimate of the overall required real-ear gain on research by Byrne and Fifield (1974) that had shown that moderate to severely hearing-impaired children preferred to use, on average, 4.6 dB of gain for each 10 dB of hearing loss. Added to this was a frequency dependent correction figure that aimed to account for loudness differences in speech across the frequency range and for the shape of the long-term speech spectrum. This approach has undergone several modifications.

In 1986, Byrne and Dillon revised the procedure as the NAL-R approach following extensive evaluation with hearing aid users fitted using the original NAL procedure. They added an X factor to take into account the slope of the audiogram and modified the formula used to calculate required gain. In 1990, the profound correction factor was added for individuals with severe and profound hearing impairments (Byrne et al., 1990) prescribing more gain overall for 60 dB+ losses and more low-frequency gain for people with a hearing impairment greater than 95 dB at 2000 Hz. In 1998, the selection of SSPL90 in the 2cc coupler was added to the NAL procedure and experimental data published on the derivation and validation of that procedure (Dillon and Storey, 1998).

A strength of the NAL-RP procedure has been its systematic validation with adults (Byrne and Dillon, 1986; Byrne et al., 1990) and to some extent with school-aged children (Ching, Newall and Wigney, 1994). Like the DSL, it can also be calculated by hand and the National Acoustic Laboratories produce a set of slide rules that can be used to select BTE, ITE and body-level hearing aids. However, the repeated modification to this prescriptive procedure has made it somewhat cumbersome and complex to calculate in this way and the NAL computer software is more user friendly. Targets for the NAL approach can be found in most real-ear measurement equipment; however, they have not always been updated to include the most recent formula modifications. Consequently, real-ear targets should be checked against those generated by NAL software or by hand. The NAL procedure is frequently used with children despite the fact it was not designed specifically for this population. This may be a disadvantage of this approach, especially when fitting hearing aids to very young children. However, there are still insufficient research data available to clearly draw this conclusion.

Both the DSL and the NAL approaches have been carefully developed to systematically prescribe hearing aids for hearing-impaired individuals. They represent two excellent theoretical models for hearing aid selection. Although some comparative studies have been published (Snik et al., 1995; Wigney, Ching and Newall, 1997), there is no conclusive evidence available to allow clinicians to confidently select one approach over the other. They must weigh up the advantages and disadvantages of each model and consider the specific population that they serve.

Whichever prescriptive approach is chosen there are some disadvantages associated with all prescriptive approaches. When a clinician selects an aid based upon a hearing aid prescription they often assume that their work is done. Once the procedure's targets have been achieved during the validation process the hearing aid fitting is seen as complete, never to be altered until some change occurs in the child's acoustic or audiological characteristics. However, although the selection and validation process is critical to the aid-fitting process, it is just the first step. All prescriptive approaches are based upon theoretical averages. On average, the targets that the audiologist seeks to achieve may be appropriate for a child with that degree of hearing impairment. However, fine tuning will be necessary to obtain an optimum match between the aid and the performance and preferences of an individual child. What is often overlooked in prescriptive procedures is the importance of feedback from the child, their parents and teachers to evaluate hearing aid benefit. Audiologists need to be willing to make some modifications to an aid fitting based upon data gathered after the aid is fitted. It is a process frequently entered into with adults but often neglected for children. Parents and teachers can play a vital role in this process, particularly if they are involved in intensive auditory habilitation with the child.

Evaluating children's performance with amplification

Ongoing evaluation is an important step in both traditional and theoretical approaches to paediatric hearing aid fitting. It is critical for initial aid fittings and also when a child is changed over to new hearing aids. Teachers and parents must work very closely with audiologists to provide the kind of feedback that the audiologist needs to judge the effectiveness of the aid fitting. This is particularly important in this new era of cochlear implants, when children are frequently undergoing hearing aid trials to assess their implant candidature.

Feedback from teachers and parents can come in several formats. For beginning listeners, their initial responses to sound may well be quite crude, gradually becoming more specific. If the child and parent or teacher is engaged in intensive auditory/oral or auditory/verbal habilitation then responses to sound and speech can be monitored closely. The development of vocalizations and speech can provide many clues about the child's access to audible speech. Older children can be observed in the pre-school or school environment to assess their responsiveness to speech and environmental sounds, their visual attention to the speaker, and their verbal repetitions. These can take the form of informal reports by teacher, parent or child or a more formalized checklist or classroom observation tool such as the Screening Instrument for Targeting Educational Risk (SIFTER) (Anderson, 1989). Self-report by older children can be very valuable. When a child is changed over to new hearing aids, gradual changes to the frequency response may be required to accommodate their listening comfort. Parents and teachers can use functional tools such as the Meaningful Auditory Integration Scale (MAIS) (Robbins, Svirsky and Kirk, 1991) to provide feedback to audiologists about the child's use of residual hearing.

At the more formal end of the spectrum, speech-perception tasks can be used to document the development of speech-perception skills. Speech-perception test results can show which sounds can be discriminated by a child and assist with a review of a child's hearing aid fitting and habilitation programme.

Processing the signal: new and old hearing aid technology

Whether hearing aid selection is based upon a theoretical approach or a traditional approach, the audiologist must make several more decisions. They must decide whether to fit binaurally, select appropriate custom-made earmoulds and select from a dazzling array of new technology that can process sound for added clarity and comfort. Since the early 1990s, hearing aid technology has become very sophisticated. The additional benefits of each new development for a child with a significant hearing impairment often remains unclear but the choices and the cost of contemporary hearing aids is impressive. This section contains a brief review of some of the choices that confront hearing professionals when they select a hearing aid for a child.

Binaural hearing aid fitting

Choosing two hearing aids for a child with a binaural hearing impairment is not new wisdom or sophisticated technology but it needs highlighting. In many ways, even considering fitting one aid to a child with a symmetrical binaural hearing impairment seems as absurd as an optometrist recommending monocles to many of their clients. As Pascoe has observed 'Hearing aids should be chosen to help restore binaural hearing. They should, in fact, be sold in pairs, just like eyeglasses' (Mueller and Hall, 1998). The advantages associated with binaural hearing aid fitting include improved sound quality, improved speech discrimination in noise, reduction of the head-shadow effect, loudness summation, sound localization and spatial balance.

Moreover, the recent research in the area of hearing aid acclimatization suggests that auditory deprivation is a real risk with monaural fittings whereby an individual will actually show decreased speech perception scores over time in the unaided ear (Byrne, Noble and LePage, 1992; Tyler and Summerfield, 1996). There is an urgent need to change the view that monaural hearing aid fitting is a legitimate way of reducing amplification costs. It should only be considered when it can be shown clearly that speech perception in one ear is so poor as to significantly decrease the overall speech intelligibility for the child

Earmould selection

Good impression taking technique and the manufacture of a well-fitting custom-made earmould is a critical component in the paediatric hearing aid fitting process. Acoustic feedback and earmould discomfort are constant problems for young soft ears. Table 17.6 contains a list of tips for obtaining a good earmould impression.

An audiologist must also select the most appropriate acoustic characteristics for the child's earmoulds. All acoustic modifications to a child's earmould will affect the gain, the frequency response and the saturation

Table 17.6. A guide to taking earmould impressions

Taking an Earmould Impression
1. Carefully inspect the ear using an otoscope.
2. Always insert a foam or cotton wool canal block into the ear canal before inserting the earmould impression material.
3. Fill the syringe with impression material and gently squeeze the plunger until a drop or two emerges from the syringe.
4. Insert the syringe into the ear canal and fill the ear canal without removing the syringe. Always keep the nozzle of the syringe buried in the impression material.
5. Fill the helix and the conch completely.
6. After a few minutes, test with a fingernail. Gently remove impression when material bounces back.
7. Inspect ear with otoscope to ensure that all material has been removed from the ear.

response (SSPL) of the hearing aid. The three main options available to a clinician are venting, damping and fitting an acoustic horn. Their impact upon hearing aid frequency response is shown in Figure 17.3.

Venting

Inserting a parallel vent into an earmould allows children to use any good low-frequency hearing they may have, reduces low-frequency real-ear gain, aerates the ear canal and relieves pressure. Vents are unlikely to be viable with severe and profound hearing impairments due to the risk of acoustic feedback.

Damping

Acoustic filters or dampers of wool or sintered metal are often used to reduce the resonant peaks created by the original response of the hearing aid earphone. In theory, dampers can be placed at various points along the tubing to damp peaks at different frequencies. In practice, with children, dampers are unlikely to stay in position unless they are placed in an ear hook. Common places are the tip or nub of the ear hook where they will have most effect around 1000 Hz. As a minimum, a low resistance damper is recommended with most hearing aid fittings to reduce some of the big peaks and troughs of the frequency response and improve the natural quality of the sound.

Acoustic horns

An acoustic horn is a stepped piece of tubing that gradually increases in diameter from 2 mm at the ear hook to 3 mm or 4 mm at the end of the sound bore. The Libby horn was patented in 1982. It works by matching the resistance of the ear canal more closely to the resistance of the

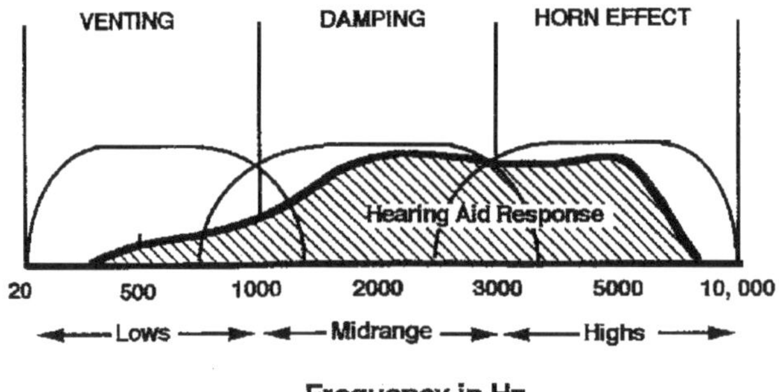

Figure 17.3. Effects of earmould acoustics on frequency. Source: from Mueller and Hall (1998) Audiologist's Desk Reference Vol II, p. 91. Reproduced with permission of Singular Publishing Group, Inc.

earphone and tubing, thus enhancing the amplification of high-frequency sounds. Table 17.7 shows the relative changes to hearing aid output that might be anticipated with a 3 mm and 4 mm acoustic horn.

Ordering an acoustic horn in a child's custom-made earmould may assist an audiologist to meet a child's high-frequency prescription targets. However, acoustic horns may not be viable for very young children. The ear canal must be able to accommodate at least a 3 mm sound bore. Acoustic feedback and loudness discomfort can also be risks, depending upon the shape of the hearing aid frequency response. The development of programmable aids with an improved high-frequency response has resulted in reduced reliance upon acoustic horns to reach prescription targets.

Table 17.7. Predicted response of Libby acoustic horns as compared to the response of 2mm constant diameter tubing

Frequency	250	500	1000	1500	2000	3000	4000	5000
Libby Horn 4mm	–1	–2	–3	0	–2	6	10	7
Libby Horn 3mm	–1	–2	–2	1	0	6	8	8

Output limiting

All hearing aids protect the hearing and comfort levels of hearing-impaired listeners by implementing a type of output limiting, usually either peak clipping or compression limiting

Peak clipping

In simple amplifiers, peak clipping limits the output of the hearing aid whenever it is driven beyond its power handling capacity or saturation point. With peak clipping amplifiers, the ratio between the sound coming into the aid and output of the aid, the input-output ratio, remains constant until the limiting level is reached. As saturation is reached, the peaks of the amplified sound signal are clipped. This results in a squaring of the waveform and adds harmonic and intermodulation distortion to the sound signal. Figure 17.4 shows the effect of peak clipping upon a sinusoidal waveform.

The distortion added to the signal by peak clipping has a significant impact upon sound quality and may also affect speech intelligibility (Dillon, 1996). Today, it is rarely the output limiting system of choice.

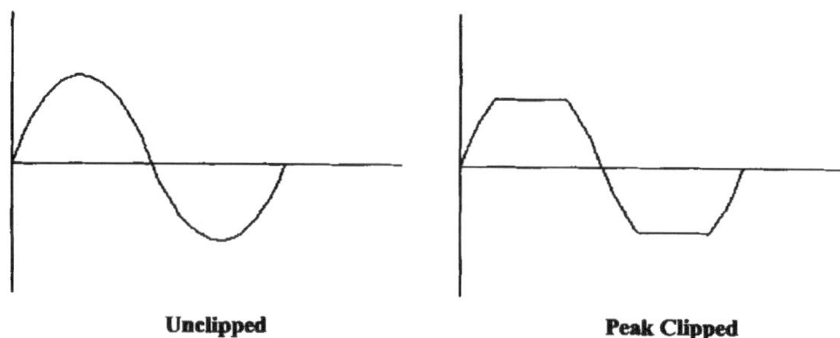

Figure 17.4. The effect of peak clipping upon a sinusoidal waveform.

Compression limiting

Automatic gain control or compression is a way of controlling the gain and output of a hearing aid. It uses an electronic feedback system to monitor either the level of the input signal (input controlled compression) or the output of the signal (output controlled compression) to prevent the signal from reaching saturation when confronted with high input levels. Most output limiting compression circuits use output controlled compression systems. When a signal is detected that exceeds a specified output level the system automatically reduces the gain of the hearing aid. When the input signal reduces below a specified level the AGC system ceases to function and the aid returns to a state of linear amplification of sound.

Several parameters can be set in output compression limiting systems. Attack time is the length of time from the point at which input exceeds the limiting level to the point at which gain is stabilized at the automatically reduced level. Attack times commonly vary from 5 ms to 100 ms. When the input level decreases, there is a short time lag from that moment to when the system returns to normal gain function. This is known as the release time. Release times in output compression systems are usually short (50–100 ms) so as to limit negative effects on speech perception. Output limiting compression systems reduce the amount of distortion added to the speech system at saturation and improve sound quality. They are superior to peak clipping systems and are generally the system of choice. However, for very profoundly deaf hearing aid users with limited dynamic range, the output compression systems may be almost constantly in saturation resulting in automatic reductions in gain. Peak clipping aids may be preferred by some of these listeners because they can provide higher output levels.

Linear and non-linear hearing aids

With linear hearing aids, the input/output (I/O) function maintains a 1:1 ratio until the limiting level is reached. Hence with every 10 dB increase in input there is a corresponding 10 dB increase in output. Hearing aids that use compression only to limit output are called linear hearing aids. Compression can also be used to alter the relationship between hearing aid input and output. With non-linear compression, the relationship between input and output is not consistent. Once the threshold at which compression is activated (kneepoint) is reached, the slope of the circuit may vary, resulting in I/O ratios of 2:1 or 5:2, 3:1, and so forth. In some circuits the I/O function is not fixed but varies with changes to input level.

Wide range dynamic compression hearing aids use a low compression kneepoint so that compression occurs over a range of inputs and a portion of the dynamic range of speech is in compression. Such systems aim to increase the listener's comfort, increase the audibility of soft phonemes, normalize loudness and reduce noise. Whole range syllabic compression circuits are similar but have a shorter release time.

Hearing aid manufacturers have been quick to adopt new compression technology and there is a vast range of different circuitry available. It seems likely that such systems can benefit many hearing-impaired listeners, however, systematic research in this area is only just starting to become available (Newman and Sandridge, 1998; Humes et al., 1999). Although it suggests that new hearing aid technologies may improve performance and satisfaction, the research needs to be carefully examined before making recommendations for young hearing-impaired children. In many environments, careful cost-effectiveness analysis may be necessary before new technology is adopted on a large scale.

Programmable hearing aids

The development of programmable hearing aids constitutes another significant advancement in hearing aid technology. Programmable hearing aids are connected to a digital programmer – either a personal computer or a dedicated device. Efficient internal adjustments can then be made to gain, output and compression parameters. Programmable devices often have multiple memories that can be accessed using a remote control unit and used for different listening situations. Many of the new signal processing strategies can only be implemented in programmable devices. Programmable hearing aids offer much greater flexibility to both clinicians and hearing-impaired listeners, including children. Some issues deserve consideration when fitting programmable devices to children. Some programmable aids use a volume-control wheel or toggle that does not display a volume setting. This can be challenging for teachers and parents because they have no way of knowing if the child has adjusted the volume unless it is locked on the recommended setting. In educational settings, where children lose hearing aids and breakdowns occur it is very difficult to set up a loaner aid system unless the school purchases a programming device and trains staff in its use.

Digital and analogue hearing aids

Although programmable hearing aids are digitally controlled devices, they are not necessarily digital hearing aids. Many programmable aids are analogue hearing aids. Truly digital hearing aids may offer the clinician and the hearing-impaired listener yet another level of flexibility and sound quality. These are a relatively recent development. Digital aids may offer children additional benefits in terms of acoustic feedback control, frequency transposition and beamforming microphone arrays, however, these aids will come at a cost. It is critical that well designed research is undertaken to evaluate the benefits of digital aid technology for children, particularly those with severe to profound hearing impairment. Only then can professionals who fit hearing aids to children weigh up the advantages of digital technology against the significant additional cost.

Listening in the real world

Hearing aids are usually selected, verified and fitted in an audiological clinic, a quiet non-reverberant world where people face each other and speak clearly. However, children have to acquire communication skills and be educated in the real world. Homes and classrooms are often characterized by reflective surfaces that absorb critical high-frequency sounds and reflect low frequencies. Background noise is always present, whether it is the hum of traffic noise or the babble of other voices. Teachers and parents speak at less-than-optimal distances and may neglect to face the child. For these reasons, hearing aids alone often cannot provide a child with a clear speech signal. An assistive device is needed that will bring the hearing aid microphone closer to the speaker and reduce the effects of background noise and reverberation.

Assistive listening devices

Assistive listening devices can include a vast array of auditory and non-auditory devices. In this chapter, the term will be used to refer to devices that work specifically to enhance the speech signal for face-to-face communication. Systems that have been used with children include hardwire systems, loop systems and FM systems. Hardwire systems can be used in special classrooms for hearing-impaired students. Each child wears a set of headphones with boom microphone, attached to a desk or console. The teacher wears a microphone linked into the amplification system. Limited adjustments can be made to individualize the headset for each child. Students receive a relatively noise-free signal from the teacher and from each other. Hardwire systems are simple and potentially inexpensive systems that can work very well with small groups of hearing-impaired students educated together. However, the trends towards integrated and more activity-based learning has made them less attractive and less viable forms of classroom amplification. Moreover, hearing aids must be removed during the time the system is used and the issue of learning to listen with two different forms of amplification has concerned educators and audiologists (Ross, 1981).

Loop systems were used briefly in classrooms as educational amplification during the 1970s. Children switched to telecoil and the teacher spoke into a microphone that sent the signal via a room loop using electromagnetic conduction. These systems fell out of favour due to the presence of dead spots in classrooms, signal overspill from room to room and alterations to the hearing aid frequency response that occurred on the telecoil setting. Since that time the FM system has become the assistive listening device most commonly used by children.

FM systems

Frequency modulated (FM) systems, also known as radio aids, radio frequency aids and FM aids, are two-part systems that use a microphone/transmitter worn by a teacher or parent and a receiver worn by the child. Sound is picked up via the microphone, worn close to the lips, and converted into frequency modulated (FM) radio waves that are transmitted on a specific frequency to a receiver. The signal is then transformed back to a speech signal and delivered to the student's hearing aids (personal FM system) or directly via button receivers (all-in-one FM aid). Sound field FM systems use a similar system but instead of personal receivers the sound is transmitted to a speaker or set of speakers set up in the classroom, thus amplifying sound throughout the whole classroom. Table 17.8 contains a brief description of FM systems currently used with children.

Selecting an FM system for a child is a complex process that requires careful pre- and post-evaluation of the child's listening situation at home or in the classroom. The goal of FM aid fitting is to allow a child to hear primary speakers (often a teacher or parent) at an enhanced signal/noise ratio so that their speech is consistently above the background noise. It is also highly desirable that children are also able to hear and monitor their own voices and hear the voices of other people who are not wearing the FM aid transmitter. This is critical for young children who are still developing their communication skills. The ease with which both goals can be achieved depends upon several factors: the child's listening environment, the FM system fitted, the coupling option selected and the child's degree of hearing impairment.

There are four possible listening modes that may be selected with different FM systems:

- FM microphone only;
- FM microphone and environmental microphone (EM) combined;
- FM plus mode or voice operated switching; and
- environmental microphone only.

In the FM-only mode, the environmental microphones are inactive and the child hears only the speaker with the FM transmitter. This mode offers the best possible S/N ratio and suits a lecture situation quite well. In a combined or FM-plus-EM listening mode both FM and EM microphones are simultaneously active. Children hear the transmitter wearer at a consistently loud level and also hear their own voices and the voices of others within hearing distance. If the listening conditions are poor, the noise entering the hearing aid microphones may significantly reduce any advantage offered by the FM system (Fabry, 1994; Hawkins, 1984). This mode is most suitable for discussion and less structured educational settings such as the pre-school setting.

An alternative to the combined setting that still offers the child some access to their own and other speakers voices is the 'FM plus' or voice-operated switching (VOX) listening mode. With this option the hearing aid or environmental microphones are attenuated by 15–30 dB only while the transmitter wearer is speaking. When the transmitter wearer stops speaking the environmental microphones are reactivated and children can hear their own voices and the voices of children around them. This option represents a compromise between the FM only and combined listening modalities. It offers a good S/N ratio without eliminating children's access to their own and other children's speech. It may not work so well in an unstructured discussion where very quick interchanges occur. There is a necessary hang time that occurs between when the transmitter wearer stops speaking and the EM is reactivated. As a consequence, the hearing-impaired child may miss the beginnings of comments made in a rapid discussion. Some FM systems also offer the option of listening via the environmental microphones alone. With most personal systems this may simply be achieved by turning or taking the FM system off. The many FM systems on the market offer different combinations of these listening modalities. It is critical, when selecting an FM system for an individual child, that the child's needs are carefully matched to the listening modes available in the FM aid selected.

Table 17.8. Brief descriptions of FM systems in use with hearing-impaired children

Types of FM systems	Description
All in one FM systems (Body worn) (Auditory trainer)	A combined body worn hearing aid and FM system usually worn with button receivers. May also be worn with lightweight headphones for students with central auditory processing disorders
Personal FM systems	A personal FM system connected to a child's personal BTE hearing aids via direct audio input or via a neckloop.
BTE FM aids	Either a combined BTE hearing aid and FM receiver or an audioshoe that attaches to a BTE hearing aid and utilizes the hearing aid battery as a power source.
Soundfield FM systems.	Utilize a conventional transmitter/microphone but sound is transmitted to a speaker or set of loudspeakers placed around the room. Many applications including classes containing children with fluctuating conductive losses, central auditory processing disorder, cochlear implants and normal hearing.
Personal sound field FM systems	Transmitter/microphone transmits teacher's speech to a portable desktop speaker. May have great application for cochlear implant users.

A simple guide to FM aid fitting and balancing

Once an FM system is selected it is necessary to set up or balance the system appropriately for the child who will wear it. As with hearing aid fitting it is critical that the FM signal is not received at a level that is either too high for comfort and clarity or too low to offer any S/N ratio benefit for the child. If the FM system is to be used in conjunction with a personal hearing aid then it is critical that the personal aid has been appropriately and individually fitted. Table 17.9 contains a brief guide to fitting FM systems.

Table 17.9. A guide to setting up FM systems with personal hearing aids

A guide to setting up FM systems
Make all measurements in dB SPL A broadband speech shaped signal is highly recommended for these measurements
1. Using a 70 dB SPL input measure the output of the child's hearing aid in dB SPL 2. Place the FM microphone in position in the test box. The hearing aid is coupled to the FM receiver and then attached to the 2cc coupler. Isolate these from the test chamber at a distance of at least 50 cm. 3. Measure the output of the FM system using an input level of 80–85 dB (chestworn microphone) or 90 dB (headworn microphone). 4. Compare the output of the aid via the FM system with the output of the aid alone. The output via the two systems should be equal, at least at 1000 Hz. The two outputs may not be perfectly matched across the entire frequency response. If the FM system is to be worn in combined mode then it is preferable to set the output received via the FM aid to be 5–10 dB higher than the output of the hearing aid. This will ensure an FM aid advantage in noise. This may not be possible with more severe and profound hearing losses. 5. Evaluate the SSPL90 of the FM system using a swept pure tone signal. Compare results to prescription targets to ensure comfort and safety when the FM aid is worn. 6. Performance of the FM system can be verified using probe tube real-ear measurement or by applying a child's individual RECD to FM aid measurements made in the hearing aid test box.

Source: Lewis D (1997) Selection and assessment of classroom amplification. In W McCracken and S Laoide-Kemp (eds.) Audiology in Education. London: Whurr Publishers Ltd and FM systems for Children: Rationale, Selection and verification strategies Phonak Focus Video: Sound Foundations. (1998). Running Time: 19 minutes.

FM aid management in the classroom, at home and at pre-school

Use of a two-part amplification system adds a degree of complexity to the communication situation that requires careful management by the child and his or her teacher or parent. The FM transmitter is worn near the teacher's or parent's lips. They cannot simply walk away from the child if they do not want to be heard. The child and the teacher must work together to ensure that the child receives relevant spoken input. In the classroom, a teacher and student may stay switched on while the teacher is addressing the class or talking to the student. However, once the class is working in groups or on individual work, it is important that students switch the receiver off so that they can focus upon their classmates or concentrate on their work. This is particularly important if the teacher is roaming the class and conversing with individual students. Similarly at home, a parent needs to view the FM aid as an aid to face-to-face conversation. It should not be used as a means of unnaturally monitoring distant behaviour or left on while the parent is having conversations with other adults. This might provide confusing spoken input that might impair the development of an already fragile construct of spoken communication.

Some of the biggest management risks are associated with FM aid use in pre-schools. Burnip and McGuire (1995) demonstrated that if a pre-school teacher were to wear the FM transmitter for a whole pre-school session, as much as 70% of the spoken language heard by a hearing-impaired child may be irrelevant. So, while young Mary is playing in the block corner with some peers, trying to negotiate the intricacies of early socialization and communication, she may be being forced to listen to her teacher telling John what a beautiful painting he has done. With such confusing input, cracking the code of spoken language may become an impossible task. Recognition of the complexities of using FM systems in pre-schools has often necessitated limited use of these aids, whereby they are only worn during group activities. For this purpose, new developments in sound field FM technology may have possibilities for pre-schools that have not yet been fully explored.

Assessing FM aid benefit and usage

A well-balanced FM system does not guarantee that students will understand the speech they hear or use and accept the aid with enthusiasm. The benefit of FM systems has been shown to vary between individuals and appears to be affected by a range of factors including listening experience, degree of hearing impairment, and auditory awareness (Ross and Giolas, 1971; Ross, Giolas and Carver, 1973; Cotton, 1988; Toe, 1998). Following electroacoustic calibration, FM benefit should be assessed in a number of ways. At a minimum, speech perception skills should be assessed with and without the FM aid using an age-appropriate standardized test. FM benefit should also be assessed in the classroom through systematic classroom observation by either an audiologist or a teacher. Self report is also a useful and often overlooked tool, empowering students at a young age to provide feedback about their own listening needs.

Hearing aid management

There seems little point in taking great care to select appropriate high-technology hearing aids for a child if little or no attention is paid to daily aid monitoring and maintenance. Over the past 35 years, a number of hearing aid performance studies have shown that hearing aids malfunction at an alarming rate. A classic study by Gaeth and Lounsbury (1966) of

134 hearing aid wearing schoolchildren showed that between 55% and 69% of hearing aids failed their evaluation procedures. In a study of a residential school, where staff had been trained to perform daily listening checks, 45% of aids failed to pass the adequate performance criteria either due to low battery voltage, acoustic feedback or inadequate volume settings (Dawson, 1987). Numerous other studies have reported similar results (Zink, 1972; Kemker et al., 1979; Robinson and Sterling, 1980; Elfenbein et al., 1988).

Although small improvements have been seen in the more recent studies and some targeted personnel training programmes have showed improved results (Kemker et al., 1979), it is clear that daily maintenance remains a substantial barrier to ensuring that children are optimally amplified. A team effort is required, with the child as the key player, developing self-management skills and good reporting strategies from an early age. Such programmes need to be well resourced. From a cost–benefit perspective there is little value in spending big money on hearing aid fitting if there is no educational audiology support for children, teachers and families to keep everything working at the coal face. Daily aid maintenance and the development of efficient repair systems are not glamorous aspects of audiology but they are critical components in the process of maximizing audibility for every child.

Conclusion

This chapter has focused upon providing a practical guide to the selection of amplification for children for audiological professionals. It has emphasized the importance of systematically selecting an aid or assistive listening device to match the audiological and acoustic characteristics of each child, particularly in an environment of rapid technological change. However, the fitting of amplification will always be but a first step in the process of audiological habilitation. Without the child's, parents' and teacher's participation in ongoing evaluation and habilitation and without dedicated management of amplification in educational settings it may be effort wasted. Only a team approach will allow every child with a hearing impairment to make maximum use of new developments in the design and fitting of hearing aids and assistive listening devices.

Resources

Software

The Desired Sensation Level Method: Version 4.1 for Windows
For computer software to implement the DSL approach to hearing aid selection contact

Hearing Health Care Research Unit
The University of Western Ontario,
Elborn College, London, Ontario, Canada
N6G 1H1
Phone: 519-661-3901
Fax: 519-661-3805
Email: dsl@audio.hhcru.uwo
Internet: http://www.uwo.ca/hhcru

National Acoustic Laboratories (NAL-RP)
Hearing aid Selection Procedure
For hearing aid fitting computer software and hearing aid selection guide slide rules to implement the NAL-RP hearing aid fitting procedure contact

Australian Hearing
National Head Office
126 Greville Street Chatswood NSW 2067
Phone: 1300 360 355 TTY: 61-2- 9412 6802
http://www.hearing.com.au

Books

Mueller HG, Hall JW (1998) Audiologists Desk Reference, Volume II: Audiologic Management, Rehabilitation and Terminology. San Diego CA: Singular Publishing Group Inc.
An excellent resource for all professionals involved in hearing aid fitting. This reference book contains excellent tables, summaries, diagrams and quick guides to every conceivable aspect of amplification.

Bess FH, Gravel JS, Tharpe AM (eds) (1996) Amplification for Children with Auditory Deficits. Nashville TN: Bill Wilkerson Center Press.
An excellent book of edited chapters covering all aspects of amplification selection for children including many innovative developments for children with a range of hearing needs.

Video resources

FM systems for Children: Rationale, Selection and Verification Strategies
Phonak Focus Video: Sound Foundations (1998). Running time: 19 minutes.
Orders: +1 (800) 777-7333.
Pediatric Hearing Instrument Fitting
Phonak Focus Video: Sound Foundations (1997).
Orders: +1 (800) 777-7333.

Chapter 18

Cochlear implants in children

R Ramsden and P Axon

Introduction

Cochlear implantation is without doubt the most exciting development in otology in recent years and many would reasonably argue of all time. During the first half of the twentieth century many of the challenges of middle-ear hearing impairment were met and to a considerable degree solved by operations such as tympanomastoidectomy and stapedectomy. With a few exceptions, however, the solutions to the problems of inner-ear deafness did not seem to lie in the surgical domain. Individuals who had lost their hearing after they had acquired speech and spoken language would have little alternative to rehabilitative strategies that relied on the use of hearing aids and lip reading. Children born with a profound hearing impairment or those developing a profound hearing impairment before the acquisition of spoken language would never be able fully to gain this skill. Education for such children has been based on either an oral tradition, employing lip reading and amplification of residual hearing, or on signing or on total communication, which uses a combination of both philosophies. Whichever educational path is followed, and however successful it might be in an individual case, the fact remains that the social, educational and psychological progress of these children is often held back and integration into the culture of normal hearing is impossible.

Cochlear implantation is based on the replacement of the lost cochlear transducer with an electrode system that delivers to the auditory pathways a processed electrical signal resembling closely the essential characteristics of speech, which the brain is capable of decoding. The development of the technique owes much to remarkable advances in a wide variety of scientific fields; engineering, microcircuitry, neurophysiology, surgery, the cognitive sciences and education. In many ways the success of cochlear implantation has been due to unique co-operation and teamwork between the scientists, manufacturers, implant clinics and educationalists. Implantation has had its opponents and controversy has often arisen as the signing deaf community has seen it as a threat to their identity. The costs incurred in the provision of cochlear implants to children and of their rehabilitation have aroused the interest of politicians who may at times be driven more by fiscal considerations than by recognition of the immense benefits that many children derive from this new technology.

History and theoretical basis of cochlear implantation

Benjamin Franklin was supposedly the first person to suggest that if an electric current was applied to the ear a sound would be heard. It is certainly true that Alessandro Volta, who was given to self-experimentation with electricity, reported to the Royal Society of London that when he placed a metal rod in each ear and connected them to his 'new electrical apparatus', the Voltaic pile, he 'experienced a commotion in my head and a few moments later I began to hear a sound or rather a noise in my ears'. It was a sort of rhythmic crackling or sizzling as though a paste or thick substance was boiling. This sound continued uninterrupted as long as the conductive circle was complete. 'The disagreeable sensation which I feared could be dangerous if the shaking in my brain meant that I did not repeat this experiment.' If one assumes that the stimulus was delivered to the organ of Corti, and not to more central structures, this graphic description is the first to show that electricity can be conducted from the periphery of the auditory system to the cortex.

The next landmark was the operation performed in Paris in 1957 by Djourno and Eyries. They placed a simple copper ball electrode on the eighth nerve of a man previously operated upon for cholesteatoma, who was undergoing further surgery for repair of his facial nerve. Electrical stimulation of this device produced an auditory percept, which the patient likened to the sound of crickets chirping or a roulette wheel. He could detect changes in the stimulus frequency up to 1000 Hz, was aware of environmental sounds and had improved recognition of the prosodic patterns of speech.

A number of workers in North America were encouraged by this case to look more methodically at the effects of electrical stimulation of the inner ear. These early workers included William House in Los Angeles, Blair Simmons at Stanford, and Robin Michelson in San Francisco. They faced opposition from basic scientists who felt that, on theoretical grounds, cochlear implantation should not work, and from sections of the deaf community who felt that the operation was unethical. Their work led to the development of an increasing number of centres throughout the world looking at experimental and clinical aspects of cochlear implantation throughout the 1970s, 1980s and 1990s. Prominent amongst these experimenters were Clark in Melbourne, Burian in Vienna, the Hochmairs in Innsbruck, Chouard in Paris, Eddington in Utah and Fraser and Douek in London. Early problems to be solved included the siting of the electrode (intracochlear or extracochlear), number of channels (single or multiple) and the signal encoding strategy (analogue or digital). Psychoacoustic tests to try to predict neuronal survival and potential benefit from implantation were studied in great depth. In addition a vast number of animal studies were necessary to establish the safety and reliability of the devices, before widespread use in humans could proceed.

The problem that cochlear implantation sets out to solve is that of severe, profound or total deafness due to partial or total absence of the organ of Corti. This loss may be congenital or acquired. The organ of Corti acts as a transducer that detects the incoming physical sound waves in the cochlear fluids and converts them into electric currents that pass down the auditory nerve and through the central auditory pathways to the primary auditory cortex in Broca's area. Association fibres project to other parts of the brain, conferring significance, meaning and an emotional overlay to the incoming signal.

The cochlear implant (CI) takes the place of the damaged organ of Corti and delivers to the inner ear a processed signal that stimulates more central neural structures, probably the spiral ganglion. In the typical CI system there is an externally worn microphone that delivers the raw electrical signal to a so-called speech processor in which the signal is manipulated to enhance speech recognition (Figure 18.1). The individual speech processing strategies vary from manufacturer to manufacturer. The refined signal is transmitted through the skin by a process of inductive coupling. The implanted component of the device decodes the incoming digitized signal and directs it as a series of discrete stimuli to the intracochlear electrode array. Currently intracochlear placement of a multichannel device is regarded as most likely to give best results (Figure 18. 2).

The implant takes advantage of several known anatomical and physiological features of the normal cochlea. The very tight tonotopic arrangement of the cochlea, with low-frequency perception at the apical end and high frequencies at the basal end, is used in the design and stimulation strategy of multichannel systems. For example, the Nucleus system features 22 intracochlear electrodes reaching from the region of the round window to the middle turn of the cochlea. In addition to tonotopic pitch perception, the so called 'place' theory, Wever's 'volley' theory proposes

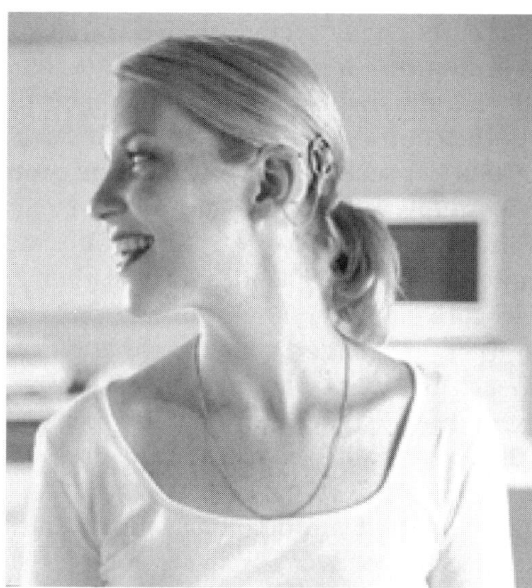

Figure 18.1. Nucleus ear level speech processor in situ.

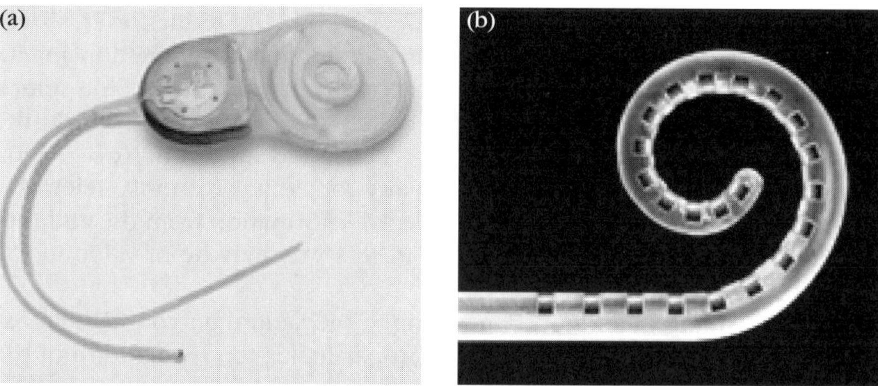

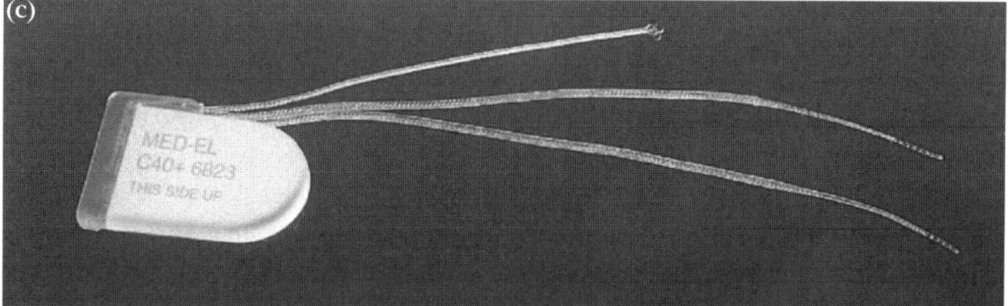

Figure 18.2. Devices (a) Nucleus CI24M with (b) magnification of electrode array. (c) Medel split electrode for use in ossified cochlea.

that up to 5000 Hz frequency recognition is at least in part related to frequency of stimulation. Most manufacturers feel that the more frequently the incoming signal is sampled the greater the fidelity of information transfer to the central nervous system, and sampling rates of up to approximately 20000 per second are possible. The problems of cross talk between electrodes at this rate of stimulation have been minimized by the strategy of continued interleaved sampling (CIS), which staggers the arrival of the stimulus at the electrodes so that they are not stimulated synchronously. An early and ingenious stimulation strategy employed by the Nucleus company depended on recognizing the specific formant frequencies of speech and extracting them from the rest of the signal. This has been superseded by a simpler strategy by means of which only the electrodes with the greatest energy peaks at any precise moment of stimulation are chosen to activate the auditory nerve. The patterns of these peaks will fluctuate rapidly from moment to moment depending on the incoming signal. Speech processing is a very complex subject and further examination of the topic is beyond the scope of this chapter.

Most of the improvements in CI performance over the past 15 years have come from refinements in signal processing rather than changes in the electrode system. A notable advance has been the reduction in size in the speech processor so that the circuitry can now be contained in an ear-level package rather than a body-worn box. In the near future it is anticipated that a totally implantable device will be available, with the microphone, processor and power source inserted surgically. New generation implant systems also have the facility for neural response telemetry (NRT), which allows the clinician to record information from the auditory nerve. It is hoped that data acquired in this way may be of value in the mapping process (see p. 374).

Understanding of auditory processing in the central nervous system has increased as a result of CI research – in particular the recognition of the complex phenomenon of neural plasticity as it relates to speech and language acquisition. The newborn child does not speak. During the first year of life its exposure to the sounds and patterns of speech is of immense significance and at about the age of 12 months babbling commences. Vocabulary and language acquisition proceed rapidly during the period between 18 months and three years in parallel with other cognitive and motor skills, and by the time the 'average' child goes to school at the age of four years it will have an unmeasurably large vocabulary and will speak fluently and more-or-less grammatically most of the time. This 'window of opportunity' for acquiring speech and language is not, however, open indefinitely. There are a few examples of children with normal hearing who have grown into adult life without hearing speech – for example, feral children or normally-hearing children of signing deaf parents. If these children are introduced to speech in their adult life they are unable to learn speech because that critical period for speech acquisition has gone. These mechanisms are highly relevant when we think about implanting individuals born deaf or becoming deaf before the language has been acquired. For such a child to have a chance of learning to speak with the implant, the device must be inserted before the window of opportunity closes. An adult born deaf is, like the normally-hearing feral child, highly unlikely to learn to assign meaning to the auditory stimuli coming from the implant and will not acquire speech. On the other hand an adult deafened in adult life will usually be a good candidate because the central auditory pathways have been previously stimulated. The auditory cortex has been previously programmed and the CI in a sense simply reawakens it from its dormant state.

Selection and assessment of children

The first recipients of cochlear implants were all adults, but as successful outcomes were obtained, and as safety and reliability were seen to be acceptable, the attention of implant teams turned to the greater challenge of children. The causes of profound hearing impairment in children have been examined in Chapter 4.

Graeme Clark's Melbourne team was the first to implant children with the multichannel cochlear implant in 1985. Since then many thousands of children have been implanted worldwide. The experience of the last decade has taught us much about the selection criteria for this operation. It is clear that these criteria are changing as time goes by and that implant teams have become less conservative as they have learned more about the cognitive processes involved in language acquisition in the young child. Diagnostic techniques have become more sophisticated, most surgical challenges have been overcome and speech-processing strategies have enhanced the fidelity of information transfer. Ethical and cultural dilemmas have been faced and largely resolved.

Children who are considered for implantation fall into two main groups. The post-lingually deafened group comprises those children who have gone deaf after the acquisition of spoken language, for example, from meningitis, head injury or from the side effects of ototoxic drugs, and those children born deaf or deafened before speech and spoken language are acquired. They will be aged three or over. In linguistic terms and in the context of post-surgical rehabilitation the post-lingually deafened child is not very different from a similarly afflicted adult. The pre-lingually deaf children include those who are born deaf, either as a result of a genetically determined abnormality or from an intrauterine event such as rubella or drug toxicity. In addition post-natal illness in the first two years of life, such as meningitis and viral damage to the cochlea, may cause a profound hearing impairment before speech has been acquired. Deafness occurring around the time that language is being learned is sometimes referred to as perilingual deafness.

Severity of hearing impairment

In the early days of adult implantation a potential patient was one with virtually no measurable hearing on pure-tone audiometry. With time it was realized that pure-tone thresholds were less important than performance on speech audiometry and at the time of writing in the UK, a maximum speech discrimination score of 20% or less is the threshold that most programmes would accept for candidacy.

With children there are of necessity a different set of values. It should be recalled that the object of the assessment process is to select for implantation children who are likely to perform better with an implant than with a conventional hearing aid, but as Dowell et al. (1997) have pointed out, it is somewhat difficult to define what the audiological profile of a child and particularly an infant should be. Clearly a speech audiogram has no place in the assessment of the pre-lingually deaf child, and even in the post-lingually deafened child there may not be enough reliable speech perception information to allow one to predict post-operative performance. Threshold assessment depends on the age of the child. In the child of nine months or over, behavioural techniques performed with meticulous care provide the most reliable estimate of threshold, and of course, threshold estimations should be made in the best aided condition as well as unaided. Auditory brainstem response (ABR) is essential and may rapidly confirm the presence of a profound hearing impairment, but there are shortcomings to the test – in particular its inability to give an accurate low-frequency threshold.

The persistence of some low-frequency hearing in a congenitally deaf child is important because it tells the surgeon that there must be an auditory nerve present. In almost all instances the child will have a trial with the most appropriate hearing aids for a period of six months and a child will commonly be referred for assessment for implantation having already had a trial with aids. It is felt that, even if the benefit has been slight, this early stimulation of the auditory pathways is of value and has a beneficial effect on outcomes with the implant. One group that is recognized as being likely to benefit from implantation is those who have previously gained some speech and language using a hearing aid but whose hearing has deteriorated to a point where powerful aids no longer help. This is known as the 'change-over' group.

Age and duration of deafness

As with adults a *post-lingually* deafened child will be implanted as soon after diagnosis and satisfactory assessment as possible. The *congenitally* deaf child will usually be about two years of age at implantation. This minimum age has come down progressively over the years as implant teams have come to realize the importance of plasticity in the auditory system and have recognized that the window of opportunity for speech and language acquisition is not large. On the other hand the process of assessment involving, as it may, a trial of hearing aids takes time as the implant team decides that implantation is the correct option for the child. Two years seems at the present time to be the optimal compromise. There is one very important exception to this rule. The child with meningitis is at risk of developing cochlear obliteration that might render the insertion of the implant impossible. These children should be implanted as soon as there is radiological evidence of this change occurring. The youngest child to be implanted so far suffered an attack of meningitis in the first week of life and was implanted at six months of age when cochlear obliteration was detected on the MR scan. At the other end of the scale, most implant teams would be reluctant to implant a congenitally deaf child over seven years old.

Speech and language ability

As the numbers of congenitally deaf or pre-lingually deafened children coming for assessment increase and the age of implantation decreases, the relevance of speech and language assessments seems to be lessening. However, many of these children have a linguistic substrate based on some form of signing strategy and this communication skill is increasingly being evaluated before implantation. In older post-lingually deafened children there are many assessment tools available to evaluate speech production skills and language performance.

Middle-ear disease

Little children with a severe sensorineural hearing impairment are no less likely to suffer from middle-ear disease than any other little children and the commonest condition to be recognized is otitis media with effusion (OME). This should be corrected and the effects of any superimposed conductive hearing impairment negated before an accurate threshold estimation is attempted, The actual presence of OME would not be seen as bar to surgery by most surgeons; indeed there is anecdotal evidence to suggest that recurrence of OME is uncommon after implantation, perhaps because of the enhanced middle-ear cleft aeration that results from the cortical mastoidectomy and posterior tympanotomy. Any more serious middle-ear condition such as perforation or cholesteatoma would require corrective surgery at a separate operation or at staged surgery before implantation could be performed. Acute otitis media, perhaps surprisingly, is not a threat to the implanted prosthesis.

Multiple handicaps

Implant teams are increasingly aware of the major problems faced by some children for whom profound deafness is just one part of a multiple disability syndrome (such as the CHARGE association). There is evidence that the existence of multiple handicaps is one of the factors that adversely affects the outcome of implantation. Nevertheless it may be that even limited benefit may be of value to these children. One particular group are children who are both deaf and blind or at risk of developing a severe visual impairment (for example Usher syndrome). Most implant teams would now be prepared to consider these children, despite the fear that, without the possibility of lip reading, performance with the implant might be less good than in sighted subjects. In fact there is evidence to suggest that these children often perform at a better level than expected. Children suspected of having major central problems that might interfere with cognition and signal processing are still a contentious group but some teams are moving cautiously to consider them.

Radiology

Radiological imaging of the inner ear is essential in the evaluation of a potential implantee to establish whether any developmental or acquired abnormality of the inner ear is present (Figure 18.3). High definition CT and MR imaging are the investigations of choice, enabling accurate delineation of cochlear anomalies. Not all dysplasias preclude implantation and Mondini's deformity, the large vestibular aqueduct syndrome and some common cavity abnormalities have all been successfully implanted. However, pre-operative diagnosis might influence the pre-operative advice given to the child's parents regarding hearing outcome. The most important anomalies to prevent implantation are total agenesis of the cochlea and agenesis of the auditory nerves (Figure 18.4). Stimulation of the auditory nerve within the modiolus is a prerequisite for cochlear implantation and the early diagnosis of agenesis of the nerve, though rare, is essential (Figure 18.5).

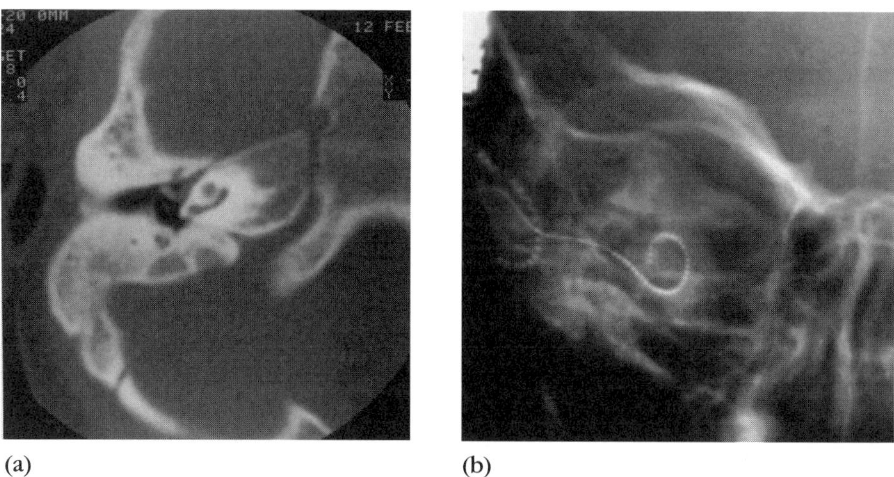

(a) (b)

Figure 18.3. (a) CT scan of normal cochlea (b) Full insertion of a multichannel electrode.

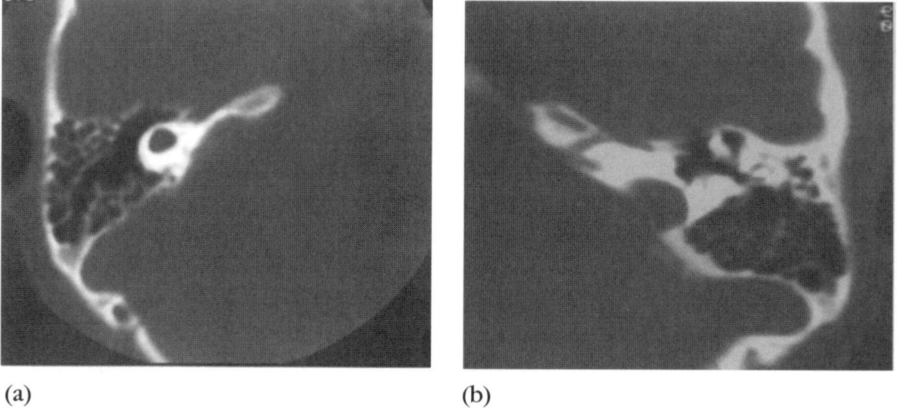

(a) (b)

Figure 18.4. CT scan showing (a) severe dysplasia (primitive otocyst) on right side and (b) total cochlear agenesis on left side (same patient).

Acquired deafness is rarely an impediment to insertion of the electrode array, but labyrinthitis ossificans after meningitis is the notable exception. Progressive ossification within the cochlear lumen can rapidly prevent full insertion of the electrode array and, although not barring surgery, can reduce implant performance (Figure 18.6). Early patient referral for radiological evaluation is paramount, enabling urgent implantation should

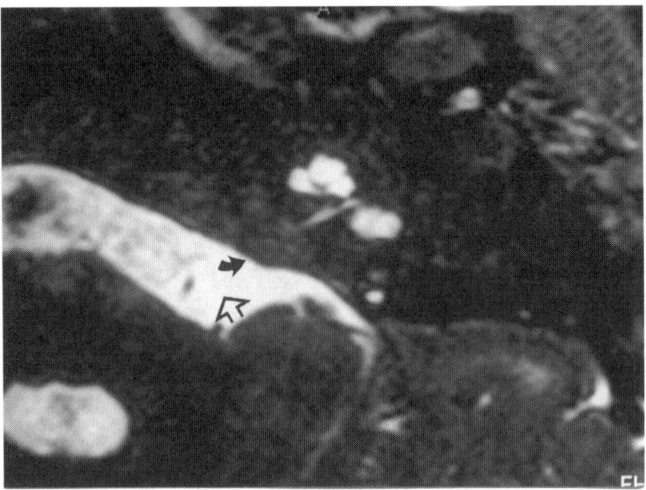

Figure 18.5. MR scan showing almost complete agenesis of the internal auditory meatus (solid arrow) and absence of cochlear nerve in the cerebello-pontine angle (open arrow).

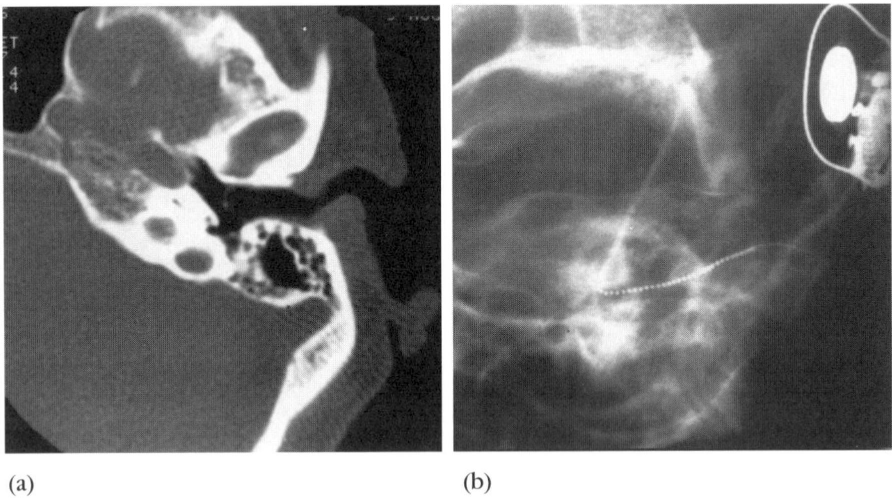

(a) (b)

Figure 18.6. (a) CT scan showing advanced obliteration of the cochlear lumen by new bone. (b) Partial electrode insertion in obliterated cochlea.

ossification be seen to be developing. Recent advances in MR imaging allow differentiation of luminal fibrosis from endolymph, which is thought a possible precursor of ossification. Three-dimensional imaging of the cochlea now allows precise localization of ossifying foci, valuable information

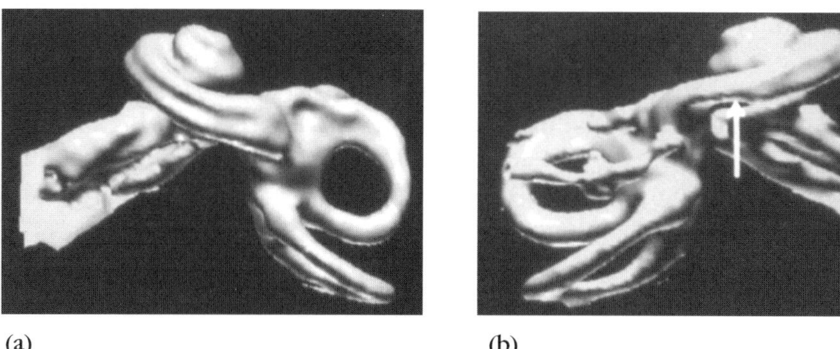

(a) (b)

Figure 18.7. 3D MR images showing (a) normal cochlea and (b) partial loss of the image from the scala tympani as a result of obliteration.

that might advise the surgeon of possible difficulties and direct him to the use of a modified electrode (Figure 18.7).

Family and psychosocial factors

Cochlear implantation is expensive. The device itself costs a lot of money (approximately £15 000). Evaluation and surgery are expensive, and rehabilitation is a very costly, labour-intensive process. It is therefore essential that the implanted child has a loving and supportive home environment, with a family that recognizes the investment in money and time and agrees to do its part in getting the most out of the technique. Parental expectations have to be carefully evaluated. There may be totally unrealistic ideas often picked from the 'gee whiz' tabloid press about how well they think their child is likely to perform with an implant. A series of counselling sessions with opportunities to meet children who have already been implanted and their parents is essential. They must realize the time scale within which progress may be expected and must be committed to long-term involvement with the child, his or her school and the implant team. The process of assessment must involve the educationalists with whom the child and family will be working and also the community paediatricians and general practitioners.

Surgery

Surgical implantation of the receiver unit and electrode array represents only a small part of the child's hearing habilitation. Nevertheless, it requires careful surgical planning and dedicated attention to detail in order to optimize implant performance while minimizing complications. The objective is to attain full insertion of the electrode array within the cochlea and placement of the subperiosteal receiver unit in a position that allows comfortable placement of the overlying magnetic transmitter coil. Fortunately the cochlea and the middle-ear structures are of adult size at birth, so there is no problem, often raised by parents and professionals alike, of having to put in a bigger implant as the child grows.

The design of the implant increasingly reflects the importance that is placed on patient comfort. The receiver unit is thin and conforms to the convexity of the skull. Its position, behind the ear, is carefully planned with post-operative placement of the magnetic transmitter coil in mind. The skin incision is remote from the receiver unit to minimize wound breakdown and the elevated skin flap is designed to incorporate a good vascular supply to minimize flap necrosis and possible implant extrusion. To gain access to the middle-ear cleft, a limited cortical mastoidectomy and posterior tympanotomy is drilled. The cortical mastoidectomy has an overhanging lip to facilitate stable placement of the electrode wires. During the child's growth, the mastoid increases in size, slowly drawing on the available slack within the mastoid bowl without displacing the electrode array. The posterior tympanotomy is performed with extreme care because the facial nerve lies in close proximity at this point in the operation. The occurrence of facial nerve injury is very rare indeed, but clearly this type of surgery should only be carried out in centres with wide otological experience. Facial nerve monitoring is recommended.

The next step is the creation of an opening into the scala tympani of the basal turn of the cochlea. Before the cochleostomy is performed, the stapes, promontory and round window niche are identified within the middle-ear cleft through the posterior tympanotomy. The cochleostomy is carefully drilled through the promontory, just in front of the round window niche and about 2 mm inferior to the stapes. A slow speed drill is used in order to minimize vibration-induced trauma to the cochlea. The endostium of the scala tympani is identified as a white membrane and is gently incised with a fine microknife. Some surgeons like to inject a small quantity of hyaluronic acid (Healon) at this stage to act as a lubricant to ease the passage of the electrode into the cochlea.

The electrode array is carefully threaded along the scala tympani with the assistance of a specially designed fine claw-like instrument. Some resistance may be met as the tip of the electrode reaches the anterior end of the basal turn but with gentle manoeuvring, sometimes with a twisting action, the whole electrode array can usually be inserted. One should never push against resistance in case of damage to the electrode array.

Electrode design varies. The Nucleus device has 22 active electrodes with 10 proximal inactive supporting bands which can be used for manipulation and instrumentation. The Medel device provides eight active electrodes and has a proximal ball-like thickening in the Silastic of the electrode array that fits snugly into the cochleostomy and helps secure the array (Figure 18.2). Alternatively a muscle plug may be inserted into the cochleostomy, to help support the array and prevent the potential for infection spreading from the middle-ear cleft. At the end of the operation it is possible to stimulate the electrode and observe an electrically evoked stapedial reflex (ESRT) (Battmer, Laszig and Lehnhardt, 1990). This tells the surgeon several things: the electrode is in the right place, the electrode is functioning, there is a functioning eighth nerve, and the facial nerve has not been damaged. Measurement of the thresholds of the ESRT has been regarded in some centres as a valuable means of predicting the settings for the system at eventual tune-up.

Ossification within the cochlear lumen after meningitis is a major consideration when planning surgery. Minor degrees of ossification in the region of the round window are common and do not present much of a problem. The cochleostomy may bypass the affected area, but if not it is a simple matter to drill past it to a clear cochlear lumen. Occasionally the scala tympani is completely obliterated by new bone formation. There are various possible solutions to this problem. One option is to attempt an insertion into the scala vestibuli, which is less likely to be affected by ossification. An alternative is to cut a gutter in the bone of the promontory and simply lay the electrode in it in the manner described by Gantz, McCabe and Tyler (1988). The manufacturers have come up with two modifications in electrode design that also address this problem. One is the compressed electrode array, which is shorter than the standard array but still has the same number of electrodes. This is clearly an advantage if there is only a very limited space in the cochlea. Alternatively one can use a so-called 'split electrode array'. There are two short arrays, each carrying half the electrodes. One is inserted into the basal turn in the usual manner and the other through a separate cochleostomy into the middle turn. The most important solution to the problem of complete ossification is avoidance if possible. This necessitates early identification of hearing loss after meningitis, and early MR imaging to pick up early ossification. Cochlear implantation may become an urgent priority for these children.

Before wound closure, the receiver unit is secured within its bony bed, flush with the outer table of the skull. In the immediate post-operative period, the correct electrode position is confirmed by plain radiograph. The slow process of hearing habilitation begins six weeks after surgery, allowing time for the surgical wound to heal.

Switch on and mapping

Before the implant system can be switched on it must be customized so that the current levels reaching each electrode during stimulation are correct for the individual patient. Each electrode has a threshold at which the stimulus just becomes audible (T level). Similarly each electrode also has a second level above which the electrical stimulus causes discomfort or pain rather than hearing (C level). The difference between the T and C levels is the dynamic range for that electrode. Stimulus levels for each electrode should lie within the dynamic range. Below the T level there will be no auditory percept. Above the C level there will be pain. T and C levels should ideally be worked out for every electrode in the array and there may be considerable variation in these levels and in the dynamic range along the array. The process of establishing these levels is known in CI jargon as *mapping*. Mapping is usually easy in linguistically competent adults who will tell you very quickly if something is audible or painful. Pre-lingually deaf children cannot do this. Furthermore, a child who associates the implant with pain or discomfort is not likely to want to wear the system and is, indeed, likely to reject the implant. Accurate mapping of a little child is one of the greatest skills in audiology, requiring expertise in conditioning and great patience. A good team will often be able to map the complete electrode array of a toddler in no more than a few sessions, although it may be felt prudent only to introduce a few electrodes at a time until the child has become accustomed to the experience of sound. Electrodes that appear to produce unwanted (non-auditory) effects can be simply left out of the map.

Work with adult CI patients has revealed a remarkably high incidence of non-auditory effects on one or two channels, and one must assume that the incidence is at least as high in children. ESRT is used by some centres as a guide to threshold setting (Battmer et al., 1990) but this has not been universal experience (Raine et al., 1997). Electrically evoked ABR recordings (EABR) may also prove of value. Once a map has been established the information has to be programmed via a computer interface into the speech processor where it will remain permanently or until the map is changed at a subsequent habilitation session. At this stage the implant system is finally switched on. At future mapping sessions T and C values are checked, additional electrodes introduced, rogue electrodes are eliminated and general fine-tuning of the system carried out. It is common to find that these psychophysical values change with time and adjustments have to be made.

Habilitation

Habilitation has been defined as 'the process by which professionals support a child and family in adapting to hearing impairment, getting used to a hearing device and developing the child's language and communication skills' (Edwards and Tyszkiewicz, 1999). This definition embodies a general principle that is as applicable to hearing aids as it is to cochlear implants. The habilitation of a child with an implant is based on this principle with modifications and additions that are specific to the use of an implant. The basic aim of habilitation is to give the child access to education through spoken language. The individuals involved in the process are the child's family, teachers of the deaf, and the audiologists, speech and language therapists and scientists on the cochlear implant team. The family has to have a realistic idea of the time frame within which progress may be expected and to structure communication strategies appropriately. For example a four-year-old who has been deaf from birth and has only had the implant for only six months will not immediately acquire the linguistic skills of a four-year-old. This may seem self-evident, but parents need to understand this and to appreciate the period of listening and learning that is essential in the process of catching up. They must know that listening and learning is a continuous process that should be integrated seamlessly into the normal day and not consigned to an allocated half hour period in the day. The child should be learning from his implant during every activity of the day, for example, dressing, eating, playing and helping in the house.

Within each of these routine activities specific linguistic goals can be set. The implant team and the teachers of the deaf need to ensure that goals are set that are appropriate to the age of the child at implantation, the duration of deafness and the length of implant use. For the child of school age it is important that these goals are incorporated into the general educational programme. The motivation of the child has to be sustained and the hope is that increased enjoyment of listening and hearing will provide that motivation rather than artificial rewards for success, which carry the negative corollary of no rewards for failure.

The implant team's involvement lies in ensuring that the device is functioning properly and is correctly programmed. It has a major role in ensuring that realistic goals are set and in liasing with teachers of the deaf and other professionals. The team will frequently visit the child in his or her domestic or educational environment and give advice and guidance to family and professionals. It provides major support to families who, despite extensive preoperative counselling, may feel that progress should be faster than it is. The team also reviews all children at regular intervals to assess progress and modify schedules as necessary.

Outcomes of cochlear implantation in children

Cochlear implantation in children has been controversial and it has certainly been expensive. From both ethical and economic standpoints it essential that the outcomes are held up to close scrutiny. Adult cochlear implantation in the UK has been the subject of a very rigorous examination by the Medical Research Council (Summerfield and Marshall, 1995). It was shown to be an effective and, indeed, cost-effective treatment for certain profoundly deafened adults. A further UK study is at present under way looking at the same issues in children.

An increasing number of reports from the large paediatric implant programmes around the world indicates favourable outcomes for well-selected deaf and deafened infants and children. The most important skills that are assessed are speech perception and speech production and language. Auditory skills may be categorized on a hierarchy of increasing difficulty: detection, discrimination, recognition and comprehension of speech. Various different types of test material are employed, which, of course, have to be appropriate to the linguistic abilities of the child. Closed set tests involve the selection of a correct choice from a limited choice of usually four pictorial options. They can be designed to assess specific information about vowel or consonant discrimination. They do not provide information about abilities to discriminate connected speech. This may be obtained from open set sentences such as BKB sentences or CID sentences or from continuous discourse tracking.

Speech perception performance at any time, as well as progress with time, may be categorized on a scoring scale. The Melbourne scale described by Dowell and Cohen (1995) has seven steps from Category 1 (detection of speech sounds only) to Category 7 (good open set speech perception >50% phoneme score). The Manchester scale recognizes 10 levels of performance. The point of entry on to the scale and the rate of progression to higher levels depend on the previous linguistic experience of the child. A post-lingually deafened child may progress to higher levels rapidly, whereas in the case of the congenitally deaf child the process may take three or four years.

There is now considerable evidence that the majority of implanted children achieve significant open set speech discrimination without lip reading. Dowell et al. (1997) found that open set speech perception should now be regarded as the norm for implanted children. There is, however, a wide scatter of performance, which can to some extent be explained by a number of factors identified as influencing outcome. The age of deafness of the congenitally deaf children and the duration of deafness of the post-lingually deafened group are strong predictors. The presence of some residual hearing, especially in the change-over group, who had previously derived benefit from hearing aids, is also a favourable indicator. An oral/aural educational strategy is also associated with better outcome. Osberger et al. (1994) assessed speech intelligibility in children with multichannel CIs and demonstrated that after 2.5 years of implant use, intelligibility was better than in children who were 'silver' hearing aid users (with pure-tone threshold of 103 dB). Higher intelligibility was also associated with an oral educational setting.

The future

The advances in cochlear implant technology in the past two decades have been spectacular but the future holds the promise of even greater things. Current developments include the ear-level speech processor, which is clearly very appealing to the patient. There are, however, still some reliability problems to be resolved. There will be improvements in the way that implant systems deliver signals to the brain. The modiolus-hugging electrode promises to improve the efficiency of signal transfer to the spiral ganglion. In the immediate future, sampling and information transfer strategies will evolve that use to the full the relatively small number of intracochlear electrodes at present at our disposal. In order to take advantage of the most efficient patterns of neural discharge, however, it may be necessary to introduce systems with considerably greater numbers of electrodes than are at present available. The totally implantable cochlear implant is almost with us. The main problems of implantation of the microphone under the skin and of recharging a totally implanted power source percutaneously are almost solved.

One of the greatest challenges, which is already being addressed, is the identification of the factors that affect the changing plasticity in the auditory pathways as the child ages. Neurotrophins are assumed to be responsible for the establishment of neural networks in the primary auditory cortex and association areas during the first few years of life. They are also assumed gradually to be switched off as the child gets older, with the result that older children and adolescents gain little speech recognition from implantation. Clark (1999) has suggested that auditory plasticity might be restored by delivery of the critical neurotrophin to the auditory system by means of the implant device itself. This might in turn trigger the release of neurotrophin in the cochlear nucleus, which might then reactivate the gene for the neurotrophin. It is envisaged that neurotrophin release might cause neural sprouting to occur at higher levels in the auditory system and encourage neural connections in the auditory pathways. If the window of opportunity could be reopened by pharmacological means, certain individuals at present debarred from implantation might once again be deemed suitable. Less ambitious might be the use of nerve growth factors or neurotrophins to increase the population of neurones in the cochlear nerve available for stimulation with the implant.

Of course, it is equally possible that a similar approach, by stimulating regeneration of the hair cells of the organ of Corti, could provide a more effective solution to the problem of sensorineural deafness than cochlear implantation itself. The experimental evidence at present suggests that limited regeneration of hair cells may be possible in the guinea-pig vestibular system, but there is no evidence to indicate that regeneration of cochlear hair cells is an imminent likelihood (Walsh, 1998)

The auditory brainstem implant (ABI) is a development from cochlear implant technology and may be indicated when total hearing impairment results from bilateral pathology that affects the auditory nerve rather than the cochlea. The electrode array is implanted on to the surface of the cochlear nucleus in the brainstem and thus stimulates the auditory pathway cranial to the damaged auditory nerves. In practice, the condition for which this device is nearly always used is neurofibromatosis type 2 (NF2), which is characterized by the occurrence of bilateral vestibular schwannomas (acoustic neuromas). The tumours themselves, or the surgery to remove them, may cause total deafness. At present this technique has only been applicable to adults. It has, however, been a matter of recent speculation as to whether the ABI might have a role in the habilitation of children born with auditory nerve agenesis.

Summary

Cochlear implanation has revolutionized the management of severe-to-profound deafness in children, whether congenital or acquired. Assuming implantation is carried out while the auditory system still retains plasticity, most children can be expected to gain open set speech discrimination and to go to mainstream schooling. Implantation is safe and the surgery is routine. Assessment and habilitation require the skills of a multidisciplinary team. It is expensive and labour intensive. It should only be available in a small number of dedicated units.

CHAPTER 19

Balance disorders

C MÖLLER

Introduction

The ability of man to walk upright on two legs and keep equilibrium is dependent on the integrity of a complex system consisting of the three major 'receptor organs'. The impulses from the vestibular part of the inner ear, the eyes and somatosensory stimuli from skin, muscles, tendons and joints are so harmoniously balanced that, under normal conditions, they are integrated subconsciously.

The first sensory organ to be formed is the inner ear, which by mid-term is fully differentiated. In fact, all the sensory systems are structurally fully developed at birth and it is just a matter of learning and adaptation that completes the maturation. At birth the newborn infant experiences a new world, where there is suddenly exposure to new kinds of movements and positions.

The task of keeping good balance is performed by three different systems.

- the vestibular system;
- the visual system;
- the somatosensory (proprioceptive) system.

The vestibular system

The vestibular system is a sensory system that has access to the cerebral cortex with conscious perception and memory, but also a motor system regulating body posture and eye position. The sensory cells of the vestibular receptors are arranged in five different formations. The utricular and saccular maculae and the three semicircular canals are orientated perpendicular to one another. In the distended part of each canal (ampullae) the sensory cells are formed to a structure called the cupula. The otolith system gives information about linear acceleration and deceleration. Head movements will, in the semicircular canals, cause an endolymph movement that will deviate the cupula. Because of the endolymph movements, the constant resting discharge will be increased or decreased depending on the direction of the flow.

The vestibular nerve forms two divisions named the inferior and superior branch. The inferior branch derives mainly from the posterior canal and the main part of the saccular macula. The superior branch supplies the cristae of the superior and horizontal canal and the utricular macular. The vestibular nuclei are located laterally below the floor of the fourth ventricle, and are partly in the pons and partly in the medulla.

From the vestibular nuclei there are two alternative pathways in which signals can be transmitted to the oculomotor nuclei and the eye muscles. The first and probably most important one is via the commissural fibres, the medial longitudinal fasciculus (MLF), and through the pontine reticular formation. The other pathway is probably through the cerebellum. From the oculomotor nuclei the impulses travel through the cranial nerves III, IV and VI and terminate in the extra-ocular muscles. The vestibular ocular reflex (VOR) and its connection are demonstrated in a very simplified way in Figure 19.1. The functional organization of the VOR responses is far more complicated than the elementary figure suggests.

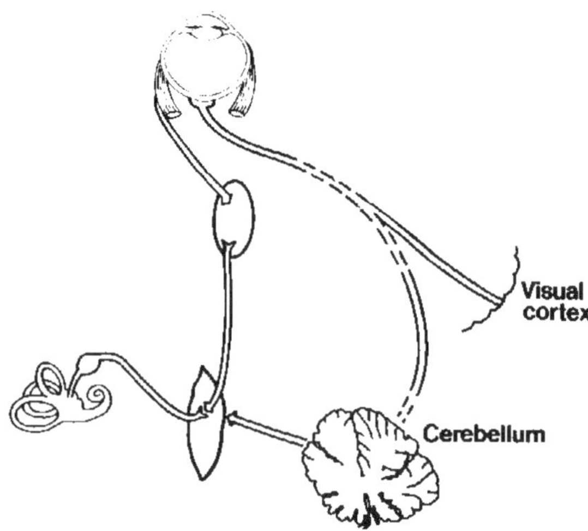

Figure 19.1. The vestibular-ocular reflex (VOR) and its connections.

The visual system

Saccades are the fastest of the eye movements, which can be executed either voluntarily or involuntarily. The aim of the saccades is to direct the gaze towards an object. The velocity of the saccade is dependent on the amplitude of the eye movement. The larger the eye movement, the greater the top speed. Recent research has emphasized the intimate relationship between oculomotor performances and the vestibular system. Even a very young child is able to execute saccadic eye movements.

Smooth pursuit refers to a tracking eye movement, stabilizing a moving target on the fovea by producing eye velocities closely matching the target velocities. Neural signals related to smooth pursuit have been found in the retina, accessory optic system, visual cortex and in the cerebral hemispheres. The exact visual pathways to the cerebellum and the brainstem are not known. Purkinje cells of the cerebellar flocculus have been found to discharge during smooth pursuit, and within the brainstem reticular formation motor neurons have been shown to encode eye position. The smooth pursuit is most effective at low frequencies (<1 Hz) and velocities (< 40°/sec). Smooth pursuit gain (eye velocity/ target velocity) depends upon a number of factors such as age, attention and motivation (Hausler et al., 1987). In daily life activities humans perform visual tracking by a combination of smooth pursuit, saccadic and vergence eye movements.

The somatosensory system

The effector organs of the somatosensory system and the vestibulo-spinal reflexes are different muscle groups such as the extensors of the neck, trunk and extremities. These reflex pathways have a high degree of complexity with contractions and relaxations in opposing muscle groups. A common finding in most of these reflexes is the automation and intimate interaction with visual and vestibular pathways, in order to maintain gait and body equilibrium.

The cerebellum

The vestibular nerves project directly and indirectly through the brainstem to flocculus, nodulus and uvula, commonly called the vestibulocerebellum. Through interactions with vision, the effect of cerebellum on the VOR seems to be mainly inhibitory.

Vestibular interaction with other systems

During head movements, gaze stabilization is maintained by vestibular, neck-somatosensory signals and visual commands. Visual information reaches the inferior olives, which will activate Purkinje cells in the cerebellum. These areas also receive vestibular information from the vestibular nuclei. The impulses from cerebellum will terminate in the reticular formation of the brainstem where a 'comparison' of the signals might be performed, and if necessary a change of the vestibular signals takes place. If the vestibular and visual information are in conflict, the visual reflexes at lower rotatory frequencies and velocities will override the vestibular reflexes, while at head movements with high velocity the VOR will dominate. Visual impulses and VOR will primarily interact to improve visual fixation of a stationary or moving target in rotations at low frequencies.

Afferent signals from all three systems convey into the brainstem, pons and cerebellum where they are processed and then transmitted through efferent nerve fibres to maintain co-ordinated movements. This interaction also is important for the development of motor milestones such as sitting unsupported, crawling and walking. Assessment of these three systems and the central integration is essential when evaluating children with balance disorders.

The anamnesis is, as in adults with balance disorders, of uttermost importance in children. It is, however, difficult to get good case histories from the child or the parents. The young child when subjected to attacks of dizziness often can respond only with crying, pallor and sleepiness. Thus it is of uttermost importance to have knowledge of normal childhood motor milestones (Table 19.1).

When a child has balance disorders it is wise to develop a strategy of 'down-to-earth questions', balance assessment and, most important, observation of the child.

Table 19.1. Early motor milestones

6 weeks	hold the head of the plane of the body
12 weeks	hold the head above the plane of the body
16 weeks	good head control
6 months	unsupported sitting
10 months	standing up with support
12 months	walking

Questions

Questions concerning a child with late motor milestones should concentrate in addressing different 'events' that the parents might remember, such as in Table 19.2. These questions might be good in sorting out symptoms such as bilateral vestibular loss or imbalance caused by central nervous deficiencies.

Table 19.2. Questions to be asked of parents

- At what age could the child lift his head, roll around ?
- At what age did the child sit unsupported ?
- At what age did the child walk unsupported ?
- Did the child experience difficulties in learning to bicycle ?
- Does the child have problems when walking in darkness and on uneven surface?
- Does the child experience motion sickness ?
- Does the child have problems in gymnastics and sport activities ?
- Is the child considered to be clumsy

When child has attacks of suspected vertigo or dizziness, a suggestion is to have the parents make a diary, where they should note the following (Table 19.3):

Table 19.3. Diary record

Symptoms
Pallor, vomiting, unsteadiness, headache, falling, etc.
Frequency of attacks
Increasing, decreasing
Duration of attacks
Hours, minutes
Time of the day
Other symptoms
Seizures, hemiparesis, etc.
Drugs, chemicals, etc.
Aminoglycosides, chemotherapeutics, diuretics, etc.

- *Balance assessment.* Balance assessment is, of course, dependent of the age of the child, but most of the tests can be performed from a very early age.
- *Observation of the child during play.* It takes time but will often give extremely useful information. A video-recording is often helpful. Important parameters to observe are patterns of locomotion. Differences when moving around during different light conditions (Figure 19.2).
- *ENT and dysmorphology examination* should be emphasized in order to detect dysmorphology of face, outer ear, ear canal, tympanic membrane and middle ear.

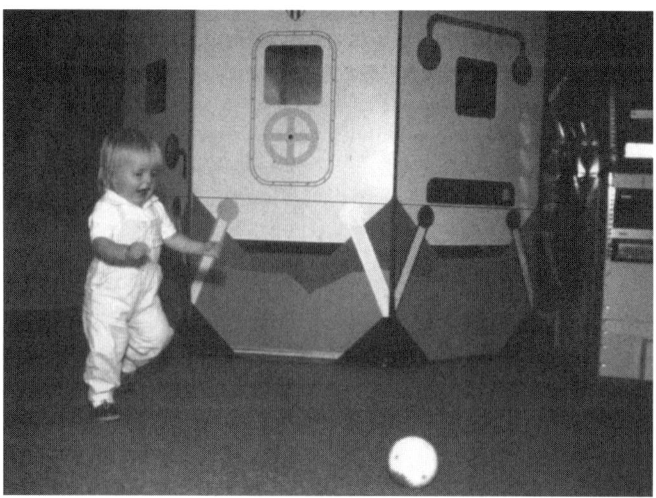

Figure 19.2. Observation of the child during play.

- *Cranial nerve tests,* deep tendon reflexes and developmental reflexes.
- *Romberg testing.* Children older than four years of age can often perform in Romberg testing, standing on one leg and so forth. The performance in younger children shows a large variation and depends on cooperation between the examiner, the child and parent.
- *Video-oculography* is a fairly new method that will give the clinician very good information concerning pathology of the vestibulo-ocular reflex noting possible spontaneous, positional and rotatory nystagmus. The easiest way to perform these tests is to have a pair of Frenzel-glasses with infra-red TV cameras in the office. By using these in the office examination it is now possible to solve many cases of childhood balance disorders. Video-oculography is not only a tool for inspection. Devices with possibilities of analysis are commercially available and will in the future probably replace electronystagmography (ENG).
- *Electronystagmography (ENG)* consists of a battery of standard neuro-otological tests. The method is based on the fact that the cornea serves as a positive pole and the retina as a negative. Electrodes are placed on the forehead, the outher canthi (for horizontal recording), above and below the eye (for vertical recording). As the eye moves horizontally or vertically, the positive pole (cornea) moves closer or further from the electrodes. ENG can be performed in small children but is subject to difficulties with calibration and irregularities of eye movements such as eye blinks. Eye movements are best recorded in darkness using the direct current (DC) electrooculography (EOG) technique.

- *Gaze (fixation) test.* The purpose of the gaze test is to identify the presence of spontaneous nystagmus during visual fixation. The child is asked to fixate or an object is in a position 30° to either side of centre gaze. With the presence of a gaze nystagmus, especially if it is present in different positions, a lesion within the brainstem cerebellum can be suspected. If, however, a unilateral gaze nystagmus is at hand, the cause might be due to an acute unilateral vestibular lesion (Figure 19.3).
- *Position tests.* Positional (dynamic) and position (static) tests are conducted to determine if changes of the head position can cause or modify a nystagmus. The tests can be performed in children either by use of video-glasses, Frenzel-glasses or ENG. They usually take some time but can be very rewarding. If a nystagmus is present in all positions it is referred to as a spontaneous nystagmus. A finding of a strong position or positional nystagmus in children can indicate both a vestibular end organ lesion as well as a CNS lesion. Specific positions and nystagmus can point towards specific diagnoses.
- *Smooth pursuit and saccade tests.* In small children these tests are best performed by direct observation of eye movements while moving toys in front of the child. With some experience there are possibilities to assess the accuracy of the saccades and smooth pursuit and whether there are any signs of eye muscle paralysis or not. ENG-recordings can be made simultaneously but are difficult to analyse. Children from the age of seven to eight years can usually perform in a regular oculo-motor test battery. The oculo-motor tests are important to assess and rule out pathological central nervous oculo-motor function.

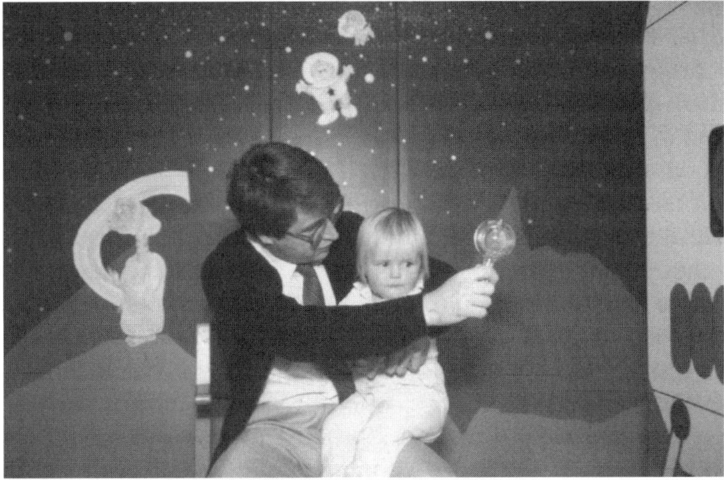

Figure 19.3. The gaze test.

- *Optokinetic test (OKN).* The function of the optokinetic system is to maintain visual fixation where the head is in motion. This system complements the vestibular system but as the smooth pursuit system it functions primarily at frequencies lower than the vestibular system. The optokinetic test can be performed at very young ages by placing the child in front of vertically or horizontally moving black and white stripes. Optokinetic abnormalities are noted in lesions affecting the visual pathways of the brainstem and cortex. The analysis of the resulting nystagmus is, however, difficult to assess and at present the test has to be considered non-specific and is replete with interpretation problems. It is not so commonly used.
- *Calorics.* The bithermal caloric test has been the mainstay of the ENG battery for many years. The induces endolymph flow in the semicircular canals (primarily the horizontal), thereby creating an excitation or inhibition of the electrical discharge. Bithermal binaural calorics should be performed with eyes open in darkness. The velocity of the slow phase is the best parameter to assess. An inter-aural difference of more than 20% is, in most laboratories, considered pathological and a total sum of four irrigations of less than 40°/sec. is considered hypoactive. Calorics can usually be performed from four or five years of age. Ice-water calorics performed binaurally (50 cc, 8 °C) can be performed in older children who do not show responses during ordinary caloric tests. This test, however, cannot be quantified but is merely a sign of some vestibular function. Caloric abnormalities usually reflect a vestibular end organ lesion but can, of course, also be seen in an isolated brainstem lesion, although this is rare.
- *Rotatory tests.* Sinusoidal rotatory chair tests are by far the best test in order to evaluate possible bilateral vestibular loss in small children. They can be performed using the EOG technique and/or infrared TV monitoring. The tests should be performed in darkness and if a vestibular function is at hand a resulting nystagmus will immediately appear. In some cases a good EOG recording is not possible and, in those cases, infrared TV monitoring focused on both the eyes of the child and the parent, will immediately show the difference in response and whether a bilateral vestibular loss is at hand. The parameters used are phase, gain and asymmetry. Some have used these parameters to diagnose a unilateral vestibular lesion. This is, however, very difficult to assess – especially when using low-frequency(<1 Hz) rotatory chairs. The rotatory test is difficult to quantify and it will not with certainty differentiate between a unilateral vestibular loss and normal bilateral function (Möller, 1996). To summarize: the strength of the rotatory

chair is to monitor change within the vestibular system, and particularly in the early detection of bilateral peripheral vestibular lesions (Figure 19.4).

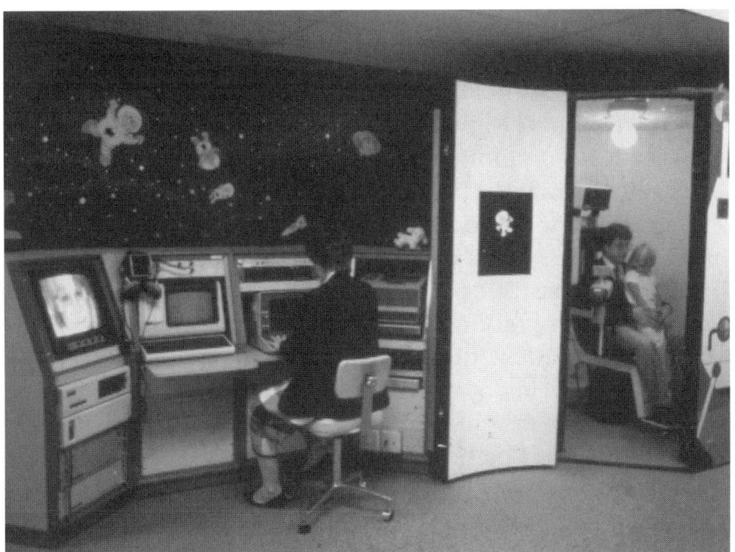

Figure 19.4. The rotatory test.

- *Dynamic posturography.* Dynamic equilibrium (balance and stability while in motion) consists of both sensory and motor components. To be in normal posture both the sensory and motor systems must be intact. Devices such as computerized dynamic posturography (Equitest) evaluates the integration of vision, somatosensory and vestibular input and the central integration resulting in different sway patterns. It uses a computer-controlled menu-driven moveable platform and visual surround. The test can help in assessing children with histories of imbalance and unsteadiness, delayed motor development, and monitoring progress or recovery. This test has large variations when used before the age of four or five years (Cyr et al., 1988).

Depending on the anamnesis, other medical and neurological test batteries such as ECG or EEG should be applied. Evaluating a child with balance disorders always involves team work where other specialists such as paediatricans, neurologists, physical therapists, and child psychiatrists might be needed.

Balance disorders

Genetic

The close proximity and the origin of the cochlea and labyrinth makes vestibular assessment in children with hearing impairments extremely important.

Deafness and severe hearing impairment due to a genetic condition constitute approximately 50% to 75% of all hearing impairments in children. Since it is common among the deaf to be 'clumsy', this is often treated as a trait of deafness and caused by the hearing impairment in itself and not by a vestibular end-organ deficiency.

As long as vision is sufficient, and in light conditions, a person with bilateral vestibular loss can perform nearly normally. On the other hand when dark, or when walking on an unsteady surface, the loss of the vestibular system can make the same person very clumsy and insecure.

The rapid discoveries of different genetic hearing deficiencies have made it necessary to differentiate between similar auditory phenotypes by using vestibular testing. In 1930, Shambaugh collected information from approximately 5000 deaf students and concluded that 70% had normal balance function, with no differences between congenital and childhood onset deafness. He did not, however, perform any vestibular tests (Shambaugh, 1930).

In 1965, Sandberg and Terkildson presented results from 57 children who underwent caloric irrigation according to present standards. They found a fair correspondence between the degree of hearing impairment and the loss of vestibular function with deficiencies in the vestibular function in 80% of the deaf population.

The author performed a balance study on 74 subjects suffering from severe or profound hearing impairment. More than 50% of all subjects displayed a walking age later than 18 months. Over 50% of the subjects displayed significant problems getting around in darkness, especially in winter. Very few had experienced any motion sickness. None reported motion sickness during car rides. A large majority (75%) remembered problems in sports and gymnastics. Many of the subjects referred spontaneously to 'I never cared because I was so clumsy.' All the subjects who displayed absent vestibular responses in the caloric and rotatory tests reported a walking age later than 18 months (Möller, 1996).

There is reason to believe that around 30% to 40% of all deaf persons suffer from bilateral vestibular areflexia. Thus it is extremely important that all children with hearing impairment have a thorough vestibular examination primarily addressing the question of whether or not there is a bilateral vestibular loss. This screening is easily done using the rotatory test with video-oculography. If the child has nystagmus we know that at least one vestibular organ is working. The other parameter to address is walking age. So far no child with congenital bilateral vestibular loss has been found walking before the age of 18 months (Möller, 1996).

Syndromal hearing impairment

Many different syndromes have been investigated concerning the vestibular function. One of the first to be characterized was Usher syndrome, where vestibular function and genetic analysis have been found to be the best discriminators between different types so far. Vestibular function in other syndromes is gradually being investigated. It is apparent that, in many syndromes, the vestibular end organ shows dysfunction expressed by the same genes that are causing the cochlear deficiency.

Usher syndrome (autosomal recessive)

Usher syndrome (hearing impairment, retinitis pigmentosa and varying vestibular function) consists of three clinical types. Usher type 1 (deafness and retinitis pigmentosa) has displayed absent bilateral vestibular function in all cases that have been genetically linked. Usher type 2 (hardness of hearing plus retinitis pigmentosa), on the other hand, has normal vestibular function bilaterally. Usher type 3 displays progressive hearing impairment and retinitis pigmentosa. The vestibular function in Usher type 3 seems to be characterized by hearing loss followed by a gradual decrease of the vestibular function.

Alström syndrome (autosomal recessive)

Alström syndrome includes early onset of retinitis pigmentosa, which will result in blindness in early teens, bilateral symmetrical progressive hearing impairment, hyperlipidemia, elevated triglycerides and onset of diabetes in early teens. The vestibular function shows a progressive decrease, which, together with the blindness, will result in severe unsteadiness especially on uneven surfaces (Möller, unpublished observation, 1999).

Alport syndrome (autosomal recessive, dominant, X-linked)

Alport syndrome has several different forms and displays progressive hearing impairment, kidney disorder and sometimes myopia. The vestibular function has been reported to be pathological.

Branchio-oto-renal syndrome (autosomal dominant)

This syndrome comprises branchial fistulas, kidney abnormalities and middle and inner-ear dysmorphology. The hearing impairment is variable but most cases known have impaired peripheral vestibular function.

Pendred syndrome (autosomal recessive)

These children have a moderate to severe hearing impairment, in teenage they develop goitre and hypothyroidism. The vestibular function can be normal or decreased (Huygen and Verhagen, 1994).

Whether or not deaf children with intact vestibular function show more clumsiness compared to normal children has also been the subject of discussion. If it is true it might be a result of the deafness in itself with lack of auditory response when crawling, walking and so forth.

Non-syndromal hearing impairment

It is likely that a phenotype reflects an underlying defect that is gene specific and from a genetic perspective, vestibular tests can discriminate otherwise similar non-syndromal deafness into two groups. Thus, hereditary deafness should always be categorized according to whether the labyrinth is involved or not. If vestibular involvement is consistent within families, then deafness with or without vestibular symptoms represents two major clinical categories of hearing impairment.

In order to study hearing disorders and to provide a better mode of classification, the vestibular function has to be evaluated in all cases of severe childhood hearing impairment and deafness.

Genetic vestibular loss

Congenital isolated vestibular loss without hearing impairment is clinically very seldom recognized. It is anyhow very likely that this occurs. The advantage of having a vestibular loss is that it can be compensated partly by vision and somato-sensation. If the vestibular loss is unilateral it is possible for the healthy side to compensate for this fully in most cases.

A progressive vestibular loss can in some cases give rise to rotatory vertigo, which in some children might be misdiagnosed as other disorders such as benign paediatric vertigo. A thorough attempt to quantify the vestibular function should therefore always be made.

Ototoxicity

There are several drugs known to be ototoxic. The most well known are antibiotics, chemotherapeutics and some diuretics. In children the most common cause of vestibular destruction and imbalance are gentamycin and cisplatinum. Both drugs are administrated intravenously.

The mechanism of ototoxicity due to gentamycin seems to be slow destruction of supporting cells, thus it is possible that damage might be apparent long after the treatment has terminated. Some families have been found to carry a gene making them more susceptible to gentamycin. The prevalence of these genes are not yet known.

The causes for vestibular damage are probably multifactorial. The doses in small children are hard to control and sometimes regular serum level measurements are not performed. The second cause is due to the fact that the vestibular part of the inner ear is much more susceptible to gentamycin compared with the cochlea.

The symptoms of ototoxicity mimic the symptoms of vestibular neuronitis and bilateral vestibular loss. Dizziness, findings of spontaneous nystagmus, unsteadiness and later if there is bilateral vestibular damage, retarded motor milestones.

These symptoms are very difficult to observe and interpret in young very sick children in bed, with high fever and vomiting. If ototoxicity is suspected, examination of spontaneous nystagmus using video or Frenzel-oculography is useful. This procedure can be performed at the bedside.

Every child who has undergone treatment with ototoxic medication should have a hearing and vestibular assessment performed.

Meningitis

Viral and bacterial meningitis is primarily a disease of early childhood (six months to 24 months). Viral meningitis does not seem to cause large damage to the inner ear, although hearing impairment and vestibular loss have been reported. Bacterial meningitis on the other hand usually gives severe vestibular lesions.

The main bacterial agents are pneumococcus, meningococcus and Haemophilus influenzae. Permanent sequelae due to meningitis are due to lesions of central nervous system (CNS) structures, cranial nerves and the inner ear. The clinical picture after CNS damage is that of mental retardation, pareses, seizures syndromes and ataxia. Central nervous system lesions have a prevalence of 1% to 10% (Salvén, Vikerfors and Olcén, 1987).

Sensorineural hearing impairment as a result of meningitis appears in approximately 20% of cases. The vestibular end organ is much more susceptible. Vestibular lesions and vertigo are frequently observed both with and without association to deafness due to meningitis. Different studies have shown the prevalence of bilateral vestibular loss after bacterial meningitis to be 40% to 80% (Möller et al., 1989; Van Rijn, 1990).

A bilateral vestibular loss can be clinically observed in many cases; this is not, however, the case of unilateral vestibular loss, which in many cases is probably not diagnosed. A child who has suffered from meningitis often has a long recovery. During that recovery it is usual to have a regression in motor milestones. Children who have been walking start to crawl again. The symptoms differ depending on whether or not the lesion is unilateral or bilateral. A child with a unilateral vestibular lesion has symptoms like a child with vestibular neuronitis – that is a spontaneous nystagmus that disappears quickly with a rapid recovery provided that there are no major CNS lesions. A child with bilateral vestibular loss does not show signs of vertigo but rather severe unsteadiness and impaired motor milestones. This is often misinterpreted as caused by the disease in itself.

Assessment of vestibular function after meningitis should be made in all cases, and if a bilateral lesion is found, appropriate balance training should be started as soon as possible (Table 19.4).

Table 19.4. Bacterial meningitis

Age of onset	**Symptoms**
usually < 2 years	vertigo, falling
increased clumsiness	
Unilateral lesion	**Bilateral lesion**
spontaneous nystagmus, vertigo	retarded motor milestones,
rapid recovery	difficulties in learning to walk

Diagnosis
observation of motor milestones
rotatory tests with video-oculography/ENG
bilateral lesion shows no rotatory nystagmus
unilateral lesion shows rotatory nystagmus

Benign paroxysmal vertigo in childhood (BPV)

This disorder is a distinct clinical entity first described by Basser in 1964. The disorder is characterized by rather alarming episodes of severe rotatory vertigo interfoliated by perfectly normal motor patterns. The disease is described in Table 19.5.

Table 19.5. Benign paroxysmal vertigo

Age of onset	**Sex**
usually < 4 years	no gender difference
Symptoms	**Frequency**
sudden onset of vertigo,	several times a week year
pallor, vomiting, nystagmus	disappears after months to years
can occur in any position,	
falling, unable to move	**Duration**
after attacks, normal activities	seconds-minutes
consciousness not impaired	

(Eeg-Olofsson et al., 1982).

The diagnosis is made by careful case history and clinical examination. It is advisable to instruct the parents to make a diary and to teach them to look for spontaneous nystagmus during the attacks. A video recording can be helpful. When examining the child there should be no hearing impairment, normal otoneurological examination and normal EEG. Thus one differential diagnosis is epilepsy (Eeg-Olofson et al., 1982). A video/electronystagmography, if possible including calorics, should be performed because some authors have reported decreased caloric responses. If the case history is not clear, the differential diagnosis of tumour and epilepsy must be ruled out.

The etiology of BPV is still unclear. The possibility of BPV being a migraine equivalent has been discussed. This has not however been confirmed. In a follow-up study (after 10 years) of children with BPV, migraine was found to be slightly more common than in a normal population. Compared to migraine patients, who often have close relatives with the same disorder, a positive family history of migraine was less common in patients who have suffered from BPV. All subjects were as adults free of vertigo and showed normal auditory and vestibular test results (Lindskog et al., 1999). After careful case history and ruling out differential diagnosis, information about the disease should be given, stressing its benign nature.

Acute vestibular loss (vestibular neuronitis)

Consulting the literature, the incidence of vestibular neuronitis in children seems to be very low. The symptoms and course of the disease are the same as in adults being an acute onset of rotatory vertigo, nausea and vomiting. No other cranial nerve symptoms should be present. The symptoms are usually quite mild in children and recovery is rapid. This implies that the real incidence of vestibular neuronitis might be higher than documented. The origin of this disease is still obscure. Some evidence supports the thought that the disease is due to viral infection of the nerve, other evidence suggest an autoimmune disorder. One can speculate if acute vestibular loss is an equivalent to sudden hearing impairment.

The child suffers from acute rotatory vertigo, nystagmus with a destruction type of nystagmus with the fast phase beating towards the healthy ear. Caloric tests show an asymmetric response. The recovery is usually very fast (two or three days), with a fast disappearance of spontaneous nystagmus, vertigo and rapidly improved balance. The child will not have any sequelae. As in adults, vestibular function might completely recover.

Migraine

The frequency of migraine in childhood is estimated to be around 4% between the ages of seven to 15 years. Around 20% of these children with migraine complain of dizziness (Prensky and Sommer, 1979). A general opinion is that the migraine with dizziness may originate within the basilar artery system. The attacks usually starts with dizziness or vertigo followed by headache and insomnia. One associated finding in children with migraine is a high incidence of motion sickness.

It is sometimes difficult to differentiate migraine from BPV. The occurrence of headache and a strong family history of migraine might help to make the diagnosis. A very rare but similar condition is paroxysmal torticollis of infancy. The symptoms are head tilting to one side with pallor and sometimes vomiting. The attacks can last minutes to days. The onset is usually around one year and the symptoms disappear within one or two years. The pathology is still unclear but due to the symptoms found one might expect dysfunction within the vestibular apparatus (Parker, 1989).

Ménière syndrome

Classical Ménière syndrome in children is rare. The symptoms of low-frequency fluctuating hearing impairment, rotatory vertigo attacks, tinnitus and fullness are the same as in adults. Auditory and vestibular findings in children with Ménière syndrome indicate the same pathology of endolymphatic hydrops as in adults (Hausler et al., 1987). The cause of Ménière syndrome is still obscure. Some families have been found to have a high incidence, suggesting a genetic factor. New discoveries in inner-ear disorders of genetic origin have demonstrated symptoms resembling Ménière syndrome. In these families with autosomal dominant fluctuating but progressive hearing impairment, the symptoms might start with rotatory vertigo. This shows the importance of performing hearing tests in children with balance disorders.

The treatment of Ménière syndrome in children has so far been the same as in adults, which includes lifestyle recommendations and a low-salt diet. The literature does not give any good statistical data concerning the course of the disease in a child, but based on results in adults one can expect a steady progress of the hearing impairment and a 20% to 30% chance of the disease being bilateral.

Trauma

A head injury in a child may result in different forms of fractures involving the petrous temporal bone. If the fracture involves the labyrinth or the vestibular nerve, a severe vertigo will result including vomiting, and unsteadiness. Even a concussion without a fracture might result in dizziness. In an acute unilateral vestibular loss a spontaneous nystagmus beating towards the healthy ear will appear. The nystagmus and the vertigo will often disappear very quickly, probably due to a rapid central compensation and large CNS plasticity. The rehabilitative treatment includes vestibular rehabilitation by a skilled physiotherapist.

Middle-ear disease

Serous otitis media is a quite common cause of vestibular disturbance in children. The symptoms found are often described as 'falling all over the place' or 'walking clumsily'. Thus the balance problems described are unsteadiness and rarely true vertigo. The cause of the problems might be attributed to pressure changes in the middle ear affecting the inner ear through the round and oval windows. The symptoms often disappear with treatment with ventilation tubes or spontaneously. It is therefore very important to examine every child with balance disorders by performing otoscopy and tympanometry.

Acute or chronic otitis media may today (in industrialized countries) in rare cases produce a secondary labyrinthitis with vertigo. If these symptoms appear with or without nystagmus, rapid treatment with intravenous antibiotics, myringotomy and sometimes mastoidectomy have to be performed.

Epilepsy

Children with epilepsy sometimes display symptoms of nausea, vomiting, loss of postural control and loss of consciousness. Most of children with dizziness associated with epilepsy do however not suffer from grand mal seizures. The epileptic foci are most often located in the temporal lobes. This condition can sometimes resemble benign paroxysmal vertigo in childhood, and thus an EEG should be performed in these cases (Eviatar and Eviatar, 1978).

Tumour

Any tumour occupying space along the vestibular system can cause vertigo and dizziness. Brainstem gliomas and cerebello-pontine angle tumours occur in childhood, but the symptoms often include other neurological abnormalities. If a tumour is located within this region, children as well as adults often show pathological smooth pursuit and/or saccadic eye movements. If a suspicion is raised a magnetic resonance imaging (MRI) should be performed.

Demyelinating disease

Demyelinating disease (multiple sclerosis) is rare in childhood. Vertigo may be a symptom if a sclerotic plaque involves the vestibular pathways. The other symptoms do not differ from those in adulthood.

Psychosomatic dizziness

The symptom of dizziness rarely occurs as an isolated entity in children with psychosomatic illness. This diagnosis should only be made when other diagnoses have been ruled out. This is one of the most difficult diagnosis to make and often requires time, certain professional skills and eventually psychological-psychiatric therapies.

Balance training programme

When suffering from a vestibular deficiency, acute or chronic, findings in recent years have stressed the fact that vestibular rehabilitation is necessary. The central nervous system seems to have a large capacity of central compensation, adaptation and plasticity but it needs 'clever' exercises.

It is important, in vestibular rehabilitation, to stimulate the vestibular, visual and somatosensory systems and their interaction. The vestibular system performs best at rather high frequencies and velocities, whereas the visual system displays a maximum capacity at lower velocity. The best rehabilitation for children is playing and sport activities. When experiencing an acute vestibular loss it is necessary to start activities as soon as possible. These can be physical activities such as using balls, walking on uneven surfaces, walking when moving the head. Other activities, depending on age, include table tennis and bicycling. If the child is fond of swimming, use goggles so that the child can use vision. Make sure that activities following a vestibular loss are carried out in sufficient light, at least in the beginning.

CHAPTER 20

Management of tinnitus in children

RS TYLER AND RJ SMITH

Introduction

In this review a general framework for understanding and treating tinnitus in children is provided. Much of what is written about tinnitus in adults is directly applicable to children. The reader is therefore referred to these reviews for further details. In this chapter, the focus is on tinnitus that is distinct to children. Studies reporting tinnitus in children are documented; the causes of tinnitus in children are discussed; and the evaluation, treatment and prevention of tinnitus are reviewed. For other summaries of tinnitus in children see Hegarty and Smith (2000) and Leonard, Black and Schramm (1983).

The existence of tinnitus in children

Studying tinnitus in children is more difficult than in adults. Tinnitus is a subjective phenomenon and children are not always good at reporting their symptoms. It is therefore difficult to obtain good estimates of the prevalence of tinnitus in children. They rarely complain of tinnitus and, when asked if they have it, they may respond positively. However, further investigation shows that they may have misunderstood the question, or they were trying to please the questioner.

Table 20.1 reviews several prevalence studies. Estimates range from 76% of hearing-impaired children to 3% of children with otitis media. In the study by Stouffer et al. (1992), additional questions were asked and hearing was measured. Their study suggested that about 6% of normal-hearing students report hearing noises in their head and ears for more than 5 minutes. In a small sample of 21 children with hearing impairment, they reported a 24% prevalence of tinnitus. These numbers are similar to those reported by Davis and El Refaie (2000) for adults with tinnitus.

Clearly, children do have tinnitus. They describe their tinnitus as ringing (Nodar, 1972), buzzing (Mills, Albert and Brain, 1986), 'beeping' or 'buzzing' (Stouffer et al., 1992), and a 'high-pitched noise' or 'whistling' (Martin, 1994). This is similar to the tinnitus described by adults. Gabriels (1996) noted that 47% (N = 21) of children surveyed with tinnitus reported concentration difficulties, 42% sleep disturbance and 33% hyperacusis.

Table 20.1. Investigations of the prevalence of tinnitus

Authors	Year	Number	Ages (yrs)	Results
Nodar	1972	2000 normal hearing	11–18	• 13% if passed hearing screen • 58% if failed screening test
Graham	1981b	74 hearing impaired	12–18	• 66% • 13% report spontaneously
Graham	1981a	158 hearing impaired		• 49%
Mills & Cherry	1984	66 with otitis media	5–15	• 29% • 3% report spontaneously
Nodar et al.	1984	37 hearing impaired		• 35%
Mills et al.	1986	93 normal hearing	5–16	• 29%
Drukier	1989	331 profoundly deaf children	6–18	• 30%
Viani	1989	102 hearing impaired	6–17	• 23%
Stouffer et al.	1992	140 normal hearing	7–10	• 36% • 6% with additional questions
		21 with hearing loss	7–10	• 76% • 24% with additional questions

Causes of tinnitus in children

Congenital tinnitus

Children with congenital tinnitus have had tinnitus since birth or infancy, and to them tinnitus can be considered 'normal'. Typically, it is not until later in life, perhaps in conversations with a friend, that they discover that not everyone has ringing in their ears (Mills and Cherry, 1984). Graham (1995) has proposed that children with congenital tinnitus can habituate to it at an early age.

Acquired tinnitus

Children who develop tinnitus later have acquired tinnitus. They are aware that the tinnitus represents a change – it was not there before. This experience is similar to what many adults experience. Like adults with tinnitus, the child could habituate to the tinnitus, or the tinnitus can become a focal issue and a handicap.

Middle-ear tinnitus

Nearly all children experience as least one episode of otitis media. Whether this infection causes tinnitus is debatable, and if tinnitus does occur, its pathophysiology is unclear. One explanation is that the associated conductive hearing impairment caused by a middle-ear effusion attenuates external sounds that normally mask low-level tinnitus. Removal of these external sounds 'unmasks' an already existing low-level tinnitus (Leonard et al., 1983).

In addition to otitis media, other middle-ear disorders can result in tinnitus in children. The list of these disorders is large and includes all tinnitus-inducing middle-ear problems of adults. Table 20.2 reports on a variety of studies in which tinnitus is mentioned. As in adults, some forms of middle-ear tinnitus can represent a more general health problem, such as an intracranial tumour. In these cases, treatment of the underlying medical condition can alleviate the tinnitus.

Table 20.2. Reports of middle-ear tinnitus in children

Etiology	*Reference*
Aberrant carotid artery	Glasscock, Seshul and Seshul, 1993
Arteriovenous fistula	Lalwani, Dowd and Halback, 1993; Cataltepe et al., 1993
Dehiscent jugular bulb	Rauch, Xu and Nadol, 1993
Glomus tumors	Bartels and Gurucharri, 1988; Jackson et al., 1996; Jacobs and Potsic, 1994; Magliulo et al., 1996; Thompson and Cohen, 1989
Palatal myoclonus	Deuschl et al., 1990; Quarry, 1972
Patulous Eustachian tube	Kavanagh and Beckford, 1988
Transmitted bruit	Levine and Snow, 1987 (adults)
Venous hums	Meador, 1982 (adults)

Sensorineural tinnitus

Tinnitus can also be associated with sensorineural hearing impairment of any cause. This is true in adults as well as in children. Table 20.3 lists some of the more common causes. Older employed children are susceptible to noise-induced tinnitus. Ototoxic drugs and recreational noise and music exposure are particularly noteworthy in children.

Table 20.3. Reports of common causes of sensorineural tinnitus in children

Etiology	*Reference*
Head trauma	Gabriels, 1996
Ménière's disease	Ménière, 1861; Hausler et al., 1987; Meyerhoff et al., 1978; Parving, 1976; Simonton, 1940; Nodar and Graham, 1965; Gabriels, 1996
Noise exposure	Davis and El Refai, 2000; Gabriels, 1996
Ototoxic drugs	
Perilymph fistula	Parnes and McCabe, 1987

Ototoxicity

Ototoxic drugs are often administered to children, including newborns. As with adults, this type of exposure is associated with a risk for hearing impairment and tinnitus. Although drug dose is adjusted for small body size, children may be particularly at risk for tinnitus.

Recreational noise- and music-induced tinnitus

Children can acquire hearing impairment and tinnitus from recreational noise, such as snowmobiles, water jet skis, gunfire or fireworks. In addition, they are often at risk for music-induced tinnitus as either players or listeners if they are exposed to intense music (>80 dB A) for long time periods (more than two or three hours) on a routine basis (more than three or four days a week). Generally, sound must be above 80 dB A for over eight hours per day to be considered potentially damaging to hearing. Exposure at higher levels for shorter durations can also cause hearing impairment. In fact, single bursts of very loud sound can damage hearing and produce tinnitus. There are no published guidelines for noise-exposure limits for tinnitus.

Musicians

Hearing impairment and tinnitus are not problems solely for rock musicians – they can occur in classical musicians as well. Risk is increased when the musician is playing next to the sound source, such as another instrument or loudspeaker, for several hours over an extended time period.

Listeners

Hearing impairment and tinnitus can occur in children who listen at rock concerts and 'dances', or through personal wearable or non-wearable sound playback systems. Rock concerts can certainly produce damaging noise levels (Clark, 1991; Yassi et al., 1993) and can last for several hours. Incredibly, Yassi et al. reported that 60% of attendees reported tinnitus immediately after a concert. Wearable headphones also produce high sound levels (Katz et al., 1982) that can produce a temporary threshold shift (Lee et al., 1985).

Evaluation

In general, the evaluation of children with tinnitus parallels that of an adult with tinnitus. There is perhaps one exception – children are frequency less verbal about their health conditions and, on questioning, they may attempt to please the healthcare worker. Therefore, open communication and caution should be exercised during the examination. Children with tinnitus can have difficulty concentrating. Academic problems, difficulty sleeping, behavioural problems and hyperacusis can ensue (Gabriels, 1996). A detailed physical and radiological evaluation has been described by Hegarty and Smith (2000) for children, and Perry and Gantz (2000) and Tyler and Babin (1993) for adults.

Treatment

Surgical treatment can be pursued for some types of middle-ear tinnitus, as is the case for adults (Tyler and Babin, 1993; Hegarty and Smith, 2000; Perry and Gantz, 2000). However, no safe medication has been shown to help large numbers of tinnitus patients in controlled investigations (Murai et al., 1992; Dobie, 1999).

Children with hearing impairment and sensorineural tinnitus should be fitted with hearing aids. Hearing aids help tinnitus because they:

- improve communication and therefore reduce the stress of listening (reducing stress helps coping with tinnitus)
- produce some background noise that facilitates masking or habituation
- amplify background noise that facilitates masking or habituation

Treatment for young children

If a young child becomes aware of sensorineural tinnitus but shows no concern, it is advisable not to create a concern. Many adults (and presumably children) have tinnitus and lead happy and productive lives.

If a young child is concerned about sensorineural tinnitus, a general discussion about the background and treatment is advisable (see Table 20.4) (Tyler, 2000). Information must be offered at an age-appropriate level for each child. Gabriels (1996) noted that the effect of tinnitus on school and social life must be considered in the management of children.

She noted one five-year-old child with tinnitus and hyperacusis who attacked a schoolmate who shouted in his ear. It also is important to engage the parents and siblings as they need to understand difficulties and problems related to tinnitus. Because tinnitus is usually subjective, in some situations it can be difficult for parents to accept their child's complaint (Gabriels, 1996).

Table 20.4. Background and treatment information that can be discussed with children

	Information area	Content
1.	Prevalence	• About 1 in every 10 adults experiences some tinnitus • About 1 in every 200 adults are severely bothered by tinnitus • Many children have tinnitus
2.	Causes	• Noise- or music-induced hearing loss • Unknown • Medications • Head injury • Almost anything that causes hearing loss
3.	Treatments	• No magic pill • Strategies to help yourself • Low-level background sound • Hearing aids, counselling, relaxation, maskers, habituation

(Adapted from Tyler, 2000)

Treatment for older children (and adults)

Tinnitus treatment for older children is similar to treatment for adults. When children do complain of tinnitus, they should be taken seriously (Hegarty and Smith, 2000). Not only can tinnitus be debilitating, but it can also reflect an underlying treatable disease. Graham (1995) noted that tinnitus can result in behavioural problems in school. Table 20.5 lists some treatments that can be helpful in adults and could be easily adapted for older children.

Prevention

Preventing tinnitus is even better than treating it. There are at least two causes of tinnitus in children that can be preventable: drug-induced tinnitus and noise-induced tinnitus. The use of ototoxic mediations

Table 20.5. Different tinnitus treatments available for adults that could be adapted for children

	Treatment	References
1.	Hearing aids	Tyler and Bentler (1987)
2.	Counselling	Tyler, Stouffer and Schum (1989) Wilson and Henry (2000)
3.	Relaxation	Erlandsson (2000)
4.	Cognitive behaviour modification	Sweetow (1986) Wilson and Henry (2000)
5.	Masking	Vernon (1998) Tyler and Bentler (1987)
6.	Habituation	Jastreboff and Hazell (1993)
7.	Sound therapy	Tyler (2000)
8.	Refocus therapy	Tyler (2000)

(Adapted from Tyler, 2000).

should be carefully monitored using drug-specific parameters and encouraging the child to report changes in hearing or the onset of tinnitus. The potentially harmful consequences of exposure to loud music and noise (continuous and impulse) can be minimized by education of the importance of hearing protection and avoidance. Modelling the judicious use of hearing protection by siblings, peers and parents is beneficial. At-risk children can also be warned of the implication of the onset of tinnitus – it may be the harbinger of permanent noise-induced hearing impairment.

Concluding remarks

Tinnitus does occur in children. In general it seems to present itself in the same fashion it does in adults, and is diagnosed and treated similarly. However, there are some differences, specifically:

- Children with tinnitus do not always report this symptom.
- When asked if they have tinnitus, children can report tinnitus because they do not understand the question or they are trying to please the examiner.
- Children with congenital tinnitus can consider this 'normal'.
- Children with tinnitus can present with academic, social, sleep and concentration difficulties.
- Children with tinnitus can have hyperacusis.
- Children are at risk for tinnitus secondary to ototoxic medications and intense noise or music.

- In a young child with tinnitus, it is important to avoid creating a significant problem if none exists.
- In managing children with tinnitus, it is important to consider the school and social environment and to engage the support of the family.
- Tinnitus in children can be prevented with education about ototoxity, hearing protection and wise listening strategies.

CHAPTER 21

Language development in hearing and deaf children

C GALLAWAY

Introduction

The general situation of deaf infants

Children generally acquire their first language in a largely trouble-free manner. Within three to four years of birth, children produce short sentences, master a large vocabulary and hold their own in conversations with other children and adults. With few exceptions, infants grow up in an environment that fosters the language-learning process. They are surrounded by caregivers and other family members who are competent users of the target language and who thus provide a model of the language and plenty of opportunities to try it out (Gallaway and Richards, 1994; Snow, 1995).

For children who are deaf, however, the process is less straightforward. Although deaf children have exactly the same linguistic potential as hearing children, they will usually face obstacles on the way to becoming competent language users. For many children with a severe or profound pre-lingual hearing loss, acquiring any language (spoken or signed) to an adequate level may prove an uphill task. There are obvious difficulties in acquiring a spoken language through the auditory channel, but there are also some rather less obvious ones implicated by a hearing loss. For a small number of children born into deaf families, the first language acquired may be a signed language. Signed languages (such as the British Sign Language(BSL)) are natural languages that exist in all deaf communities, and for children born into signing families the acquisition of a signed language proceeds in a similar way to that of spoken language (Woll, 1998). However, fewer than 5% of pre-lingually deaf children have signing deaf parents. The great majority, then, are born into a situation where there is a mismatch of hearing status between child and parents. In these circumstances, the fostering and facilitation of spoken or signed language requires strategic and often intensive intervention.

Severe to profound hearing loss poses the biggest obstacle to language development, but children with mild to moderate sensorineural hearing losses will also have difficulties (Quigley, 1978; Davis et al., 1986). Diminished access to the language causes delay. The aim of this chapter is to explain how the child's capacities and developing abilities and the environment interact in the language-acquisition process. A description that is chiefly process-oriented enables us to understand better the particular hurdles faced by the deaf child acquiring spoken language. For professionals dealing with deaf children, it is crucial to appreciate the nature of the task faced by children when they acquire their language and the events, conditions and milestones that constitute this process.

The structure of language

The apparent ease of the language-acquisition process belies the complexity of language. Languages consist of several interrelated and highly complex structural systems, and the learning of our first language has been labelled by one linguist as the 'greatest intellectual feat any one of us is ever required to perform' (Bloomfield, 1933). Language users have to develop competence at several linguistic levels. They must master the phonological system, which entails discriminating between, and producing accurately, a number of sounds (about 44 in British English), and using correct stress and intonation patterns. Developing a vocabulary means knowing between 50 000 and 250 000 words (Aitchison, 1987). Grammar is the complex system of rules that enables us to put words together meaningfully. Even word order is a significant feature in English (with 'cat eats mouse' having a different meaning from 'mouse eats cat'). Finally, language has to be used appropriately for the situation. Any successful language interaction involves implicit knowledge at all these levels.

This description of language fits natural signed languages such as BSL, which have the same abstract structural characteristics as spoken languages (Sutton-Spence and Woll, 1999) but, of course, differ in some respects due to their modality. For instance, the system of sounds (the phonological structure of the language) is replaced by a similarly highly constrained and analysable structure consisting of handshapes, hand movements and facial expressions. Therefore, learning a signed language is a task that is comparable in complexity to learning a spoken language. Other systems exist for developing languages in deaf children that are not natural languages but mixed systems contrived by hearing people in varyingly successful attempts to make spoken language more accessible to deaf people (see Chapter 24 of this volume).

Human infants are born without specific linguistic skills but with a range of innate capacities that are useful for the acquisition of a language. The actual substance of the language – sounds, words, grammar, social-linguistic conventions – is acquired from what children hear around them. The hearing child experiences a constant flow of language and can extract useful information, appropriate to its stage of development. The existence of any sort of hearing impairment can potentially restrict this free-flowing stream of linguistic information, and the most overarching general difficulty for the deaf child learning spoken language is simply that much less language will be experienced compared to the hearing child. In other words, the deaf child suffers 'depletion of sensory input'.

For instance, children with normal hearing learn some of their language skills from overhearing others. They certainly learn a good deal about conversations, not just from language addressed to them but also from the conversations they hear others constructing all around them. Language 'out there' – not directly addressed to the child – is less easy for deaf and hard-of-hearing children to access and so some of the opportunities for picking up useful linguistic information (for example, how answers follow questions) are generally less available. Language acquisition is a robust or 'well-buffered' process (Snow, 1994); that is, in normal circumstances, the child has almost no chance of hearing insufficient language for it to develop its own linguistic system. For deaf children, however, the quantity and quality of spoken language experienced is reduced, thus making it more difficult for the child to get whatever information it needs to trigger the acquisition of the system.

The first year of life: pre-linguistic development

Innate capacities

The physical and cognitive capacities that the child brings to the language learning task are not of themselves linguistic but must be developed in the context of the child's maturing communicative skills. We now consider what these capacities are. The first point applies to children with normal hearing and the remainder to all children. First, hearing infants are born with fine auditory-perceptual discrimination: they can discriminate between speech sounds with only tiny differences, such as /p/ and /b/. Second, all children have complex articulatory organs that enable them to produce the finely contrasting sounds of speech (unlike, for instance, apes and chimpanzees). Third, they have an overriding desire to communicate with those around them. Fourth, their aim is to imitate and acquire behavioural patterns like those around them so as to eventually become adults and take their role in human society. Fifth, they can use gaze and gesture as communicative tools.

During the first year of the baby's life, all these capacities are increasingly turned to communicative purposes. This is often referred to as 'prelinguistic development' or the 'precursors of language'. Infants experience language from their birth onwards and from then essential foundations are laid for the development of the adult language system. They gradually learn to communicate using a variety of means: gaze, gesture and voice.

Hearing sounds

Infants display formidable discriminatory abilities at or very soon after birth. Eimas et al. (1971) showed that babies of one and four months could discriminate between /p/ and /b/. Questions asked since this classic discovery have been whether, first, this capacity is confined to humans and, second, whether it constitutes a specific linguistic ability. In fact, chinchillas show similar discriminatory abilities (Kuhl and Miller, 1975); human infants, however, need to learn which contrasts are relevant in their language. For instance, the sound that classes as /p/ has some different acoustic properties depending on where it occurs in combination with other sounds, whether it is spoken by a male or a female voice, and so on. In other words, what is phonologically equivalent may be acoustically different. In fact, babies are classing acoustically different but phonologically equivalent sounds together by six months of age (Hoff-Ginsberg, 1997). This, then, becomes speech perception rather than simply auditory perception.

Jusczyk (1997) has postulated that the first year is a particularly fertile period for infants learning about the structural organization of sound patterns in their native language, and that this is because 'sound patterns constitute the most perceptibly transparent information in the signal'. However, learning about phonology may have an importance reaching beyond the level of the sound system. It may also play a role in learning about higher level features of language, such as word segmentation and even some aspects of grammar (Morgan and Demuth, 1996; Jusczyk, 1997). If this is so – and evidence is beginning to come down in heavily in its favour – then developments in speech perception in the first six months of life form indispensable underpinnings for language acquisition. According to Markides (1986) and Yoshinaga-Itano et al. (1998) there is a significant advantage in speech development for oral children diagnosed and aided before six months, rather than at any later point. In the view of the current writer, these two sets of findings – one from the field of speech perception and one from the field of deaf children's speech development – are almost certainly linked but, as far as we are aware, the connection has not yet been made; it has most certainly not yet been investigated.

Producing sounds

Hearing children will have already been vocalizing for about six months before their first word is produced. This babble, which, apparently, is the practising of speech sounds, has been thought important for later vocal development, although there has been a good deal of debate about its precise role (Hoff-Ginsberg, 1997). The vocal babble of deaf children is similar, but not identical, to that of hearing children (Stoel-Gammon and Otomo, 1986; Oller and Eilers, 1988). This has implications for social-conversational development. Mothers react to their infants' babble in a conversational way, and if the vocalizations are not very speechlike then there is a danger that they are less likely to chat with their infants (Cheskin, 1982). However, with respect to the development of speech, it remains unclear how important this stage is for deaf children (Marschark, 1993). Deaf children receiving implants or aids may begin to hear and produce words without having first shown canonical babble patterns (Yoshinaga-Itano, personal communication). Thus, it seems, the babbling stage may be bypassed without detriment to the eventual development of clear speech.

Gesture

In the second half of year one, infants are just embarking on intentional communication. Gaze and gesture are important adjuncts to early vocalizations: in particular, pointing, a gesture found only in human beings, is an essential part of development in all children. As single words and then, eventually, word combinations appear, so reliance on gesture diminishes for hearing children (although, of course, adults may still use gesture occasionally). By the age of three, when hearing children will have mostly dropped the use of gesture as a primary communicative tool, oral deaf children may still be relying on it to a large extent (Nicholas and Geers, 1997; Lederberg and Everhart, 1998). This is not surprising as children (and indeed adults) will use whatever means they can to communicate successfully – but there is evidence from these studies and others that a lower reliance on gestures at this age predicts better progress in oral language development.

This should not be taken to imply that oral deaf children should be discouraged from using gestures. Rejection of any aspect of a child's communicative offerings could have harmful consequences, and there is evidence that gestures play a more important part in oral deaf children's communicative development overall (De Villiers et al., 1993; Volterra, Beronesi and Massoni, 1990). However, for oral deaf children, professionals and parents must be committed to facilitating the child's spoken language to a level where it becomes the preferred and primary mode of communication.

For deaf children acquiring a signed language, early gestures come to have a linguistic significance. Early attempts at signs will emerge, and constitute 'sign babble' (Petitto and Marentette, 1991) akin to vocal babble. Given the low incidence of native signing families, early acquisition of a signed language will often require the introduction of deaf signing adults into the child's environment (Young, 1997). Whichever route is taken, it is of crucial importance that the child must be enabled to develop a full linguistic system – that is, a language – and must not be allowed to rely permanently on temporary, piecemeal and *ad hoc* communicative strategies as does the developing toddler.

Gaze, attention management and the emergence of reference

Infants are not born with the knowledge that words refer to things. They have to learn this basic symbolic function of language, a procedure that is facilitated by the nature of maternal language. Mothers spend a great deal of time talking about objects that are of interest to their infants – for instance, those being manipulated by them (Messer, 1978). Hearing children experience the world simultaneously through sound and vision.

Eventually, therefore, they realize that the word and the thing being talked about are connected (Sachs, 1997). This realization, which is called the 'naming insight', emerges at around one year and is a prerequisite for language development. Wood and his colleagues (Wood, 1982; Wood et al., 1986) pointed out that deaf children may have to experience words and the objects they refer to sequentially rather than simultaneously. If the word is signed then they must look at the sign and object in sequence; if it is spoken then they may need to look at mother's face in order to lip read. This division of attention may delay the acquisition of the naming insight.

Recently, there has been closer investigation of shared attentional contexts and other aspects of early interaction between deaf infants and both hearing and deaf mothers during the first 18 months (see, for example, Adamson, Bakeman and Smith, 1990; Harris and Mohay, 1997; Meadow-Orlans, 1997; Waxman and Spencer, 1997; Koester, Karkowski and Traci, 1998; Prezbindowski, Adamson and Lederberg, 1998). Deaf mothers may employ more successful strategies than hearing mothers for managing a deaf infant's attention (Kyle, 1990) but this comparison may be simplistic as both deaf and hearing mothers' behaviours are quite heterogeneous (Harris and Mohay, 1997). Sensitivity to the deaf infant's particular needs may be displayed by both deaf and hearing mothers. Undoubtedly, we have learned and will continue to learn a great deal from observing deaf mother–child dyads.

The features discussed are not the only factors contributing to success in early interactions. We now turn to the broad issue of language used by adults to children.

Early interaction: conversations with small children

General characteristics

Language directed at small children generally facilitates the participation of the young speaker. Children are encouraged to speak and they are supported in their attempts to do so by those around them by a variety of linguistic means and conversational strategies. In very early interaction, this support has to do with maternal strategies for attention management and their attentional focus as discussed, which is based on mothers' sensitivity to their child's interactional needs. As children grow older, language addressed to them is characteristically modified, producing a type of language often called 'motherese', and more recently, 'caregiver speech'. Not only mothers but all adults and older children modify their speech when talking to toddlers. There is nothing mysterious about this because tailoring language to a listener's needs is a normal component of any speaker's conversational skill. However, since the modifications are potentially helpful to the young language learner, the whole issue becomes critical when considered in the context of the language-acquisition process.

When compared with speech addressed to adults, child-directed speech has been observed to:

- display exaggerated intonation and high pitch;
- be simpler, with shorter sentences and less complex grammatical structures;
- be more repetitive (more redundant);
- be concerned much more with the 'here and now';
- contain more questions and imperatives;
- contain expansions and reformulations, or recasts, of the child's immature utterances.

It has proved quite difficult to pinpoint exactly how far the existence of any, or all, of these features is a necessary or sufficient condition for language learning. Caregiver modifications are not identical across all cultures (Lieven, 1994) although the use of some kind of 'baby talk' (an earlier term: Ferguson, 1964) appears to be universal. No linguistic community has yet been discovered without it, and as we might expect, child-adapted signing can be observed in mothers who sign to their children. One useful approach has been to take each feature and investigate what its purpose might be; another is to test, via intervention studies, whether this or that type of linguistic input facilitates learning. With respect to children with a hearing impairment, the questions become more complex. For neither oral deaf nor signing children can it be assumed, *a priori,* that caregiver modifications will be the same, nor that they will have the same effect. However, knowing that some modification generally takes place is a good basis for looking further at how interaction works. We now consider some of these characteristics.

Exaggerated intonation and pitch

Firmly established as part of English caregiver speech (Snow and Ferguson, 1977), it does not play a role everywhere (Pye, 1986; Lieven, 1994) and is thought to have an attention-managing purpose. Language addressed to children who are not paying attention is not very useful. For all deaf children, this is a crucial matter. Oral deaf children have to learn how to listen, and parents have to work on engaging their attention. Signing children have to learn how to watch the signer in order to receive the message. For parents of both oral and signing children, the act of engaging attention will involve the visual channel and also physical activities at some stage. For instance, deaf adults tap infants or wave their hand in front of deaf children (Harris et al., 1989; Smith, 1996; Waxman and Spencer, 1997).

This issue of attention sheds light on the apparently unrelated research finding that quantity of language addressed to the child correlates positively with future language development (Ellis and Wells, 1980): roughly, the more language young children hear, the faster their speech develops. However, with deaf children, rather than quantity of language per se, quantity of language addressed when they are attending is more likely to be crucial. For instance, deaf mothers tend not to sign to their children unless they are watching. Spencer (1993) found relatively low quantities of maternal language but nevertheless age-appropriate signing skills in a group of deaf infants aged 12–18 months with deaf mothers. The message here for hearing mothers of deaf children is that they should certainly address plenty of language to their child but in the context of the child's interest and attention, with extra effort put in to manage the latter where necessary.

Simple and repetitive language, and the 'here and now'

The notion that the use of simplified language or baby words is detrimental to a child's linguistic development (sometimes found in western cultures in middle-class families) is a view entirely without foundation and based on a lack of understanding of the language-acquisition process. Other types of linguistic behaviour, such as lack of encouragement or ignoring the child's imperfect communicative attempts, or over-zealous correction, are far more likely to cause problems.

As soon as children start to speak, caregivers of hearing children seem to pitch their language at a level a little beyond the child's own output (Snow, 1995). That is, to a child using predominantly two-word utterances, parents will typically use four-to-six word utterances, and the majority of words used will mirror the child's use to a great extent. Parental language will not contain a high density of words new to the child, nor abstract ideas, nor cognitively complex verb tenses. However, this adjustment concerns the child's cognitive maturity as well as his or her language level. It is often more difficult for adults to tune their language level appropriately to a deaf child because in the case of spoken language delay, cognition and language output are mismatched, and the speaker may feel ill at ease addressing 'baby' language to a much older child.

Language concerning the 'here and now' – in other words, firmly based in the current extralinguistic context – is easier to understand than language that is not. For instance, the meaning of everyday transactional language such as that dealing with food, shopping, meals, etc. can often be guessed at quite successfully even if the language is unknown. This context-bound nature of early language is an essential plank in the infant language-learning process; vocabulary and grammatical structure is not taught, but learnt from the obvious contexts in which language happens.

Interrogatives (questions) and imperatives

A frequent theme in the research on caregiver speech is that an over-controlling parental interaction style does not foster language development in the child. As early as the 1970s, both mothers and teachers of deaf children were accused of too much control and directiveness and a lack of sensitivity in response (see Gallaway and Woll, 1994 for a range of references). One feature of 'controlling' interaction is a large number of closed questions (those which can only be answered by 'yes' or 'no') and another is a high proportion of imperatives ('do that now!'). The use of both structures in maternal speech however is accepted as relating positively to language gain in the literature on language acquisition (Ellis and Wells, 1980; Richards, 1994).

Reasons for this apparent lack of consensus are, first, that language in school and at home is not designed for the same functions nor addressed to children at the same developmental level; second, that some language structures have been taken too readily as controlling when they are not; and third, that the type of language used to children is most often determined by their language level – so empirical studies of longitudinal design are needed to show whether various interaction styles facilitate development or not. Finally – and this is often the case in research about deaf children – some still-quoted early research was carried out either before modern findings were available or by researchers who were not familiar with relevant research about child language development. Here, the reader is referred to discussions elsewhere (Gallaway and Lewis, 1993; Gallaway and Woll, 1994; Gallaway, 1998) and this section continues with a description of how questions and imperatives work in conversation.

Questions are not used solely, or even primarily, to seek factual information. Their functions are many and complex: as invitations/offers ('would you like to go out/ a biscuit?'), as requests/instructions ('can you shut that window?'), requests to a previous speaker for clarification or repetition ('what?'), or to seek agreement as in tag questions ('that was surprising, wasn't it?'). Imperatives are more straightforward and are used to adults indicating a direct order or prohibition ('come here!' 'don't touch that!'). The relatively high proportion of both these structures in speech to toddlers arises quite naturally from the primary purposes of talking to them: to manage their behaviour and keep them safe from harm, to comment on their current actions, to give them a chance to participate in the conversational exchange, and to seek clarification of their immature utterances.

Imperatives are used frequently to very young hearing children: 'eat your peas!' 'Don't touch!' They give way to question forms that might have the same function as the child advances linguistically (Bellinger, 1979): 'aren't you going to eat your peas?' It has also been widely observed that parents often comment on current actions using imperative forms (Caissie and Cole, 1993; Gallaway and Lewis, 1993): 'that's right!' 'Put the little man on the horse!' These utterances, which are imperatives in form, function as comments and could equally well be expressed in some other grammatical form, for example 'let's put the little man on the horse!'

In short, caregiver speech should and usually does contain a variety of different grammatical structures that contribute to language appropriate for the child's communicative needs at any particular stage. An interpretation of the research, which was oversimplified to the point of absurdity, has led to some professionals suggesting adults should avoid questions and imperatives so as not to be too 'controlling'. This is completely erroneous; interactions can not be judged as 'controlling' on the basis of the occurrence of particular structures and any conscious attempts to modify language input to children along these lines should be avoided. Advice about responding to children's early language should concentrate on what parents (and teachers perhaps) should do (be responsive and sensitive to their children's attempts at communication) and not what they should not do, because this could result in misleading and possibly undermining advice.

Recasts

These are responses from an adult which take the child's immature utterance and recast it in a correct form:

Child: that duck
Adult: that's a duck yes

Both naturalistic and experimental data show that children who are developing normally gain benefit from this kind of response (Nelson, Loncke and Camarata, 1993; Saxton, 1997). Virtually no research has been carried out with deaf children on this topic.

Summary

In summary, then, there is a good deal of evidence, that language addressed to hearing infants and toddlers is structured in a way that supports their language-learning processes. Identifying which characteristics are helpful, why they are helpful and at what stage, however, has proved a long task, but it is a necessary one before we can begin to understand the situation with respect to young deaf children. Much headway has been made in understanding attentional processes, but very little in understanding specific spoken language adjustments. Earlier studies investigated similarities and differences between language addressed to deaf children and language addressed to hearing children of either the same chronological age or a similar language level. Differences tended to be labelled as deficiencies, and thus it was suggested that mothers were not always providing the best linguistic environment for their deaf children. Such claims were at best premature and at worst vacuous in the absence of an adequate theoretical model and in the almost total absence of longitudinal studies that properly examined the effects of types of interaction on language development (see discussion in Gallaway and Woll, 1994).

Recently, a significant step forward in developing a theoretical position on the input-output debate with respect to deaf children has been achieved by Nelson et al. (1993). With regard to empirical evidence, it is still lacking and likely to remain so, if viewed from a perspective comparable to the general 'motherese' research. This is because, with deaf children, there are so many variables affecting their language development that isolating parental interaction styles in correlational studies is impractical as well as possibly inappropriate. Different methods, and probably more qualitative and small-scale studies, are needed to investigate the nature of interaction, its success or lack of it, and the long-term effects on the child's developing linguistic system.

We now turn to the issue of child-adjusted signing. As far as we know, mothers provide signed language to their infants, which is modified in similar ways in order to facilitate communication and which is likely to support language learning. The visual-spatial nature of signed languages determines that some of the realizations of these adjustments will be entirely different (hence the need for a clear understanding of exactly what purposes caregiver modifications serve). Some strategies used to ensure the visibility and clarity of signs to the child are: signing in the child's space, signing on a child's body (Maestas y Moores, 1980; Harris et al., 1989) and signing slowly (Maestas y Moores, 1980). Signs might be exaggerated in size and shape (Harris et al., 1989; Erting et al., 1990) and may be reduplicated (Gallaway and Woll, 1994). However, as in any spoken language, such adjustments can only be appropriately made by a competent language user (readers doubting this can put it to the test by choosing a language in which they are not perfectly fluent and then trying to converse with a three year old). For deaf children of hearing parents, those parents will themselves be sign-language learners, so the linguistic model they provide needs to be supplemented by deaf signing adults (Young, 1997).

Vocabulary

At around one year, hearing infants start producing recurring sound clusters with meanings. These 'words' are only vaguely similar to adult words. Here are some examples:

odi something like 'oh dear' – used when something falls on the floor;
tat the family cat – but not pictures of cats;
de said when pointing to various objects.

Over a few months, the child gradually acquires more of these expressions and the words become more recognizable and adult like. Over the next few years, thousands of words will be acquired: not consciously taught by adults, but acquired by the child understanding words heard in context and deducing their meanings. Later, new aspects of the meanings of words already in use will be added to the child's mental lexicon. For instance, body parts are learned rather early, but metaphorical extensions such as 'the head girl' and 'the foot of a mountain' are added later.

Words for concrete objects and activities are easier to learn than abstract words and metaphorical uses. The possible number of all such words in a language is infinite ('open') and we continue adding to our vocabulary throughout our lives. However, any language also has a finite stock of grammatical, or 'closed' class words. Examples in English are 'in', 'the', 'to', 'and'. They are not labels, and cannot be learned or taught by giving definitions or pointing to objects, but only by experiencing the word on thousands of occasions in appropriate contexts. As one would expect, the reduced linguistic experience of oral deaf children often causes delay in acquiring both function words and metaphorical extensions (Webster and Wood, 1989).

Currently, very little is known about deaf children's early vocabulary learning. Large-scale studies assessing deaf children's linguistic competence rely on standardized measures, and almost no work has been done from a developmental psycholinguistic perspective. Two early studies reported more personal-social words than referential words being used by oral deaf infants and their mothers than by hearing infants and their mothers (Gregory and Mogford, 1981; Meadow et al., 1981). This would be consistent with the notion that oral deaf children experience delay in grasping the symbolic function of language, but the evidence is not substantial. A more recent study (Stokes and Bamford, 1990) showed vocabulary acquisition proceeding in a near-normal fashion. Some researchers report a 'sign advantage', that is, that young signing children acquire a larger vocabulary faster than hearing children do in their language (see Marschark, 1993); however, Harris (1992), discussing the emergence of first signs, shows, and explains why, the acquisition of a sign lexicon appeared to proceed very slowly in some cases.

The relatively small amount of reliable facts in this area draws attention to the general difficulties of researching with deaf children. First, deaf children constitute a far more heterogeneous population than hearing children in terms of their development (Marschark, 1993), which limits the validity of findings. Second, carrying out intensive research on language development in families with very young deaf children (in addition to already detailed intervention and management processes) is often inappropriate and/or unwished for. Third, much of the child's putative linguistic output may be unintelligible. The study of early words and signs is particularly intensive and difficult and has to rely heavily on both parental observation and experimenters' interpretation.

Finally, there has now been some investigation of vocabulary acquisition by children with cochlear implants, using standardized tests (for example, Miyamoto et al., 1992; Willis and Edwards, 1996). Willis and Edwards (1996) report one child's development of vocabulary as faster than hearing-age peers. This pinpoints an additional difficulty in the research. Currently, more detailed and focused monitoring is given to children with cochlear implants than has ever been given to children with hearing aids, and comparisons and broad overviews of developmental levels are extremely difficult to make.

The acquisition of grammar

Early word combinations

At around two years old, hearing children progress from single-word utterances to word combinations. This begins the move into acquiring gradually, over the next few years, the rules of grammar. Between about two and four, word combinations become longer; grammatical endings, tenses and different sentence structures (such as questions) begin to appear in the child's speech.

Here are some examples of typical utterances from infants aged between two and three-and-a-half years old.

baby drink
more biscuit
mummy tired
that a car
Lucy's pussycat
my want ice cream
Mummy you go swings
I been to the sweetie shop
want that ice cream grandad bought
I maked it with water

Children have to learn how to form questions ('can you do that?' 'do you want that?') and negatives ('I can't do that', 'I don't want that') and how to structure phrases ('the big black cat', 'not even that one', 'some of the others') and express complex strings of ideas ('can we go to the park if Grandad gets here before lunch?'). There is much individual variation with respect to likely ages for developments. For instance, some children appear to rely extensively on imitation of whole phrases whereas others are more analytical and build up their sentences gradually. The range of normal variation for acquiring grammatical rules may be as much as two years. Many overgeneralization errors and omissions occur in toddlers' speech, such as in the list above.

Corrections

How do hearing children acquire the rules of grammar? We know that they are not explicitly taught. In the early stages, all children make grammatical errors, such as this: 'I maked it with water.' These errors disappear as the child's grammatical system matures. Brown and Hanlon (1970) showed that explicit corrections do not generally follow children's ungrammatical utterances and, broadly speaking, this fact has held up in subsequent studies. Additionally, when such errors are explicitly corrected, toddlers rarely pay attention to the correction they are offered. However, a lack of explicit corrections does not mean the child receives no corrective feedback at all. Adults frequently model the correct version of their child's immature utterances (Saxton and Gallaway, 1998)

Child: I chooseded one.
Adult: You chose one.

There is evidence from studies of naturally-occurring conversation and experimental studies that such corrective feedback is helpful and plays a role in the language-learning process (Saxton, 1997). For deaf children, as the amount of spoken language they take in may be gravely reduced, the amount of correct modelling available is also reduced, and the information needed to speed along acquisition of correct forms is less accessible.

Deaf children's grammar

Discussions of deaf children's acquisition of grammar have often been based on research carried out on written language rather than spoken, and frequently make reference to the 'delay or deviance' debate (Bamford and Saunders, 1991). Deaf children often do not develop age-appropriate grammatical skills in spoken language (although some do). This is hardly surprising as most deaf children lack sufficient exposure to the spoken input language and in particular, the critical features which would enable them to formulate functional categories (De Villiers, de Villiers and Hoban, 1994). In particular, unstressed grammatical elements such as tense markers, inflections, relative pronouns and other functional markers are both difficult to hear and linguistically complex, and deaf students are indeed reported as having difficulties with auxiliaries, tense and complex sentences (De Villiers et al., 1994).

Although all children have the same potential to develop grammar, deaf children's language may display structural features that resemble those of second-language learners rather than simply delayed younger learners. In hearing infants, linguistic skills develop alongside increasing cognitive maturity. There is not generally a huge mismatch, therefore, between what the child wants to express and how it can be said; that is, short sentences, concrete words and simple sentences are enough till the next stage. However, with deaf children, if their expressive language skills are seriously delayed, cognition and communicative needs will outgrow the means to express them adequately. For this reason, many advocate the use of sign language or mixed systems at an early stage, if spoken language is not developing commensurate with the child's needs.

There is another reason: exposure to a signed language may enable a very deaf child to 'hook in' to a structural linguistic system and start this cognitive-linguistic part of the brain working on language structures. If the child cannot make sense of the sounds of speech, then the grammatical system as encoded in spoken language will remain a mystery. However, this only applies if we are considering a natural signed language, and not a 'pidgin' version or any artificially built-up system.

Speech intelligibility

The intelligibility of deaf children's speech has always been a central – and problematic – issue. Producing intelligible speech involves not only reasonably accurate reproduction of the sound repertoire, both vowels and consonants, but also stress and intonation patterns, and appropriate voice quality and pitch. Too much technical detail would be required to describe here how these features interact in the production of intelligible speech; suffice it to note that distortion in any, some or all of these areas may result in 'deaf speech' which lay people find difficult to follow (Bench, 1992). Children with mild to moderate hearing impairments generally have no difficulty with developing relatively normal-sounding speech but may have difficulty with particular sounds (Bench, 1992).

For both hearing and deaf infants, the sounds of speech are acquired primarily by auditory means but this is supplemented by the visual perception of speech movements; this visual aspect probably contributes more to the procedure for deaf children (Mogford, 1988). Visual aspects of sound production are used extensively in some intervention programmes and probably serve as a natural strategy for profoundly deaf children but, the visual aspects of speech alone (such as the closing and opening of the lips to produce /b/ and /p/, the rounding of lips to produce oo, and so on), are not sufficient to guarantee accurate production.

A difficult question is how far speech training and the conversational use of language can converge. For some profoundly deaf children, the recognition and production of sounds is arduous and requires intensive training. Although such training has positive results in terms of conscious sound production, achieving intelligibility during natural conversation may still be an elusive goal. However, both early diagnosis and cochlear implants are likely to provide a significant step forward; at the time of writing this, it is still too early to evaluate the evidence and judge the long-term consequences (but see Yoshinaga-Itano et al., 1998).

Language use

Knowing the components of a language is not enough to guarantee its efficient use, just as knowing how to steer and change gear is not enough to guarantee a safe drive through traffic. Language speakers must have practical communicative competence in an everyday world. This entails not only formal language structure but a mastery of many complex pragmatic and sociolinguistic features. An important feature of successful conversation is that both the listener and the speaker must recognize when a conversational breakdown occurs and know how to retrieve it. One essential type of conversational repair is a clarification request. If the speaker presumes too much knowledge on the part of the listener, then the listener has to ask for clarification. The speaker may then embark on revision behaviour to clarify:

A: Are you coming to the party?
B: Which party? (clarification request)
A: There's one at number fifteen tonight. (revision)

Hearing children start developing these conversation management strategies (at least in a rudimentary fashion) as early as their second year (Lloyd, 1999). Studies that have been carried out so far with (mainly older) hearing-impaired children are inconclusive, but the general trend suggests that the development of successful conversational repair strategies is likely to be delayed or, possibly, to proceed somewhat differently for them (Lloyd, 1999). This is an extremely important dimension of language skills and must not be overlooked.

Conclusion

Whether a profoundly deaf child will be successful in acquiring spoken language is not entirely predictable and it is commonplace to describe children with similar hearing losses but widely divergent levels of competence in spoken language. A wealth of research seeking predictive factors has not provided clear-cut answers. Until recently, research was dominated by studies arguing the case for one or other communication system; more recently, many other factors are included in such studies. Musselman and Kirçali-Iftar (1996) adopted a retrospective approach to investigate 'unexplained variance' in two groups of deaf children with unusually poor or unusually good spoken language. Factors associated with success were: earlier use of aids, more highly educated mothers, auditory-oral instruction, reliance on spoken language, individualized instruction, integration and structured teaching by parents. Yoshinaga-Itano et al. (1998) took two groups of children who were early- and later-identified (before and after six months) and found a significant advantage in language development for the early-identified group, regardless of other potentially influential factors.

Much more information is available than was even five years ago, but it is vital that research continues to work assiduously at defining which factors cause one child to thrive in language development where another does not. However, recent advances on several fronts are likely to cause radical changes and have far-reaching consequences. First, children with hearing losses should have a better chance than ever before of making sense of the sounds of speech. Hearing aid technology continues to improve, but cochlear implants are becoming widespread as a means of providing consistent access to sound. Secondly, neonatal screening programmes and early aiding are well under way in some areas, allowing infants to get a much-needed early start on the language learning process. Thirdly, the psycholinguistic and socio-cultural features of sign languages are increasingly studied and understood. Professionals should increasingly be able to understand the implications and consequences of various types of intervention and linguistic choice, so that deaf infants and children have an optimal chance of fulfilling their linguistic potential.

CHAPTER 22

Delay and disorder in speech and language

G BAIRD

Introduction

Many clinicians make a distinction between language delay and language disorder. The term *disorder* implies an abnormal pattern of development not normally seen in normal language acquisition. This is contrasted with delay, which is regarded as language acquisition proceeding along normal lines but more slowly than expected. Many children with problems have mixtures of delay and disorder.

Severe delays in one part of the linguistic system may result in uneven progressions, which resemble 'disorder'. Some researchers have proposed that disorders are extremes of patterns found in normal development; for instance, very late talkers are an extreme of the normal gap between comprehension and expression. Others insist that 'disorder' is a pattern not found in normal development. In practice delay and disorders are commonly found together and *impairment* (which may lead to disability or handicap) is the preferred term.

Specific speech and/or language impairment (SLI) is defined as a problem in acquiring the skill in the absence of obvious hearing, neurological or learning impairment. It is generally a diagnosis of exclusion. There is less agreement about positive inclusion criteria and many researchers are looking for diagnostic markers of SLI in the grammatical system (Rice, 1997) or the phonological system (Bishop et al., 1996). In most studies, the definition of SLI is reached by comparison of speech or language level and chronological age and for some definitions by comparison with cognitive age. The suggestion is that cognitive level should be one of the descriptors, not an exclusion factor.

These methods do not necessarily define stable groups of children or the same groups of children. Changes of category and description can occur with age (Cole et al., 1995).

Describing speech and language impairments

The current International Classification System (ICD 10) uses the headings of:

- specific speech articulation disorder;
- expressive language disorder;
- receptive language disorder;
- acquired aphasia with epilepsy.

Speech language and communication learning involves integration of several systems, viz. the phonological components (the perception and production of sounds to words and sentences), semantics and syntax (words, their meaning, the morphemes and rules combining words in sentences – that is the structures of language) and pragmatics (the understanding and use of language in context). Many children have problems in all areas (Conti-Ramsden, Crutchley and Botting, 1997). Rapin and Allen (1987), among others, have proposed clinical subtypes. A problem affecting speech or expressive language only is generally regarded as being less severe in terms of long-term significance compared with comprehension impairment. The view that expressive disorders all have normal receptive skills is less tenable, with increasing research showing often subtle problems not previously found on cruder tests.

Expressive and speech subtypes

- Phonological programming deficits leading to a variably severe speech impairment.
- Verbal dyspraxia (originally conceived as a motor-programming deficit in automaticity of speech production). Some have such extreme speech production difficulty as to be almost apraxic and some dysarthria may be found.
- Mixtures of problems are common.

Receptive-expressive subtypes

The development of first words, learning vocabulary, grammar and phonology are all delayed. The following patterns are seen:

- Severe receptive-expressive subtype: verbal auditory agnosia. Comprehension of environmental sounds and even awareness may be affected. Particularly seen in acquired aphasias due to epilepsy.
- Moderate receptive-expressive subtypes in two forms:

Phonological syntactic problems	Lexical-syntactic problems
Dysfluency	Variable fluency
Short sentence length	Short sentences
Function words omitted	Immature syntax
Word endings omitted	Severe word-finding problems
Problems with articulation	Articulation clear
Often delayed verbal comprehension	Often delayed verbal comprehension

Possible underlying mechanisms affecting development of the structures of language and speech

Problems of auditory-processing affecting how the linguistic system learns to decode, encode and produce speech can affect any or all of comprehension, expressive language and speech. They are associated with poor auditory memory, poor vocabulary and word learning (Rice, Buhr and Nemeth, 1990), grammar errors, sequencing problems, difficulties with processing quantities of information at speed and problems in formulation and production of expressive language or speech all to varying degrees functionally and in tests. In contrast, tests that require knowledge of meaning, especially integrating other cues, may be better and the skills of non-verbal communication and social interaction are usually intact. The most severe speech-auditory processing problems are seen in acquired epileptic aphasias (Deonna, 1991).

One postulated underlying developmental deficit (Tallal et al., 1993) is temporal decoding where the crucial factor is the ability to decode speech sounds at less than 100 ms stimulus intervals – the phonemic level, a process even more impaired by the acoustic environment (tested using a masking sound). Replication is needed to assess how universal this deficit is in speech-impaired children. Tallal and colleagues have proposed modified speech input for children at risk – FastForWord (1996). There might also be impairments in touch or visual stimuli processing.

Other postulated deficits arise in segmenting speech (Bird and Bishop, 1992) – for example, a problem in phonemic segmentation (dividing up words into different component sounds) can result in difficulty in acquiring vocabulary, inconsistent speech sound production and poor phonological awareness (knowledge of sounds linking to written symbols), which is linked to reading problems. Gathercole and Baddeley (1993) have postulated a phonological memory defect shown not only in limited rote memory for digits but also by difficulty in repeating accurately non-words. The non-word repetition test appears sensitive even to a history of speech and language impairment and may be a useful marker in family studies (Bishop et al., 1996).

Slowness in information processing is a common feature of some children with language impairments and can also affect other modalities of processing.

The omission of grammatical markers, especially tense markers, are a consistent feature of children with structural SLI (Leonard, Black and Schramm, 1992; Leonard, 1997). Leonard has shown the cross-cultural differences that exist depending on which language is being learned. He proposes that the strong-weak prosodic sequence assists the child to perceive the salience of the morpheme and that those grammatical markers omitted are weaker – another example of misperception by some children of input features of language (Bedore and Leonard, 1998). The ability to work out meaning from the relationships of words within a sentence depends upon the speed and efficiency with which a child can process that information. Being unable to analyse a sentence as it is spoken by relating one part to another can result in grammatical comprehension errors particularly of embedded clauses – for example, the 'car that hit the bus was black' is understood as saying that the bus was black.

Many children with speech production difficulties have delayed articulation; some have variable production of speech sounds with poor oro-motor skills and general clumsiness. Besides specific linguistic processing problems it is postulated that efficient automatic motor programming is delayed and 'developmental verbal dyspraxia' is the terminology used (reserving phonological impairment for the group who are motorically normal). This terminology is unsatisfactory because there is a variable mix of language and speech problems (including prosody, rhythm and intonation problems), the oro-motor component is variable and the motoric problems can be difficult to clearly distinguish from dysarthria on the one hand and delayed motor maturation on the other (Stackhouse, 1992).

Metacognitive impairments (higher-order language problems)

Metalinguistic problems

Children must acquire a knowledge of the connection between sounds and written symbols, and an awareness of the segmentation of words into syllables and basic rhythms because this is required for reading, writing and spelling. This more advanced aspect of language processing leading to phonological awareness has been called metalinguistics. Problems are associated with delayed literacy (Goswani and Bryant, 1990).

Semantic-pragmatic problems

Another kind of metacognitive skill is to know what someone else is talking about and be able to monitor this in conversation. In some situations meaning is obvious because it can be seen in concrete terms. In other situations information may not be visually obvious and the speaker's intentions must be inferred. The recipient understands the intended meaning by selecting what is relevant on the basis of both received and previous information and the result of his or her own cognitive processes (Sperber and Wilson, 1986).

Some children have a particular difficulty in understanding what people are talking about or referring to; such children may also be poor at making clear to the listener what they are talking about; in very young children this may mean that they are poor at communicating their own social intentions. Children with 'pragmatic' problems may present as fluent speakers but may lack flexibility of meaning and have problems with social appropriateness and learning the social rules of discourse and conversation. For example, they may wish to talk about only one topic, ask too many questions and fail to appreciate the partner's needs in a conversation. Frequently such children have non-verbal communication, play and other social deficits. There continues to be debate about whether this is a problem of speech and language understanding and usage alone (a pragmatic impairment of language), which can be clearly separated from the social inappropriateness and lack of reciprocity of the autistic spectrum disorders. This is because both problems probably derive from difficulties with social cognitive and communicative learning but vary in associated features including co-morbidities (Bishop and Rosenbloom, 1987; Bishop, 1989, 1997).

Features of a 'pragmatic' language impairment

- stereotyped well-formed sentences;
- limited initiative in conversation or asks questions all the time;
- fails to take account of partner's need for information;
- gives too much detail;
- abnormal prosody;
- odd associations of thought, literal interpretation and difficulty following others;

- referent; misinterpretation of situations, perseveration;
- poor use of facial expression;
- word-finding problems;
- difficulty sequencing ideas;
- problems with inferring people's feelings, situations beyond the here and now, difficulty with 'why?' question words;
- social-emotional dysfunction with poor peer interaction and lack of awareness of personal space;
- sharing and game playing difficult;
- poor imaginative play;
- may show preference for adults and liking for routines.

Other speech problems

- dysfluency (children often have other language problems);
- mutism, a common transient phenomenon in normal children but also associated with speech and language disorders and other psychiatric co-morbidities.

Prevalence of speech and language problems

The exact definition of 'language delay' and what is a 'case' is still a matter for debate. Some studies use precise definitions based on tests that provide scores in terms of standard deviations from the mean. Many clinicians use simple rules, such as having less than eight words by the age of two or no word combinations by two-and-a-quarter (10% of the population in the MacArthur study – Fenson et al., 1993), or not producing four syllable phrases by the age of three. There is reason for concern whenever a child is not socially communicating at any age and in any situation where a parent or other adult thinks the child is not understanding what is being said when others of the same age do. A *clinical* view of delay causing concern may be less stringent than that proposed for research studies (<–2 SD compared with chronological age) and depend upon a variety of circumstances including parental views, availability of resources and the effect of the problem on child and family.

Several large research studies in the 1970s and 1980s that investigated language delay in pre-school children varied in exact prevalence figures depending on the *definition* of speech or language problem used and the *age* and *demographic variables* of the population studied. The generally accepted range is between 3% and 10%, although a smaller proportion has severe and persistent problems. Expressive language and speech problems are more common than receptive problems in all these studies.

A more recent epidemiological study explores the relationship between speech delay and language impairment (Shriberg and Tomblin, 1999). Over 7000 kindergarten children were screened; 7.4% showed specific language impairment compared with chronological and non-verbal mental age (8% boys and 6% girls) – many of them previously undetected; 3.8% had speech delay; less than 2% had overlapping speech and language delay. Boys were 1.5 times more likely to have speech delay.

Prevalence figures of language and speech delay vary according to the age of the child and a child described as speech or language delayed at one point in time may not be later and vice versa. For example, 9% to 17% of two-year-olds, 3% to 8% of three-year-olds, and 1% to 3% of five-year-olds are said to show speech delay, indicating a degree of catch up or difficulty in assessment at younger ages or both.

Risk factors for or common associations with speech and language delays

A number of factors within the child and external to the child affect or are associated with slow speech and language development and interact with each other. One factor on its own may be insufficient to cause impairment in language and speech development. In combination they may each be significant contributors:

- male sex;
- family history of speech or language delay;
- learning delay/reading problems;
- large families;
- twins and other multiple pregnancies;
- glue ear;
- behaviour problems;
- attention difficulties;
- motor clumsiness;
- environmental deprivation;
- low level of parental education;
- adverse maternal mental health including depression.

Gender and genetics

There is a strong male predominance in language impairment, with a male:female ratio of 4:1 as in many other developmental disorders. Despite ingenious theories, particularly involving testosterone, there is no clear reason for this. There is often a positive family history of language impairments, or reading or spelling difficulties, in other family members.

Tomblin, Smith and Zhang (1997) found that maternal educational status and a positive paternal history of speech and learning problems were associated with SLI. Genetic influences can be expressed either directly or through the environment. The degree of heritability may vary for different subtypes of language impairment – for example speech problem versus comprehension/expression problem (Bishop, North and Donlan, 1995).

In twin studies the concordance rates for monozygotic twins is high, suggesting strong genetic influence. The genetic influence on language development may be more marked in severe delay and may be greater for girls than boys. At the age of two years in normal development heritability accounts for 25% of the variance in language and shared environment 65% (Dale et al., 1998). The influence of genetics increases with age.

Specific gene sites relevant to language and speech are now being identified. One large family with complex speech and language impairments has shown linkage to a region of chromosome 7q31 (Fisher et al., 1998). Tomblin et al. (1999) have recently reported links to a similar site in a large group of unrelated children with SLI.

In SLI, a chromosome test is usually indicated but usually normal, although there is an increased incidence of language problems in children with sex chromosome disorders. The fragile-X syndrome should be excluded.

Pre- and perinatal influences

Several risk factors that may damage the central nervous system will also produce language impairment – for example, cytomegalovirus and rubella. Tomblin et al. (1997) reviewed the literature and compared pre- and perinatal factors that could be specific risks for SLI in a control and population sample. He concluded that 'SLI was associated with risk factors pertaining to parental status prior to conception rather than risk factors occurring during foetal development or the perinatal period.' Breast feeding was a protective factor for SLI, possibly for general cognitive or other reasons. Low birth weight is a risk factor for more general cognitive difficulty of perceptuo-motor impairments with a lack of agreement for specific SLI effect.

Hearing impairment

Sensorineural hearing impairment will clearly have an effect upon the reception of auditory information, which can be substantially ameliorated by early diagnosis and a rehabilitation programme including hearing aids, skilled teaching and cochlear implants for the profoundly impaired where the auditory nerve is intact. There is more controversy about the importance of secretory or serous otitis media (otitis media with effusion – OME). This is extremely common – 50% or more of all children will have at least one attack and 10% of children under five will have OME at any one time, a prevalence rate that will rise to over 50% in day nurseries during the winter months. Otitis media with effusion is very rarely the primary or sole cause of significant language impairment but, in some children, it may be a substantial contributory factor (Bishop and Edmundson, 1986). Persistent hearing impairment associated with OME and frequent recurrent attacks may be particularly important to identify (Roberts, Wallace and Hendersen, 1997). Hearing should be tested in every child with a speech and language impairment.

The language environment

It is obvious that a child would not learn to speak unless exposed to some spoken language. Environmental influences have attracted particular attention and language delays are more common in families where there are several children, multiple births and higher levels of stressful family problems including parental mental health (Stevenson and Richman, 1978). Studies of children brought up in situations of extreme deprivation show the adverse effects on language skills but emphasize the variability even for later adoptees (Croft et al., 1999).

Studies on the ways in which parents normally talk to their children have emphasized that language acquisition can be made easier by adult behaviours that use contingent responding (following the child's interests) or predictable routines. The optimum environment for language learning is affectively warm with mutual parent–child responsiveness. Parents who are depressed are less able to respond in conversation even with a baby, who soon looks upset and becomes silent (Tronick et al., 1982). Language development is particularly sensitive to abusive environments. In the study by Culp et al. (1991), neglect, as opposed to physical abuse, had the greatest affect on language. The critical level of input is unknown.

Throughout language learning, parents help the process by correcting the child's use of language, paying particular attention to meaning rather than pronunciation or grammar. They do this by using 'motherese' (baby talk), repeating key words, recasting (putting words in different forms) and emphasizing above all the context (linking words to actions, objects, people and events). Ward (1992) has shown an effect on language development through a scheme of enhancing language input in babies.

Cross-cultural studies show that although language is usually simplified to children (child-directed speech – motherese), that cultures vary widely on the age at which they expect children to be intentional communicators and conversational partners and that this does not have a major effect on grammar development. Although there is no doubt that seriously neglected and abused children show communicative impairment, an inadequate environment is not the primary cause of most cases of language impairment. Although parents do, in general, communicate and participate less with the language-impaired child, this is probably the result of the child's difficulties rather than the cause. In children with language problems the way that mothers speak changes; it becomes more directive and less contingent. The number of 'recasts' is reduced. This may be a response to the child with delayed language.

Brain structure and function

Brain–behaviour relationships have been most studied in acquired disorders in adults and children. Although closely connected, different parts of the brain may be important in understanding a word (temporal-parietal lobe) and speaking it (frontal lobe). In studies of children with congenital and early unilateral lesions in either hemisphere, the striking finding is that, although there may be some delay in early language milestones, most children have language in the normal range. Certainly if the brain damage has occurred before six years of age their difficulties are very mild compared with children with specific language impairments.

There is some suggestion that the type of language problem depends on whether the left or right hemisphere is damaged. For example, left-hemisphere damage is more likely to lead to expressive language problems and right-side damage is more likely to lead to receptive problems. Adult right- or left-hemisphere damage results in predictable patterns.

Language deficits after left-hemisphere damage

Damage to Broca's area (left frontal)

- Slow and hesitant speech.
- Poor production of the sounds of language.
- Lack of grammatical features – for example, prepositions and conjunctions.
- Agrammatical writing.
- Comprehension intact and the patient can sing.

Damage to Wernicke's area

- Word-finding difficulties and imprecise referents.
- Paraphasias or incorrect word use.
- Can speak fluently with good grammar and melody.

Other possible features

- Word blindness with or without agraphia.
- Pure agraphia.

Language deficits after right-hemisphere damage

- Lexical-semantic processing.
- Metaphorical language.
- Comprehension of humour.
- Context and conversation.
- Prosody and stress.
- Emotional language.

As the child grows through childhood to adult life, increased cerebral differentiation becomes more marked. After the age of six, damage in either hemisphere will show an increasingly adult pattern with loss of language skills if they are sited in a damaged left hemisphere as the right hemisphere becomes increasingly committed to other tasks. It has been postulated that certain developmental speech and language disorders may be related to particular hemispheric dysfunction, for example phonological-syntactic problems in the left hemisphere and semantic-pragmatic problems in the right hemisphere. Involvement of the frontal lobes has also been suggested because loss of executive function skills, planning, goal setting, inhibiting behaviours and anticipating outcomes especially in social matters follow damage in these areas.

Reading delays are more common in left-hemisphere lesions although comprehension deficits may occur in right-sided damage. One of the few PET studies in children with specific language impairment showed lower flow in the left hemisphere, pre-frontal and perisylvian regions. Magnetic resonance imaging (MRI) studies (Jernigan et al., 1991) have shown a lack of the usual brain asymmetry of normal development indicating that in some children there may be pre-natal influences on developing brain anatomy. Lack of perisylvian asymmetry has not been a consistent finding (Plante, 1996). Specific speech impairments, which are severe and associated with oro-motor impairments, as in Worster-Drought syndrome and pseudo-bulbar cerebral palsy, may be caused by an underlying cortical dysplasia apparent on MRI scan. In summary, it is most unlikely that localized brain injury is responsible for developmental language impairments which are more likely to involve bilateral dysfunction.

Epilepsy

Increased epilepsy is found in children with speech and language impairments. (Robinson, 1987). Two recognizable epileptic syndromes show acquired speech and language disorders as symptoms. One is the syndrome of autosomal dominant rolandic epilepsy and the other is the Landau-Kleffner syndrome (Landau and Kleffner, 1957). Loss of language skill can happen with more generalized epilepsy when other features of general development are usually affected as well (Deonna, 1991).

Localized areas of dysfunction occur in the Landau-Kleffner syndrome (acquired receptive aphasia with epilepsy). This syndrome has a typical onset between the ages of three and seven years; the child loses language previously acquired over a period of days or weeks, the course fluctuates and slow progress is made for a few years. Many children never have a fit but the EEG in the initial stages is typical with continuous spike wave (SSPS) in sleep. Some children recover reasonable language skills; others do not and rely on signing. The length of time the SSPS has lasted is important in prognosis as the presence of the epileptic discharge seems causative. Some children's electrical status is steroid sensitive; in others anti-epileptic drugs may help. Surgery may have a place (sub-pial resection) in resistant abnormality.

An EEG is indicated if there has been loss of language skill or any suggestion that there may be fits, particularly, nocturnal epilepsy. Epilepsy and abnormalities on EEG are more common in children with receptive language problems. Recent studies have been conflicting with variable abnormalities most commonly seen in sleep – 50% had an abnormal EEG even without obvious seizures (Tuchman, 1994; Picard et al., 1998), although this is also true of healthy adults – and a non-significant association in a recent Australian study (Collins et al., 1999). Whether it is causative or an epiphenomenon remains uncertain, except in a few children where variability of language remains the most helpful clinical guide to whether further investigation is needed.

Other neurological disorders that affect brain development will clearly have an influence on language development, for example, any cause of mental retardation, intra-uterine infections, chromosome abnormalities, and so forth, are all likely to be associated with delayed language. Disorders such as Duchenne muscular dystrophy are recognized and associated with other learning problems, particularly language delay, and this may be the presenting factor, making it necessary for the clinician to do a full physical examination, paying particular attention to motor skills and measuring the CPK in young boys with language delay and any suggestion of motor delay.

Soft neurological signs (Robinson 1987) tend to be increased in children with language delays and disorders. The head circumference of children with semantic-pragmatic and autistic spectrum disorders tends to be above the mean (Woodhouse et al., 1996). Medical investigations in general give a very low yield and brain scans are only indicated in specific circumstances or research projects.

General learning difficulties

The most important influence on the rate of language acquisition is that of general (cognition) learning. Children with general learning difficulties have delayed language to varying degrees. In some children the language impairment seems disproportionate – for example, speech difficulty in Down's syndrome. Other groups of children with severe learning problems have disproportionately good linguistic skills, for example Williams syndrome.

In structural abnormalities of palate, for example in cleft palate, there is a very important association with glue ear, which is persistent and thus may cause a consistent low-frequency hearing impairment.

Cerebral palsy

Children with significant brain abnormalities resulting in, for example, cerebral palsy, will have language problems affecting particularly speech output. Like children with structural abnormalities of the palate and other lower motor neurone disorders, aspects of receptive language may be perfectly normally developed in line with general learning. The children are very frustrated by inabilities to use spoken language and sometimes even gestural language, depending on how severely affected their limbs are. Some children have a more localized bulbar or pseudo-bulbar cerebral palsy with relative preservation of the limbs known as the Worster-Drought syndrome, involving the perisylvian regions. Such children need alternative techniques for both communication and recording skills.

Co-morbidities

Although theories of modularity of brain development might suggest that speech and language impairments are isolated problems, the common clinical experience is that children have functional impairments in other areas of development more commonly than children without speech and language problems.

Specific cognitive impairments

Many of the children with language impairment have subtle difficulties in high-level problem solving and thinking and it is difficult to know whether it is these problems, rather the language impairment per se, which might be responsible for some of the later deficits in educational skills (Johnston, 1994). Many non-verbal thinking tasks may be language mediated mentally. Inner language and verbal working memory are used in verbal reasoning, which is increasingly abstract, for mental computation, and literacy skills, and for non-verbal reasoning – especially tasks involving integrating information from pictures, possibly even design copying and visuo-spatial construction.

Early language delay is a risk factor for later reading problems and also maths. This risk is greatest:

- when there is a general impairment in all areas of speech and language, and
- in those children where the language problem persists beyond the age of five years.

Skill in reading in the general population is predicted by short-term memory phonological awareness (for example, the skill of being able to delete a phoneme from a word like 'bus' to say 'us' and the ability to generate rhyme such as 'hat, mat' at the age of four or five years correlates with later reading skills) and letter recognition (Hatcher, Hulme and Ellis, 1994). However, once the decoding skills are acquired, comprehension of what is being read is increasingly important and additionally impaired in language impairments (Snowling, Bishop and Stothard, 2000). Children with semantic pragmatic problems may show hyperlexia – advanced mechanical reading skills – but may not necessarily understand the meaning of what they are reading. Increasing research interest is now being focused on the maths problems of language-impaired children.

General motor skills and oral function

A number of children with language impairment also have impaired control of mouth movements, chewing and swallowing, with an increase in dribbling. Where eating has been a significant mechanical problem, speech is likely to be affected, for example, poor sucking, chewing and facial movements to command. Food down the nose rather than the gullet may indicate palatal dysfunction such as a sub-mucous cleft.

A generalized clumsiness may be associated particularly with expressive and speech delay; children may show slowness on other movement tasks, such as moving pegs around a board and in daily tasks of using cutlery and ball skills. Learning a sequence of motor skills may be a particular problem and has also been found in adults with dyslexia; suggestions of cerebellar dysfunction have been made. This might represent a generalized neurological immaturity that improves with time, or it might be part of a slowness in processing sequentially delivered information and developing rapidly automated movement patterns.

Behaviour

There are strong associations between language impairment and behavioural difficulties. In one study of three-year-olds with language delay, 58% had behaviour problems against a base rate of 14%. Non-compliance and temper tantrums are common; so also is immaturity of attention control with distractability and impulsivity. Some children have increased anxiety.

Psychiatric disorders are highest in children with receptive language problems as opposed to those with speech problems (Baker and Cantwell, 1982). To some extent, non-compliance and tempers might be explained by frustration: the child knows what he or she wants to say but lacks the ability to articulate clearly and, in addition, may have problems in understanding and acting upon instructions. Nevertheless, this may be an over-simplification of a complex association. Elective mutism is common in most children when they start school but quickly disappears. Mutism that persists is more likely to be associated with additional speech and language problems and social difficulties.

Communication and social interaction impairments

Children with language delay and disorder show increased problems with social relationships. The social impairment is particularly marked when comprehension of language is affected (and the cause is not hearing impairment) and can be a mixture of delay in maturity and features such as inappropriateness either of content or context and failure to understand social cues. Children with receptive language problems are more likely to be delayed in their understanding and use of non-verbal communication (Thal, Tobias and Morrison, 1991) and to initiate communication less frequently when younger with less joint attention with an adult. Showing and directing attention, socially directed gaze and range of facial expression plus repetitive behaviours are not necessarily the result of language delay (Lord and Pickles, 1996). Follow-up studies, especially of receptive disorders, highlight the continuing social impairments of this group (Howlin, Mawhood and Rutter, 2000).

There continues to be debate about whether, in some children with receptive language delay (especially where semantics and context are involved), there is an underlying functional deficit that might cause both the language problem and the social learning difficulty, either a general information processing problem or specific social cognitive impairment. An alternative explanation is that the presence of speech and language impairment has consequent implications for socialization. A group of children learning English as a second language as well as a group with SLI were both found to have lower social status among peers and to initiate less interactions with peers (Rice, Hadley and Alexander, 1993). Thus even young pre-schoolers are aware of other children's communicative skills and rank them socially. This has implications for placement. The debate about overlaps with the pervasive developmental disorders and the possible shared social cognitive impairment continues.

Autism and the autistic continuum

Significant deficits of social interactive and communicative learning (autism and the autistic continuum) form part of the differential diagnosis of language impairments. Language delay is common in childhood autism, whereas normal language milestones are one of the diagnostic criteria of Asperger syndrome. Severe receptive and expressive delays, often with early apparent deafness, are common, as are semantic pragmatic impairments. Problems involving the structure of language and speech articulation problems can also occur.

The social communication deficits in the autistic continuum disorders are also characterized by a failure to use non-verbal communication including facial expression and gestures such as pointing to share interests, and a tendency to use communication to have needs met, rather than for the purposes of sharing interest.

Wing (1988) has summarized the impairments of the autistic spectrum disorders:

- impairment of quality of social interaction;
- impairment of social communication and lack of reciprocity;
- impairment of social understanding and imagination, lack of or repetitive pretend play;
- limited pattern of self-chosen activities.

These features can occur in varying levels of severity; for example, no speech and direct use of hands to talking a lot but without reciprocity. Underlying theories focus on 'mentalizing as in a theory of mind', a lack of central coherence of cognition, and specific impairments in perception of social information or ability to use such information – an executive deficit. For further discussion see Happe, 1994 (autism), Astington and Jenkins (1995), Dunn (1995).

In Asperger syndrome there are normal speech milestones, a normal range of intelligence but social interaction impairments and over-intense interests. For some clinicians, clumsiness is also part of the syndrome. Absolute clarity on the separation of Asperger and high-functioning autism is the subject of ongoing debate as several diagnostic schema are in use which do not necessarily coincide. Suggestions have been made that Asperger syndrome may be a 'right hemisphere syndrome' (Klin et al., 1995).

Prognosis and outcome of speech and language impairments

Do children with speech and/or language delay catch up? Children with marked language delays at age three in the Dunedin (Silva, 1987) longitudinal study, were found to have a higher frequency of learning and behaviour problems in school compared with the control group. It is now clear that many of these children had additional learning problems beyond their language problems. Approximately 70% had a low IQ compared with 8% of the controls. The language delay was therefore a symptom, a first sign that there might be more significant problems interfering with the developmental progression.

In a follow-up of the pupils from special speech and language schools, two-thirds had reasonable comprehension and approximately half had adequate language production but still a significant continuing functional problem (Haynes and Naidoo, 1991).

Whether there is a speech or expressive problem only or a problem in comprehension is also important. In one study of two-year-olds with expressive language delay only (late talkers), at follow-up at six years most had 'caught up' to within the normal range but still had subtle problems in short-term memory, word finding and complex language production (Rescorla and Schwartz, 1990). Whitehurst and Fischel (1994) did not find lasting problems from a group of speech-delayed two-year-olds unless, crucially, their comprehension of language was also affected.

Another long-term study (Stothard et al., 1998) of pre-school children with significant language delay examined a sample of four-year-olds with speech and language delay and has recently published outcome at 15 years indicating the value of a sufficiently long-term follow up. At 5.6 years of age, 44% of the children had language in the normal range, were thought to have caught up, and when reassessed at age eight years had normal range reading and spelling. In those who did not, receptive language was more likely to be affected than expressive and several aspects of language, rather than one, were involved. A problem restricted to articulation had a good prognosis (Bishop and Edmundson, 1987a and b). However when the young people were seen again at age 15 years, even the apparently recovered group scored a lower composite score on the WORD tests of reading and on tests of short-term auditory memory and phonological skills than the control group. The persistently delayed speech and language group at five years and eight years still showed functionally disabling delay in verbal comprehension and expression as well as literary tasks at age 15 years (Snowling et al., 2000). Bishop concluded 'If a child's language difficulties are still present by 5.6 years, there is a high risk of continuing language, literacy and educational difficulties throughout childhood, even in children with normal initial non-verbal IQ.'

Rutter and Mahwood (1991) followed up to adult life a group of children with severe receptive language problems. As adults 70% showed persistent social impairments despite language improvements. All aspects of literacy were impaired in the majority. Two had developed psychoses (Howlin et al., 2000).

In summary, the outcome of children with significant problems in speech and language is variable and is worse if there is involvement of receptive as well as other aspects of language that persists beyond 5.6 years. Even in those who apparently recover by this age, there may be subtle persistent difficulties.

Screening

In view of the difficulties in determining the level or age at which language delay should be regarded as significant, it is not surprising that there have been difficulties in deciding whether population screening for language problems is advisable, but significant delays in language development should be regarded as a symptom that needs evaluating and a differential diagnosis. The success of screening programmes is judged by well-known criteria.

Several screening tests have been devised for different age groups, for example using 'no babble and apparent deafness' under one year of age (Ward, 1992). The CHAT screen (Baron-Cohen et al., 1996; Baird et al., 2000) at 18 months is designed to look at early communicative behaviour, particularly imaginative play and pointing behaviours, which might be early indicators of autism. The positive predictive value of a persistent impairment at 18 months is high, as is specificity, but sensitivity is low. Law et al.

(1998) have described a language speech screening test set at < –1.5 SD at two-and-a-half years of age. Developmental tests such as Denver and the Schedule of Growing Skills also include language. Language screening for the whole population is currently not recommended (Hall, 1996; Law et al., 1998).

Assessment

The assessment of a child with speech and language impairment is a multidisciplinary task and the paediatrician needs to be involved in planning referral pathways for children with speech and language problems. If the problem is confined to speech and language, the speech and language therapist should usually manage the child. If, however, a more wide-ranging developmental delay is suspected or if there are concerns about social and communicative skills, the child should be referred to the multidisciplinary assessment child development team. In either situation, audiological assessment will be required. The paediatrician should ask about current behaviour and the development of skills in each of the behavioural areas outlined:

- signs of general developmental delay especially behaviours that should have disappeared, such as mouthing;
- the communicative environment and any social interaction problems between mother and child;
- the opportunity to play with peers and any problems which arise;
- behaviour, remembering that the outcome generally for speech and language problems accompanied by behaviour problems is less good;
- any unusual behaviours;
- understanding and expression of language, speech, play, communication, behaviour;
- motor and co-ordination skills;
- family history of speech and literacy, regression epilepsy and other general health aspects including hearing.

Parents are reliable if asked the right questions. Asking open questions, for example, allows a judgement to be made about the behaviour. If the parent says ‘he understands everything we say’, an example ensures that the child is not using situational cues. Structured history-taking schedules have been developed that focus on social and communicative behaviours, for example the ADI (Le Couteur et al., 1989) and the DISCO (Wing, 1988).

A friendly and informal atmosphere should be arranged where child and parent feel relaxed and where there are suitable toys for the age of the child. Full assessment of complex problems needs time.

Non-directive play techniques may be employed, occasional imitation of the child's actions or sounds is a useful technique, but in this setting there should be two aims:

- to see what the child can generate in terms of social communicative play and language behaviour, and
- what is possible with some 'scaffolding' from the professional.

For many children the gap between elicited behaviour and actual behaviour is very significant. Some children with language and communication problems are able to achieve skills in a structured situation with a helpful adult that they cannot achieve 'in real life' especially with peers. Informal and formal assessment of all behaviours listed are needed. It may be helpful to arrange a school or nursery visit as part of the assessment.

As with any developmental assessment one should then check whether the assessment matches the parents' or teacher's perception. How the child actually functions in real life may be better (if the child is good at general inference) or worse (if it is not). In structured assessment:

1. Test the hearing.
2. Check useful functional vision.
3. Assess language and speech. It is difficult even for the very experienced professional to guess accurately a child's comprehension. This should be formally assessed. When testing expressive language look at length of sentences using words assessed in comprehension. Note especially the difference, if any, between the fluency children can use when talking about their own ideas and the fluency to confrontational demand – to someone else's ideas, which may show up a formulation problem. Pragmatic problems may be much more apparent in open conversation and play than formal tests. Receptive language is usually in advance of expressive and the opposite is seen in language problems like semantic-pragmatic or autistic spectrum problems. There are many tests of speech and language available. The clinician should be aware that they all measure slightly different functions and one child can achieve different scores on each test especially on tests reliant on single word identification (using either equivalent age or standard score) (Howlin and Kendall, 1991). Until recently many tests had used small samples for standardization. A range of language assessments that are suitable for very young children are the Reynell, the Pre-school

Language Scales and Pre-school CELF and the CELF for children of five to 12 years and over (Sewel et al., 1987). These tests are fast becoming the standard in-depth assessment used for children in child development centres and speech units. (Most have UK norms.) As a test of global language and speech functioning, the Bus story for children of three-and-a-half years in which the adult tells a story with pictures and the child retells it, is excellent and a very good guide to the overall severity of the problem. Speech assessments, and specific phonological tests are also available. Stackhouse and Wells describe a logical psycholinguistic approach to assessment of a speech production problem that looks at input to output skills in a series of steps (Stackhouse and Wells, 1993). All of these tests allow retest and therefore comparison over time. The Children's Communicative Checklist (Bishop, 1998) measures qualitative aspects of children's communication and can be used by parents or teachers. Most paediatricians will work with speech and language therapists who will use these tests, but it is useful to have watched them administered. Anyone administering tests should have been trained in and understand the basic principles of psychometrics.

4. Assess the cognitive skills. As discussed above many non-verbal thinking tasks may be language-mediated mentally. The British Ability scales and the WISC have performance tasks that are suitable. The Leiter and Snijders-Ooman require no speech for their administration.
5. Motor skills – gross and fine. Problems with co-ordination are common, there are varying reasons, maturity of motor precision, planning problems and in some children, impairment of spatial awareness. The occupational therapist is a helpful member of the assessment team for these problems especially as they affect recording skills and those of daily living.
6. Assessment of social communication looking for:
   - the reasons for and methods of communication – for example, eye gaze, gestures, speech/needs only or sharing interests (Stone et al., 1994);
   - the frequency of communicative behaviours both initiated and responsive – for example, looking at people, which is child-initiated. The drawing of social attention to self by coming close to the parent is a social behaviour but does not indicate shared interests and may be of normal frequency in autism.

   A standard instrument has been developed, the ADOS (Lord et al., 1989).
7. Assessment of play, looking for the degree of sociability, organization, complexity and variety of play ideas. Children with new ideas, social communication and autistic spectrum problems may produce chunks

of video-learned play but lack variety and new ideas. Stages of play are:

- sensorimotor;
- definition by use;
- pretend.

8. Assessment of attention:
   - 0–1 distractable;
   - 1–2 own choice of activity;
   - 2–4 single channel but increasingly easy to direct by adult and shift attention to self;
   - 4–6 integrated attention increasingly sustained.

   General problems of attention with impulsivity, physical hyperactivity, poor persistence or attention to task and distractability need to be distinguished from those joint attention deficits where the child does not share interests but can sustain superb attention for his or her own interests. Specific attentional problems for auditory information may indicate a problem with short-term memory and auditory processing.
9. Physical examination. Check the speech production apparatus, remember the possibility of sub-mucous cleft and the possibility that a speech problem may be part of a more widespread neurological abnormality. Look for neuro-cutaneous syndromes. A full formal neurological examination will not normally be necessary but should be undertaken if there is any other suggestion of neurological dysfunction or a deteriorating condition. Soft neurological signs are more marked in language problems. An EEG is important if there is a clear loss of language/speech skills beyond the first 10-word stage. Chromosome analysis, indicated especially in wider ranging problems, gives a low yield and should be audited.
10. Note any unusual behaviours – either persistence of an earlier and therefore immature behaviour such as mouthing, or motor mannerisms.

Intervention in speech and language problems

Every parent and whole family faces a difficult adjustment when a child has significant developmental problem but there are special difficulties in coping with a communication disorder, one of the most fundamental aspects of humanness. This aspect of therapeutic need should not be neglected nor the effect on the children themselves forgotten. After every assessment, parents should be given all information including a written report and informed of the parents' association relevant to their child's needs (such as AFASIC for speech and language-impaired children).

Studies on speech and language therapy have shown that individual language processes *can* be improved by therapy in the short term. Long-term benefits are harder to disentangle from natural history. Many children with speech and language impairments will have special educational needs requiring the health services to liaise with the education authorities at the earliest opportunity.

Therapies either are aimed at specific deficits uncovered by assessment, or general measures designed to emphasize aspects of input occurring in normal development, such as recasts, or specific modifications for presumed underlying deficits, for example 'FastForWord' or using strengths to compensate for weaknesses.

Children with severe problems may need alternative communication systems – the earlier the better. Parents are often concerned that teaching children signs will stop them talking. The reverse is true if speech and signs are used together. Signs or picture symbols can be useful in a variety of ways. For children who are finding it difficult to focus on what someone is talking about, a picture makes that clearer. Some children find it easier to think in terms of pictures not words and yet others find it easier to learn gestures than spoken words. Cued speech can help speech clarity of sounds.

The poorer outcome for children with comprehension problems suggest that this is the group (with its several co-morbidities) that should be identified early. The evaluation of procedures to screen comprehension deficits are needed.

The Hanen programme, which is a parent programme focusing on the parent–child interactional environment for language learning and using videos to teach skills, is currently very popular.

Clinical experience suggests that co-morbidity and secondary communication and behaviour problems can be helped by strategic intervention. It is of particular importance that behaviour problems are given a very high priority, and that whichever professional has the lead role with speech and language problems should feel confident in this management task. This may mean that speech therapists should have substantial training in this area as well paediatricians. The behaviour should be tackled as a problem in its own right and not seen as secondary to the speech and language even though there is likely to be a close association. Parents whose children are having severe behaviour problems and are demoralized in this parenting role cannot manage complex language interventions and need to regain their confidence in handling the child alongside any speech and language tasks.

Outcome should be judged on prevention of secondary problems such as social communication and behaviour as well as language. One important factor seldom measured in outcome studies is self-esteem; the factors that promote this will vary from child to child but may be crucial in choosing the correct educational placement.

Chapter 23

Psychological effects of hearing impairment

S Palmer

Introduction

One of the major influences on the psychological development of the hearing-impaired child is the age at which the diagnosis is made. More than 90% of hearing-impaired children are born into hearing families and, unless there are other handicaps that might prompt early hearing screening, many hearing-impaired children are not diagnosed for anything up to three years. Such a late discovery of a hearing impairment can have a significant and far-reaching impact on the children, their parents, and on the relationships between them.

The discovery that their child is deaf may be greeted with feelings of relief by some parents. Other parents have a very difficult time adjusting to the idea that their 'perfect' baby is no longer perfect. In either case there is likely to be a period of grief. Such grief follows a natural course beginning with a period of denial and searching for miracle cures or plea bargaining. This phase is often replaced with a period of anger. Anger towards themselves, the medical profession, God or even towards the baby itself. This in itself can have very negative effects on relationships. Anger may eventually give way to guilt and parents, especially the mother, blaming themselves or others. It is only in the final phase of grieving, acceptance, that the parents can begin to reconstruct their lives to accommodate their child's needs.

Most families with a deaf child function quite normally after a period of adjustment. However, some professionals suggest that such families should be considered 'at-risk' due to the potentially increased level of stress. The most significant factor in the family's ability to cope is the amount of positive practical and emotional support the family receives from friends and family. In addition, the child's social and emotional development depends on parental attitude towards the diagnosis and the adjustment of the quality and quantity of interaction between the child and his parents, peers and family.

Pre-natal and early post-natal experience

Pre-natal auditory experiences can affect later learning and perception and they can play an important role in early bonding between the hearing infant and its mother. During the last trimester, the baby's head usually rests against the mother's pelvis. Through bony conduction, the baby can hear and react to the mother's voice as well as her heartbeat. Within hours of birth, babies are able to distinguish their mother's voice from any other female's and show a preference for it (DeCasper and Fifer, 1980; DeCasper and Spence, 1986). In addition, DeCasper and Spence (1986) have shown that babies can remember and show preference for rhythmic sounds structures, such as stories read by their mothers, heard antenatally. The hearing-impaired child does not have this early start in his social development.

Babies' perceptual skills are particularly well adapted for interacting with the people in their world. They hear best in the range of the human voice; they can discriminate their mother from others on the basis of smell (Cernoch and Porter, 1985), sight (Walton, Bower and Bower, 1992), and sound (DeCasper and Fifer, 1980); their eyes focus best at the feeding distance; they have a built-in preference for the human face. However, interaction is a two-way thing. Just as babies are likely to respond positively to the familiar sight and sound of the mother, so mothers are likely to respond positively to an infant who smiles and looks at her face in response to her voice.

The role of parenthood is a learned one, often by trial and error on the job. This is particularly true for the mother, who more often than not has the main nurturing responsibility. One of the important influences in her adjustment to her new role is the appearance and behaviour of the baby. The early developmental behaviour of the hearing-impaired child may not deviate significantly from that of his hearing peers and thus the parent-baby interaction patterns evolve naturally. However, normal mother-baby interactions become attuned through the development of synchronization of actions and reciprocal behaviour (Brazelton, 1982). The actions of the baby and mother are mutually reinforcing. They stimulate each other and respond to each other. These early interactions provide the roots for later attachment and emotional bonding between mother and child and form the foundations for language development.

The baby with a severe hearing impairment will not orient to the mother's voice, nor become quieter at the sound of her approach. In time some parents can feel rejected, deprived and anxious about their child's lack of reciprocity. They can feel that they are the only partners in the interaction and that it may be their inadequacies that are causing the lack of response from the baby. Consequently, the parent's social behaviour will change to accommodate this lack of response causing idiosyncratic interaction strategies to develop in the baby.

Children born with a hearing impairment are not aware of their handicap and will confront the tasks of their development with the same enthusiasm as any other infant. The only tool they lack for the job is audition. Deafness is an invisible handicap. Sensory deprivation limits the world of experience; unfortunately deafness can cut a person off from the world of people. Out of sight really can be out of mind and can limit the baby's anticipatory reactions to the presence of his parents.

Parents often use vocalizations to soothe a fractious baby especially if they are at a distance from their baby. With hearing-impaired children this may be impossible. Although vocalizations can be replaced by rhythmic tactile behaviour, for the majority of hearing-impaired children, their parents have no idea of their hearing impairment and thus do not attempt to compensate for the lack of hearing with increased touching or increased visual communication.

Attachment

We assume that the infant's psychological state is initially one of undifferentiation. He is at one with the world, unaware of where he ends and it begins. His expressions of discomfort bring relief magically. His only tool for adaptation lies in his helplessness and the response it evokes. Crying, smiling and babbling are all proximity promoting behaviours for the caregiver. The baby does not mind at this point who brings care and comfort as long as he is kept clean, dry, fed, warm and entertained. Most adults will automatically display a distinctive and universal pattern of behaviours in response to their babies' demands.

We can perform these behaviours with any baby, but we rely on the development of synchronization to form a bond with them. This takes time and many rehearsals and some infants and parents are more skilful or learn faster than others. A hearing impairment can limit the opportunity to develop synchrony and thus can affect the early bonding experience, especially when parents have no idea that their baby is deaf and so make no allowances or compensations.

By about three months, the baby begins to respond more discriminantly. His biggest smiles are reserved for familiar faces. His longest vocalizations are held with those closest to him. At this stage he still does not mind other people 'talking' to him or smiling at him or even cuddling him, but he is most comfortable with those he sees most often. No one person has yet become a safe base. Children at this stage show little anxiety at being separated from their parents and no fear of strangers (Bowlby, 1980). Hearing-impaired children will act no differently from normally-hearing children except in their lack of response to vocal stimulation. However, even at this early stage they may have adapted their behaviour to respond to non-verbal signals giving the impression that they are responding to verbal communication. They babble and smile in the same way as their normally-hearing peers. This may delay parents seeking advice about their child's hearing impairment.

Three or four months later we see the beginnings of attachment proper. Most babies become partly mobile and so instead of proximity-promoting behaviours they can now indulge in proximity-seeking behaviours. If mum moves away, they can follow. At this stage we see the baby using mum as a safe base from which to explore the world around her. At the same time they begin to show separation anxiety and fear of strangers. When reunited with their mother, children who have warm and secure attachments will greet them and seek comfort from them. In contrast, children with less secure attachments will not approach their mother on her return or will do so but will not be comforted and may react negatively by throwing a temper tantrum.

It is often claimed that deaf children are less securely attached to their mothers compared to hearing children. This has never been backed up by research per se, but we do know that the strength and stability of attachment of deaf children and their mothers, irrespective of the mother's hearing status, is a function of the mother's communicative efficiency (Marschark, 1997). Hearing mothers of deaf children are often described as being intrusive and over-controlling and that it is this that causes insecure attachments. However, what we must bear in mind is that, for the majority of hearing-impaired children, their impairment is often undiagnosed at this stage and that when mother's attention is withdrawn from her deaf child, from the child's perspective the change may be greater than for the hearing child, and the consequent reaction may appear to be more extreme. Alternatively, the child may welcome less control and intrusion and may therefore appear to be less upset than his hearing peers. Ignoring the mother or increased fussiness on her return may be as a result of them not noticing her arrival and then surprise in seeing her rather than a reflection of the security of attachment.

Although hearing children may understand little of the mother's speech at first, by the time they reach eight or nine months, they typically have a large receptive vocabulary that will include a variety of words to indicate that mum is taking temporary leave. Mum will often tell the child in the cot or the playpen that she is going into the kitchen to make his dinner. While the mother is away the hearing child can keep tabs as she moves around the house by following her sounds. This monitoring may not be available to the hearing-impaired child and, unless the mother and baby have developed a signing vocabulary, the added information will not be available so that the baby may not register in advance that the mother is leaving. As soon as the mother moves out of his line of vision, she has left him as far as he is concerned, unless they develop a system of communicating movement, which may make him feel less insecure.

Consequences of attachment development

Once a child has developed clear attachments several other behaviours also appear. One of these is social referencing whereby babies will respond to faces displaying different emotions, as well as voices speaking with varying emotional tones. Infants may use such emotional cues to help them figure out what to do in a novel situation such as when a stranger comes to visit, or in a doctor's surgery. Babies of this age will look at mum or dad's face and listen to his or her tone of voice to check for the adult's emotional expression. If mum looks and sounds happy the baby is likely to be at ease or accept the stranger with less fuss. If mum looks or sounds frightened or concerned, the baby responds to these cues and reacts with equivalent fear or concern. Because of the limited vocal input, the hearing-impaired child often finds it more difficult to interpret facial expressions alone. It may be then that even if the content of language does not play a primary role in attachment, it may have secondary effects on the emotional development of the child.

Although virtually all children go through the sequence from pre-attachment to attachment, the quality of the attachment they form differs from one infant to the next. They create internal working models of their relationships with key others. This internal working model of attachment relationships includes such elements as the child's confidence, or lack of it, that the attachment figure will be available or reliable, the child's expectation of rebuff or affection, and the child's sense of assurance that the other really is a safe base for exploration.

Internal working models begin to develop from about one year old, becoming increasingly elaborated and firm until by about five years old most children have clear internal models of their relationship with the mother or other caregiver. In addition a self-model and a generalized relationship model that mirrors the degree of attachment of the original model also develops. Once formed, such models shape and explain experiences and affect memory and attention. We notice and remember experiences that fit our models, and miss or forget experiences that do not match. These models also affect a child's future behaviour as they tend to recreate in each new relationship the patterns with which the child is familiar. Children who have loving secure relationships with their parents will go on to develop strong friendships and secure adult relationships easier than those whose early relationships were less secure.

Mothers of hearing-impaired children who have established an effective reciprocal style of communication, or have attended early intervention classes, have less need to control especially by the use of physical means. They are also more likely to develop secure attachment bonds and thus facilitate later social development by providing more explicit social information (Ledderberg and Mobley, 1990). Any factor that decreases the availability of mothers to meet their child's needs has the potential to result in underlying mistrust or doubt as the child reflects on the attachment bond. The quality of attachment is predictive of later individual differences in social ability. Suboptimal communication abilities of parents can disrupt the development of secure attachments in hearing-impaired children and thus may have consequences for later social and emotional development.

Among hearing children, insecure early attachment has been linked with later behavioural problems. Such behavioural problems include low frustration thresholds, aggression and emotional distancing. These characteristics are very similar to those frequently used to describe young deaf children of hearing parents especially where there are low levels of communication that disturbs the availability and responsiveness of the mother.

Development of the sense of self

During the same time that the child is developing an attachment to his parents and creating an initial primitive internal working model of attachment, he is also developing a model of self. Both Freud and Piaget have influenced our thinking of the emerging sense of self. Freud emphasized the symbolic relationship between the mother and the young infant. He believed that the infant did not understand himself to be separate from the mother. Piaget (1964) emphasized that the child's understanding of the basic concept of object permanence was a necessary precursor for the child's attaining a sense of self as a stable continuing entity.

The subjective self, or 'I', develops as a child realizes there is a basic distinction between himself and everything else. This arises from the interactions the baby has with people and objects and leads to understanding that he can have an effect on things. When the child touches a mobile it moves; when he cries, someone appears to comfort him; when he smiles, others smile back. This sense of self develops over the first three or four months but it is not until about eight to 12 months that he will realize that mum and dad continue to exist when they are out of sight.

This timetable happens quite naturally with the hearing child as he can hear his parents go about their business in another part of the house. However, the hearing-impaired child does not always have this added comfort or reassurance. It may therefore take longer for the hearing-impaired child to develop a sense of person permanence and hence may take longer to develop a sense of confidence that he is not being abandoned.

Just as important as developing a realization that the baby exists as a separate entity is the development of understanding that the baby is also an object that has properties or qualities such as gender, size, a name, confidence and shyness. This development of self-awareness might begin when the baby is put in front of a mirror. Most babies will look at their reflection, make faces at their reflection or even try to interact with the baby in the mirror. This emerging self-awareness may also be seen in a range of other behaviours such as insisting upon doing things for themselves or showing ownership of toys.

The child is creating an internal working model of self. He first learns of his separate existence, then realizes that he can affect the world and finally realizes that he has certain qualities. The toddler is therefore already building up a picture of himself, his qualities and abilities. This model will affect the choices a toddler makes such as friends, toys and activities. At the same time, this internal model will influence the way the toddler interprets his experiences so that the model is strengthened and carried forward. Hence it is important that the toddler is given every opportunity to develop a positive self-image at this stage as it may be difficult to change a strong negative image later. This can lead to all sorts of problems due to lack of confidence. It is important from this point of view that the hearing-impaired child is given the same sort of opportunity to develop individuality as his hearing peers and the same chance to build a positive self-esteem and high sense of self-efficacy. Parents who show negative reactions to a diagnosis of deafness, or embarrassment about the child having to wear hearing aids, will not help the development a positive self-image and may be impeding the child's acceptance of himself as a member of the deaf community.

The key to this period is finding the right balance between the child's emerging skills and his desire for autonomy, and the parent's need to protect and control his behaviour. In the early years, the parent's task is to provide enough warmth, predictability and responsiveness to foster a secure attachment. Once the child becomes physically and cognitively more independent, the need for control becomes a central aspect of the parent's task. Too much control, and the child will not have sufficient opportunity to explore; too little control and the child will become unmanageable and fail to learn the social skills he needs to get along with his peers as well as adults.

Children need to develop a mixture of instrumental and emotional independence blended with self-reliance, assertiveness and a need for achievement. The hearing-impaired child's need for greater instrumental assistance for safety's sake frequently leads to overprotection by the parent creating impediments to social and emotional independence. However, most hearing-impaired children are quite able to do tasks that others often do for them. The narrow range of tasks that they cannot do are often overgeneralized so that their parents do far too much. This in turn leads to a self-fulfilling prophecy and eventually the child gives up even trying to do things for himself. Lack of experience, lack of opportunity to practise and lack of time and patience by the parents all contribute to learned helplessness.

> Parents and teachers of hearing impaired children think for them, anticipate and avoid errors, and prevent the child from learning through trial and error. The justification is that there is so little time to learn so much – the hearing impaired child grows up without the experience he needs to attack new problems without fear of making mistakes.
>
> (Lane et al., 1976)

It may take extra time for the hearing-impaired child to understand instructions and therefore additional time to understand what is expected and necessary for performance of even fairly simple tasks. But it is important for later development to be given this extra time at a young age to foster the confidence to tackle more complex tasks. There is a strong relationship between the degree to which parents promote social independence in pre-schoolers and the extent to which older children are socially outgoing, spontaneous and motivated (Schlesinger and Meadow, 1972)

Emergence of self-control

Along with self concept, the pre-schooler must also develop self-control. Toddlers live in the here and now. When they want something they want it immediately. When they are tired they cry. When they are hungry they want food straight away. They are bad at waiting or working towards distant goals and they find it hard to resist temptation. To function acceptably as social beings they must learn self-control.

Hearing-impaired children are often seen as being more impulsive in their behaviour than their hearing peers. This may be due in part to poorer communication skills leading to parents being unable to adequately explain the need for delayed gratification. Hearing parents of hearing-impaired children frequently give in to demands for attention and assistance to avoid temper tantrums. Without the ability to explain past present and future, these parents may be teaching their children that emotional and instrumental dependence is immediately rewarded, which can lead to emotional difficulties.

The process of acquiring such self-control is basically one of shifting control from the parents to the child. With toddlers, parents provide most of the control through the use of prohibitions and requests. Over the preschool years the child gradually internalizes the various standards and expectations and takes on much of the control for himself. Such internalization and the resultant improvement in self-control is built on the development of language. From about two years we can hear children using 'private speech' to help control or monitor their own behaviour. The improvement of linguistic skills also makes it easier for parents to communicate with their child so they can explain rules of behaviour, which in turn can be internalized and practised. Internalization of such rules is brought about by parental warmth, sensitivity, responsiveness, levels of expectation, clarity and consistency of rules, and child-centred methods of control.

A variety of studies involving hearing mothers have reported that they tend to be more directing, tense and controlling in their verbal and non-verbal interactions with their hearing-impaired children (Power, Wood and Wood, 1990; Spencer and Gutfreund, 1990). Hearing mothers tend to be the initiators of interactions and tend to control the turn taking and topics of attention. Maternal intrusiveness and directiveness can impede the development of independence and autonomy. Mothers who have established an effective channel of communication would have less need for such control, especially physical control. The establishment of good social communication skills within the family are necessary for venturing out into the social world. Failure to establish good channels of communication can lead to feelings of frustration and a reduction in parent's responsiveness to affective cues from their children.

As children grow older, linguistic interaction becomes even more necessary for social and emotional development as parents communicate social norms, behavioural rules and the reasons for observed and imminent social events. Effective modes of communication provide for more rapid and detailed transmission of social information, both implicitly and explicitly. Lack of such communication has been shown to be linked to impulsive behaviour, poorer self image, more disruptive behaviour and an external locus of control on the part of the hearing-impaired child. For their parents, ineffective communication tends to result in less satisfying interactions and the use of more physical control and punishment.

Effective communication plays an essential role in development. Age appropriate social and emotional development is inversely related to the degree of hearing impairment. There is a need for parents and children to develop reciprocity in their visually based interactions, through attention switching and turn taking. The importance of mothers being able to control the flow of interactions during the first year when infants lack the strategies for doing so themselves must be gradually replaced by fading that control so that children can develop the ability to participate as full partners. Adults seem less ready to give over control to hearing-impaired than hearing children.

Peer relationships

If hearing-impaired children are to be integrated into a nursery school, they need to be able to cope with all types of behaviour from other children. Some parents of hearing-impaired children hope that their children will 'learn' from other hearing children by them modelling relatively more advanced social and linguistic behaviours (Spencer, Stafford and Meadow-Orlans, 1994). However, the communication needs of the hearing-impaired child may create a major challenge for complete integration. Most nursery-age children are unable to adapt their communication to meet the visual needs of their hearing-impaired peers creating many barriers to free interaction. Communication by hearing children directed toward the hearing-impaired child are often presented vocally or by gesture outside the line of vision without first gaining the visual attention of the hearing-impaired child. Hearing children might feel that their attempts at communication have been rejected, which may lead to the rejection of the hearing-impaired child.

Research has shown that hearing-impaired children do not interact with, nor become accepted by their hearing peers simply by being placed in an integrated setting (Antia, 1982). Peer interactions are important for the formation of peer relationships. Communication with peers becomes part of the child's pattern of interpersonal behaviour and interpersonal relationships. Children are developmentally at risk when they do not experience successful encounters with peers. Social communication behaviours learned through interaction with adults do not automatically generalize to peers. Adults will often take the major responsibility for initiating and maintaining interactions by questioning, commenting and expanding on the child's communication. In contrast, peer interactions require the child to assume responsibility for initiating and maintaining the interaction.

Children who are hearing-impaired may find themselves at a disadvantage in developing peer relationships because of their poorer communication skills and lack of experience in playgroups with other young children. Early intervention programmes are frequently structured around interaction with adults with little emphasis on playing with peers. Educators may find it worthwhile to implement strategies that promote interaction between children who are hearing-impaired and their peers. Promoting positive peer interaction should be one of the goals of an educational programme for young hearing-impaired children because early peer relationships can affect social acceptance, self-esteem and the ability to form later social relationships (Antia, 1994).

Cognitive development

According to Piaget, babies engage in an adaptive process trying to make sense of the world. They assimilate incoming information to the limited array of schemas they are born with, and accommodate those schemas based on experience. This is the starting point for cognitive development in which the primitive form of thinking is a sensorimotor intelligence. In contrast to Piaget's thought about the way an infant develops, learning theorists argue that a child's behaviour and characteristics are a product of experience. The question of whether very young infants learn from experience is also important from a practical point of view. It affects the sort of advice we should give to parents about suitable stimulation for their child.

If a child's perceptual abilities develop largely through maturation rather than learning, we would be less likely to advise parents to buy mobiles to hang above the baby's cot. However, if learning is possible from the earliest days then various kinds of enrichment would be beneficial. Repeated exposure to a stimulus allows expectancies to develop through schematic learning. Once formed they can help the baby to distinguish between the familiar and the unfamiliar. This is important in both social and cognitive development.

Childhood cognition is a mixture of competence and limitations and this is particularly so during the stage of pre-operational development. The defining characteristics of the movement from sensorimotor to pre-operational thinking is the onset of representational ability or symbolic function. According to Piaget, children of about two years begin to use symbols – images, words or actions – to stand for something else in their play and communications. At the same time we see an improving ability to manipulate these symbols internally in such things as improving memory and systematic searching.

Representational, in the head, problem solving is superior to sensorimotor problem solving in several ways. It is faster and more efficient and allows a child to test out ideas using inner thought rather than literal action. Representational thought is more mobile and not limited to the here and now. Because of the emergence of language it is socially shareable allowing the child to share and receive ideas in ways that are not possible without language.

During this period children acquire qualitative identity – the realization that the nature of something is not changed by a change in its appearance – although it is not until the age of about five or six that they begin to understand quantitative identity. Piagetian tasks such as conservation of number, liquid or mass are impossible until the child can focus his attention on more than one aspect of a problem at a time.

The hearing-impaired child may be at a particular disadvantage relative to his normally hearing peers. Young hearing-impaired children are more restrained in their experiences, their language and by their frequently over-controlling parents (Piaget, 1964; Rittenhouse and Kenyon, 1996). Their lack of hearing could be an impediment to a child's recognition of constancy during perceived changes as they do not have the benefit of parental description accompanying the perceptual changes, or the verbal rationale underlying qualitative changes in the environment. Conservation entails not only the understanding of the quantitative measure and the ability to ignore changes in shape that do not affect quantity, but also an understanding of the comparative words such as 'more than', 'less than', 'heavier', 'lighter', or 'the same as'. To the extent that hearing-impaired children are more reliant on perceptual observations rather than conceptual understanding than their hearing age mates, we might expect them to perform less well.

In looking at the normal course of development, much has been said about the active problem-solving enquiries of children as they test out their environment with the support of a facilitating adult. At the heart of learning is the nature of the adult–child collaboration, dependent on the motivation of the child to initiate interaction with partners, and the sensitivity of adults as they respond. Both are required to be negotiators, without a sense of the adult dominating or over-directing the child. Unfortunately, the consequences of hearing impairment appear to be that the child becomes a more passive learner, difficult to engage and the adult also becomes less facilitative.

Developmental psychologists such as Vygotsky and Bruner have explored the idea that children negotiate meaning and understanding in a social context. The child develops repertoires of shared meaning even before language, starting with phenomena such as joint attention. With language, the child gains a much more powerful entry point into images, the metaphors, the ways of interpreting events, which are distinctive to his own environment. These are social representations that give the child a framework for constructing knowledge. As a result of the social interactions between the growing child and other members of that child's community, the child acquires the tools of thinking and learning. It is out of this co-operative process of engaging in mutual activities with more expert others that the child becomes more knowledgeable. Instruction is at the heart of learning. You do not have to wait for the child to be ready to learn. Children learn from others who are more knowledgeable than themselves. 'Expert' intervention should be at a level beyond the child's existing developmental level so that it provides some challenge but not too far ahead, so that it is still comprehensible and the child can accomplish something he could not do alone, whilst still learning from the experience.

Theory of mind

Minds are the main difference between people and other entities. Children cannot make much progress toward understanding everyday events involving other people until they have some understanding of the mind. A child watching a friend rummaging through a toy box can only make sense of the friend's actions by assuming that a particular toy is wanted, believes it can be found there, intends to play with it, will feel sad if it is not found, and so forth. These implicit notions are called the child's *theory of mind.*

Research on the child's ability to take others' perspectives shows that children as young as two or three have at least some ability to understand that other people see or experience things differently from the way they do. Children will adapt their play to the demands of their companion although such understanding is not perfect at this young age. At level one, usually between two and three, a child recognizes that human beings are feeling, thinking beings. Precursors to this knowledge include the use of social referencing, intentional communication and the early use of pretence.

At stage two, by about four or five, they do know that not everyone has the same knowledge to act on and can also differentiate emotional states of desire and belief caused by external events. They can distinguish between appearance and reality for both objects and people and can realize that people may react differently to the same stimulus. Knowing that what you see may not be what you get has an adaptive purpose. Young children need to know not to eat plastic food, or to walk through a clear glass door. Even adults need to be aware of misleading appearances, such as what looks like an adult in the distance when driving might turn out to be a child who is much closer.

In the case of a hearing-impaired child, conversational deprivation early in life is a likely contributor to delayed understanding of mental states. One of the main problems is that conversation tends to be confined to concrete visible topics. The children are not likely to be exposed to the kind of spontaneous conversations at home that appear to be associated with development of a theory of mind (Marschark, 1993). Children whose actions are constrained by mothers who take on an educational role rather than a playful one, may be delayed in development of pretend play (Courtin and Melot, 1998) and pretend play is important in developing perspective taking and appearance-reality distinction. It has been shown that deaf children are up to six years behind their hearing peers in the development of theory of mind but that these results are dependent of hearing status of the parents and mode of communication (Peterson and Seigal, 1995; Courtin and Melot, 1998).

Play

Play provides the opportunity to strengthen the body, improve the mind, develop the personality and acquire social competence. It is thus as necessary for the child as is food, warmth and protective care. It represents, for the child, practice in independent living, opportunity to research and explore, relief from boredom, and simple fun and enjoyment. Different types of play emerge in a sequence as the child learns to use his sensory and motor abilities to their best advantage. Children's playtime accomplishments closely reflect their normal cognitive and social developmental progress. By monitoring children's progress in play we can indirectly monitor their cognitive and social development.

During the first six months, babies develop hand–eye co-ordination. They will explore objects most often by putting them into their mouth. In this way they learn about the way things feel, their size, colour and shape, how they sound and so on. In this way they learn primitive categorization. By about six months their neuromuscular control, manipulation, stereoscopic vision and hand–eye co-ordination are so advanced that they can reach out for any size or shaped object within arm's length. They will have also learned to accommodate for different sizes, shapes and textures sometimes using the feet as auxiliary graspers to help with larger objects. Although at this stage many children have learned about person permanence, they have still not developed object permanence. When a toy falls from his hand, unless it is within his continuing range of vision, it ceases to exist for him.

As babies become more mobile, their range of vision increases. In this way they quickly learn about object permanence, beginning to look for hidden toys and enlisting the help of others in an active way to retrieve toys that have fallen from the high chair. At the same time, infant–adult communication patterns are becoming established. We see babies enjoying turn taking games such as 'clap hands' and 'peek-a-boo'. This encourages the baby to listen to sounds and rhythm and to make a set response in return. Such turn taking is a prerequisite for taking turns in later conversations. Although turn taking has been in evidence since the babbling stage, up until this point it has been adult controlled. By about six or seven months we see the baby making an equal contribution.

During this period language becomes increasingly important. Babies begin to find meaning in their world. They like to watch and listen to familiar adults as they go about their daily routines and enjoy periodically to be touched, talked to and played with as they pass. Babies' early learning depends on the quality and quantity of this affectionate one-to-one mother teaching. Their attentions, relationships and play are still mainly at the level of ongoing perceptions rather than concepts, but their brief imitations indicate that they have come into possession of a short-term memory and are developing long-term memory banks.

Adults bring objects and events to the notice of the child. More often however, the adult will follow the child's gaze and mirror the child's visual exploration, giving a label or an explanation to the object of the child's attention. Shared attention, and shared visual experience of the world is tied to patterns of language used to explain it. In this way the adult can help to link together the child's experience with language and emphasize the relationship between speech sounds and events. Both the baby and the adult are capable of reading intentions in each other's behaviour and respond to many features of a context, not just the sounds or the words.

At home, children must learn to balance their need to be close to their mothers with their need to explore. In doing so they integrate motor activity with sensory alertness and emotional satisfaction. They also learn that in the home things are more consistent than in the park, for instance. In the kitchen, mother is less likely to suddenly disappear and therefore children can tolerate extending time and distance intervals between themselves and their mothers. However, this depends on the child's safety needs being met. For the hearing-impaired child this may necessitate a much closer physical proximity as the mother cannot give verbal warnings so easily.

However, mothers of hearing-impaired children must allow their child the same amount of independence that is given to hearing children, otherwise they will never develop initiative. Children without other handicaps must be given the same chance to explore, undress and play. Mothers often need reminding that it is only the hearing that is impaired and not the ability to play.

Hearing-impaired children must come to terms with people and learn about the world they live in mainly through looking, touching, smelling, exploring and exploiting the environment, and communicating with people in any way that is open to them. They are at a major disadvantage however, because they cannot divide their attention between the toy they are playing with and communication with the mother. As all communication involves their vision, whether speech reading or signing, it is not surprising that some babies create a fuss when their mother interrupts their play to 'talk' to them. Hearing children do not have this problem as they can concentrate visually on the toy whilst listening to their mother's voice. As learning and communication is primarily through one sensory mode, the child will necessarily need to periodically break off attention as their concentration span is limited.

Conclusions

In laying the foundations of language, the types of exchanges between infants and adults are very important. Adults scaffold their interactions with very young children by joint attention and turn taking, with the adults leaving long pauses after their vocalizations to allow the child to respond. Adults are quick to respond when a child vocalizes, treating the child as if he or she was a competent conversational partner. This eventually leads to genuine turn taking in interaction stimulating the giving and receiving of messages. The hearing-impaired child needs these 'proto conversations' just as much as the hearing child. Mutual attention, joint referencing, turn taking and contingent responses are more difficult for the adult to establish with the hearing-impaired child. However, it is possible if the correct strategies are used. These could include sharing picture books, turn-taking games, imitative play such as dressing up, shop, and house, creating opportunities for joint referencing such as finger puppets, construction toys, jigsaws or responding contingently to the child's glances, gestures or vocalizations.

The hearing-impaired child has to learn how to divide his attention between the person addressing them, the object of attention and what is being said. Initially the child may be unaware that anything is being said and his attention may wander from one thing to another. Parallel play with the adult alongside, commenting on the child's actions, will give the adult opportunity to follow the child's gaze and introduce the appropriate language.

Familiar play routines may establish turn taking and interaction. The idea is to teach the child that communicative acts produce anticipated responses. The adult should respond immediately to any of the child's actions that may be construed as having communicative intent. Nursery rhymes with movement such as *Ring-o-Roses* or *Insy Winsy Spider* give the child the opportunity to anticipate and join in. Mutual understanding is easier with shared experiences. This applies to language as well as play. By structuring the child's language and play environment so that routine and familiarity is established, the child can build up a 'vocabulary' of actions and words. Talking with and not at the child is as important as sharing relevant and meaningful activities. Giving the child time to respond before the adult intervenes and keeping the activities short with few distractions until the child's attention span develops is also important.

Constant sympathetic, but non-stressful adult encouragement to engage in all types of spontaneous play is essential to both the contentment of children and their fundamental learning experience. From their use of playthings that they can grasp, bang, poke, throw and so forth, until they can incorporate them into imaginative play, children first discover through their visual, auditory and tactile perceptions what they are and what special properties they possess. They then go on to discover what they can do with them and, finally, how they can adapt them to their own needs.

Detailed studies of communication between deaf children and hearing adults are rare. One of the main problems that hearing people face in communicating with hearing-impaired children, no matter what their mode of communication, is too much control. High adult control results in low child initiative and short child utterances. These children are rarely exposed to communications that involve speculation, hypothesis testing, imagination or negotiation. In such cases children receive a meagre linguistic diet and little space to develop flexibility, creativity and self-expression (Wood, 1996).

Intervention studies have shown that the amount of control used can be changed and that, when it is, children respond by showing more initiative in communication. However, what we have to bear in mind is that the hearing-impaired child faces additional cognitive demands if his or her main mode of monitoring is visual. If we say something to a deaf child, he must look away from the object of communication to what is being communicated. There may be frequent dislocations of mutual understanding because adults may start to communicate before they have the child's full attention. Some adults, in trying to minimize this problem, may try to force the child's attention. In doing so they might leave the child with the problem of working out the meaning of what they are trying to do. If such experiences are commonplace then it is not surprising that the hearing-impaired child experiences experiential deficits and cognitive delay.

Experience is necessary for children and adults to acquire expertise in most intellectual, social and physical skills. Children typically acquire expertise through repeated interactions with stimuli in their environment. However, sometimes children are unable to profit from their experiences. Sometimes they are not ready to learn a concept or to develop a certain skill. We must take into consideration the processing demands of a task. Working memory allocates cognitive energy to both processing and storage and if processing takes up too much energy and space there will be little or none left over for storage. Keeping this in mind is important when planning a learning experience for a hearing-impaired child – especially a child who has to devote a lot of energy to lip reading or sign interpretation. The key to learning and memory is to make the steps small; set achievable goals; give support, help and encouragement; and give plenty of praise when goals are achieved.

Chapter 24

Choosing between alternative communication approaches

W Lynas

Introduction

A diagnosis of profound bilateral deafness, whether at three weeks, six months, nine months or later, is a shock to parents and generates questions that reflect their feelings of deep anxiety and uncertainty about the prospects for their child. Will he or she talk? How will we talk with him or her? Must we learn sign language? And so forth. Unfortunately parental anxiety about their children's communication is rarely met with firm reassurances regarding their deaf child's potential ability to acquire language and become literate. Parents know from the outset that deafness from birth imposes a severe threat to the development of language and communication and they want to do the best thing for their children. But they do not know how to unlock the barrier to communication associated with their child's deafness. Even when they are ready to make serious enquiries about the best form of communication for their child, they will in all likelihood meet with confusing and conflicting advice, not least because of the partisan politics of deaf education. For example, they may be advised by 'oralists' to follow a strict auditory-oral approach, using speech and no signs and to prepare themselves for the possibility of a cochlear implant operation for their child at the age of around two years. They may be told to make sure that the child is fitted with the best possible amplification but at the same time to do 'what comes naturally' from a communication point of view, using gesture and signs with speech as 'total communication' on the grounds that making use of all modalities will help move forward the development of communication. They may, on the other hand, be advised by pro-signers that they are blessed with a child with special features that are not the same as those possessed by a hearing child; that their child's natural language as a deaf child is sign language and that preparation for the world of the culturally deaf through a sign bilingual approach is what the child needs. This approach requires, as a first step, that they and other members of their family must start to learn sign language.

Parents cannot deal with the quandary raised by conflicting advice by putting into practice all the aforementioned methods of communication because the different approaches are so incompatible. Moreover, the more they investigate the more they will realize that the professionals, whose role it is to serve their needs as parents of a deaf child, have different views as to what is best for their particular deaf child and favour different incompatible communication approaches. In any event, leaving the decision to 'experts' is inadvisable because parents will feel undermined if they do not play a major role in the decision making. It is parents who must decide and parents must, therefore, be empowered to do the best thing for their children. No educational method is going to work well unless parents freely choose it and take responsibility for it. In these circumstances 'doing the best thing' for their deaf child means getting to know as much as possible about the nature and implications of the available communication approaches so as to make an informed choice. Parents need to be able to understand the advantages and disadvantages of different approaches and to really *see* the applicability to their own child. Parents are the key stakeholders in the deaf child's education and future life and professionals, whatever their own stance might be, should warn parents to arm themselves against biased opinion and partisan advice.

There are no absolutely clear solutions to the problem of giving deaf children communication and language nor in providing them with educational opportunities equal to those of similar children with full unaided hearing capacity. Nor are there any certain ways of knowing how young deaf children, as future adults, will want to live their lives. Yet a choice of communication approach has to be made, and it is present-day adults who must make the decisions on behalf of deaf children. Because the approaches are, for the most part, mutually exclusive and because decisions are so consequential and fateful, it is the duty of all concerned to examine the best available evidence before the choice of communication option is made.

The aim of this chapter is to offer information in as clear and impartial way as possible to help clarify issues and claims made on behalf of different communication approaches in order that professionals can help parents arrive at their own solutions. The three major communication options – total communication, sign bilingualism and auditory-oral – will in turn be examined in order to reveal the arguments used to support each particular method and to examine its practical implications together with the most recent available educational outcome evidence. The choice of options that are likely to be available in any particular child's local area will also be considered.

The methodological controversy – historical background

To understand why there are very marked distinctions in communication approaches available to deaf children at the turn of the century, it is helpful to look back at the historical antecedents to the different communication methods.

Ever since attempts have been made to give a means of communication to the deaf, there have been 'oralists' and 'manualists'. 'Oralists' believe that deaf children could and should be made to be as 'normal' as possible by being taught to speak and understand the speech of others. 'Manualists' believe that the barrier to communication caused by deafness can be circumvented through the use of manual-visual signs: this approach relies on the use of hands to produce communication symbols and on vision to perceive those symbols. Faulty or defective hearing is thus supplemented or bypassed.

Both 'oralism' and 'manualism' were to be found in different institutions for deaf children and adults in nineteenth century Europe and North America (Bender, 1981) yet neither method could claim successful outcomes on a large scale in terms of educational or linguistic standards; the majority of deaf children failed to achieve even basic literacy. However, by the beginning of the twentieth century there was concern on both sides of the Atlantic, even from 'manualists' themselves, that signs were being overused. Gallaudet, the founding father of 'manualism' in the US, expressed the view that excessive use of signs interfered with the mastery of English (Gallaudet, 1997). Hence the oral method prevailed for most of the twentieth century supported in part by the 'discovery' that almost all deaf children had residual hearing and by the invention of electronic hearing aids which could boost residual hearing.

However, in the latter part of the twentieth century, 'oralism' came under severe criticism, and major government reports in the US and in Britain in the 1960s (Babbidge, 1965; DES (The Lewis Report), 1968), revealed dispiritingly low educational outcomes for the majority of deaf school leavers despite technological advances (Conrad, 1979), and relatively generous educational and health service provisions in post-war expanding economies. Added to that, was a concern about social and emotional consequences of a 'failed' oral education: oral failure and emotional failure were perceived as going hand-in-hand (Mindel and

Vernon, 1971; Denmark, 1994). Oralism, particularly in the US, was further undermined by a much-publicized study from the US by Stuckless and Birch (1966) that revealed that deaf children of deaf parents, exposed to early manual communication, were superior to the control group of deaf children of hearing parents on measures of reading and writing, suggesting therefore that the early use of signs did not interfere with the later development of verbal language.

That 'pure oralism' was failing most children in terms of their academic achievements led to the development of *total communication* (TC), an approach that involves the use of signs with speech. By the 1980s almost all profoundly deaf children in the US, and a smaller but significant proportion of deaf children in the UK, were being educated through a communication approach that made explicit and extensive use of signs. By the 1990s, however, there was a shift of emphasis: a new and radically different form of 'manualism', sign bilingualism, was introduced, which prescribes that sign language, unaccompanied by speech, should be offered deaf children as their first language and verbal language, such as English, as a second language. The trend towards sign bilingualism has reduced the popularity of TC as an alternative to oral approaches, but the use of speech alongside signs is still regarded as a sensible option for some children at some stages in their development and education. Despite the growth of sign alternatives, oral approaches have by no means disappeared: the auditory-oral approach remains the preferred option for many deaf children in many parts of the UK and elsewhere, with a recent boost from ever-advancing audiological technology.

The theory and practice of total communication will be examined first because it was a major challenge to the oral approach in the 1970s and 1980s. Then, sign bilingualism – the approach that took root in the UK in the 1990s – will be described and evaluated. Finally, the current auditory-oral approach will be considered, particularly in light of new developments in technology.

Total communication

Total communication (TC) sounds a very attractive proposition. It involves the use of *all* methods of communication – sign, gesture, finger spelling, speech, hearing, lip movements and facial expression. It is not intended that signs, finger spelling, and so forth, will *replace* speech: the use of hearing and making maximum use of residual hearing using the best possible amplification is essential in TC. The idea is that visual communication will *support* audition and speech.

Those who introduced TC believed that it was unfair to expect deaf children to perceive spoken language through the auditory channel alone and this belief was supported by the low educational and linguistic standards associated with oral methods during the greater part of the twentieth century. Speech and signs, sight and hearing, it is claimed, work together in a TC approach and the deaf child thereby gets 'the best of all worlds' from a communication point of view.

The signs used in a TC approach are taken from the sign languages used by members of the deaf community in a particular country. So, for example, in the UK the signs are drawn from British Sign Language (BSL) and in the US from American Sign Language (ASL). The sign system in a TC approach, however, differs from BSL in significant ways: BSL has evolved over the years within the British deaf community and has a very different structure from the structure of English or any verbal language. It is not a manual-visual form of English and cannot, therefore, be used simultaneously with speech. The signing used in TC, however, *is* a signed form of English, termed Signed English or Signs Supporting English, and, in theory, can be used simultaneously with spoken English. It is a contrived system, therefore, which takes signs from BSL but presents them in English word order. There are additional invented signs to represent English syntactic features, for example verb inflections such as '-ing', '-ed', and function words such 'the', 'as', 'of'. Where there is no BSL sign corresponding to a word in English, finger spelling is used to supplement signs.

It is easy to see the appeal of TC: signs are 100% accessible to the deaf child, whereas speech is always heard imperfectly. The TC approach appears to offer a deaf child easy communication and access to verbal symbols through sign whilst making use of whatever residual hearing the deaf child has.

Total communication is considered by many current advocates as a crucial means of establishing communication in deaf infants: deaf infants, like any other, use their eyes to scan the environment, to notice objects and events. If caregivers can offer signs and gestures in response to the infant's visual attention, they not only develop satisfying interaction and communication but provide readily accessible linguistic symbols. As the infant is wearing a hearing aid, speech signals can be perceived. Supporters of TC claim that, far from detracting from the development of spoken language, the early use of signs facilitates speech communication. The pressure to use and receive speech, and only speech, is removed: by being able to use sign and gesture in the early years, it is claimed, the deaf child gains confidence in communication and is better able to cope with the difficult task of receiving and producing speech. Parents and members of the family need to learn some signs, but the task of learning the signs of Signed English is nowhere as demanding as that of learning a natural sign language such as BSL, which has a structure that is very different from any spoken language.

Total communication used in schools by teachers of the deaf, support assistants or interpreters, will ensure, so advocates of TC claim, continued development of language and full access to the curriculum. Presenters of signs in accompaniment to speech, must, of course, be competent signers and have a sufficiently rich sign vocabulary to offer an enriched language input.

An evaluation of the TC approach

There have been many years of experience of TC practice, both in the US and the UK, so it should be possible to judge the effectiveness of the approach. Examination of practice, however, suggests that TC does not live up to all of its claims.

Some research in the UK indicates that gesture and sign may have a constructive role to play in the deaf child's progression to speech (Robinshaw, 1992, 1995). Robinshaw examined the transition from non-communicative behaviour to language production in deaf and hearing infants. For all the infants, deaf and hearing, the use of communicative gesture formed an important step from pre-symbolic to symbolic language. The deaf infant's use of gesture as a primary means of communication continued over a longer period compared with the hearing infants. The deaf children's use of gesture did decline towards the end of the period of study as their auditory perception improved and their attempts at speech became more intelligible to caregivers. She concluded, furthermore, that the use of gestures and signs with deaf infants is particularly helpful in promoting mutual communication between deaf child and caregiver at a time when interpreting the vocalizations of the deaf child is difficult. She speculates, however, that once the deaf child begins to perceive and discriminate auditorily the continued use of sign and gesture would have a detrimental effect on the development of auditory discrimination and vocal/verbal development.

Robinshaw's suggestion that the use of signs and speech beyond the early stages of communication development undermines the acquisition of verbal language, literacy and intelligible speech is confirmed by several research studies (Bornstein and Saulnier, 1981; Geers et al., 1984; Markides, 1988). The several large-scale studies of the attainments of deaf children and young people in the US offer perhaps the most serious indictment of the use of TC during the school years. The surveys, which involve thousands of deaf children and young people, indicate that TC-educated young people are leaving school with standards of literacy and speech achievements that are no higher than those of deaf young people leaving school in the 1950s and 1960s – that is, before the introduction of TC (Schildroth and Hotto, 1991).

Research work in the late 1970s and 1980s offer reasons why the appealing idea of TC is difficult to put into practice. A signed form of English takes about twice as long as the spoken form to articulate. Transcripts of speech-and-signs indicate distortions to speech, which is slowed down and over-simplified, and distortions to the signed component where signs are typically omitted, especially 'difficult' vocabulary and signs conveying grammatical information (Baker, 1978; Kluwin, 1981; Newton, 1985; Wood and Wood, 1992). Total communication has been shown, therefore, to be doing the very opposite of what is often claimed – ensuring 'total' linguistic information.

There is, then, some qualified support for the use of TC – that is, gestures, speech and signs, as a route into verbal language at the early stages of communication. But if practised throughout the school years, TC seems to lead to reading ages of between eight and nine years and poor speech (Schildroth and Hotto, 1991): we have come no closer to our goal of offering language and literacy to the vast majority of deaf children. Many people who believed that a combination of speech and signs would provide a solution to the problem of giving language to deaf children became fiercely critical of TC (for example, Hansen, 1990; Lane et al., 1996).

The emergence of sign bilingualism

The growing disillusion with TC during the 1980s did not, however, lead in the 1990s to a full-scale return to oralism. A new voice has emerged from those who might describe themselves as the 'culturally deaf', which has come to be extremely powerful in the education of deaf children. The deaf community offers a perspective on deafness that rejects the idea of deafness as a medical condition that requires correction and invites us to see deafness as a cultural difference that needs to be respected (Bouvet, 1990). The culturally deaf are supported by many idealists who espouse the social model of disability and the notion that disability is a difference not a defect. They argue that in order for deaf children to be assured full human rights and equal opportunities, they should be offered their natural language, sign language, as a first language. The natural sign languages that have developed over the years within deaf communities have been analysed by linguists and judged to be 'proper' languages, in contrast with the 'unnatural' contrived sign system used in TC. A sign language such as BSL, therefore, has the same capacity as any verbal language for the expression of ideas (Stokoe, 1960). Where speech is the medium of exchange, the deaf individual can never be equal and in the past, it is argued, deaf children have been disabled by hearing educators who have sought to impose on them their hearing-speaking norms. Deaf children who are offered sign language as their first language can communicate as effectively as anyone else, so bilingualists claim, and are thus free from disability. With sign language, children can develop pride in a distinct deaf identity as a member of a cultural and linguistic minority (Lane et al., 1996). Moreover, any educational approach that does not reflect the necessity of sign language as a first language constitutes a violation of the human rights of deaf children (BDA, 1996).

The approach incorporating natural sign language, known in Britain as sign bilingualism, demands that BSL should begin as soon as the infant's deafness has been identified and that English should be learned later as a second language. Deaf children, so it is claimed, if given sufficient sign language experience in the early years, will acquire language as readily as a hearing child acquires spoken language and hence deaf children can thus begin their formal education on an equal footing with hearing children. The majority of children born with severe and profound hearing impairments have hearing parents – around 90% in Britain – who are unlikely to know sign language. Parents need, therefore, considerable support and guidance in order to facilitate their deaf child's sign-language acquisition (Mahshie, 1995). Classes in BSL may be available in their local area. Deaf signing adults can play a crucial role in enabling parents in their learning of sign language and in offering helpful interaction in sign with the young deaf child. If parents have selected a sign approach they will, so it is claimed, be naturally well motivated to learn sign language themselves. Furthermore, it is argued that when the deaf child starts to communicate in sign, parents will become even more enthusiastic in developing their sign language skills (Bouvet, 1990).

Sign bilingualists argue that once formal schooling has begun, deaf children, through the medium of sign language, can be offered the full curriculum and have the same opportunity as the hearing child to acquire knowledge and 'achieve' academically. Whether in a special or mainstream school, the deaf child needs a generous supply of trained signing teachers, including deaf teachers, signing interpreters, signing classroom assistants. With such provision the deaf child will have the same opportunity as the hearing child to acquire knowledge and 'achieve' academically. It is considered important that the deaf child should have access to a variety of sign users, children and adults, during the course of the day in order to sustain language growth. This is taken to mean, in Scandinavian countries, where there is around 20 years experience of offering a bilingual approach to deaf children, that deaf children should be educated in special schools for the deaf (Bergman and Wallin, 1994). However, given that there is a strong tradition in the UK of educating deaf children in the mainstream, UK bilingualists do not necessarily believe that a special school is essential (Pickersgill, 1997). However, for deaf children to receive sufficient input of sign language, with maximum use made of the scarce resources of deaf signing adults, interpreters, and signing teachers, it is considered important that they are grouped together in a unit or resource centre within a mainstream school (BDA, 1996). This also gives the deaf child access to a deaf peer group (Pickersgill, 1997).

With the bilingual approach, the goal of literacy in English has to be achieved by teaching the deaf child English as a second language. Bilingualists acknowledge that making the transition between BSL and written English, which has a completely different structure from that of any sign language, is not easy to achieve (Pickersgill, 1997). However, there are some ideas about how to bridge the gap between sign language and the majority verbal language (Mahshie, 1995; Strong, 1995; Pickersgill, 1997). Pickersgill (1997), for example, suggests that manually coded English can play a role in translating BSL into English. Furthermore, it is believed that children of school age are capable of analysing the structure of their own language use and are thus in a position to understand the structure of another language. The principle of developing an understanding of the structure of one's first language in order to facilitate the learning of another is well accepted in second language teaching (Cummins and Swain, 1986; Ahlgren, 1994; Strong, 1995).

There seem to be differences of opinion, or at least emphasis, amongst sign bilingualists concerning the development of speech in deaf children. For some, time spent on developing speech is considered 'time wasted' because the goal of speech is judged to be 'virtually impossible' (Johnson, Liddell and Erting, 1989). In Britain, the most commonly expressed view is that 'live' English as well as written English should be a target language (Pickersgill, 1997). Most deaf children will move in both the hearing-speaking world and the deaf-signing world. It is considered to be a very important principle, however, that the two forms of communication should be separated: sign language should be used in contexts where sign is the primary means of communication and spoken language should be associated with speaking people (Jansma, Knoors and Baker, 1997). Deaf children, like other bilingual children the world over, will become sociolinguistically competent (Volterra and Taeschner, 1978) and appreciate when sign is required and when it is appropriate to use oral communication. However, we have no evidence to date from educators advocating and using a sign bilingual approach about the competence and intelligibility of the speech of sign bilingually educated deaf children.

An evaluation of the sign bilingual approach

Sign bilingualism has a strong ideological underpinning and few would quarrel with the principle of respect for cultural and linguistic diversity. The sign languages developed by deaf people the world over are testimony to remarkable human linguistic creativity. That deaf people can express ideas and communicate with others in a manner that does not depend on hearing is something that we acknowledge and in which we rejoice. That deaf people have acquired self-confidence not as a dependent disabled category but as a group with a distinct identity has helped us all in the process of shedding our disablist notions. Few would question the right of deaf people to become stakeholders in the education of deaf children.

However, to acknowledge the validity of sign language as a means of expressing the most complex of ideas does not inexorably lead to support for a sign bilingual approach in the education of all deaf children. Sign bilingual education for deaf children in the UK is in its relatively early days and research evidence relating to outcomes from anywhere is sparse (Luterman et al., 1999). There has nonetheless been some critical appraisal of the principles of the approach (Lynas, 1994; Luterman et al., 1999) and much careful reflection on the practice (Luterman, 1995; Strong, 1995; Moores, 1996; BATOD, 1997).

Are the goals of sign bilingualism achievable?

Given that the majority of deaf children are born into a home environment where communication is through speaking, there is a serious problem in offering the deaf infant and young child sufficient sign language input in the crucial early years of language acquisition. However enthusiastic parents might be about learning sign language, the task for hearing people in learning sign is at least as difficult as learning Russian and therefore not lightly accomplished. The task of providing sign language input to the young deaf child could be given over to those outside the home who can sign fluently, but this could undermine the bonds between the deaf children and their families. A recent longitudinal study in Bristol of deaf children educated bilingually indicates that, for the hearing parents, 'It is difficult to learn to sign. It is difficult to accept the otherness of one's child' (Ackerman, Sutherland and Young, 1997).

The promise of age-appropriate language in sign on reaching school age is an appealing feature of the sign bilingual approach. The question is, can this promise be fulfilled? Some research undertaken in Britain (Harris et al., 1989; Harris and Mahoney, 1997) throws doubt on whether deaf children exposed to sign language in the early years develop sign language as quickly as hearing children acquire spoken language, even when the parents are themselves deaf and use sign. One investigation involving four deaf mothers with their young, very early diagnosed deaf children indicated that all of the children were, for their age, considerably behind what is average in spoken language development for children with normal hearing (Harris et al., 1989). A further study of hearing mothers using sign with their young deaf children revealed difficulties in establishing interaction through sign (Harris and Mahoney, 1997).

The achievement of literacy is an established goal of sign bilingualism. Despite around a decade of experience of the use of a sign bilingual approach in parts of the UK, data on literacy achievements do not exist. Furthermore, with around 20 years of experience of a bilingual approach in Denmark and Sweden, we do not have evidence from large-scale studies of literacy attainments. Knoors (1997), reviewing a book based on a conference in Sweden on bilingualism in deaf education, notes an absence of contributions based on achievement data: 'Alas, there were virtually no data, and far too much rhetoric.' So far, then, we cannot say with confidence that learning verbal language through sign language *is* possible for the majority of deaf children.

We can accept that the deaf child who is given sign language as a first language has mastery of the means of expressing ideas and has communication, but can we accept that the deaf individual without literacy is truly enabled? Can we accept that making a decision to undermine the deaf child's ability to use spoken language as an adult is not a restriction rather than an enhancement of educational opportunity? If the decision is made to immerse the deaf child in sign so that sign language becomes the mother tongue can we be confident that the child would have chosen that option? The ability of the deaf child educated through a sign bilingual approach to acquire speech and verbal language later on is, to say the very least, uncertain. We do know, however, that orally educated deaf young people and adults can choose to learn sign language and, if well motivated, have done so, some choosing as adults to communicate primarily through sign (Winston, 1990; Luterman et al., 1999).

The moral issues and practical issues associated with a bilingual approach seem as great as those associated with the use of an oral-only approach in the past. Disillusion with oral practice and oral outcomes earlier this century did not, however, result in universal rejection of the oral approach: in Britain and in North America an auditory-oral approach continues to be considered by many to be the approach that offers the deaf child the greatest potential for linguistic, social and educational development. Now, more than ever before, oralists believe that technological advances have secured for even the profoundly deaf child a hearing, speaking future.

The case for the auditory-oral approach

The ideological position behind the present-day, auditory-oral approach is, as it has been with any oral approach at any time, that verbal communication, particularly spoken communication, is the predominant medium of social exchange. Deaf people are surrounded most of the time by normally-hearing people, and the demands of everyday life necessitate a considerable amount of exchange with people who speak and do not sign. Without the ability to speak and understand the speech of others, the individual's links with wider society are severely restricted. Those who currently advocate an auditory-oral approach argue that it is not only desirable but possible to enable even severely and profoundly deaf children to talk and to acquire language through the medium of spoken exchange. The poor educational attainments reported during the 1960s reflect an era when hearing aids were not as effective or readily available; when even severe or profound hearing impairment might not be identified until two years or later; when cochlear implants were not available to deaf children; when professionals and parents were not as competent at managing hearing aids as they are today. Where the auditory-oral method is practised competently, where available technology is used to its potential and where parents receive well-informed, sensitive support in managing linguistic interaction with their deaf child, then educational achievements are much closer to what we would like them to be.

In the UK generally, however, the academic achievements of deaf children continue to be disappointing and considerably lower than for children with normal hearing (Powers, 1996; 1998). Powers' survey of the GCSE attainments of two cohorts of school leavers in England, 344 in 1995 and 403 in 1996 indicated that only 14% in 1995, and 18% in 1996, achieved five or more GCSE grades A–C compared with the national average of 44% and 45% respectively. The young people's hearing impairments ranged from moderate to profound and they had been educated through a variety of communication approaches, although these were not specified. However, studies of children and young people educated consistently through an auditory-oral approach from the US (for example, Geers and Moog, 1989) and from the UK (for example, Harrison et al., 1991; Lewis, 1996; Lewis and Hostler, 1998) give heartening evidence of more positive educational outcomes in relation to academic achievements.

For example, the study by Lewis and Hostler (1998), on behalf of the Ewing Foundation, involved *complete* populations of severely and profoundly deaf young people in five local education authorities (LEAs) in England and provide encouraging data on GCSE results. All the 28 young people had received a natural aural education in mainstream schools. The

GCSE examination results for 1995–7 indicated that 50% of the deaf pupils achieved five or more GCSE grades A–C or above, compared with the national average of 45% for those years. Furthermore, taking into account 'school' and 'social class' factors, 22 out of the 28 achieved the same or better than their peers and 12 out of 16 achieved as well as or better than siblings. The sample is small, too small for sweeping generalizations to be made and 'factors other than communication approach' may have been operating. Nonetheless, it can be said with certainty that these 'successful' pupils had an education that did not include signs or sign language.

Audiological technology has been advancing steadily from the days of reported 'oral failure', as have educational practices towards more natural language experience (Clark, 1989) and more natural language environments in mainstream schools (Lynas, 1986). Those advocating an auditory-oral approach claim that the fruits of improved technology and educational practice can already be seen in the outcomes reported by the Ewing study (Lewis and Hostler, 1998). This is despite the fact that even 10 years ago, technology was not as effective in exploiting and augmenting residual hearing as is it is now.

The current auditory-oral position stakes its claim primarily on the fact that all children have residual hearing and, with the aid of recent technology, hearing can be harnessed and enhanced to provide sufficient auditory information to the deaf child's brain to enable speech to be perceived and produced. There have been enormous technological breakthroughs over the last decade and oralists argue that technology, if employed properly, can minimize the negative consequences of deafness: 'oral failure' should be seen as a thing of the past.

Advances in technology

The major breakthroughs that give the present-day oralist so much confidence are:

- Digital, programmable, 'smart' hearing aids that give a clear speech signal, which reduce background noise and which are customized to suit the needs of an individual hearing impairment (Ross, 1997).
- The prospect in the very near future in the UK of universal neonatal screening for hearing impairment (Davis et al., 1997). This means that sensorineural hearing impairment can be detected at birth and hearing aids fitted within the first month after detection. The importance of amplifying the hearing of severely and profoundly deaf children during the first six months cannot be underestimated: the first months of life has been shown by scientists to be crucial to the development of the

auditory processing mechanisms of the brain (Jusczyk, 1997). If the deaf child's auditory mechanisms can be activated during this early period, when hearing aid rejection is unlikely, then the foundations for speech discrimination are laid in a similar way to those of hearing children. Indeed research from the US on the speech perception and speech production of deaf children diagnosed and fitted with hearing aids before six months offers the remarkable but welcome finding that age-appropriate spoken language reception and production can be expected for most deaf children (Yoshinago-Itano, 1998).

- The growth in availability of cochlear implantation for young deaf children (Edwards and Tyszkiewicz, 1999). The success of cochlear implantation in significantly improving the hearing capacity of deaf adults and older deaf children has led to greater confidence in the use of this surgical procedure with young children. Implantation is now widely available to profoundly deaf children in the UK at the age of around two years. Luterman et al. (1999), writing in the US, claims that 'cochlear implants . . . are producing a new kind of child – "the hard of hearing deaf child".' Furthermore, he claims that improved technology will further enhance the effectiveness of cochlear implants in the future.

If deaf children can be enabled to hear from an early age and are offered sensitive spoken language input then they should be able to acquire spoken language during the language-sensitive first five years. They should, with appropriate support, be able to attend their local mainstream school and achieve according to their intellectual potential. Whilst 'technology changes everything', according to current auditory-oral thinking, hearing aids and implants remain complex, fiddly devices that are capable of breaking down. Survey after survey of hearing aid use in schools indicates under-utilization of technology (Ross, 1992). In the UK, however, the expectations of standards of audiological management required of professionals continue to rise (NDCS, 1998; Davis, Gregory and Bamford, 1999) and this includes enabling parents and deaf children themselves to take responsibility for good audiological care. It is perhaps more crucial than ever before that professionals working in the health services, particularly in audiology, work closely with professionals in education if the potential benefits to deaf children of current technology are to be realized.

According to Luterman et al. (1999) the 'technological revolution we are currently experiencing . . . will tip the balance in favour of' the oralists. He believes that the 'bilingual/bicultural movement' will decline in influence and popularity: 'They are fighting yesterday's wars.' However, this does not mean that there is no need for sign language in a deaf individual's life nor that a signing deaf community has no place. Orally educated deaf young people may derive strength from their affiliations at deaf clubs and many learn signs during the latter years at school or on leaving school (Gregory et al., 1995). Furthermore, success in spoken language does not guarantee deaf children a future that is problem free.

A deaf individual, however successful in acquiring verbal language, intelligible speech and literacy, remains deaf. The deaf child and the deaf adult who resides in the mainstream of the hearing-speaking world will experience day-in, day-out problems in grasping all that is said, particularly in informal social situations. It takes strength and a high degree of self-confidence to know and accept the real limitations of a substantial hearing impairment and rise above them. A deaf child might have that confidence as a child in the context of the support and protection offered by families and the professionals whose job it is to promote access to education and a healthy self-image. However, that same deaf individual in the less-protected world of adulthood may lose confidence. As Ross (1992) has insightfully commented, deaf 'audiologic successes' might 'eventually come to an identity crisis which they must painfully resolve'.

The pure auditory-oral approach, then, has its problems but advocates would argue that it is the best option 'on balance' and the one that offers the deaf individual the greater opportunities and choice in life. 'There is more to life than being deaf', so it is argued, and the use of an auditory-oral approach allows the deaf individual participation in the wider society and all the very many cultural and interest groups that exist within a diverse society such as Britain. There are plenty of opportunities for deaf individuals to become part of the 'deaf world' if they want to do so. No one is stopping deaf children/young people learning sign language or joining the local deaf club when they are of an age to make that choice for themselves. Deaf children reared and educated in environments where sign language predominates, so oralists would argue, are in danger of losing for ever the opportunity to perceive speech and learn to talk. Deaf children, especially those with the greater hearing impairments, who have sign language as a first language selected for them may not have much choice as adults except to have a social identity as a deaf person.

Choice in communication approach

That 'good achievement' during the school years can, by and large, be predicted for most deaf children through an auditory-oral approach does not of itself prescribe an oral approach for all deaf children at all stages of their education. Children, with disorders over and above deafness may not benefit from modern technology however up-to-date and well managed.

Some parents, whether themselves deaf or hearing, may prefer their deaf child to have access to a signing deaf culture from an early age in order to establish their child's right to a deaf identity. Some children may show a persistent preference for communication through visual signs rather than speech. At the secondary and post-16 stage of education, for some deaf students in some teaching contexts, it might be more effective to deliver information through sign language than through spoken language. For reasons of physiology, not all deaf children can have cochlear implants and for reasons not yet known, a tiny minority of deaf children appear to gain no benefits to audition having had an implant (Edwards and Tyszkiewicz, 1999). There will always be some deaf children who do not have their hearing impairments detected early despite 'universal' neonatal screening.

So, if all deaf children are to have access to the fundamental right to communication, and if parents are to have real choices, it is to be welcomed that there are, within the UK, communication options. Local education authority services in the UK are increasingly offering more than just one communication approach (Eatough, 1995), but it is *not* the case that all three approaches are available in each LEA area. What is 'standard practice' in one LEA, or district within an LEA, may be unobtainable in another area. For example, in many LEAs, an auditory-oral education for profoundly deaf children is not available because *all* profoundly deaf children are believed to need sign support or sign language. In some LEAs sign language options are not available in the local area, though may be available 'out of district'. It is equally important that parents and professionals who do not work in the education service are aware that there are discrepancies between the communication 'options' offered and the *quality* of that provision. That communication options are 'available' does not mean that the different approaches are being delivered effectively. The bilingual option particularly, has very difficult and demanding requirements and it is acknowledged by some bilingualists that this approach will fail if not properly implemented or thought through (Pickersgill, 1997). That different communication options for deaf children appear to be available should not delude anyone into thinking that what is actually on offer is necessarily a faithful realization of a particular approach.

Parents who are unhappy with the advice they receive from the professionals in their local area, or the educational practices they observe, can be advised to seek a second opinion. If parents feel that a sign approach is being 'foisted' on them, then DELTA, the Deaf Education through Listening and Talking Association, or the Ewing Foundation, might be approached to offer advice. If parents believe that the auditory-oral approach offered is not suitable for their child, then NDCS, the National Deaf Children's Society, can offer a range of alternative advice.

Decisions about selection of communication approach are determined as much by the ideas of adults as by intrinsic, unalterable features of the child. It would be so much easier if it were otherwise and the approach selected could be dictated simply by the 'needs' of the child. The most important factor, perhaps, is which of the alternative options available to the young child will be least constraining and which will leave most options open to the deaf child on becoming an adult. It is this consideration that should be uppermost in the minds of those making the choice on behalf of the deaf infant.

CHAPTER 25

Education of the hearing-impaired child

C POWELL AND I TUCKER

Introduction

At the beginning of the new millennium, we can be confident that the revolution in the education of deaf children that has taken place during the past quarter of a century will continue for several more decades. It is likely that by the year 2050 childhood deafness will remain a significant problem only in the developing countries of the world. However, even in the West, we still have to manage several generations of deaf children before we reach that stage.

The field is still riven by controversy. No chapter on the current-day education of deaf children can ignore the centuries' old division between those who favour the use of manual sign systems as the principle medium through which the curriculum should be delivered and those who favour an auditory/oral approach and spoken language. But the argument is rapidly changing to one that is essentially political rather than educational. It is now more about the rights of minority groups, in this case the deaf community, and respect for their language and culture rather than educational achievement. Former claims that deaf children educated in systems that use signs (such as total communication and bilingualism) will reach a higher level of educational attainment and literacy than those following sign-free approaches are less widely heard, because they have not been borne out by the findings of research. On the contrary, the most recent evidence, certainly in the UK, shows that, by the time they reach the end of their period of compulsory education, deaf pupils educated in a system that focuses on the use of the spoken word, backed up by appropriate and consistent use of the latest technology and with some regard to the acoustic environment, are the highest achieving group of deaf pupils. In many cases their attainments are as high as those of their hearing peers, who have not had to deal with a profound or severe hearing impairment.

Education systems vary from country to country and each is subject to periods of vigorous change, followed by periods of relative stability. There are marked differences between some countries and great similarities amongst others. This chapter draws primarily on the current situation in the UK, because, in its diversity, this reflects most of the major issues that face those involved in the education of deaf children today.

Definitions

The word 'deaf' encompasses all degrees of hearing impairment, from the mildest of conditions where a person may have some difficulty in discriminating speech in some situations for some of the time, to those very rare occurrences where there is a total absence of hearing. Clearly, in children, the degree of hearing impairment is a major consideration when determining the type of educational management that would be most beneficial. It is important, therefore, that the adjectives used to describe the degree of deafness should be precise so that, if need be, accurate comparisons can be made. In Britain the following definitions have been adopted by the principal professional organizations concerned with hearing impairment:

Mild: <40 dB HL average.
Moderate: 41–70 dB HL average.
Severe: 71–95 dB HL average.
Profound: >96 dB HL average.

Values are derived from a conventional pure-tone audiogram and are calculated by taking the average of the levels found at the five octave frequencies, 250 Hz–4 kHz. If there is a 'no response' at any of these five frequencies the arbitrary value of 130 dB HL is substituted for the basis of the calculation. The degree of hearing impairment is recorded as that of the better ear – the ear with the lower calculated value. So a person with no measurable hearing in one ear and an average of 43 dB HL in the other would be defined as having a 'moderate' hearing impairment. Note that the British system takes the average of five frequency values rather than the three values of the Fletcher Index that is frequently used in the US. As hearing-impaired people usually have more hearing in the lower frequencies, the effect of this difference in calculation method is for the Fletcher Index to record a slightly greater degree of loss than when using the British method. Also the boundary for profound hearing impairment is higher in Britain at 96 dB HL, compared to 90 dB SPL usually used in the US.

The problem

As a result of medical advances the numbers of children being born severely or profoundly deaf, or who develop deafness before spoken language is established – the pre-lingually deaf – reduced considerably during the latter part of the twentieth century. Immunization against rubella in young women and the virtual elimination of deafness resulting from rhesus incompatibility, coupled with more advanced special care baby units for babies who have problems at birth (and better ante-natal care generally) have had a considerable impact. The numbers of deaf babies have reduced significantly, but the number whose deafness is genetic in origin, especially an autosomal recessive type, has probably remained relatively unchanged. As a consequence the proportion of children born with deafness from a genetic origin has increased, and this is now the major cause of deafness in children in Britain.

The great majority of congenitally deaf children, probably now more than 95%, are born into families where both parents are hearing, and where spoken language is used in the home. Congenital deafness also seems to affect all sections of society equally, and, with the exception of babies from an Asian background where it is significantly greater, the prevalence amongst ethnic minority groups appears to reflect that of society as a whole.

Total numbers are small. Evidence collected in a recent survey of prevalence (Davis et al., 1997) suggests that only about 350 children are born each year in the UK with a severe or a profound hearing impairment (more or less equally divided between the two categories suggesting a prevalence of 0.47 per 1000 live births). If one includes those with moderate hearing impairment, the figure rises to 840. In January 1998 (BATOD, 1998) there were just over 4400 children with severe and profound hearing impairments undergoing their 11 years of compulsory education in England. This gives an average yearly cohort size of approximately 400, but of course this includes those whose hearing impairment was not congenital but acquired. Just under one-third of these pupils attended special schools for the deaf, and of these just under 28% were severely deaf, the remainder having a profound hearing impairment. Those not attending a special school were being educated either wholly in mainstream classes supported by peripatetic teachers of the deaf, or in mainstream schools that incorporated special units for hearing-impaired pupils where additional support could be given.

With such a low incidence of disability it is clearly impractical for the whole range of educational provision to be supported in each locality. This can cause difficulties if the type of programme the child needs, or that the parents are seeking, is not available locally, for example, for a deaf child of deaf parents who wish their child to be educated through the use of British Sign Language. In such circumstances the only viable solution may be for the child to live away from home in a specialist boarding school.

Role of the parent and parental wishes

It has long been accepted that parents have an important role to play in the education of their children. This role becomes crucially important where the children are deaf, particularly in respect of the pre-school acquisition of the language of the home by the child. It is, however, salutary to remember that only 30 years ago the practice was to place severely and profoundly deaf pupils in special schools for the deaf, many of them from the age of two, and many of them in boarding schools. There was a shortage of places and there was a national campaign to increase the number of nursery class places available in special schools. The prevailing view was that teaching language to a severely or profoundly deaf child was such a difficult and onerous task that it could be entrusted only to those who had received specialist training as teachers of the deaf. Lacking the necessary training, parents were not up to the task.

However opinions were changing rapidly. Parent guidance programmes, which had been pioneered by Professor Sir Alexander Ewing and his first wife Lady Irene Ewing at Manchester University were bearing fruit, demonstrating that, providing they were given regular support and appropriate training, parents were more effective 'teachers' of their children as far as language development was concerned than those who were professionally qualified. The demand for nursery places in special schools, especially residential places, fell away. Some new purpose-built nursery departments attached to special schools were never occupied by the pupils for whom they were intended. Formal recognition of the vital role of parents came with the publication in 1978 of the Government 'Report of the Committee of Enquiry into the Education of Handicapped Children and Young People' – the Warnock Report (HMSO, 1978). Paragraph 5.3 states: 'In the earliest years parents rather than teachers should be regarded wherever possible as the main educators of their children.' However the report recognized that most parents would not have all the necessary skills and suggested ways in which they could be helped to develop them. It called for the further development of peripatetic teaching services for children of pre-school age with teachers working with parents in their homes. Interestingly the unique nature of sensory disability was recognized and this is reflected in paragraph 5.37 where the Committee writes 'in view of the specific skills required for their teaching, children with sensory disabilities should be visited by teachers with related expertise'.

For the first time, the report gave official sanction to the concept of parents as partners in the education of their children. 'We have insisted throughout this report that the successful education of children with special educational needs depends upon the full involvement of their parents: indeed, unless their parents are seen as equal partners in the educational process the purpose of our report will be frustrated' (HMSO, 1978). Notice the use of the word 'equal' partners. This theme of partnership has been re-iterated since the Warnock Report in many government publications, culminating in the Education Acts 1981 and 1993 – the later Act establishing the current framework for special education. Referring to this Act the updated parents' charter, *Our Children's Education*, published by the Department for Education in 1994 says, 'These changes will benefit children with special needs, promoting partnership between their parents and all those involved in special education.'

Slowly the influence of parents increased as they gradually grew into their role as partners, and in time this extended to the assessment of their child's special educational needs and the educational provision that is required to ensure that those needs are met. Following the publication of the Warnock Report, the Education Act 1981 laid down that the special educational needs of children with handicapping conditions that resulted in learning difficulties should be recorded in a 'statement of special educational needs'. The process was refined by the Education Act 1993, which also established the Special Educational Needs Tribunal, an independent body to which parents in dispute with their local education authority (LEA) in respect of their child's special educational needs could appeal. The 1993 Act also required the Secretary of State for Education to issue a 'Code of Practice' (DFE, 1994a) to provide guidance to all LEAs and governing bodies of schools on their responsibilities to children with special educational needs. The code advises that 'children with special educational needs require the greatest access to a broad and balanced education, including the National Curriculum'. At the time of writing this Code, published in 1994, is undergoing revision.

The statement of special educational needs, which has legal status, is drawn up following a period of multidisciplinary assessment of the child's special needs. Parents are involved throughout this process, contributing as they feel appropriate. The 'statement' has several parts but the key ones are Parts 2, 3 and 4, which are the description of the child's learning difficulties and special educational needs, the educational provision that should be made to ensure that these identified needs are met, and the school or educational establishment where this provision can be made. Parents have a right to state a preference for the school that they wish their child to attend, and the local educational authority must comply with that request unless

- the school is unsuitable to the child's age, ability, aptitude and special educational needs;
- the placement would be incompatible with the efficient education of the other children with whom the child would be educated;
- the placement is incompatible with the efficient use of resources.

Notice that parents are not able to choose a school for their child; they have a right only to state a preference. If the local educational authority does not agree with this preference and refuses to place the child at the school chosen by the parents, parents have the right to appeal to a Special Educational Needs Tribunal, the independent body set up by the government, to adjudicate between the two parties. Parents also have a right to appeal against Parts 2 and 3 of the 'statement' if they believe that their child's strengths, weaknesses and special needs have not been properly described, or if they believe that the provision set out to meet those needs is not appropriate.

Segregation, integration, inclusion

For many years, in developed countries, there has been pressure to educate children with disabilities in ordinary schools, and in respect of deafness this gathered pace in the 1950s with the setting up of special units sited within ordinary schools. This movement has now taken on a political dimension with government policies actively seeking the 'inclusion' of people on the margins of society, the poor, the unemployed and including those with disabilities. Indeed the British government has set up a high-level unit attached to the Cabinet Office, The Social Exclusion Unit, to try to ensure that nobody is shut out from the mainstream of society (*The Economist,* 8 January 2000).

In education then the political definition of 'inclusion'/'integration' refers to the right of all children regardless of level of disability to attend mainstream schools. Special schools then become defined as 'segregated' (second class) provision. The whole issue is closely linked to human rights with the clear implication that denial of a mainstream place would be denial of a human right. Farrell (2000) argues that the aforementioned does not sit easily with the 'right' of parents to 'continue to have a right to express a preference for a special school where they consider this appropriate to their child's need' (DfEE Chapter 4, Paragraph 4) or the intention expressed in *Meeting Special Educational Needs: a Programme for Action* (DfEE, 1998) of 'promoting inclusion within mainstream schools where parents want it and appropriate support can be provided' (DfEE Chapter 3, Paragraph 1).

Farrell then asks which parents would wish to choose a placement for their child if it overlooks a 'human right'? The present authors believe that parents are far more pragmatic than politicians and that they would wish to choose the mode of educational delivery that they believed offered the child the greatest opportunities for making educational and social progress and the best chances either now or in the future of inclusion into mainstream society.

Farrell goes on to argue that education in the mainstream is not a human right and presses that the term 'educational inclusion' is what we should be seeking. This would give equal value to the different venues of education and the measure of success would become the educational appropriateness of the placement. This view is in line with the thinking within the special needs profession and there have been many attempts to establish a definition of inclusion that reflects this.

The National Deaf Children's Society *Quality Standards in Education for England* (1999) defines inclusion in the following terms:

> Inclusion is best seen as a set of principles or a statement of values and attitudes that:
>
> - assume that all pupils have a right to be educated in their local school but
> - promote the whole society approach to disability and difference that transcends concerns with schools and education in a search to create an inclusive society
> - seek to maximise opportunity, independence, participation and achievement for all pupils according to individual needs and wishes
> - recognise that, as well as concerns for the need of individual children, there are also concerns for the needs of society and the community (including the school).

The first bullet point is at odds with Farrell's view and we would take the line that parents have the right to have the special educational needs of their children met, but that the venue is only one issue of many which need to be debated in coming to that view.

In our view a more rounded definition is that of National Association of Special Educational Needs (NASEN), which defines 'inclusion' as follows:

> Inclusion is not a simple concept, restricted to issues of placement. Its definition has to encompass broad notions of educational access and recognise the importance of catering for diverse needs. Moreover, inclusive principles highlight the importance of meeting children's individual needs, of working in partnership with pupils and their parents/carers and of involving teachers and schools in the development of more inclusive approaches. Inclusion is a *process* not a state.

Clearly the attitudes of those who manage and teach in the mainstream are a key contributor to the success of pupils with disability who are educated in the mainstream.

Special school versus mainstream

Whilst recognizing a continuing need for some children to be educated in special schools, we have shown that legislation and government publications in recent years have all stressed the desirability of children with special educational needs being educated alongside ordinary children in mainstream schools. As a result there has been a thrust by LEAs to place children with hearing impairment in ordinary schools and, because this is usually a cheaper option, this thrust has been strongly reinforced by financial considerations. In 1993 the Education Act formally laid a qualified duty on LEAs to secure education of children with special educational needs in ordinary schools. The political 'buzz word' changed from 'integration' to 'inclusion' and we have commented on this in more detail above. However the absence of a suitable and agreed definition of 'inclusion' has meant that many LEAs simply, and conveniently, regard it as a synonym for integration! Interestingly in 1994 UNESCO issued a statement on special needs education that has become known as the Salamanca Agreement (UNESCO, 1994). The government of the day was a signatory to that agreement, which strongly promotes the concept of inclusion *except for deaf and deaf/blind persons:* 'Owing to the particular communication needs of deaf and deaf/blind persons, their education may be more suitably provided in schools for such persons or special classes and units in mainstream schools.' As in the Warnock Report, the World Conference recognized the unique nature of deafness as an obstacle to education.

As a result of these influences there has been a strong trend away from placing deaf children in special schools for their education. Apart from a small number of deaf children attending special schools catering for learning difficulties other than those caused by deafness, the survey of deaf children in England carried out in 1998 by the British Association of Teachers of the Deaf (BATOD 1998), only 32% of those with a profound or severe hearing impairment attended a special school for the deaf. The remaining 68% were all receiving their education in ordinary schools, although two-thirds of these schools had special units attached to them. Only a very small number of children with a moderate hearing impairment attend a special school for the deaf.

The type of provision made by special schools for the deaf is fairly straightforward. Children are educated in small classes of usually no more than 10 pupils, taught by specialist teachers of the deaf. Regardless of the communication approach being used, the classrooms are usually well treated acoustically, with reverberation and noise levels carefully controlled so that hearing aids can be used effectively. The use of personal hearing aids is also frequently supplemented with the use of radio hearing aid systems or headphone amplification systems such as auditory training units or group hearing aids. The latter provide the best form of amplification available, because all children are able to hear themselves and every other child in the class at optimum listening levels. There is also considerably less distortion with these systems. Because of the low incidence of severe and profound deafness, most special schools for the deaf have residential provision, consequently there is the problem of being segregated from society at large. However, special schools are aware of this danger and some go to great lengths to combat it. This is clearly more difficult where some form of manual communication is adopted by the school for its teaching. Only large cities are able to run a viable day school for the deaf, and even where this is the case, the numbers on roll are small. Several special school closures have occurred during the past decade as a result of falling rolls, and in 1998 there were only 40 special schools for the deaf in the whole of the UK.

Types of mainstream placement are more varied. There is a range of options, for example:

- Complete integration or mainstreaming within the ordinary class without any supportive help.
- Mainstreaming with varying levels of individual support.
- Basing the child in a resource room or base unit and integrating the child on a part-time basis into the ordinary class. The subjects for which the child integrates can also vary.
- Team teaching by the ordinary teacher and a teacher of the deaf of an integrated class into which is placed one hearing-impaired child or more.
- Reversed mainstreaming where normal-hearing pupils become part of a class of hearing-impaired pupils. This is less common, but seems to be done more frequently at the nursery end where the educators of the

hearing-impaired place high value on the influence of ordinary children and set up a nursery to attract in ordinary children to mix with the hearing-impaired. Nursery places are difficult to find in many areas and this seems to be a successful route to integration of such children.

- Self-contained classes or units from which pupils go to ordinary classes for one or more specific academic subjects.
- Self-contained classes or units from which pupils go to ordinary classes for one or more non-academic activities.
- Completely self-contained classes or units with little or no contact with normal-hearing peers.

Of these options, mainstreaming with varying levels of support, and the 'resource', or 'base', unit are becoming the most popular. Both offer a level of flexibility that enables an individual programme to be changed as the child's individual special needs change. It also allows planners to be more flexible in their use of resources. The problem presented by resource units is that often the child has to make a considerable journey away from his home area in order to attend. This usually entails a taxi journey and this can often make it difficult for the child to participate in after school extra-curricular activities. Also of course, when he gets home there are no school friends to play with. This can lead to social isolation in the home area, unless positive steps are taken to overcome this. The advantages are that there is usually a teacher of the deaf on the premises who is able to provide intensive help and follow-up work with language development and in areas of the curriculum with which the child is having some difficulty. This teacher is also able to check and ensure that the amplification equipment used by the child is in good working order, or if not arrange for it to be repaired. The specialist resource-base classroom is also often acoustically treated, making it easier for the child to use his hearing aids more effectively. Mainstream classrooms are generally not acoustically treated and even when using a radio aid system the child will have difficulty in following what is happening in the classroom if background noise levels are not very carefully controlled by the teacher.

Where there is no specialist resource base in school it may be difficult for a teacher of the deaf supporting a child to find an area that is sufficiently quiet for intensive work to take place. Usually the support from a teacher of the deaf comes from a peripatetic teacher who visits the child in school on a regular basis. The frequency and duration of these visits will vary according to a child's individual needs (and resources available). Some children will receive daily visits and some only one a term. Part 3 of a child's statement of special educational needs, which outlines the provision required, should be 'specific, detailed and quantified' and should record the frequency and duration of such visits, or the total time allocation per week or per term.

Most children who spend the majority of their time in mainstream classrooms will be provided with some form of individual support either from teachers who are not qualified to teach deaf children, or more usually from classroom support assistants. A number of different nomenclatures are used to describe such personnel, from 'special needs assistant' to 'human aids to communication' but their role is essentially the same. It is to facilitate access to the curriculum for the child. The method of facilitation will vary from child to child and may take the form of simple note taking, lip speaking or a signed commentary on the content of the lesson. The support assistant will also provide differing degrees of help in completing the tasks that children are set. The problem inherent in this system is that the child may have more difficulty developing independent learning skills and may become overly dependent on his support assistant. It can also mean that the child does not access the curriculum directly for himself, but through an intermediary who may know little of the subject matter being taught, which in the secondary school curriculum can be very wide ranging – anything from Spanish to physics to economics.

A further problem that severely and profoundly deaf children have to overcome in mainstream classes is how to participate in the classroom discussions that today have an important place in the curriculum. Most such children place considerable reliance on their lip reading ability. However, during classroom discussion sessions they will have difficulty in locating the speaker because the amplification equipment they use provides very little directional information. The speaker's voice could be coming from anywhere. Once they have located the speaker, the moment may have passed. But even if the speaker can be located in time, lip reading may be difficult because of distance, lighting or angle of view. If the children's own speech is sometimes difficult for their classmates to understand, they may be discouraged from participating actively in the proceedings. There may be strategies that the teacher can adopt to help overcome this problem but they tend to interfere with the pace of the lesson and to destroy its spontaneity.

A big advantage of provision in the neighbourhood mainstream school is that the child has more opportunity to be part of the local community. If he has been successful in establishing friendships at school, these friends will be probably be around after school. Participation in after school activities is likely to be less of a problem and local events that so frequently figure in playground chatter will be more meaningful. *However this does depend on the attitudes of the mainstream schools towards inclusion.*

Communication approaches

The chapter by Lynas earlier in this volume provides a detailed and excellent evidence base for making choices in communication methodology. However, it would be remiss of us not to briefly consider this area and interpret it in the light of current approaches being used in the practice of education with deaf children. As Lynas outlines there are now three broad categories of communication approach used with young deaf children, the auditory/oral approaches, sign bilingualism and total communication. Each of these groups has variations within it.

Total communication (TC), which its advocates prefer to refer to as a philosophy rather than an approach or method, is a loose conglomerate of practices that vary from school to school, class to class and child to child. However 'TC as generally practised involves the use of speech simultaneously with a sign version of all or part of the spoken utterance' (Lynas, 1995). Total communication is intended to foster the development of spoken English, and the signs that accompany it may be drawn from an established sign language, such as British Sign Language (BSL), but they are used in the same word order as English. The intention is to provide additional information that the child can use to decode the message and to provide a crutch that will facilitate language acquisition. However, unfortunately, the general goal of TC seems not to have been realized. It has been suggested that this is due to the interference of the signing that accompanies speech with the spoken pattern, and speech interfering with the fluency and synchronicity of the signing. Because the two stimuli, speech and signs, do not seem to fuse well together, the child receives two discrete signals each of which is more deficient of information than if either speech or sign were used on its own. The vital acoustic patterns of speech are distorted, and the comprehensiveness of the sign is lacking. A large survey by Allen (1986) in the US demonstrated that in spite of the huge amount of energy that went into the TC programme in the US, the standard of education achieved by students completing their education was no higher than it had been a decade or so earlier, before the introduction of TC.

Although the BATOD (1998) survey indicates that there are still large numbers of severely and profoundly deaf pupils in the UK following TC programmes (43.8%), the approach is now largely discredited as an educational solution to the problems of educating deaf children. Very few TC-educated pupils have successfully developed intelligible spoken language and their reading ability and educational attainments as indicated by public examination results are poor. 'Condemnation based on the overall failure of TC to raise the educational standards of deaf children and young people is shared by all critics' (Lynas, 1995). However, perhaps they have developed the skills needed to be part of the deaf community, and perhaps this is considered to be the most appropriate goal by deaf people themselves.

However, not all critics of TC believe that an auditory/oral approach should be used instead. Many 'believe that signs should be used in the education of deaf children, but not in combination with speech' (Lynas, 1995). The alternative that is being proposed is bilingualism or now more commonly 'sign bilingualism'. Under this system a natural sign language, such as British Sign Language (BSL) is used in the early stages of language development, until a measure of fluency is achieved. Then English is taught as a second language. It is however conceded that it may be extremely difficult for a severely or profoundly deaf child who has developed sign language as his first language to be given sufficient opportunity to develop his hearing well enough for spoken English to be a realistic goal. Therefore, for many deaf children written English, rather than spoken English, becomes the second language aim. Of course, competence in written English is an essential educational goal, since sign language itself does not have a written form, and the ability to read is crucial if the school curriculum is to be accessed effectively.

It is too early to judge the outcomes of bilingual programmes in this country but there is no evidence so far that, in terms of educational attainments or English literacy levels, such programmes are any more successful than TC programmes. Some studies (Weisel, Dromi and Dor, 1990; Gallaway and Woll, 1994) have indicated that many hearing parents have problems in learning sign and interacting effectively with their children through its means. Young children who attend specialized facilities where sign language is used may quickly come to outstrip their hearing parents in sign-language competence. In the home the key to the quality of the linguistic interaction that takes place is the competence of the weakest communicator. It seems inevitable that, in practice, hearing parents will quickly become the weaker linguistic members of the group, a situation that reverses the natural order of things. How important this is for the linguistic and more general development of the child has yet to be shown. The figures currently available indicate that 7.5% of severely and profoundly deaf children are following either BSL or sign bilingual programmes in the UK. There is as yet no indication that this number is growing, but such is the political thrust with which bilingualism is being promoted that it seems likely that it will.

The great majority of congenitally deaf children (95%) are born to hearing parents and the great majority of these parents would prefer their children to be able to talk and understand spoken language. It is not surprising therefore that the most commonly used communication approach in the UK is natural auralism, which is followed by 44.2% of the severely and profoundly deaf population of schoolchildren. It is used almost exclusively with children with more hearing than this. This far exceeds the use of other auditory/oral approaches such as the Structured Oral, or Maternal Reflective approaches, which between them are used with less than 3% of the population.

The natural aural approach concentrates on hearing and listening, and the use of natural spoken English. The approach has developed from the growth of knowledge, from the mid-1950s onwards, of acoustic phonetics and the normal processes of language acquisition in children. It is now widely held that if, from the moment of diagnosis, deaf children are given consistent and appropriate amplification, and a facilitatory linguistic environment where there is frequent exposure to meaningful spoken language, they will become very competent English language users by the end of their period of compulsory education. This view is borne out by the evidence of the educational achievements of children educated in this way. In terms of their literacy they outperform pupils educated through other approaches (Lewis, 1996); for pupils in special schools the attainments in public examinations, such as GCSE, of those being educated in auditory/oral schools is markedly better than those attending schools that use TC or bilingualism (DfEE, 1994 to 1998); and a recently executed but as yet unpublished research study by the Ewing Foundation has shown that severely and profoundly deaf pupils who have followed a natural aural approach in mainstream schools achieve GCSE examination results that are on a par with those of hearing children, and that their reading levels are very close to their chronological ages. The educational case for natural auralism is therefore a strong one, and has been enhanced by recent developments in amplification technology, which enables any residual hearing that a child may have to be exploited to the full. There is also the strong sociological argument that if deaf children can be educated in a way that enables them to use spoken English fluently as a means of communication, then social, educational and vocational opportunities are greatly increased.

Pre-school education

Regardless of the communication approach that parents choose to use with their offspring, the help and support that they receive during the pre-school years are crucial. In many LEAs, parents of young deaf children are visited regularly in their homes by peripatetic teachers of the deaf who seek to help parents create a language environment from which the child can benefit. Parents are shown how to check and maintain hearing aids, how to talk to their child, what to say and how to involve all members of the family so that as much interaction as possible takes place. Such work demands a high level of skill. Once the child is of nursery age, he might be placed in a nursery class. There still are special nursery classes for deaf children but the trend is very much for these children to be placed in the normal nursery or playgroup setting and be supported there by peripatetic teachers of the deaf and special needs support assistants. In many cases visits to the parents' home would still continue during this period, because it is recognized that parents have a vital role to play at this phase.

The National Curriculum: constraints opportunities and accountability

The National Curriculum, which was designed to help raise education standards, was first introduced into schools in England in 1989. It lays down the subject matter that must be covered for all ages of schoolchildren and the standards that they are expected to reach in each. In addition to requiring that the curriculum be broad and balanced, it recognizes the importance of three core subjects, English, mathematics and science. The attainments of all pupils in these core subjects are regularly assessed by the government-administered Standard Assessment Tests (SATs). All schoolchildren have a right to the National Curriculum, and this includes children with all degrees of deafness. However, in certain circumstances the National Curriculum may be modified for individual children, or they may even be excluded (disapplied) from part or all of it.

The government of the day recognized that if standards were to be raised they would need to be carefully monitored, so in addition to the specially designed SATs, results of the performance of the pupils in individual schools are published annually. This is part of a programme to make schools more accountable for the standard of education that they offered. Of course, some schools are more advantaged than others in terms of the quality of the intake of their pupils. Schools serving suburban middle-class areas would be expected to achieve better results in the tests than those in inner-city areas. To take account of these differences the government publishes historical data showing by how much a school has improved or deteriorated over a period of time. It is also currently investigating ways of recording 'value added' – the amount by which schools are able to increase the attainments of their pupils from a given baseline compared to national averages. It is perhaps interesting that in the first pilot survey of 'value added' by the DfEE the school that outperformed every other school in England was a special school for the deaf – Mary Hare Grammar School.

A further thrust towards ensuring greater accountability has been the reform of the system of school inspection with the creation of the Office for Standards in Education (OFSTED) (HMSO, 1992). All schools, including special schools, are now regularly inspected as part of a rolling programme. Unlike the DfEE School Inspectors, who had an advisory role as well as an inspectorial role, the newly created OFSTED inspectors have a duty simply to inspect and to publish their findings.

In the opinion of most commentators, the National Curriculum and the 'accountability' measures being undertaken are contributing to raising standards generally, and this is certainly true for deaf children. Regrettably the process frequently highlights the degree of underachievement of some of our deaf children. This may be uncomfortable knowledge for some of our teachers, but at least it raises awareness of the shortcomings of individual schools and the need for improvements to be made!

Post-compulsory education – college and university

Despite the lead given in the early part of the twentieth century by luminaries such as Thomas Arnold and his pupil Abraham Farrar, the entry into higher education by deaf people was slow in coming. It was really the vision of a famous teacher, Miss Mary Hare, who having developed a very successful private school, bequeathed in her will all her property, to be used for the establishment of a national grammar school for deaf children, that provided the breakthrough. Following her death, a school bearing her name was established in 1946. Since that time Mary Hare Grammar School for the Deaf has striven for academic excellence and today over three-quarters of its students gain places at British universities for undergraduate courses of study. Many continue to take higher degrees and other post-graduate qualifications. With the growth of numbers of deaf people with such qualifications, the opportunities for careers of a professional nature have greatly increased.

A number of LEAs and ordinary schools are now following the lead that Mary Hare has given, and although it is still not commonplace, there are individuals with a severe or profound hearing impairment who have attended mainstream schools and then carried on to university for a degree course. However, many mainstream schools do not have sixth forms where advanced study can be undertaken. The route for deaf students in these circumstances is through sixth-form colleges or colleges of further education, which although providing adult education generally, are set up to cater particularly for the needs of the 16–19 age group.

The nature and degree of support that deaf students receive when they attend university or other colleges varies considerably according to their individual needs. But the general principle is that grants of money are made available to the student to purchase any specialized equipment that may be necessary, and to pay for any support needed in terms of human aids to communication (note takers, sign language interpreters, and so forth).

Whatever the drawbacks of this system, there can be no doubt that the number of deaf people graduating each year from British universities is increasing steadily. We are moving into an age where increasingly well-qualified and well-educated deaf people are starting to occupy more prominent positions not only in the workplace but in society as a whole.

Advances in technology and medicine

Technological and medical developments that are currently taking place are likely to have an enormous impact on the educational consequences of deafness in children. The improvement in the performance of personal hearing aids has already had an impact. Very high-power hearing aids brought new listening experiences to deaf children. These will be augmented in the very near future by the introduction of high-power digital hearing aids, which will be able to process the signal in a way that should benefit the individual listener, and with the introduction of a programmable directional microphone option that will avoid the poorer low-frequency response often associated with directional microphones. Both of these developments should enhance the signal-to-noise ratio experienced by the hearing aid user. It has been claimed that for some systems this could lead to an improvement in the S/N ratio of as much as 10 dB. This will mean that listening through hearing aids in less-than-ideal acoustic conditions will be considerably easier.

Another development that has already had a dramatic effect is the cochlear implant. By implanting an electrode array directly into the cochlea it is possible to bypass damaged hair cells and trigger the afferent nerve cells directly by electrical stimulation. Where the neural pathways are intact this has resulted in subjects being able to detect sounds in the high frequencies that would be unavailable to them through conventional hearing aids. This has made a huge difference to some children implanted in infancy. There are cases of profoundly deaf children entering primary school at five with language development that is within normal limits – a situation unheard of a decade ago. In good listening conditions many are able to hold a social conversation without needing to lip read, and their own spoken language reflects the niceties and phatic communion that epitomizes human speech. Many are also able to use the telephone successfully. However, not all situations are favourable to the use of cochlear implants – users are just as vulnerable to the deleterious effects of background noise, and a good acoustic environment is necessary to ensure that the S/N ratio is good if they are to be used effectively.

Apart from paying greater attention to the acoustic treatment of rooms, another development that is being used in an attempt to enhance S/N ratios is sound field amplification. This system is designed primarily for hearing children and is essentially sound distribution equipment, similar to a public address system, which is installed in an ordinary classroom. The teacher wears a radio microphone and her amplified speech is transmitted to a number of loudspeakers strategically placed throughout the room. It is claimed that this enables pupils in the classroom to hear their teacher better and a consequence is that noise levels generally are reduced, further enhancing the S/N ratio. Currently trials of this system are taking place in mainstream classes where deaf children are placed. It seems unlikely that this will be as effective as full-scale acoustic-room treatment because it only enhances the teacher's voice, but it may be an acceptable compromise.

The development of universal neonatal screening programmes will also have an impact. Currently most congenitally deaf children are diagnosed between the ages of six months and three years. With the now realistic possibility of being able to identify deafness in newborn children within the first few days of life, the doors will be opened to much earlier intervention both in terms of amplification and training parents.

However, potentially the greatest advances will probably come from the medical field. Whilst it is still in its infancy, it seems likely that genetic engineering will have a major contribution to make. At the time of writing it seems likely that before the first quarter of the next millennium is over there will be a 'cure' for most forms of congenital deafness of genetic origin.

Conclusion

There is every reason to be optimistic as far as the education of deaf children is concerned. There have been many developments during the past half-century that have changed the education of deaf children out of all recognition. Our growth in knowledge of the language acquisition process, of acoustic phonetics and how even very tiny amounts of residual hearing can be effectively harnessed; medical advances in the prevention of childhood deafness caused by the rubella virus, by rhesus incompatibility, difficult births and a greater awareness of ototoxic drugs; the impact of technology with the development of sophisticated amplification systems and the introduction of cochlear implantation; our understanding of the critical importance of the acoustic environment and the establishment of the role of parents as partners in the educational process, have all resulted in more effective educational management of deaf children. The major distraction of the long-standing debate regarding methods of communication, whilst still vigorous, is nearing its end as spoken language, used in conjunction with the latest technology, linguistic knowledge and the latest educational practices, asserts itself as the more effective way to educate deaf children, as well as being more in keeping with the wishes of parents. The future for deaf children today is brighter than it has ever been, and the century that has just begun will undoubtedly see an end to deafness as a major barrier to education.

References

Abdelhak S, Kalatzis V, Heilig R et al. (1997) A human homologue of the drosophila eyes absent gene underlies branchio-oto-renal (BOR) syndrome and identifies a novel gene family. Nature Genetics 15: 157–64.

Abramovitch SJ, Gregory S, Slemick M, Stewart A (1979) Hearing loss in very low birth-weight infants treated with neonatal intensive care. Archives of Diseases in Childhood 54: 421–6.

Ackerman J, Sutherland H, Young A (1997) A practice report: bilingual/bicultural workshops for hearing families. Deafness and Education 21: 58–61.

Adamson LB, Bakeman R, Smith CB (1990) Gestures, words and early object sharing. In Volterra V, Erting CJ (eds) From Gesture to Language in Hearing and Deaf Children. Heidelberg: Springer-Verlag.

Ahlgren I (1994) Sign language as the first language. In Ahlgren I, Hyltenstam K (eds) Bilingualism in Deaf Education: Proceedings of the international conference on bilingualism in deaf education, Stockholm, Sweden. International studies on sign language and communication of the deaf, Vol.27. Hamburg, Germany: Signum-Verlag Press.

Aitchison J (1987) Words in the Mind. Oxford: Blackwell.

Alberti PW (1995) The effect of noise on children and adolescents. Journal of Audiological Medicine 4: ii–viii.

Alberti PW, Hyde ML Corbin H et al. (1983) An evaluation of BERA for hearing screening in high risk neonates. Laryngoscope 93: 1115–121.

Alford CA, Stagno S, Pass RF, Britt WJ (1990) Congenital and perinatal cytomegalovirus infection. Review of Infectious Diseases 12: S745–S753.

Allen SE, Dyar D (1997) Profiling linguistic outcomes in young children after cochlear implantation. American Journal of Otology 18 (Suppl. 6): S127–8.

Allen T (1986) Patterns of academic achievement among hearing-impaired students: 1974 and 1983. In Schildroth A, Karchnmer M (eds) Deaf Children in America. San Diego, CA: College-Hill Press.

Alvarez LS, Navascues J (1990) Shaping, invagination and closure of the chick embryo otic vesicle: scanning electron microscopic and quantitative study. The Anatomical Record 228: 315–26.

American Academy of Pediatrics. (1997) Committee on Environmental Health. Pediatrics 100: 724–7.

American Academy of Pediatrics Task Force on Newborn and Infant Hearing (1999) Newborn and infant hearing loss: Detection and intervention. Pediatrics 103: 527–9.

Anand NK, Gupta AK, Raj H (1991) Auditory brainstem response in neonates with hypoxic-ischemic-encephalopathy following perinatal asphyxia. Indian Pediatrics 28: 901–7.

Anastasi A (1982) Psychological Testing. New York: Macmillan.

Anderson K (1989) Screening Instrument for Targeting Educational Risk (SIFTER). Little Rock AR: Educational Audiology Association Products Manager.

Anderson KL (1992) Keys to effective hearing conservation programs: hearing status of school age children. In Cherow E (ed.) Proceedings of the ASHA Audiology Superconference. ASHA 21: 38–47.

Aniansson G, Alm B, Andersson D et al.(1994) A prospective cohort study on breast feeding and otitis media in Swedish infants. Pediatric Infectious Disease Journal 13: 183–88.

Aniko M, Sobin A (1987) Ethacrynic acid effects on the isolated inner ear: evaluation of the ototoxic potential in an organ culture system. American Journal of Otolaryngology 8: 48–62.

Anson BJ, Donaldson JA (1981) Surgical Anatomy of the Temporal Bone. Philadelphia, PA: WB Saunders Co.

Antia S (1982) Social interaction of partially mainstreamed hearing impaired children. American Annals of the Deaf 127: 18–25.

Antia S (1994) Strategies to develop peer interaction in young hearing impaired children. Volta Review 96: 277–90.

Anvar B, Mencher GT, Keet SJ (1984) Hearing loss and congenital rubella in Atlantic Canada. Ear and Hearing 5: 340–5.

Arcand P, Desrosiers M, Dube J, Abela A (1991) The large vestibular aqueduct syndrome and sensorineural hearing loss in the paediatric population. Journal of Otolaryngology 20: 247–50.

Arlinger SD, Billermark E (1997) Hearing threshold for speech using insert earphones and supra-aural earphones. Scandinavian Audiology 26: 151-4.

Arnold P (1982) Oralism and the deaf child's brain: a reply to Dr Conrad. International Journal of Pediatric Otorhinolaryngology 4: 275–86.

Arthur RM, Pfeiffer RR, Suga N (1971) Properties of 'two-tone inhibition' in primary auditory neurones. Journal of Physiology 212: 593–609.

ASHA (1994) Joint Committee on Infant Hearing 1994 Position Statement. ASHA 38–41.

ASHA (1996) American Speech Language Hearing Association. Task Force on Central Auditory Processing Consensus Development. American Journal of Audiology 5: 41–54.

Astington JW, Jenkins JM (1995) Theory of mind development and social understanding. In Connections between Emotions and Understanding in Development. Hove: Lawrence Erlbaum Associates.

Atlas MD, Chai F, Boscato L (1998) Ménière's disease: evidence of an immune process. American Journal of Otology 19: 628–31.

Azema B, Virole V, Huyghe V et al. (1994) Effect of a hearing aid on progressive hearing loss. Annals Otolaryngologie Chirurgie Cervicofaciale 111: 239–47.

Babbidge HS (1965) Education of the Deaf. A Report to the Secretary of Health, Education, and Welfare by his Advisory Committee on the Education of the Deaf. Washington, DC: US Government Printing Office 0-765-119.

Bachmann KR, Hall JW III (1998) Pediatric auditory brainstem response assessment: The cross-check principle 20 years later. Seminars in Hearing 19: 41–60.

Bachor E, Karmody C (1995) Endolymphatic hydrops in children. Otorhinolaryngology 57: 129–34.

Bailey ML, Kirkpatrick CMJ, Begg EJ (1999) Once daily aminoglycoside therapy. Clinical Pharmacokinetics 36: 89–98.

Baird G, Charman T, Baron-Cohen S et al. (2000) A screening instrument for autism at 18 months of age: a 6 year follow-up study. Journal of the American Academy of Child and Adolescent Psychiatry 39: 694–703.

Baker C (1978) How does 'sim-com' fit into a bilingual approach to education? In Caccamise F, Hicks D (eds) American Sign Language in a Bilingual Context: Proceedings of the second national symposium on sign language research and teaching. Silver Spring, MD: National Association of the Deaf.

Baker L, Cantwell DP (1982) Psychiatric disorder in children with different types of communication disorder. Journal of Communication Disorders 15: 113–26.

Balcarek KB, Warren W, Smith RJ et al. (1993) Neonatal screening for congenital cytomegalovirus infection by detection of virus in saliva. Journal of Infectious Diseases 167: 1433–6.

Baldwin CT, Hoth CF, Amos JA et al. (1992) An exonic mutation in the HuP2 paired domain gene causes Waardenburg's syndrome. Nature 355: 637–8.

Baldwin M, Watkin P (1992) The clinical applications of oo-acoustic emissions in paediatric audiological assessment. The Journal of Laryngology and Otology 106: 301–6.

Baldwin RL, Sweitzer RS, Friend DB (1985) Meningitis and sensorineural hearing loss. Laryngoscope 95: 802–5.

Baldwin S, Whitley RJ (1989) Teratogen update: Intrauterine herpes simplex virus infection. Teratology 39: 1–10.

Bamford J, McSporran E (1993) Evoked visual reinforcement audiometry. In McCormick B (ed.) Paediatric Audiology 0–5 years. 2 edn. London: Whurr Publishers.

Bamford JM, Saunders E (1991) Hearing Impairment, Auditory Perception and Language Disability. 2 edn. London: Whurr Publishers.

Baraff LJ, Lee SI, Schriger DL (1993) Outcomes of bacterial meningitis in children: a meta-analysis. Paediatric Infectious Diseases Journal 12: 389–94.

Baran JA, Musiek FE (1991) Behavioral assessment of the central auditory nervous system. In Rintleman WF (ed.) Hearing Assessment. 2 edn. Austin, TX: Pro-Ed.

Barclay ML, Kirkpatrick CMJ, Begg EJ (1999) Once daily dosage of aminoglycosides. Clinical Pharmacokinetics 36: 89–98.

Barker DF, Denison JC, Atkin CL, Gregory MC (1997) Common ancestry of three Ashkenazi-American families with Alport syndrome and COL4A5 R1677Q. Human Genetics 99: 681–4.

Baron-Cohen S, Cox AD, Baird G et al. (1996) Psychological markers in the detection of autism in infancy in a large population. British Journal of Psychiatry 168: 158–63.

Barr B, Wedenberg E (1965) Perceptive hearing loss in children with respect to genesis and the use of hearing aid. Annals of Otolaryngology and Rhinology 59: 462–74.

Bartels LJ, Gurucharri M (1988) Pediatric glomus tumors. Otolaryngology, Head and Neck Surgery 99: 392–5.

Basser L (1964) Benign paroxysmal vertigo of childhood. Brain 87: 141–6.

Bast TH, Anson BJ (1949) The Temporal Bone and the Ear. Philadelphia, PA: WB Saunders Co.

Bast TH, Anson BJ, Gardner WD (1947) The developmental course of the human auditory vesicle. Anatomical Record 99: 55 –74.

Batchava Y (1993) Antecedents of self-esteem in deaf people: a meta-analytic review. Rehabilitative Psychology 38: 221–34.

BATOD (British Association of Teachers of the Deaf) (1997) Deafness and Education 21: 3.

BATOD (British Association of Teachers of the Deaf) (1998) Deaf Children in England, Wales, Scotland, Northern Ireland. British Association of Teachers of the Deaf.

Battmer R-D, Laszig R, Lehnhardt E (1990) Electrically elicited stapedial reflex in cochlear implant patients. Ear and Hearing 11: 370–4.

Baumann NM, Kirby Keyser LJ, Dolan KD et al. (1994) Mondini dysplasia and congenital cytomegalovirus infection. Journal of Pediatrics 124: 71–8.

BDA (British Deaf Association) (1996) The Right to be Equal. British Deaf Association Education Policy Statement. London: British Deaf Association.

Bedore LM, Leonard LB (1998) Specific language impairment and grammatical morphology: a discriminant function analysis. Journal of Speech, Language and Hearing Research 41: 1185–92.

Belenky WM, Madgy DN, Leider JS et al. (1993) The enlarged vestibular aqueduct syndrome (EVA Syndrome). Ear, Nose and Throat Journal 72: 746–51.

Bellinger D (1979) Changes in the explicitness of mothers' directiveness as children age. Journal of Child Language 6: 443–58.

Bellis TJ (ed.) (1996) Central auditory processing disorders in the educational setting. San Diego, CA: Singular Publishing Group.

Bellman S (1987) Hearing disorders in children. British Medical Bulletin 43: 966–82.

Bellman S (1998) The effect of cochlear implantation on paediatric audiology. Seventh David Edward Hughes Lecture. May 29.

Bellman S, Marcuson M (1991) A new toy test to investigate the hearing status of young children who have English as a second language: A preliminary report. British Journal of Audiology 25: 317–22.

Bench R, Bamford J (1979) The Spoken Language of Hearing Impaired Children. London: Academic Press.

Bench RJ (1992) Communication Skills in Hearing-impaired Children. London: Whurr Publishers.

Bench RJ, Boscak N (1970) Some applications of signal detection theory to paedo-audiology. Sound 4: 58–61.

Bender R (1981) The Conquest of Deafness. Danville, IL: Interstate Publishers.

Bennett K, Haggard MP (1999) Behaviour and cognitive outcomes from middle ear disease. Archives of Disease in Childhood 80: 28–35.

Bennett MJ (1975) The auditory response cradle: A device for the objective assessment of auditory state in neonates. Symposium of the Zoological Society of London 37: 291–305.

Berg FS (1972) Educational Audiology: Hearing and speech management. New York: Grune & Stratton.

Bergman B, Wallin L (1994) Swedish sign language and society. In Erting CJ, Johnson RC, Smith DL, Snyder BD (eds) The Deaf Way: Perspectives from the international conference on deaf culture. Washington, DC: Gallaudet University Press.

Bergman I, Hirsch RP, Fria TJ, Shapiro SM, Holzman I, Painter MJ (1985) Cause of hearing loss in the high-risk premature infant. The Journal of Pediatrics 106: 95–101.

Bergstrom L, Hemenway WG, Downs MP (1971) A high risk registry to find congenital deafness. Otolaryngologic Clinics of North America 4: 369–99.

Bergstrom L, Nebleth LM, Hemenway WG (1972) Otologic manifestations of acrocephalosyndactyly. Archives of Otolaryngology 96: 117–23.

Berlin CI, Bordelon J, St John P et al. (1998) Reversing click polarity may uncover auditory neuropathy in infants. Ear and Hearing 19: 37–47.

Berrettini S, Ravecca F, Sellari-Franceschini S et al. (1999) Progressive sensorineural hearing loss in childhood. Pediatric Neurology 20: 130–6.

Berry GA (1889) Note on a congenital defect (coloboma?) of the lower lid. Royal London Ophthalmic Hospital Reports 12: 255–7.

Bess FH (1982) Children with unilateral hearing loss. Journal of the Academy of Rehabilitative Audiology 20: 131.

Bess FH (1986) Children with unilateral hearing loss. Ear and Hearing 7: 2–54.

Bess F, Dodd-Murphy J, Parker R (1998) Children with minimal sensorineural hearing loss: Prevalence, educational performance and functional status. Ear and Hearing 19: 339–54.

Bess FH, Gravel JS, Tharpe AM (eds) (1996) Amplification for Children with Auditory Deficits. Nashville, TN: Bill Wilkerson Center Press.

Bess FH, McConnell FE (eds) (1981) Audiology, Education and the Hearing Impaired Child. St Louis, MO: CV Mosby.

Bess FH, Murphy JD, Parker RA (1998) Children with minimal sensorineural hearing loss: Educational performance and functional status. Ear and Hearing 19: 339–54.

Bess FH, Paradise JL (1994) Universal screening for infant hearing impairment: Not simple, not risk-free, not necessarily beneficial, and not presently justified. Pediatrics 93: 330–4.

Bess FH, Tharpe AM (1984) Unilateral hearing impairment in children. Pediatrics 74: 206–16.

Bess FH, Tharpe AM (1986) Case history data on unilaterally hearing impaired children. Ear and Hearing 7: 14–19.

Bess FH, Tharpe AM (1999) Minimal, progressive and fluctuating hearing losses in children. Characteristics, identification and management. Pediatric Clinics of North America 4: 65–78.

Bess FH, Tharpe AM, Gibler A (1986) Auditory performance of children with unilateral sensorineural hearing impairment. Ear and Hearing 7: 20–6.

Best JM, Banatvala JE (2000) Rubella. In Zuckermann AJ, Banatvala JE, Pattison JR (eds) Principles and Practice of Clinical Virology. 4 edn. Chichester: John Wiley & Sons.

Bhatt SM, Cabellos C, Nadol JB Jr et al. (1995) The impact of dexamethasone on hearing loss in experimental pneumococcal meningitis. Pediatric Infectious Diseases Journal 14: 93–6.

Bhatt SM, Halpin C, Hsu W (1991) Hearing loss and pneumococcal meningitis: an animal model. Laryngoscope 101: 1285–92.

Bhatt SM, Lauretano A, Cabellos C Jr et al. (1993) Progression of hearing loss in experimental pneumococcal meningitis: correlation with cerebrospinal fluid cytochemistry. Journal of Infectious Diseases 67: 675–83.

Bird J, Bishop D (1992) Perception and awareness of phonemes in phonologically impaired children. European Journal of Disorders of Communication 127: 289–313.

Bishop DVM (1989) Autism, Asperger's syndrome and semantic-pragmatic disorder: Where are the boundaries? British Journal of Disorders of Communication 24: 231–63.

Bishop DVM (1997) Uncommon understanding. Development and Disorders of Language Comprehension in Children. Psychology Press.

Bishop DVM (1998) Development of the children's communication checklist (CCC). Journal of Child Psychology and Psychiatry 39: 879–92.

Bishop DVM, Edmundson A (1986) Is otitis media a major cause of specific developmental language disorders? British Journal of Disorders of Communication 21: 321–38.

Bishop DVM, Edmundson A (1987a) Language impaired four-year-olds: Distinguishing transient from persistent impairment. Journal of Speech and Hearing Disorders 52: 156–73.

Bishop DVM, Edmundson A (1987b) Specific language impairment as a maturational lag: Evidence from longitudinal data on language and motor development. Developmental Medicine and Child Neurology 29: 442–59.

Bishop DVM, North T, Donlan C (1995) Genetic basis of specific language impairment: evidence from a twin study. Developmental Medicine and Child Neurology 37: 56–71.

Bishop DVM, North T, Donlan C (1996) Non-word repetition as a behavioural marker for inherited language impairment: evidence from a twin study. Journal of Psychology and Psychiatry 37: 391–404.

Bishop DVM, Rosenbloom L (1987) Classification of children with language disorders. In Yule W, Rutter M (eds) Language Development and Disorders. Clinics in Developmental Medicine Nos.101 and 102 London: MacKeith Press.

Bitner-Glindzicz M, de Kok Y, Summers D et al.(1994) Close linkage of a gene for X linked deafness to three microsatellite repeats at Xq21 in radiologically normal and abnormal families. Journal of Medical Genetics 31: 916–21.

Blair JC (1985) Effects of amplification, speech reading and classroom environments on reception of speech. Volta Review 79: 443–9.

Bleischmidt E (1961) The Stages of Human Development before Birth. Philadelphia, PA: WB Saunders Co.

Bloomfield L (1933) Language. British revised edition (first published by Holt, 1933). London: George Allen & Unwin.

Bocca E, Calearo C, Cassinari V (1954) A new method for testing hearing in temporal lobe tumor. Acta Otolaryngologica 44: 219–21.

Boedts D (1967) Stapes chirurgie in Crouzon syndrome. Acta Otolaryngologica Belgica 21: 143–55.

Bohme G (1985) Progression of early childhood sensorineural hearing damage. Laryngorhinootologie 64: 470–2.

Boney S, Bess FH (1984) Noise and Reverberation Effects on Speech Recognition in Children with Minimal Hearing Loss. Paper presented at the American Speech-Language-Hearing Association, November, San Francisco, CA.

Bonfils P, Uziel A (1989) Clinical applications of evoked acoustic emissions: results in normally hearing and hearing -impaired subjects. Annals of Otology, Rhinology and Laryngology 98: 326–31.

Boothman R, Orr N (1978) Value of screening for deafness in the first year of life. Archives of Disease in Childhood 53: 570–3.

Boothroyd A (1968) Developments in speech audiometry. Sound 2: 3–10.

Boothroyd A (1986) A Three Interval, Forced-choice Test of Speech Pattern Contrast Perception. New York: City University and Lexington Center.

Bopanna SB, Pass RF, Britt WJ et al. (1992) Symptomatic congenital cytomegalovirus infection: neonatal morbidity and mortality. Pediatric Infectious Diseases Journal 11: 93–9.

Bordley JE , Kapur YP (1977) Histopathologic changes in the temporal bone resulting from measles infection. Archives of Otolaryngology 103: 162–8.

Borg E (1997) Perinatal asphyxia, hypoxia, ischemia and hearing loss. An overview. Scandinavian Audiology 26: 77–91.

Bornstein H, Saulnier K (1981) Signed English: a brief follow-up to the first evaluation. American Annals of the Deaf 126: 69–72.

Bornstein SP, Wilson RH, Cambron NK et al. (1994) Low- and high-pass filtered Northwestern University auditory test No. 6 for monaural and binaural evaluation. Journal of the American Academy of Audiology 5: 259–64.

Borradori C, Fawer CL, Buclin T, Calame A (1997) Risk factors of sensorineural hearing loss in preterm infants. Biology of the Neonate 71: 1–10.

Bosher SK, Warren RL (1978) Very low calcium content of cochlear endolymph, an extracellular fluid. Nature 273: 377–8.

Bourguet J, Mazeas R, le Huérou Y (1996) De láttente des deux premiers fentes et des deux premiers arcs branchiaux. Revue Neuro-Ophthalmologie 38: 161–75.

Bouvet D (1990) The Path to Language: Bilingual education for deaf children. Clevedon: Multilingual Matters.

Bovo R, Martini A, Agnoletto M et al. (1988) Auditory and academic performance of children with unilateral hearing loss. Scandinavian Audiology 30 (Suppl.) 71–4.

Bowlby J (1980) A Secure Base. New York: Basic Books.

Boyd SF (1974) Hearing Loss: Its educationally measurable effects on achievement [Master's degree requirement]. Department of Education. Carbondale, IL: Southern Illinois University.

Bradford BC, Baudin J, Conway MJ et al. (1985) Identification of sensory neural hearing loss in very preterm infants by brainstem auditory evoked potentials. Archives of Disease in Childhood 60: 105–9.

Brasier VJ (1974) Pitfalls in audiometry. Public Health 39: 31–8.

Brass DP et al. (1994) Assessment of an implementation of a narrow-band, neonatal otoacoustic emission screening method. Ear and Hearing 15: 467–75.

Brazelton T (1982) Joint regulation of neonate behaviour. In Tronick EZ (ed.) Social Interchange in Infancy. Baltimore, MD: University Press.

Britt WJ, Alford CA (1996) Cytomegalovirus. In Field BN, Knipe DM, Howley PM (eds) Fields Virology. 3 edn. Philadelphia, PA: Lippincott-Raven Publishers.

Brodal A (1981) Neurological Anatomy in Relation to Clinical Medicine. 3 edn. Oxford: Oxford University Press.

Brodie HA, Chole RA, Griffin GC, White JG (1992) Macrothrombocytopenia and progressive deafness: a new genetic syndrome. American Journal of Otology 13: 507–11.

Brookhouser PE, Auslander MC, Meskan ME (1988) The pattern and stability of post-meningitic hearing loss in children. Laryngoscope 98: 940–8.

Brookhouser PE, Worthington DW, Kelly WJ (1991) Unilateral hearing loss in children. Laryngoscope 101: 1264–72.

Brookhouser PE, Worthington DW, Kelly WJ (1994) Fluctuating and /or progressive hearing loss in children. Laryngoscope 104: 958–64.

Brown DP, Israel SM (1991) Audiological findings in a set of fraternal twins with CHARGE association. Journal of the American Academy of Audiology 2: 183–8.

Brown DR, Watcho JF, Sabo D (1991) Neonatal sensorineural hearing loss associated with furosemide: a case controlled study. Developmental Medicine and Child Neurology 33: 816–23.

Brown MR, Tomec MS, van Laer L et al. (1997) A novel locus for autosomal dominant non syndromic hearing loss, DFNA13, maps to chromosome 6p. American Journal of Human Genetics 61: 924–7.

Brown MT, Cunningham MJ, Ingelfinger JR, Becker AM (1993) Progressive sensorineural hearing loss in association with distal renal tubular acidosis. Archives of Otolaryngology Head and Neck Surgery 119: 458–60.

Brown R, Hanlon C (1970) Derivational complexity and order of acquisition in child speech. In Hayes J (ed.) Cognition and the Development of Language. New York: Wiley.

Brownell WE, Bader CR, Bertrand D, Ribaupierre Y (1985) Evoked mechanical responses of isolated cochlear outer hair cells. Science 227: 194–6.

Brucher JM, Dom R, Lombart A, Carton H (1981) Progressive pontobulbar palsy with deafness: Clinical and pathology study of two cases. Archives of Neurology 38: 186–90.

Brunner HG (1996) Alport Syndrome. In Martini A, Read A, Stephens D (eds) Genetics and Hearing Impairment. London: Whurr Publishers.

Brusis T (1974) Gleichzeitiges Vorkommen von degenrativer Innenohrschwerhorigkeit, Vestibularisstorung, beiderseitigen Ohr-und laterale Halsfistelnbei mehreren Mitgliedern einer Familie. Laryng Rhinol 53: 131–9.

BSA (British Society of Audiology) (1981) Recommended procedures for pure tone audiometry using a manually operated instrument. British Journal of Audiology 15: 213–16.

BSA (British Society of Audiology) (1985) Recommended procedures for pure tone bone conduction audiometry without masking using a manually operated instrument. British Journal of Audiology 19: 281–2.

BSA (British Society of Audiology) (1986) Recommendations for masking in pure tone threshold audiometry. British Journal of Audiology 20: 265–6.

Buchanan LH (1990) Early onset of presbyacusis in Down's Syndrome. Scandinavian Audiology 19: 103–10.

Burd L, Fisher W (1986) Central auditory processing disorder or attention deficit disorder? Journal of Developmental and Behavioral Pediatrics 1: 215–16.

Burnip L, McGuire B (1995) FM amplification in the preschool: Investigation of the FM signal and child attention. Australian Journal of Audiology 17: 123–9.

Butler K (1981) Language processing disorders: Factors in remediation. In Keith RW (ed) Central Auditory and Language Disorders in Children. Houston, Texas: College Hill Press.

Byrne D, Ching TYC (1997) Optimising amplification for hearing-impaired children: issues and procedures. Australian Journal of Education of the Deaf 3: 21–8.

Byrne D, Dillon H (1986) The National Acoustic Laboratories (NAL) new procedure for electing the gain and frequency response of a hearing aid. Ear and Hearing 7: 257–65.

Byrne D, Fifield D (1974) Evaluation of hearing aid fittings for infants. British Journal of Audiology 8: 47–54.

Byrne D, Noble W, Le Page E (1992) Effects of long term bilateral and unilateral fitting of different hearing aid types on the ability to localise sounds. Journal of American Audiology 3: 369–82.

Byrne D, Parkinson A, Newall P (1990) Hearing aid gain and frequency response requirements of the severely/profoundly hearing-impaired. Ear and Hearing 11: 40–9.

Byrne D, Tonnison W (1976) Selecting the gain of hearing aids for persons with sensorineural hearing losses. Scandinavian Audiology 5: 51–9.

Bysshe J (1995) Deafness in childhood: Are deaf children getting the education they need? Professional Care of Mother and Child 5: 1–13.

Caird D (1991) Processing in the colliculi. In Altschuler RA, Bobbin RP, Clopton BM, Hoffman DW (eds) The Central Auditory System. New York: Raven Press.

Caissie R, Cole EB (1993) Mothers and hearing-impaired children: Directiveness reconsidered. Volta Review 95: 49–59.

Carhart R (1965) Monaural and binaural discrimination against competing sentences. International Audiology 4: 5–10.

Carlson DL, Reeh HL (1993) X-linked mixed hearing loss with stapes fixation: Case reports. Journal of the American Academy of Audiology 4: 420–5.

Carney AE, Moeller MP (1998) Treatment efficacy: Hearing loss in children. Journal of Speech, Language and Hearing Research. 41: S61–84.

Casselman JW, Kuhweide R, Deimling M et al. (1994) Constructive interference in steady stage-3DFT MR imaging of the inner ear and cerebellopontine angle. American Journal of Neuroradiology 4: 47–57.

Cataltepe O, Berker M, Gurcay O, Erbengi A (1993) An unusual dural arteriovenous fistula in an infant. Neuroradiology 35: 394–7.

CDC (Centers for Disease Control and Prevention) (1997) Measles eradication: Recommendations from a meeting co–sponsored by the World Health Organisation, the Pan American Health Organisation, and CDC. Morbidity and Mortality Weekly Report 46: 1–20.

CDSC (Communicable Disease Surveillance Centre) (1996) HIV, AIDS and sexually transmitted infections: Global epidemiology, impact and prevention. Health and Population occasional paper. Sexual Health and Care. London: Overseas Development Agency.

Cernoch J, Porter R (1985) Recognition of maternal auxiliary odours by infants. Child Development 56: 1593–6.

Ceruti S, Stinckens C, Casselman JW et al. (2001) Temporal bone malformations in the branchio-oto-renal (BOR) syndrome: detailed Otology and Neuro-otology CT and MRI findings. Submitted.

Chaib H, Lina-Granade G, Guilford P et al. (1994) A gene responsible for a dominant form of neurosensory non-syndromic deafness maps to the NSRD1 recessive deafness gene interval. Human Molecular Genetics 3: 2219–22.

Chalmers D, Stewart I, Silva P, Mulvena A (1989) Otitis Media with Effusion – The Dunedin Study. Clinics in Developmental Medicine No 108. London: Mackeith Press.

Cheatham MA, Dallos P (1993) Longitudinal comparisons of IHC ac and dc receptor potentials recorded from the guinea pig cochlea. Hearing Research 68: 107–14.

Chen A, Francis M, Ni L et al. (1995) Phenotypic manifestations of branchio-oto-renal syndrome. American Journal of Medical Genetics 58: 365–70.

Chen TC, Maceri DR, Giannotta SL et al. (1992) Unilateral acoustic neuromas in childhood without evidence of neurofibromatosis: case reports and review of the literature. American Journal of Otology 13: 318–22.

Chermak GD, Musiek F (1992) Managing central auditory processing disorders in children and youth. American Journal of Audiology 1: 61–5.

Chermak GD, Musiek FE (eds) (1997) Central Auditory Processing Disorders: New perspectives. San Diego, CA: Singular Publishing Group.

Chermak G, Vonhof M, Bendel R et al. (1989) Word identification performance in the presence of competing speech and noise in learning disabled adults. Ear and Hearing 10: 90–3.

Chermak GD, Somers EK, Seikel JA et al.(1998) Behavioral signs of central auditory processing disorder and attention deficit hyperactivity disorder. Journal of the American Academy of Audiology 9: 78–84.

Cheskin A (1982) The use of language by hearing mothers of deaf children. Journal of Communication Disorders 15: 145–53.

Cheung PY, Haluschak MM, Finer NN, Robertson CMT (1996) Sensorineural hearing loss in survivors of neonatal ECMO. Early Human Development 44: 225–33.

Childs F, Aukett A, Darbyshire P et al. (1997) Dietary education and iron deficiency anaemia in the inner city. Archives of Diseases of Childhood 76: 144–7.

Ching TYC, Newall P, Wigney D (1994) Audio-visual and auditory paired comparison judgements by severely and profoundly hearing impaired children: Reliability and frequency response preferences. Australian Journal of Audiology 16: 99–106.

Chisaka O, Musci TS, Capecchi MR (1992) Developmental defects of the ear, cranial nerves and hindbrain, resulting from targetted disruption of the mouse homeobox gene Hox-1.6. Nature 355: 88–9.

Cinque P, Cleator GM, Weber T et al. (1998) Diagnosis and clinical management of neurological disorders caused by cytomegalovirus in AIDS patients. Journal of Neurovirology 4: 120–32.

Cizman M, Rakar R, Zakotnik B et al. (1999) Severe forms of tick-borne encephalitis in children. Wiener Kliner Wochenschrifte 111: 484–7.

Clark AD, Richards CJ (1966) Auditory discrimination among economically disadvantaged and non-disadvantaged pre-school children. Exceptional Children 33: 259–62.

Clark GM (1999) Cochlear implants in the third millennium. American Journal of Otology 20: 4–8.

Clark M (1989) Language through Living for Hearing-impaired Children. London: Hodder & Stoughton.

Clark WF (1991) Noise exposure from leisure activities: A review. Journal of Acoustical Society of America 90: 175–81.

Coggon D, Rose G, Barker D (1993) Epidemiology for the Uninitiated. London: British Medical Journal.

Cole K, Schwartz I, Notari A et al. (1995) Examination of the stability of two methods of defining specific language impairment. Applied Linguistics 16: 103–23.

Collins K, Parry-Fielder B, Anderson V et al. (1999) Case control study of prevalence of epileptiform electroencephalograms in developmental dysphasia. Afasic Third International Symposium.

Comis SD, Osborne MP, Stephen J et al. (1993) Cytotoxic effects on hair cells of guinea pig cochlea produced by pneumolysin, the thiol activated toxin of Streptococcus pneumoniae. Acta Otolaryngologica 113: 152–9.

Connexin-deafness homepage: http: //www.iro.es/cx26deaf.html

Conrad R (1979) The Deaf Schoolchild. London: Harper & Row.

Conti-Ramsden G, Crutchley A, Botting N (1997)The extent to which psychometric tests differentiate subgroups of children with SLI. Journal of Speech, Language and Hearing Research. 40: 765–77.

Conyn-Van Spaendonck MAE , Van Knapen F (1992) Choice in preventive strategies: Experience with the prevention of congenital toxoplasmosis in the Netherlands. Scandinavian Journal of Infectious Diseases 84: 51–8.

Cooper LZ, Preblud SR, Alford CA (1995) Rubella. In Remington JS, Klein JO (eds) Infectious Diseases of the Fetus and Newborn Infant. 4 edn. Philadelphia, PA: WB Saunders.

Cordes SP, Barsh GS (1994) The mouse segmentation gene kr encodes a novel basic domain-leucine zipper transcription factor. Cell 79: 1025–34.

Corey DP, Breakefield XO (1994) Transcription factors in inner ear development. Proceedings of the National Academy of Sciences, USA 91: 433–6.

Cosgrove K, Hickson F (1996) Sound localisation in profoundly deaf children. Journal of British Association of Teachers of the Deaf 20: 42–9.

Costello MR (1977) Evaluation of auditory behavior of children using the Flowers-Costello test of central auditory abilities In Keith RW (ed.) Central Auditory Dysfunction. New York: Grune & Stratton.

Cotter CS, Singleton GT, Corman LC (1994) Immune-mediated inner ear disease and parvovirus B19 Laryngoscope 104: 1235–9.

Cotton S (1988) Evaluation of FM fittings. Unpublished master's thesis, Macquarie University, New South Wales, Australia.

Courtin C, Melot A-M (1998) Development of theories of mind in deaf children. In Marschark M (ed.) Psychological Perspectives on Deafness Volume 2. New Jersey: LEA.

Couvreur J (1999) Problems of congenital toxoplasmosis. Evolution over four decades. Presse Medicale 28: 753–7.

Crandell CC (1993) Speech recognition in noise by children with minimal degrees of sensorineural hearing loss. Ear and Hearing 14: 210–16.

Crandell CC, Smaldino JJ, Flexer C (1995). Sound-field FM Amplification – Theory and Practical Applications. San Diego, CA: Singular Publishing Group.

Crann SA, Schacht J (1996) Activation of aminoglycoside antibiotics to cytotoxins. Audiology and Neuro-Otology 1: 80–5.

Cremers CWRJ (1981) Hearing loss in Pfeiffer's syndrome. International Journal of Pediatric Otorhinolaryngology 3: 343–53.

Cremers CWRJ (1985) Meatal atresia and hearing loss. Autosomal dominant and autosomal recessive inheritance. International Journal of Pediatric Otorhinolaryngology 8: 211–13.

Cremers CWRJ, Bolder C, Admiral RJ et al. (1998) Progressive sensorineural hearing loss and a widened vestibular aqueduct in Pendred syndrome. Archives of Otolaryngology, Head and Neck Surgery 124: 501–5.

Cremers CWRJ, Fikkers-van Noord M (1980) The earpits deafness syndrome. Clinical and genetic aspects. International Journal of Pediatric Otorhinolaryngology 2: 309–22.

Cremers CWRJ, Marres HAM, Brunner H (1993) Neo-oval window technique in the BOR syndrome and myringo-chorda-vestibulopexy. Laryngoscope 103: 1186–9.

Cremers CWRJ, Thijssen HOM, Fischer AJEM, Marres EHMA (1981) Otological aspects of the earpit-deafness syndrome. Otorhinolaryngology 43: 223–39.

Cremers FPM, Bitner-Glindzicz M, Pembrey ME, Ropers H-H (1995) Mapping and cloning hereditary deafness genes. Current Opinion in Genetics and Development 5: 371–5.

Croft C, Andersen-Wood and the English and Romanian study team, Institute of Psychiatry (1999) Language development following severe early deprivation. Afasic, Third International Symposium.

Culbertson JL, Gilbert LE (1986) Children with unilateral sensorineural hearing loss: cognitive, academic, and social development. Ear and Hearing 7: 38–42.

Cullington HE, Brown EJ (1998) Bilateral otoacoustic emission pass in a baby with Mondini deformity and subsequently confirmed profound bilateral hearing loss. British Journal of Audiology 32: 249–53.

Culp R, Watkins RV, Lawrence H et al. (1991) Maltreated children's language and speech development: abused, neglected, and abused and neglected. First Language 11: 377–91.

Culpepper B, Thompson G (1994) Effects of reinforcer duration on the response behavior of preterm two-year-olds in visual reinforcement audiometry. Ear and Hearing 15: 161–7.

Cummins J, Swain M (1986) Bilingualism in Education: Aspects of theory, research and practice. Harlow: Longman.

Cutts FT, Robertson SE, Diaz-Ortega JL, Samuel R (1997) Control of rubella and congenital rubella syndrome (CRS) in developing countries, Part 1: Burden of disease from CRS. Bulletin of the World Health Organization 75: 55–68.

Cyr D, Moore G, Möller C (1988) Clinical application of computerised dynamic posturography. ENT Journal (Suppl.) September 36–47.

Daffos F, Forestier F, Capella-Pavlovsky M et al. 1988) Prenatal management of 746 pregnancies at risk for congenital toxoplasmosis. New England Journal of Medicine 318: 271–5.

Dagillas A, Antoniades K, Palasis S, Aidonis A (1992) Branchio-oto-renal dysplasia associated with tetralogy of Fallot. Head and Neck 14: 139–42.

Dahle AJ, McCollister FP, Stagno S et al. (1979) Progressive hearing impairment in children with congenital cytomegalovirus infection. Journal of Speech and Hearing Disorders 44: 220–9.

Dahlen RT, Harnsberger HR, Gray SD et al. (1997) Overlapping thin-section fast spin-echo MR of the large vestibular aqueduct syndrome. American Journal of Neuroradiology 18: 67–75.

Dale P, Simonoff E, Bishop D et al. (1998) Genetic influence on language delay in two-year old children. Nature Neuroscience 1: 324–8.

Dalebout SD, Stach JW (1999) Mismatch negativity to acoustic differences not differentiated behaviorally. Journal of American Academy of Audiology 10: 388–99.

Dallos P, Cheatham MA (1976) Production of cochlear potentials by inner and outer hair cells. Journal of the Acoustical Society of America 60: 510–12.

Dallos P, Schoeny ZG, Cheatham MA (1972) Cochlear summating potentials: Descriptive aspects. Acta Otolaryngologica (Suppl.302): 1–46.

Darlow BA, Harwood LJ, Mogridge N, Clemett RS (1997) Prospective study of New Zealand very low birthweight infants and outcome at 7–8 years. Journal of Pediatrics and Child Health 33: 47–51.

Das VK (1988) Aetiology of bilateral sensorineural deafness in children. Scandinavian Audiology (Suppl. 30): 8107–593.

Das VK (1990) Prevalence of otitis media with effusion in children with bilateral sensory hearing loss. Archives of Disease in Childhood 65: 757–9.

Das VK (1991) Adverse perinatal factors in the causation of sensorineural hearing impairment in young children. International Journal of Pediatric Otorhinolaryngology 21: 121–5.

Das VK (1996) Aetiology of bilateral sensorineural hearing impairment in children: a 10 year study. Archives of Disease in Childhood 74: 8–12.

Davidson J, Hyde ML, Alberti PW (1988) Epidemiology of hearing impairment in childhood. Scandinavian Audiology (Suppl. 30): 13–20.

Davidson J, Hyde ML, Alberti PW (1989) Epidemiologic patterns in childhood hearing loss: A review. International Journal of Pediatric Otorhinolaryngology 17: 239–66.

Davies B (1988) Auditory disorders in Down's Syndrome. Scandinavian Audiology (Suppl. 30): 65–8.

Davis A (1988) Response times as an indicator of access to frequency-resolved information. British Journal of Audiology 22: 305–8.

Davis A (1990) What are the prerequisites for identifying priorities in social science research and deafness? Paper presented at RNID Seminar.

Davis AC (1993a) The prevalence of deafness. In Ballantyne J, Martin A, Martin M (eds) Deafness. London: Whurr Publishers.

Davis AC (1993b) A public health perspective on childhood hearing impairment. In McCormick B (ed.) Paediatric Audiology 0–5. 2 edn. London: Whurr Publishers.

Davis A, Bamford J, Wilson I et al. (1997) A critical review of the role of neonatal screening in the detection of congenital hearing impairment. Health Technology Assessment 1–10.

Davis A, El Refaie A (2000) Epidemiology. In Tyler RS (ed.) Handbook on Tinnitus. San Diego, CA: Singular Publishing Group.

Davis A, Gregory S, Bamford J (1999) Paediatric Audiology Service Index (PASI); Deaf Education Early Service Index (DEESI). Personal Communication.

Davis A, Parving A (1994) Towards appropriate epidemiological data on childhood hearing disability: A comparative European study of birth cohorts 1982–88. Journal of Audiological Medicine 3: 35–47.

Davis A, Sancho J (1988) Screening for hearing impairment in children: A review of current practice in the UK with special reference to the screening of babies from special baby units for severe/profound impairments. In Gerber SE, Mencher GT (eds) International Perspectives on Communication Disorders. Washington, DC: Gallaudet University Press 237–75.

Davis A, Wood S (1992) The epidemiology of childhood hearing impairment: Factors relevant to planning services. British Journal of Audiology 26: 77–90.

Davis A, Wood S, Healy R et al. (1995) Risk factors for hearing disorders: epidemiological evidence of change over time in the UK. Journal of American Academy of Audiology 6: 365–70.

Davis AC (1993) A public health perspective on childhood hearing impairment. In McCormick B (ed.) Paediatric Audiology 0–5. 2 edn. London: Whurr Publishers.

Davis AC, Wharrad JH, Sancho J, Marshall D H (1991) Early detection of hearing impairment – what role is there for behavioural methods in the neonatal period. Acta Otolaryngologica (Suppl.) (Stockholm) 482: 103–10.

Davis A, Wood S (1992) The epidemiology of childhood hearing impairment: Factors relevant to planning services. British Journal of Audiology 26: 77–90.

Davis A, Wood S, Healy R et al. (1995) Risk factors for hearing disorders: Epidemiological evidence of change over time in the UK. Journal of American Academy of Audiology 6: 365–70.

Davis GL (1969) Cytomegalovirus in the inner ear. Annals of Otology, Rhinology and Laryngology 78: 1179–88.

Davis JM, Elfenbein J, Schum R, Bentler RA (1986) Effects of mild and moderate hearing impairments on language, educational, and psychosocial behavior of children. Journal of Speech and Hearing Disorder 51: 53–62.

Davis LE, James CG, Fiber F, McLaren LC (1979) Cytomegalovirus isolation from the human inner ear. Annals of Otology, Rhinology and Laryngology 88: 424–6.

Davis LE, Johnsson LG, Kornfeld M (1981) Cytomegalovirus labyrinthitis in an infant: Morphological, virological, and immunofluorescent studies. Journal of Neuropathology and Experimental Neurology 40: 9–19.

Dawson KG, Emerson JC, Burns JL (1999) Fifteen years of experience with bacterial meningitis. Pediatric Infectious Disease Journal 18: 816–22.

Dawson P (1987) A hearing aid performance study. Australian Journal of Audiology 9: 49–54.

Deayton J, French P (1997) Incidence of early syphilis acquired in former Soviet Union is increasing. British Medical Journal 315: 1018–19.

DeCasper A, Fifer W (1980) Of human bonding: Newborns prefer their mother's voices. Science 208: 1174–6.

DeCasper A, Spence M (1986) Prenatal maternal speech influences new borns' perception of speech sounds. Infant Behaviour and Development 9: 133–50.

Dechesne CJ (1992) The development of vestibular sensory organs in human. In Romand R (ed.) Development of Auditory and Vestibular systems 2. New York: Academic Press.

Dee A, Rapin I, Ruben RJ (1982) Speech and language development in a parent-infant total communication program. Annals of Otology, Rhinology and Laryngology (Suppl. 97): 62–72.

Deitrich KN, Succop PA, Berger OG et al. (1992) Lead exposure and the central auditory processing abilities and cognitive development of urban children: The Cincinnati Lead Study cohort at age 5 years. Neurotoxicology and Teratology 14: 51–6.

De Kok YJ, Bom SJ, Brunt TM et al. (1999) A Pro51Ser mutation in the COCH gene is associated with late onset autosomal dominant progressive sensorineural hearing loss with vestibular defects. Human Molecular Genetics 8: 361–6.

De la Mata I, De Wals P (1988) Policies for immunisation against rubella in European countries. European Journal of Epidemiology 4: 175–80.

Denmark J (1994) Deafness and Mental Health. London: Jessica Kingsley.

Denoyelle F, Marlin S, Weil D et al. (1999) Clinical features of the prevalent form of childhood deafness, DFNB1, due to a connexin-26 gene defect: Implications for genetic counselling. Lancet 353: 1298–303.

Dent CT (1897) Case of fragilitas ossium. Transaction of the Medical Society of London 20: 339–42.

Deol MS (1966) Influence of the neural tube on the differentiation of the inner ear in the mammalian embryo. Nature 209: 219–20.

Deonna TW (1991) Acquired epileptiform aphasia in children (Llandau-Kleffner syndrome). Journal of Clinical Neurophysiology 8: 288–98.

DES (Department for Education and Science) (1968) The Education of Deaf Children: The Possible Place of Finger Spelling and Signing (The Lewis Report). London: Her Majesty's Stationery Office.

Desmontes G, Couvreur J (1974) Congenital toxoplasmosis: A prospective study of 378 pregnancies. New England Journal of Medicine 290: 1110–16.

Deuschl G, Mischke G, Schenck E et al. (1990) Symptomatic and essential rhythmic palatal myoclonus. Brain 113: 1645–72.

De Villiers F, Bibier L, Ramos E, Gatty F (1993) Gestural communication in oral deaf mother-child pairs: Language with a helping hand? Applied Psycholinguistics 14: 319–48.

De Villiers J, de Villiers P, Hoban E (1994) The central problem of functional categories of English syntax of oral deaf children. In Tager-Flusberg H (ed.) Constraints on Language Acquisition: Studies of atypical children. Hove, UK: Lawrence Erlbaum Associates.

De Villiers PA (1992) Educational implications of deafness – language and literacy. In Eavey RD, Klein JO (eds) Hearing Loss in Childhood: In: 102nd Ross Conference on Pediatric Research – Hearing Loss in Childhood: A primer. Ross Laboratories.

DFE (1994a) Code of Practice on the identification and assessment of special educational needs. London: The Stationery Office Ltd.

DFE (1994b) Our Children's Education: The updated parent's charter. London: The Stationery Office Ltd.

DfEE (1994 to 1998) Secondary School Performance Tables. London: DfEE.

DfEE (1998) Meeting Special Educational Needs: A programme for action. London: DfEE.

Dias O (1990) Childhood deafness in Portugal: Aetiological factors and diagnosis of hearing loss. International Journal of Pediatric Otolaryngology 18: 247–55.

Dillon H (1996) Tutorial: Compression? Yes, but for low or high frequencies, for low or high intensities and with what response times? Ear and Hearing 17: 287–307.

Dillon H, Storey L (1998) The National Acoustic Laboratories' procedure for selecting the saturation sound pressure level of hearing aids: Theoretical derivation. Ear and Hearing 19: 255–66.

Dingle AF, Flood LM, Kumar BU, Hampal S (1993) The mini-grommet in tympanosclerosis; results at 2 years. Journal of Laryngology and Otology 107: 108–10.

Dixon J, Edwards SJ, Gladwin AJ et al. (1996) Positional cloning of a gene involved in the pathogenesis of Treacher Collins syndrome. Nature Genetics 12: 130–6.

Dobbins JG, Stewart JA, Demmler GJ (1992) Surveillance of congenital cytomegalovirus disease, 1990–1991. Collaborating Registry Group. Morbidity and Mortality Weekly Report 41: 35–9.

Dobie RA (1999) A review of randomized clinical trials in tinnitus. Laryngoscope 109: 1202–11.

Dodge PR, Davis H, Feigin RD et al. (1984) Prospective evaluation of hearing impairment as a sequela of acute bacterial meningitis. New England Journal of Medicine 311: 869–74.

Dodson EE, Hishasaki GT, Todd C et al. (1998) Intact canal wall mastoidectomy with tympanoplasty for cholesteatoma in children. Laryngoscope 108: 977–83.

Domenech J, Santabarbara P, Carulla M, Trassera J (1988) Sudden hearing loss in an adolescent following a single dose of Cisplatin. Journal of Otorhinolaryngology and Related Specialties 50: 405–8.

Douek E, Dodson HC, Bannister Lhet al. (1976) Effects of incubator noise on the cochlea of the newborn. Lancet ii: 1110–13.

Dowell RC, Blamey PJ, Clark GM (1997) Factors affecting outcome in children with cochlear implants. In Clark GM (ed.) Cochlear Implants. XVI World Congress of Otolaryngology Head and Neck Surgery, Sydney, Australia 2–7 March 1997. Bologna, Italy: Monduzzi Editore.

Dowell RC, Cowan RSC (1995) Evaluation of benefit: infants and children. In Clark GM, Cowan RSC, Dowell RC (eds) Cochlear Implantation for Infants and Children. San Diego, London: Singular Publishing Group.

Downs DW, Crum MA (1978) Processing demands during auditory learning under listening conditions. Journal of Speech and Hearing Research 21: 702–14.

Downs MP, Sterritt GM (1964) Identification audiometry for neonates: A preliminary report. Journal of Auditory Research 4: 69–80.

Doyle LW (1995) Outcome to five years of age of children born 24–26 weeks gestational age in Victoria. The Victorian Study Group. Medical Journal of Australia 163: 11–14.

Drukier G (1989) The prevalence and characteristics of tinnitus with profound sensorineural hearing impairment. American Annals of the Deaf 134: 260–4.

D'Souza SW, McCartney, Nolan M, Taylor IG (1981) Hearing, speech and language in survivors of severe perinatal asphyxia. Archives of Disease in Childhood 56: 245–52.

Duara S, Suter CM, Bessard KK, Gutberlet RL (1986) Neonatal screening with auditory brainstem responses: Results of follow-up audiometry and risk factor evaluation. The Journal of Pediatrics 108: 276–81.

Duffy LC, Faden H, Wasielewski R et al. (1997) Exclusive breastfeeding protects against bacterial colonisation and day care exposure to otitis media. Pediatrics 100 E7.

Dunn J (1995) Children as psychologists: The later correlates of individual differences in understanding of emotions and other minds. In Connections Between Emotion and Understanding in Development. Hove, UK: Lawrence Ehrlbaum Associates.

Eatough M (1995) BATOD Survey 1994; England. Journal of the British Association of Teachers of the Deaf 19: 142–60.

Edwards J, Tyszkwiewicz E (1999) Cochlear implants. In Stokes J (ed.) Hearing Impaired Infants: Support in the first eighteen months. London: Whurr Publishers.

EEC (1998) European Consensus Statement on Neonatal Hearing Screening. European consensus development conference on neonatal screening. Milan, May 1998.

Eeg-Olofsson O, Ödkvist L, Lindskog U, Andersson B (1982) Benign paroxysmal vertigo in childhood. Acta Otolaryngologica 93: 283–9.

Ehret G (1997) The auditory cortex. Journal of Comparative Physiology 181: 547–57.

Eimas PD (1974) Auditory and linguistic units of processing cues for place of articulation by infants. Perception and Psychophysics 16: 513–21.

Eimas PD (1975a) Developmental studies of speech perception. In Cohen LB, Salaptek P (eds) Infant Perception: From sensation to cognition. New York: Academic Press.

Eimas PD (1975b) Auditory and phonetic coding of the cues for speech: Discrimination of the r-l distinction by young infants. Perception and Pyschophysics 18: 341–7.

Eimas PD, Siqueland ER, Jusczyk PW, Vigorito J (1971) Speech perception in infants. Science 171: 303–306.

Eiser C (1990) Chronic Childhood Disease. Cambridge: Cambridge University Press.

Elfenbein J, Bentler R, Davis J, Niebuhr D (1988) Status of school children's hearing aids relative to monitoring practices. Ear and Hearing 9: 212–17.

Elliott LL, Hammer MA, Scholl ME (1989) Fine-grained auditory discrimination in normal children and children with language-learning problems. Journal of Speech and Hearing Research 32: 112–19.

Ellis R, Wells CG (1980) Enabling factors in adult-child discourse. First Language 1: 46–62.

Elssan SF, Matkin ND, Sabo MP (1987) Early identification of congenital sensorineural hearing impairment. The Hearing Journal 40: 13–17.

Ensink RJH, Camp GV, Cremers CWRJ (1998) Mitochondrial inherited hearing loss. Clinical Otolaryngology 23: 3–8.

Epstein CJ, Sahud MA, Piel CF et al. (1972) Hereditary macrothrombocytopathia, nephritis and deafness. American Journal of Medical Genetics 52: 299–310.

Erlandsson S (2000) Psychologic profiles. In Tyler RS (ed.) Handbook on Tinnitus. San Diego, CA: Singular Publishing Group.

Erting CJ, Prezioso C, O'Grady, Hymes M (1990) The interactional context of deaf-mother communication. In Volterra V, Erting CJ (eds) From Gesture to Language in Hearing and Deaf Children. Heidelberg: Springer Verlag.

Ertl T, Hadzsiev K, Vincze O, Pytel J, Szabo I, Sulyok E (2001) Hyponatremia and sensorineural hearing loss in preterm infants. Biology of the neonate 79: 109–12.

Estivill X, Fortina P, Surrey S et al. (1998a) Connexin-26 mutations in sporadic and inherited sensorineural deafness. Lancet 351: 394–8.

Estivill X, Govea N, Barceló A et al. (1998b) Familial progressive sensorineural deafness is mainly due to the mtDNA A1555G mutation and is enhanced by treatment with aminoglycosides. American Journal of Human Genetics 62: 27–35.

Evenberg G (1957) Deafness following mumps. Acta Otolaryngologica 48: 397–403.

Evenburg G (1960) Etiology of unilateral total deafness. Annals of Otology, Rhinology, and Laryngology 69: 711–30.

Evenhuis HM, van Zanten GA, Brocaar MP, Roerdinkholder WH (1992) Hearing loss in middle-aged persons with Down's Syndrome. American Journal of Mental Retardation 97: 47–56.

Eviatar L, Eviatar A (1978) Neurovestibular examination of infants and children. Advances in Oto-Rhino-Laryngology 23: 169–91.

Ewing Foundation (1998) Some Outcomes of Mainstream Education. Manchester: Ewing Foundation, Centre for Human Communication and Deafness, University of Manchester.

Ewing IR, Ewing AWG (1944) The ascertainment of deafness in infancy and early childhood. Journal of Laryngology and Otology 59: 309–38.

Fabry DA (1994) Noise reduction with FM systems in FM/EM mode. Ear and Hearing 15: 82–6.

Fageeh NA, Schloss MD, Elahi MM et al. (1999) Surgical treatment of cholesteatoma in children. Journal of Otolaryngology 28: 309–12.

Fallis-Cunningham R, Keith RW (1998) Auditory testing for temporal processing disorders. Los Angeles, CA: Presentation to the Annual Meeting of the American Auditory Society.

Farrell M (2000) Educational inclusion and raising standards. British Journal of Special Education 27: 1.

Farrugia D, Austin GF (1980) A study of the social-emotional adjustment patterns of hearing-impaired students in different educational settings. American Annals of the Deaf 25: 535–41.

Feigin JA, Kopun JG, Stelmachowicz PG, Gorga MP (1989) Probe tube microphone measures of ear canal sound pressure levels in infants and children. Ear and Hearing 10: 254–8.

Feinmesser M, Tell L (1976) Neonatal screening for detection of hearing loss. Archives of Otolaryngology 102: 297–9.

Feinmesser M, Tell L, Levi H (1986) Etiology of childhood deafness with reference to the group of unknown cause. Audiology 25: 65–9.

Feinmesser M, Tell L, Levi H (1990) Decline in the prevalence of childhood deafness in the Jewish population of Jerusalem: Ethnic and genetic aspects. Journal of Laryngology and Otology 104: 675–7.

Fenson L, Dale PS, Resnick JS et al. (1993) MacArthur's Communicative Development Inventories. San Diego, CA: Singular Publishing.

Ferguson CA (1964) Baby talk in six languages. American Anthropologist 66: 103–14.

Fernandez C, Goldberg JM (1971) Physiology of peripheral neurons innervating semicircular canals of the squirrel monkey II. The response to sinusoidal stimulation and dynamics of the peripheral vestibular system. Journal of Neurophysiology 34: 661–5.

Fifer RC, Sierra- Irizammy B (1988) Clinical applications of the auditory middle latency response. American Journal of Otology 9 Suppl: 47–56.

Finitzo-Hieber T, Tilman TW (1978) Room acoustics effects on monosyllabic word discrimination ability for normal and hearing impaired children. Journal of Speech and Hearing Research 21: 440–58.

Finsnes KA (1973) Lethal intracranial complication following air insufflation with pneumatic otoscope. Acta Otolaryngologica (Stockholm) 75: 436.

Fisch L, Osborne DA (1955) Congenital deafness and haemolytic disease of the newborn. Archives of Disease in Childhood 29: 309–16.

Fisch U (1983) Management of sudden deafness. Otolaryngology, Head and Neck Surgery 91: 3–8.

Fischel-Ghodsian (1996) Mitochondrially determined hearing impairment. In Martini A, Read A, Stephens D (eds) Genetics and Hearing Impairment. London: Whurr Publishers.

Fisher LI (1976) Auditory Problems Checklist. Bemidji, MN: Life Products.

Fisher S, Vargha-Khadem F, Watkins K et al. (1998) Localisation of a gene implicated in a severe speech and language disorder. Nature Genetics 18: 168–70.

Fitch N, Lindsay JR, Srolovitz H (1976) The temporal bone in the preauricular pit, cervical fistula hearing loss syndrome. Annals of Otology 85: 268–75.

Fiumara NJ, Lessell S (1970). Manifestations of late congenital syphilis. Analysis of 271 patients. Archives of Dermatology 102: 78–83.

Fletcher HF, Munson WA (1933) Loudness, its definition, measurement, and calculation. Journal of the American Acoustical Society 5: 82–108.

Flexer CA (1996) Amplification for children with minimal hearing loss. In Bess FH, Gravel JS, Tharpe AM (eds) Amplification for Children with Auditory Deficits. Nashville, TN: Bill Wilkerson Center Press.

Flock A (1971) Sensory transduction in hair cells. In Lowenstein WR (ed.) Handbook of Sensory Physiology. Principles of receptor physiology Vol 1. Berlin: Springer-Verlag.

Fonseca S, Forsyth H, Grigor J et al. (1999) Identification of permanent hearing loss in children: Are the targets for the outcome measures attainable? British Journal of Audiology 33: 135–43.

Fortnum H, Davis A (1993) Hearing impairment of children after bacterial meningitis; incidence and resource implications. British Journal of Audiology 27: 43–52.

Fortnum H, Davis A (1997) Epidemiology of permanent childhood hearing impairment in Trent region, 1985–1993. British Journal of Audiology 31: 409–46.

Fortnum H, Hull D (1992) Is hearing assessed after bacterial meningitis? Archives of Disease in Childhood 67: 1111–12.

Fourman P, Fourman J (1955) Hereditary deafness in family with earpits (fistula auris congenita). British Medical Journal 2: 1354–6.

Fowler KB, McCollister FP, Dahle AJ et al. (1997) Progressive and fluctuating sensorineural hearing loss in children with asymptomatic cytomegalovirus infection. Journal of Pediatrics 130: 624–30.

Franceschetti A, Zwahlen P (1944) Un syndrome nouveau: LA dysostose mandibulofaciale. Bull Schweiz Akad Med Wiss 1: 60–6.

Francois M, Laccourreye L, Huy ETB, Narcy P (1997) Hearing impairment in infants after meningitis: Detection by transient evoked otoacoustic emissions. Journal of Pediatrics 130: 712–17.

Fraser FC, Ling D, Clogg D, Nogrady B (1978) Genetic aspects of the BOR syndrome – branchial fistulas, earpits, hearing loss and renal anomalies. American Journal of Medical Genetics 2: 241–52.

Fraser G (1976) The Causes of Profound Deafness in Children. Baltimore, MD: John Hopkins University Press.

Freemantle N et al. (1992) The Treatment of Persistent Glue Ear in Children. Effective health care. Leeds: University of Leeds.

Froding CA (1960) Acoustic investigation of newborn infants. Acta Otolaryngologica 52: 31–41.

Fukushima Y, Ohashi H, Wakui K et al. (1995) De novo apparently balanced reciprocal translocation between 5q11.2 and 17q23 associated with Klippel-feil anomaly and type A1 brachydactyly. American Journal of Medical Genetics 57: 447–9.

Gabriels P (1996) Children with tinnitus. In Reich GE, Vernon JA (eds) Proceedings of the Fifth International Tinnitus Seminar. Portland, OR: American Tinnitus Association.

Gaeth JH, Lounsbury E (1966) Hearing aids and children in elementary schools. Journal of Speech and Hearing Disorders 31: 283–9.

Galambos R, Hicks GE, Wilson MJ (1984) The auditory brain stem response reliably predicts hearing loss in graduates of a tertiary intensive care nursery. Ear and Hearing 5: 254–60.

Galambos R, Wilson MJ, Silva DP (1994) Identifying hearing loss in the intensive care nursery: A twenty year summary. Journal of the American Academy of Audiology 5: 141–5.

Gale JE, Ashmore JA (1997) An intrinsic frequency limit to the cochlear amplifier. Nature 389: 63–7.

Gallaudet EM (1997) Is the sign language used to excess in the teaching of deaf mutes? American Annals of the Deaf 142: 21–3.

Gallaway C (1998) Early interaction. In Gregory S, Knight P, McCracken W, Powers S, Watson L (eds) Issues in Deaf Education. London: David Fulton Publishers Ltd.

Gallaway C, Lewis S (1993) Talking to children. Part One: Fact and fiction. Research Journal of the British Association of Teachers of the Deaf 17: 137–42.

Gallaway C, Nunes A, Johnston M (1994) Spoken language development in hearing impaired children: A bibliography covering research from 1996-present. Manchester: Centre for Audiology, Education of the Deaf and Speech Pathology, University of Manchester.

Gallaway C, Richards BJ (eds) (1994) Input and Interaction in Language Acquisition. Cambridge: Cambridge University Press.

Gallaway C, Woll B (1994) Interaction and childhood deafness. In Gallaway C, Richards BJ (eds) Input and Interaction in Language Acquisition. Cambridge: Cambridge University Press.

Gans DP (1987) Improving behavioural observation audiometry testing and scoring procedure. Ear and Hearing 8: 92–100.

Gans D, Gans KD (1993) Development of a hearing test protocol for profoundly involved multi-handicapped children. Ear and Hearing 14: 128–40.

Gantz BJ, McCabe BF, Tyler RS (1988) Use of multichannel cochlear implants in obstructed and obliterated cochleas. Otolaryngology, Head and Neck Surgery 98: 72–81.

Gardner MB, Gardner RS (1973) Problem of localization in the median plane: Effect of pinna cavity occlusion. Journal of Acoustical Society of America 53: 400–8.

Gascon G, Johnson R, Burd L et al. (1986) Central auditory processing in attention deficit disorders. Journal of Child Neurology 1: 27-33.

Gat I, Keith RW (1978) An effect of linguistic experience: Auditory word discrimination by native and non-native speakers of English. Audiology 17: 339.

Gathercole SE, Baddeley AD (1993) Working Memory and Language. Hove, UK: Lawrence Erlbaum Associates.

Geers A, Moog J (1989) Factors predictive of the development of literacy in profoundly hearing-impaired adolescents. Volta Review 91: 69–86.

Geers A, Moog J, Schick B (1984) Acquisition of spoken and signed English by profoundly deaf children. Journal of Speech and Hearing Disorders 49: 378–88.

Geffner DS, Levitt H, Freeman LR, Gafney R (1978) Speech and language assessment scales of deaf children. Journal of Communication Disorders 11: 215–26.

Gengel R, Pascoe DP, Shore I (1971) A frequency-response procedure for evaluating and selecting hearing aids for children with severe hearing impairment. Journal of Speech and Hearing Disorders 36: 341–53.

Gerber SE (1990) Review of a high risk register for congenital or early onset deafness. British Journal of Audiology 24: 345–56.

Gerber SE (ed.)(1996) The Handbook of Pediatric Audiology. Washington, DC: Gallaudet University Press.

Gerkin KP (1984) The high risk register for deafness. ASHA 26(3): 17–23.

Gerkin KP (1986) The development and outcome of the high risk register. In Swigart ET (ed.) Neonatal Hearing Screening. Philadelphia, PA: Taylor & Francis.

Gershon AA (1995) Chickenpox, Measles and Mumps. In Remington JS, Klein JO (eds) Infectious Diseases of the Fetus and Newborn Infant. 4 edn. Philadelphia, PA: WB Saunders.

Gibbin KP (1988) Otological considerations in the first five years of life. In McCormick B (ed.) Paediatric Audiology, 0–5 years. London: Taylor & Francis.

Gillet P (1993) Auditory Processes. Novato, CA: Academic Therapy Publications.

Gimsing S, Dyrmorse J (1986) Branchio-oto-renal dysplasia in three families. Annals of Otology Rhinology and Laryngology 4: 421–6.

Givens KT, Lee DA, Jones T, Ilstrup DM (1993) Congenital rubella syndrome: Ophthalmic manifestations and associated systemic disorders. British Journal of Ophthalmology 77: 358–63.

Glasscock ME, Seshul M, Seshul MB (1993) Bilateral aberrant internal carotid artery – case presentation. Archives of Otolaryngology Head and Neck Surgery 119: 335–9.

Goetzinger CP (1962) Effects of small perceptual losses on language and on speech discrimination. Volta Review 64: 408–14.

Gold E, Nankervis GA (1982) Cytomegalovirus. In Evans AS (ed.) Viral Infections of Humans: Epidemiology and control. 2 edn. New York: Elsevier.

Gold M, Rapin I (1994) Non-Mendelian mitochondrial inheritance as a cause of progressive genetic sensorineural hearing loss. International Journal of Pediatric Otorhinolaryngology 30: 91–104.

Goldberg JM, Fernandez C (1971) Physiology of peripheral neurons innervating semicircular canals of the squirrel monkey I. Resting discharge and responses to constant angular accelerations. Journal of Neurophysiology 34: 635–60.

Goldin-Meadow S, Mylander C (1984) Gestural communication in deaf children: The effects and noneffects of parental input on early language development. Monographs of the Society for Research in Child Development 49: 1–151.

Good C, Phelps PD, Lim DP (1995) Case report: Greatly enlarged jugular fossa with progressive sensorineural hearing loss. Journal of Laryngology and Otology 109: 350–2.

Gorga MP, Reiland JK, Beauchaine KA et al. (1987) Auditory brainstem responses from graduates of an intensive care nursery: Normal patterns of response. Journal of Speech and Hearing Research 30: 311–18.

Gorlin RJ (1995) Genetic hearing loss asssociated with endocrine and metabolic disorders. In Gorlin RJ, Toriello HV, Cohen MM (eds) Hereditary Hearing Loss and its Syndromes. Oxford: Oxford University Press.

Gorlin RJ, Toriello HV, Cohen MM (eds) (1995) Hereditary Hearing Loss and its Syndromes. Oxford monograms on medical genetics No. 28 Oxford: Oxford University Press.

Goswani U, Bryant P (1990) Phonological Skills and Learning to Read. Hove: Lawrence Erlbaum Associates.

Gottschlich S, Billings PB, Keithley EM et al. (1995) Assessment of serum antibodies in patients with rapidly progressive sensorineural hearing loss and Ménière's Disease. Laryngoscope 105: 1347–52.

Goulding MD, Chalepakis G, Deutsch U et al. (1991) Pax-3, a novel murine DNA binding protein expressed during early neurogenesis. EMBO Journal 10: 1135–47.

Graham J (1981a) Tinnitus in children with hearing loss. In: CIBA foundation symposium. Pitman Books Ltd: London 85: 172–92.

Graham J (1981b) Pediatric tinnitus. Journal of Laryngology and Otology 4: 117–120.

Graham JM (1995) Tinnitus in children with hearing loss. In Vernon JA, Moller AR (eds) Mechanisms of Tinnitus. Needham Heights: Simon & Schuster.

Grantham DW (1995) Spatial hearing and related phenomena. In Moore BCJ (ed.) Handbook of Perception and Cognition: Hearing. San Diego, CA: Academic Press.

Gravel J, Ellis MA (1995) The auditory consequences of otitis media with effusion: The audiogram and beyond. Seminars in Hearing 16: 44–58.

Gravel JS, Traquina DN (1992) Experience with the audiological assessment of infants and toddlers. International Journal of Pediatric Otolaryngology 23: 59–71.

Graziani LJ, Baumgart S, Desai S et al. (1997) Clinical antecedents of neurologic and audiologic abnormalities in survivors of neonatal ECMO. Journal of Child Neurology 12: 415–22.

Green RH, Balsamo MR, Giles JP et al. (1965) Studies of the natural history and prevention of rubella. American Journal of Diseases of Childhood 110: 348–65.

Gregg NM (1941) Congenital cataract following German measles in the mother. Transactions of the Ophthalmic Society of Australia 3: 35–46.

Gregory S (1995) Deaf Children and their Families. Cambridge: Cambridge University Press.

Gregory S, Bishop J, Sheldon L (1995) Deaf Young People and their Families. Cambridge: Cambridge University Press.

Gregory S, Mogford K (1981) Early language development in deaf children. In Woll B, Kyle J, Deuchar M (eds) Perspectives on British Sign Language and Deafness. London: Croom Helm.

Griffiths PD (2000) Cytomegalovirus. In Zuckermann AJ, Banatvala JE, Pattison JR (eds) Principles and Practice of Clinical Virology. 4 edn. Chichester: John Wiley & Sons.

Grundfast KM (1996) Infant hearing screening. Practical Reviews. Otolaryngology, Head and Neck Surgery 3: 1–4.

Grundfast KM, Lalwani AK (1992) Practical approach to diagnosis and management of hereditary hearing impairment (HHI). Ear Nose Throat Journal 71: 479–93.

Gustafson PA, Boyle DW (1995) Bilirubin index: A new standard for intervention? Medical Hypotheses 45: 409–16.

Guyot JP, Vibert D (1999) Patients with Charge association: A model to study saccular function in the human. Annals of Otology Rhinology and Laryngology 108: 151–5.

Hack M, Fanaraff AA (1999) Outcomes of children of extremely low birthweight and gestational age in the 1990s. Early Human Development 53: 193–218.

Haggard MP, Hughes E, (1991) Screening Children's Hearing. London: HMSO.

Hall D (1996) Health for all Children. London: HMSO.

Hall JW III (1992) Handbook of Auditory Evoked Responses. Needham Heights, MA: Allyn & Bacon.

Hall JW III (1999) CAPD in Y2K: An introduction to audiologic assessment and management. The Hearing Journal 52: 35–42.

Hall JW III (2000) Handbook of Otoacoustic Emissions. San Diego, CA: Singular Publishing Group.

Hall JW III, Kileny PR, Ruth RA (1987) Clinical validation study of the ALGO-1 automated hearing screener. Paper presented at the 10th International Evoked Response Audiometry Study Group Meeting, Charlottesville, Virginia.

Hall JW III, Mueller HG III (1997) Audiologists' Desk Reference. Volume I. San Diego, CA: Singular Publishing Group.

Halpern J, Hosford-Dunn H, Malachowski N (1987) Four factors that accurately predict hearing loss in 'high risk' neonates. Ear and Hearing 8: 21–5.

Hampal S, Flood LM, Kumar BU (1991) The mini-grommet in tympanosclerosis. Journal of Laryngology and Otology 105: 161–4.

Hanid TK (1976) Hypothyroidism in congenital rubella. Lancet 2: 854.

Hansen B (1990) Trends in the Progress Towards Bilingual Education for Deaf Children in Denmark. Copenhagen: Centre of Total Communication.

Hanshaw JB, Dudgeon JA, Marshall WC (1985) Viral Diseases of the Fetus and Newborn. 2 edn. Philadelphia, PA: WB Saunders.

Happe F (1994) Autism: An Introduction to Psychological Theory. London: University College London Press.

Harkness P, Topham J (1998) Classification of otitis media. Laryngoscope 108: 1539–43.

Harris JD (1965) A factor analytic study of three signal detection abilities. Journal of Speech and Hearing Research 7: 71–8.

Harris JP, Fan JT, Keithley FM (1990) Immunologic responses in experimental labyrinthitis. American Journal of Otolaryngology 11: 304–8.

Harris M (1992) Language Experience and Early Language Development. Hove: Psychology Press.

Harris M, Clibbens J, Chasin J, Tibbitts R (1989) The social context of early sign language development. First Language 9: 81–97.

Harris M, Mahoney H (1997) Learning to look in the right place: A comparison of attentional behaviour in deaf children with deaf and hearing mothers. Journal of Deaf Studies and Deaf Education 2: 95–103.

Harrison D, Simpson P, Stuart A (1991) The development of written language in a population of hearing-impaired children. Journal of the British Association of Teachers of the Deaf 15: 76–85.

Hashim FA, Ahmed AE, el Hassan M et al. (1995) Neurologic changes in visceral leishmaniasis. American Journal of Tropical Medical and Hygiene 52: 149–54.

Hatcher PJ, Hulme C, Ellis AW (1994) Ameliorating early reading failure by integrating the teaching of reading and phonological skills: The phonological linkage hypothesis. Child Development 65: 41–58.

Hausler R, Toupet M, Guidetti G et al. (1987) Ménière's disease in children. American Journal of Otolaryngology 8: 187–93.

Hawkins DB (1984) Comparisons of speech recognition in noise by mildly to moderately hearing impaired children using hearing aids and FM systems. Journal of Speech and Hearing Disorders 49: 409–18.

Hawkins DB, Montgomery AA, Prosek RA, Walden BE (1987) Examination of two issues concerning functional gain measurements with children. Journal of Speech and Hearing Disorders 52: 56–63.

Hayes E, Babin R, Platz C (1980) The otologic manifestations of mucopolysaccharidoses. American Journal of Otology 2: 65–9.

Haynes C, Naidoo S (1991) Children with specific speech and language impairment. Clinics in Developmental Medicine No.119 Oxford: Blackwell.

Hecox K, Galambos R (1974) Brainstem auditory evoked responses in human infants and adults. Archives of Otolaryngology 99: 30–3.

Hedley-Williams A, Tharpe A, Bess FH (1996) Fitting hearing aids in the pediatric population: A survey of practice procedures. In Bess F, Gravel J, Tharpe A (eds) Amplification for Children with Auditory Deficits. Nashville, TN: Bill Wilkerson Center Press.

Hegarty JL, Smith R (2000) Tinnitus in children. In Tyler RS (ed.) Handbook on Tinnitus. San Diego, CA: Singular Publishing Group.

Hendershot EL (1978) Luetic deafness. Otolaryngology Clinics of North America 11: 43–7.

Henley CM, Rybak LP (1995) Ototoxicity in developing mammals. Brain Research Reviews 20: 68–90.

Hereditary Hearing Loss Homepage. Internet database freely accessible at http://dnalab-www.uia.ac.be/dnalab/hhh/

Hess M, Finckh-Kramer U, Bartsch M et al. (1998). Hearing screening in at-risk neonatal cohort. International Journal of Pediatric Otorhinolaryngology 46: 81–9.

Hicks T, Fowler K, Richardson M et al. (1993) Congenital cytomegalovirus infection and neonatal auditory screening. Journal of Pediatrics 123: 779–82.

Hickson FS (1987) The Manchester Picture Test (1984): A summary. Journal of the British Association of Teachers of the Deaf 11: 161–6.

Hickson LM, Alcock D (1991) Progressive hearing loss in children with congenital cytomegalovirus. Journal of Paediatrics and Child Health 27: 105–7.

Hildebrand M (1982) Analysis of Vertebrate Structure. 2 edn. New York: John Wiley & Sons.

Hildesheimer M, Maayan Z, Muchnik C et al. (1989) Auditory and vestibular findings in Waardenburg's type ll syndrome. Journal of Laryngology and Otology 103: 1130–3.

Hillier SL, Nugent RP, Eschenbach DA et al. (1995) Association between bacterial vaginosis and preterm delivery of a low-birth weight infant: The vaginal infections and prematurity study group. New England Journal of Medicine 333: 1737–42.

Hiltunen-Back E, Haikala O, Koskela P, Reunala T (1996) Increase of syphilis in Finland related to the Russian epidemic. Eurosurveillance 1: 1–2.

Hind SE, Atkins RL, Haggard MP et al. (1999) Alternatives in screening at school entry: Comparison of the childhood middle ear disease and hearing questionnaire (CMEDHQ) and the pure tone sweep. British Journal of Audiology 33: 403–14.

Hindley P, Parkes R (1999) Speaking sign language from birth can make deaf children confident. British Medical Journal 318: 1491 (letter).

Hindley PA, Hill PD, McGuigan S, Kitson N (1994) Psychiatric disorders in deaf and hard of hearing young people. Journal of Child Psychology and Psychiatry 34: 917–34.

Hinman AR, Hersh BS, de Quadros CA (1998) Rational use of rubella vaccine for prevention of congenital rubella syndrome in the Americas. Pan American Journal of Public Health 4: 156–60.

Hirsh IJ, Pollack I (1948) The role of interaural phase in loudness. Journal of the Acoustical Society of America 20: 761–6.

Hisashi K, Komune S, Taira T et al. (1993) Anticardiolipin antibody-induced sudden profound sensorineural hearing loss. American Journal of Otorhinolaryngology 14: 275–7.

HMSO (1975) Hearing handicapped children. In The School Health Service 1908–1974. London: HMSO, pp. 15–18.

HMSO (1978) Report of the Committee of Enquiry into the Education of Handicapped Children and Young People. London: The Stationery Office Ltd.

HMSO (1992) Education (Schools) Act 1992 (c.38). London: The Stationery Office.

HMSO (1993) Education Act 1993. London: The Stationery Office.

Hoff-Ginsberg E (1997) Language Development. Pacific Grove, CA: Brooks/Cole.

Holt JA (1993) Stanford Achievement Test – 8th Edition: reading comprehension subgroup results. American Annals of the Deaf 138: 172–5.

Hood JD (1960) The principles and practice of bone conduction audiometry. Laryngoscope LXX: 1211–28.

Hood LJ (1998) An overview of neural function and feedback control in human communication. Journal of Communication Disorders 31: 461–9.

House JW, Sheehy JL (1980) Cholesteotoma with intact tympanic membrane: A report of 41 cases. The Laryngoscope 90: 70–6.

Howe DT, Gornall R, Wellesley D et al. (2000) Six year survey of screening for Down's Syndrome by maternal age and mid-trimester ultrasound scans. British Medical Journal 320: 606–10.

Howlin P, Kendall L (1991) Assessing children with language tests –which tests to use? British Journal of Disorders of Communication 26: 355–69.

Howlin P, Mawhood L, Rutter M (2000) Autism and developmental receptive language disorder – a comparative follow-up in early adult life. Social, behavioural and psychiatric outcomes. Journal of Child Psychology and Psychiatry 41: 561–78.

Hu DN, Qui WQ, Wu BT et al. (1991) Genetic aspects of antibiotic induced deafness: Mitochondrial inheritance. Journal of Medical Genetics 28: 79–83.

Hudspeth AJ , Corey DP (1977) Sensitivity, polarity, and conductance change in the response of vertebrate hair cells to controlled mechanical stimuli. Proceedings of the National Academy of Science USA 74: 2407–11.

Hudspeth AJ, Gillespie PG (1994) Pulling springs to tune transduction: Adaptation by hair cells. Neuron 12: 1–9.

Hughes DC (1997) Paradigms and paradoxes: mouse (and human) models of genetic deafness. Audiology and Neuro-otology 2: 3–11.

Hui CC, Joyner AL (1993) A Mouse model of Greig cephalopolysyndactly: The extra toes mutation contains an intragenic deletion of the Gli3 gene. Nature Genetics 3: 241–6.

Hultcrantz M, Sylven L (1997) Turner's Syndrome and hearing disorders in women aged 16–34. Hearing Research 103: 69–74.

Hultcrantz M, Sylven L, Borg E (1994) Era and hearing problems in 44 middle-aged women with Turner's Syndrome. Hearing Research 76: 127–32.

Humes LE, Allen SK, Bess FH (1980) Horizontal sound localization skills of unilaterally hearing impaired children. Audiology 19: 508–18.

Humes LE, Christenson L, Thomas T et al. (1999) A comparison of the aided performance and benefit provided by a linear and a two channel wide dynamic range compression hearing aid. Journal of Speech, Language and Hearing Research 42: 65–79.

Hunter LL, Margolis RH, Rykken JR et al. (1996) High frequency hearing loss associated with otitis media. Ear and Hearing 17: 1–11.

Hurley RM, Museik FM (1997) Effectiveness of three central auditory processing (CAP) tests in identifying cerebral lesions. Journal of the American Academy of Audiology 8: 257–62.

Hurst JA, Meinecke P, Baraitser M (1991) Balanced t(6;8) (6p8p; 6q8q) and the CHARGE association. Journal of Medical Genetics 28: 54–5.

Huygen PL, Verhagen WL (1994) Peripheral vestibular and vestibulo-cochlear dysfunction in hereditary disorders. Review of the literature and a report on some findings. Journal of Vestibular Research 4: 81–104.

Huygen PL, Admiraal RJ (1996) Audiovestibular sequelae of congenital cytomegalovirus infection in three children presumably representing three symptomatically different types of delayed endolymphatic hydrops. International Journal of Pediatric Otorhinolaryngology 35: 143–54.

Huygen, PL, Cremers CW, Verhagen WI, Joosten FB (1996) Camurati Engelmann disease presenting as 'Juvenile otosclerosis'. International Journal of Pediatric Otorhinolaryngology 37: 129–41.

Hyde ML, Malizia K, Riko K, Alberti PW (1991) Audiometric estimation error with the ABR in high risk infants. Acta Otolaryngologica 111: 212–19.

Hyde ML, Riko K, Corbin H et al. (1984) A neonatal hearing screening research program using the brainstem electric response. Journal of Otolaryngology 13: 49–54.

Igarashi M, Schuknecht HF (1962) Pneumococcic otitis media, meningitis and labyrinthitis: a human temporal bone report. Archives of Otolaryngology 76: 126–30.

Irvine DRF (1986) The auditory brainstem. In Ottoson D (ed.) Progress in Sensory Physiology 7. Berlin: Springer-Verlag.

Ishikawa K, Yasui N, Monoh K et al. (1997) Unilateral acoustic neuroma in childhood. Auris Nasus Larynx 24: 99–104.

Ising H, Babisch W, Hanee J, Kruppa B (1997) Loud music and hearing risk. Journal of Audiological Medicine 6: 123–33.

ISO (1991) Acoustics – Standard Reference Zero for the calibration of pure tone air conduction audiometers, ISO 389. Geneva: International Organization for Standardization.

ISO (1992) Audiometric test methods – Part 2: Sound-field audiometry with pure tone and narrow band signals. ISO 8253-2. Geneva: International Organization for Standardization.

ISO (1993) Draft International Standard 389–7, ISO 389–7 Geneva: International Organization for Standardization.

Jackler RK, de la Cruz A (1989) The large vestibular aqueduct syndrome. Laryngoscope 99: 1238–43.

Jackson CG, Pappas DG Jr., Manolidis S et al. (1996) Pediatric neurotologic skull base surgery Laryngoscope 106: 1205–9.

Jacobs IN, Potsic WP (1994) Glomus tympanicum in infancy. Archives of Otolaryngology, Head and Neck Surgery 120: 203–5.

Jansma S, Knoors H, Baker A (1997) Sign language assessment: A Dutch project. Deafness and Education 21: 39–46.

Jastreboff PJ, Hazell JWP (1993) A neurophysiological approach to tinnitus: Clinical implications. British Journal of Audiology 27: 7–17.

JCIH (Joint Committee on Infant Hearing) 1994 Position Statement (1994a) Audiology Today 6: 6–9.

JCIH (Joint Committee on Infant Hearing) 1994 Position Statement (1994b) Pediatrics 95: 1–5.

JCIH (Joint Committee on Infant Hearing) High Risk Register for Identification of Hearing Impairment (2000). Principles and guidelines for early intervention programs: Year 2000 position statement. See www.audiology.org and/or www.asha.org.

Jensen JH, Borre S, Johansen PA (1989a) Unilateral sensorineural hearing loss in children: Cognitive abilities with respect to right/left ear differences. British Journal of Audiology 23: 215–20.

Jensen JH, Johansen PA, Børre S (1989b) Unilateral sensorineural hearing loss in children and auditory performance with respect to right/left ear differences. British Journal of Audiology 23: 207–13.

Jerger J, Jerger S, Pirozzolo F et al. (1989) Speech understanding in the elderly. Ear and Hearing 10: 79–89.

Jerger J, Oliver T, Chmiel R et al. (1988) The auditory middle latency response. Seminars in Hearing 9: 75–85.

Jerger JF, Hayes D (1976) The cross-check principle in paediatric audiometry. Archives of Otolaryngology 102: 614–20.

Jerger S (1987) Validation of the Pediatric Speech Intelligibility Test in children with central nervous system lesions. Audiology 26: 298–311.

Jerger S, Allen JS (1998) How behavioral tests of central auditory processing may complicate management. In Bess F (ed.) Children with Hearing Impairment: Contemporary Trends. Nashville, TN: Vanderbilt Bill Wilkerson Center Press.

Jerger S, Jerger J (1985) Audiologic applications of early, middle, and late auditory-evoked potentials. The Hearing Journal: 31–3.

Jernigan T, Hesselink JR, Sowell E, Tallal P (1991) Cerebral structure on magnetic resonance imaging in language and learning impaired children. Archives of Neurology 48: 539–45.

Jewett DL, Williston JS (1971) Auditory evoked far fields averaged from the scalp of humans. Brain 4: 681–96.

Jiang ZD (1995) Long-term effect of perinatal and postnatal asphyxia on developing human auditory brainstem responses: Peripheral hearing loss. International Journal of Pediatric Otorhinolaryngology 33: 225–38.

Johnsen NJ, Bagi P, Elberling C (1983) Evoked acoustic emissions from the human ear III. Findings in neonates. Scandinavian Audiology 12: 17–24.

Johnsen N, Bagi P, Parbo J, Elberling C (1988) Evoked acoustic emissions from the human ear IV. Final results in 100 neonates. Scandinavian Audiology 17: 27–34.

Johnson DR (1967) Extra toes: a new mutant gene causing multiple abnormalities in the mouse. Journal of Embryology and Experimental Morphology 17: 543 –81.

Johnson GD, Harbaugh RE, Lenz SB (1994) Surgical decompression of Chiari I malformation for isolated progressive sensorineural hearing loss. American Journal of Otology 15: 634–8.

Johnson RE, Liddell SK, Erting CJ (1989) Unlocking the curriculum: Principles for achieving access in deaf education. Gallaudet Research Institute Working Paper 89–3. Washington, DC: Gallaudet University.

Johnston J (1994) Cognitive Abilities of children with language impairment. In Watkins R, Rice M (eds) Specific Language Impairments in Children. Baltimore, MD: Paul Brooks.

Jordt J, Ching TYC, Byrne D et al. (1997) Optimising amplification for hearing-impaired children: II. Aided speech audiogram. Australian Journal of Education of the Deaf 3: 29–33.

Jusczyk PW (1997) The Discovery of Spoken Language. Cambridge, MA: MIT Press.

Kacser H, Mya KM, Duncker M et al. (1977) Maternal histidine metabolism and its effect on fetal development in the mouse. Nature 265: 262–6.

Kahlmeter G, Dahlager JII (1984) Aminoglycoside toxicity – a review of clinical studies published between 1975 and 1982. Journal of Antimicrobial Chemotherapy (Suppl. A): 9–22.

Kanagasuntheram R (1967) A note on the development of the tubotympanic recess in the human embryo. Journal of Anatomy 101: 731–41.

Kaplan DM, Fliss DM, Kraus M et al. (1996) Audiometric findings in children with chronic suppurative otitis media without cholesteatoma. International Journal of Pediatric Otorhinolaryngology 35: 89–96.

Kaplan M, Beutler E, Vreman HJ et al. (1999) Neonatal hyperbilirubinaemia in Glucose-6-Phosphate Dehydrogenase-deficient heterozygotes. Pediatrics 104: 68–74.

Kaplan SL, Caitlin FI, Weaver T, Feigin RD (1984) Onset of hearing loss in children with bacterial meningitis. Pediatrics 73: 575–8.

Kaplan SL, Hawkins EP, Kline MW et al. (1989) Invasion of the inner ear by Haemophilus influenzae type b in experimental meningitis. Journal of Infectious Diseases 159: 923–30.

Karchmer MA (1991) Causal factors and concomitant impairment. In Matz GJ (ed.) Early identification of hearing impairment in infants and young children: NIH Consensus Development Conference. Bethesda, MD: National Institute of Hearing.

Karma PH, Sapela MM, Cataja MJ, Penttila MA (1993) Pneumatic otoscopy in otitis media. Value of different tympanic membrane findings and their combinations. In Lim DJ, Bluestone CD, Klein JO, Nelson JD, Ogra PL (eds) Recent advances in otitis media. Proceedings of the Fifth International Symposium. Hamilton, Canada: Decker Periodicals.

Karmody CS, Schuknecht HF (1966) Deafness in congenital syphilis. Archives of Otolaryngology 83: 18–27.

Kasman-Kellner B, Weindler J, Pfau B, Ruprecht KW (1999) Ocular changes in mucopolysaccharidosis IVA (Morquio A syndrome) and long term results of perforating keratoplasty. Ophthalmologica 213: 200–5.

Katona G, Buki B, Farkas Z et al. (1993) Transitory evoked otoacoustic emissions (TEOAE) in a child with profound hearing loss. International Journal of Pediatric Otorhinolaryngology 26: 263–7.

Katz AE, Gerstman HI, Sanderson RG, Buchanan R (1982) Stereo earphones and hearing loss. New England Journal of Medicine 307: 1460–1.

Katz J (1962) The use of staggered spondaic words for assessing the integrity of the central auditory nervous system. Journal of Auditory Research 2: 327–37.

Katz J (1983) Phonemic synthesis. In Lasky EZ, Katz J (eds) Central Auditory Processing Disorders: Problems of speech language and learning. Baltimore, MD: University Park Press.

Katz J, Stecker N, Henderson D et al. (1992) Central Auditory Processing: A transdisciplinary view. St. Louis, MO: Mosby Year Book.

Kavanagh KT, Beckford NS (1988) Adenotonsillectomy in children: Indications and contraindications. Southern Medical Journal 81: 507–14.

Kay R (1991) The site of the lesion causing hearing loss in bacterial meningitis: A study of experimental streptococcal meningitis in guinea pigs. Neuropathology and Applied Neurobiology 17: 485–93.

Kayan A (1990) Bilateral sensorineural hearing loss due to mumps. British Journal of Clinical Practice 44: 757–9.

Keeney G, Gebarski SS, Brunberg JA (1992) CT of severe inner ear anomalies including aplasia in a case of Wildervanck syndrome. American Journal of Neuroradiology 13: 201–2.

Keibel F, Mall FP (1912) Manual of Human Embryology Vol II. Philadelphia, PA: JB Lipincott.

Keith RW (1986) SCAN: Screening Test for Auditory Processing Disorders in Children. San Antonio, TX: The Psychological Corporation.

Keith RW (1994) SCAN-A: Test of Auditory Processing Abilities for Use with Adolescents and Adults. San Antonio TX: The Psychological Corporation.

Keith RW (1999) Diagnosing central auditory processing disorders in children. In Roeser R, Hosford-Dunn H, Valente M (eds) Audiology: Diagnosis, treatment strategies, and practice management. New York: Thieme Medical and Scientific Publishers.

Keith RW (2000) SCAN-C: Test of Auditory Processing Abilities in Children – Revised. San Antonio, TX: The Psychological Corporation.

Keith RW, Fallis R (1998) How behavioural tests of central auditory processing influence management. In Bess F (ed) Children with Hearing Impairment. Nashville, TN: Vanderbilt Bill Wilkerson Center Press.

Keith RW, Farrer S (1981) Filtered word testing in the assessment of children with central auditory disorders. Ear and Hearing 12: 267–89.

Keith RW, Jacobson J (1994) Physiological responses in multiple sclerosis and other demyelinating diseases. In Jacobson J (ed.) Principles and Applications in Auditory Evoked Potentials. San Diego, CA: Allyn & Bacon.

Keith RW, Katbamna B, Tawfik S et al. (1987) The effect of linguistic background on Staggered Spondaic Word and Dichotic Consonant Vowel Scores. British Journal of Audiology 21: 21.

Keith RW, Tallis HP (1970) The use of noise in speech audiometry. Journal of Auditory Research 10: 201–4.

Keleman G (1958) Toxoplasmosis and congenital deafness. Archives of Otolaryngology 68: 547–61.

Keller WD (1992) Auditory processing disorder or attention deficit? In Katz J, Stecker N, Henderson D (eds) Central Auditory Processing: A transdisciplinary view. St. Louis: Mosby Yearbook.

Kelley PM, Harris DJ, Corner BC et al. (1998) Novel mutations in the connexin 26 gene (GJB2) that cause autosomal recessive (DFNB1) hearing loss. American Journal of Human Genetics 62: 792–9.

Kelly DA (1995) Central Auditory Processing Disorder: Strategies for use with children and adolescents. San Antonio, Texas: Communication Skill Builders.

Kemker FJ, McConnell F, Logan SA, Green BW (1979) A field study of children's hearing aids in a school environment. Language Speech and Hearing Services in the Schools 10: 47–53.

Kemp D (1978) Stimulated acoustic emissions from within the human auditory system. Journal of the Acoustical Society of America 64: 1386–91.

Kemp D (1998) Otoacoustic emissions – distorted echoes of the cochlea's travelling wave. In Berlin C (ed.) Otoacoustic Emissions – Basic Science and Clinical Application. London: Singular Publishing Group ISBN 1-56593-975-1.

Kemp D, Ryan S (1995) The use of transient evoked otoacoustic emissions in neonatal hearing screening programs. Seminars in Hearing 14: 30–45.

Kemperman MH, Koch SMP, Joosten FBM et al. (2001) Inner ear anomalies, frequent but non-obligatory features of the Branchio-Oto-Renal syndrome. Archives of Otolaryngology Head and Neck Surgery. submitted.

Kennedy DW, Hoffer ME, Holliday M (1993) The effects of etidronate sodium on progressive hearing loss from otosclerosis. Otolaryngology, Head and Neck Surgery 109: 461–7.

Kenworthy OT, Klee T, Tharpe AM (1990) Speech recognition ability of children with unilateral sensorineural hearing loss as a function of amplification, speech stimuli and listening condition. Ear and Hearing 11: 224–70.

Khetarpal U, Schuknett HF, Gacek RR, Holmes LB (1991) Autosomal dominant sensorineural hearing loss. Pedigrees, audiological findings and temporal bone findings in two kindreds. Archives of Otolaryngology, Head and Neck Surgery 117: 1032–42.

Kiang NYS, Watanabe T, Thomas EC, Clark LF (1965) Discharge patterns of single fibers in the cat's auditory nerve. Research Monograph No. 35. Cambridge, MA: MIT Press.

Kileny P (1985) Middle latency (MLR) and late vertex auditory evoked responses in central auditory dysfunction. In Pinheiro M, Musiek F (eds) Assessment of Kluwin T (1981) A rationale for modifying classroom signing systems. Sign language studies 31: 179–97.

Kileny PR, Boerst A, Zwolan T (1997) Cognitive evoked potentials to speech and tonal stimuli in children with implants. Otolaryngology, Head and Neck Surgery 117: 161–9.

Kimberling WJ, Möller C (1995) Clinical and molecular genetics of Usher syndrome. Journal of the American Academy of Audiology 6: 63–72.

Kinney CE (1953) Hearing impairments in children. Laryngoscope 63: 220–6.

Kittrell AP, Arjmand EM (1997) The age of diagnosis of sensorineural hearing loss in children. International Journal of Paediatric Otorhinolaryngology 40: 97–106.

Klapper PE, Morris DJ (1990) Screening for viral and protozoal infections in pregnancy. A review. British Journal of Obstetrics and Gynaecology 97: 974–83.

Klin A, Volkmar FR, Sparrow SS et al. (1995) Validity and neuropsychological characterisation of Asperger syndrome: Convergence with non-verbal learning disabilities syndrome. Journal of Child Psychology and Psychiatry 36: 1127–41.

Kluwin T (1981) A rationale for modifying classroom signing systems. Sign Language Studies 31: 179–97.

Kluyskens P, Verstraete W, Ringoir S, Daneels R (1966) Beschrijving van een nieuwfamiliaal voorkomende associatie van oor- en nierpathologie.Verh Vlaam Akad Geneeskunde Belg. 28: 241–65.

Knell SM, Klonoff EA (1983) Language sampling in deaf children: A comparison of oral and signed communication modes. Journal of Communication Disorders 16: 435–47.

Knoors H (1997) Book review on bilingualism in deaf education. In Ahlgren I, Hylenstam K (eds) Deafness and Education 21: 53–4.

Knox C, Roeser RJ (1980) Cerebral dominance in normal and dyslexic children. Seminars in speech, language, and hearing 1: 181–94.

Kobayashi H, Suzuki A, Nomura Y (1994) Unilateral hearing loss following rubella infection in an adult. Acta Otolaryngologica (Suppl.) 514: 49–51.

Koch SMP, Kumar S, Cremers CWRJ (2000) Autosomal dominant inherited dysmorphic small auricles, lip pits and congenital conductive hearing impairment. Archives of Otolaryngology.

Koester LS, Karkowski AM, Traci MA. (1998) How do deaf and hearing mothers regain eye contact when their infants look away? American Annals of the Deaf 143: 5–13.

Kohut RI, Hinojosa R, Ryu JH (1996) Update on idiopathic perilymph fistulas. Otolaryngologic Clinics of North America 29: 343–52.

Kok M, van Zanten , Brocaar M , Wallenburg H (1993) Click-evoked oto-acoustic emissions in 1036 ears of healthy newborns. Audiology 32: 213–24.

Konkle D, Schwartz D (1981) Binaural amplification: A paradox. In Bess FB, Freeman BA, Sinclair S (eds) Amplification in Education, Washington, DC.

Konkle DF, Knightley CA (1993) Delayed onset hearing loss in RDS: Case reports. Journal American Academy of Audiology 4: 351–4.

Konradsson KS (1996) Bilaterally preserved otoacoustic emissions in four children with profound idiopathic unilateral sensorineural hearing loss. Audiology 35: 217–27.

Kornhuber HH (1974) Handbook of Sensory Physiology Vol. VI/I Vestibular System part 1: Basic Mechanisms and part 2 Psychophysics, Applied Aspects and General Interpretations. Berlin: Springer-Verlag.

Kountakis SE, Psifidis A, Chang CJ, Stiernberg CM (1997) Risk factors associated with hearing loss in neonates. American Journal of Otolaryngology 18: 90–3.

Kraus N, McGee T, Carrell TD, Sharma A (1995) Neurophysiologic basis of speech discrimination. Ear and Hearing 16: 19–37.

Kraus N, McGee T, Comperatore C (1989) MLRs in children are consistently present during wakefulness, Stage 1, and REM sleep. Ear and Hearing 10: 339–45.

Kraus N, Ozdamar O, Hier D, Stein L et al. (1982) Auditory middle latency responses (MLRs). Patients with Cortical Lesions. Electroencephalography and Clinical Neurophysiology 54: 275–87.

Kraus N, Smith E, Reed N et al. (1985) Auditory middle latency responses in children: Effects of age and diagnostic category. Electroencephalography and Clinical Neurophysiology 62: 343–51.

Kros C (1996) Physiology of mammalian cochlear hair cells. In Popper AN, Fay RR (eds) The Cochlea: Springer Handbook of Auditory Research. New York: Springer.

Kuhl PK, Miller JD (1975) Speech perception by the chinchilla: Voiced-voiceless distinction in alveolar-plosive consonants. Science 190: 69–72.

Kumar S, Deffenbacher K, Marres HAM et al. (2000) Genomewide search and genetic localization of a second gene associated with autosomal dominant branchio-oto-renal syndrome: Clinical and genetic implications. American Journal of Human Genetics 66: 1715–20.

Kumar S, Kimberling WJ, Marres HJ, Cremers CW (1999) Genetic heterogeneity associated with branchio-oto-renal syndrome. American Journal of Medical Genetics 83: 207–8.

Kumar S, Kimberling WJ, Weston MD et al. (1998a) Identification of three novel mutations in human EyA1 protein associated with branchio-oto-renal syndrome. Human Mutation 11: 443–9.

Kumar S, Marres HAM, Cremers CWRJ, Kimberling WJ (1998b) Autosomal dominant branchio-oto (BO) syndrome is not allelic to the branchio-oto-renal (BOR) gene at 18q13. American Journal of Human Genetics 76: 395–401.

Kurihara Y, Kurihara H, Suzuki H et al. (1994) Elevated blood pressure and craniofacial abnormalities in mice deficient in endothelin-1. Nature 368: 703–10.

Kyle J (1990) From gesture to sign to speech. Final Report to the Economic and Social Research Council. University of Bristol.

Laccourreye L, Francois M, Tran Ba Huy E, Narcy P Bilateral evoked otoacoustic emissions in a child with bilateral profound hearing loss. Annals of Otology, Rhinology and Laryngology 105: 286–8.

Lalwani AK, Dowd CF, Halbach VV (1993) Grading venous restrictive disease in patients with dural arteriovenous fistulas of the transverse/sigmoid sinus. Journal of Neurosurgery 79: 11–15.

Lalwani AK, Linthicum FH, Wilcox ER et al. (1997) A five-generation family with late-onset progressive hereditary hearing impairment due to cochleosaccular degeneration. Audiology and Neuro-Otology 2: 139–52.

Lalwani AK, Sooy CD (1992) Otologic and neurotologic manifestations of acquired immune deficiency syndrome. Otolaryngologic Clinics of North America 25: 1183–7.

Landau W, Kleffner FR (1957) Syndrome of acquired aphasia with convulsive disorder in children. Neurology 7: 523—30.

Lane H, Bahan B (1998) Ethics of cochlear implantation in young children: a review and reply from the Deaf-World perspective. Otolaryngology – Head and Neck Surgery 119: 297–313.

Lane H, Boyes-Braem P, Bellugi U (1976) Preliminaries to a distinctive feature analysis of handshapes in ASL. Cognitive Psychology 8: 263–89.

Lane H, Hoffmeister R, Bahan B (1996) A Journey into the Deaf-World. San Diego, CA: Dawn Sign Press.

Langenbeck B (1935) Das symmetriegesetz der erblichen taubheit. Zeitschrift fur Ohrenheilkunde. 223: 261.

Langhendries JP, Battisti O, Bertrand JM et al. (1998) Adaptation in neonatology of the once-daily concept of aminoglycoside administration: Evaluation of a dosing chart for amikacin in an intensive care unit. Biology of the Neonate 74: 351–62.

Laurenzi C, Monteiro B (1997) Mental health and deafness – the forgotten specialism. ENT News: 6: 22–4.

Law J (1994) Before School: A handbook of approaches to intervention with preschool language impaired children. London: AFASIC.

Law J, Boyle J, Harris F et al. (1998) Screening for speech and language delay: A systematic review of the literature. Health Technology Assessment 2 (9).

Leavitt R, Flexer C (1991) Speech degradation as measured by the Rapid Speech Transmission Index (RASTI). Ear and Hearing 12: 115–18.

Le Couteur, A Rutter, M Lord et al. (1989) Autism diagnostic interview: A standard investigator-based instrument. Journal of Autism and Developmental Disorders 23: 323–39.

Lederberg A, Mobley C (1990) The effects of hearing impairment on the quality of attachment and mother-child interaction. Child Development 61: 1596–604.

Lederberg AR, Everhart VS (1998) Communication between deaf children and their hearing mothers: The role of language gesture and vocalisations. Journal of Speech, Language and Hearing Research 41: 887–99.

Lee PC, Senders CW, Gantz BJ, Otto SR (1985) Transient sensorineural hearing loss after overuse of portable headphone cassette radios. Otolaryngology, Head and Neck Surgery 93: 622–5.

Lenars T (1997) Cochlear implants: what can be achieved? American Journal of Otology (Suppl. 18): S2–3.

Lenneberg EH, Rebelsky GF, Nichols IA (1965) The vocalisation of infants born to deaf and to hearing parents. Human Development 8: 23–37.

Leon P, Bonilla J, Sanchez JR et al. (1981) Low frequency heriditary deafness in man with childhood onset. American Journal of Human Genetics 33: 209–14.

Leon PE, Raventos H, Lynch E et al. (1993) Clinical evaluation of autosomal dominant post lingual deafness and a genetic map of the DFNA1 region of 5q31. American Journal of Human Genetics (Suppl. 53): Abstract 1031.

Leonard G, Black FO, Schramm VL (1983) Tinnitus in children. In Bluestone CD, Stool SE (eds) Pediatric Otolaryngology. Philadelphia, PA: WB Saunders.

Leonard L, McGregor K, Allen G (1992) Grammatical morphology and speech perception in children with specific language impairment. Journal of Speech and Hearing Research 35: 1076–85.

Leonard LB (1997) Children with Specific Language Impairments. Cambridge, MA: MIT Press.

Lesperance MM, Hall JW, Bess FH et al. (1995) A gene for autosomal dominant hereditary hearing impairment maps to 4p16.3. Human Molecular Genetics 4: 1967–72.

Levenson MJ, Parisier SC, Jacobs M, Edelstein DR (1989) The large vestibular aqueduct syndrome in children. Archives of Otology, Head and Neck Surgery 115: 54–8.

Levi H, Tell L, Feinmeisser M (1993) Progressive hearing loss in hard-of-hearing children. Audiology 32: 132–6.

Levin BA, Shelton C, Berliner KL (1989) Sensorineural loss in chronic otitis. Archives of Otolaryngology, Head and Neck Surgery 115: 814–16.

Levine SB, Snow B (1987) Pulsatile tinnitus. Laryngoscope 97: 401–6.

Levitt H, McGarr N, Geffner D (1987). Development of language and communication in hearing impaired children. ASHA: Monograph 26: 9–24.

Lewis D (1997) Selection and assessment of classroom amplification. In McCracken W, Laoide-Kemp S (eds) Audiology in Education. London: Whurr Publishers.

Lewis S (1996) The reading achievements of a group of severely and profoundly hearing-impaired school leavers educated within a natural aural approach. Journal of the British Association of Teachers of the Deaf 20: 1–7.

Lewis S, Hostler M (1998) Some outcomes of mainstream education, A Ewing Foundation Study. Paper presented to the Conference for Heads of Schools and Services for the Hearing Impaired. Hull, November, 1998.

Liberman MC (1982) The cochlear frequency map for the cat: Labeling auditory-nerve fibers of known characteristic frequency. Journal of Acoustical Society of America 72: 1441–9.

Licklider J (1948) The influence of interaural phase relations upon the masking of speech by white noise. Journal of the Acoustical Society of America 20: 213–32.

Liebreich R (1861) Abkunft und Ehen unter Blutsverwandten als Grund von Retinitis Pigmentosa. Dtsch Arch Klin Med 13: 53–5.

Lieven EVM (1994) Crosslinguistic and crosscultural aspects of language addressed to children. In Gallaway C, Richards BJ (eds) Input and Interaction in Language Acquisition. Cambridge: Cambridge University Press.

Lim DJ, Rueda J (1992) Structural development of the cochlea. In Romand R (ed.) Development of Auditory and Vestibular Systems 2. New York: Academic Press.

Lindsay JR (1973) Profound childhood deafness: Inner ear pathology. Annals of Otology, Rhinology and Laryngology (Suppl. 82): 88–102.

Lindsay JR, Davey PR, Ward PH (1960) Inner ear pathology in deafness due to mumps. Annals of Otology, Rhinology and Laryngology 69: 918–35.

Lindsay JR, Hemenway WG (1954a) The pathology of rubella deafness. Journal of Laryngology and Otology 68: 461–4.

Lindsay JR, Hemenway WG (1954b) Inner ear pathology due to measles. Annals of Otology, Rhinology and Laryngology 63: 754–71.

Lindskog U, Ödkvist L, Noaksson L, Wallquist J (1999) Benign paroxysmal vertigo in childhood: A long-term follow up. Headache 39: 33–7.

Ling D , Nienhuys TG (1983) The deaf child: Habilitation with and without a cochlear implant. Annals of Otology, Rhinology and Laryngology 92: 593–8.

Linglof T (1995) Rapid increase of syphilis and gonorrhoea in parts of the former USSR. Sexually Transmitted Diseases 22: 160–1.

Lins OG, Picton P, Picton TW et al. (1995) Auditory steady-state responses to tones amplitude-modulated at 80–110 Hz. Journal of the Acoustical Society of America 97: 3051–63.

Linthicum FH, Galey R (1981) Computer aided reconstruction of the endolymphatic sac. Acta Otolaryngologica 91: 423–9.

Lippy WH, Burkey JN, Schuring AG, Rizer FM (1998) Short- and long-term results of stapedectomy in children. Laryngoscope 108: 569–72.

Littmann TA, Magruder A, Strother DR (1998) Monitoring and predicting ototoxic damage using distortion product otoacoustic emissions: Pediatric case study. Journal of the American Academy of Audiology 9: 257–62.

Liu X, Xu L (1994) Nonsyndromic hearing loss: An analysis of audiograms. Annals of Otology, Rhinology and Laryngology 103: 428–33.

Lloyd J (1999) Hearing impaired children's strategies for managing communication breakdown. Deafness and Education International 1: 188–99.

Logigian EL, Kaplan RF, Steere AC (1990) Chronic neurologic manifestations of Lyme disease. New England Journal of Medicine 323: 1438–44.

Lord C, Pickles A (1996) Language level and non-verbal social-communicative behaviours in autistic and language delayed children. Journal of American Academy of Child and Adolescent Psychiatry 35: 1542–50.

Lord C, Rutter M, Goode S et al. (1989) Autism diagnostic observational schedule: A standardised observation of communicative and social behaviour. Journal of Autism and Developmental Disorders 19: 185–212.

Lowenstein O, Sand A (1940a) Mechanisms of semicircular canal responses of single fibre preparations to angular accelerations and to rotation of constant speed. Proceedings of the Royal Society 129B: 256–75.

Lowenstein O, Sand A (1940b) The individual and integrated activity of the semicircular canals of the elasmobranch labyrinth. Journal of Physiology 99: 98–101.

Lufkin T, Dierich A, LeMeur M et al. (1991) Disruption of the Hox 1.6 homeobox gene results in defects in a region corresponding to its rostral domain of expression. Cell 66: 1105–19.

Luotonen M, Uhari M, Aitola L et al. (1998) A nation-wide population-based survey of otitis media and school achievement. International Journal of Pediatric Otorhinolaryngology 43: 41–51.

Luterman D (1995) Counselling for parents of children with auditory disorders. In Roeser R, Downs M (eds) Auditory Disorders in School Children. New York: Thieme Publishers.

Luterman D, Kurtzer-White E, Seewald RC (1999) The Young Deaf Child. Baltimore, MD: York Press.

Lutman ME, Mason SM, Sheppard S, Gibbin KP (1989) Differential diagnostic potential of oto-acoustic emissions: A case study. Audiology 28: 205–10.

Lutman ME, Davis AC, Fortnum HM, Wood S (1997) Field sensitivity of targeted neonatal hearing screening by transient-evoked otoacoustic emissions. Ear and Hearing 18: 265–76.

Luxon L (1998) Toys and games: Poorly recognised hearing hazards? European case ascertainment will help to confirm the association (editorial). British Medical Journal 316: 1473.

Lynas W (1986) Integrating the Handicapped into Ordinary Schools: A study of hearing-impaired pupils. London: Croom Helm.

Lynas W (1994) Communication Options in the Education of Deaf Children. London: Whurr Publishers.

Lynas W (1995) A current review of approaches to communication in the education of deaf children. Manchester: Ewing Foundation Publication, Centre for Audiology, Education of the Deaf and Speech Pathology, University of Manchester.

Lynn GE, Cullis PA, Gilroy J et al. (1983) Olivopontocerebellar degeneration: Effects on auditory brainstem responses. Seminars in Hearing 4: 375–84.

Lyons Jones K (ed.) (1997) Smith – Recognizable Patterns of Human Malformation. New York: WB Saunders.

Lyos AT, Marsh MA, Jenkins HA, Coker NJ (1995) Progressive hearing loss after transverse temporal bone fracture. Archives of Otolaryngology, Head and Neck Surgery 121: 795–9.

MacKeith NW, Coles RRA (1971) Binaural advantages in hearing of speech. Journal of Laryngology and Otology 85: 213–32.

Macrae J (1982) Invalid aided thresholds. Hearing Instruments 33: 20–2.

MacRae MJ (1979) Bonding in a sea of silence. American Journal of Maternal Child Nursing 4: 29–34.

Madell JR, Sculerati N (1991) Non-congenital hereditary hearing loss in children. Archives Otolaryngology, Head and Neck Surgery 117: 332–5.

Madriz JJ, Herrera G (1995) Human immuno-deficiency virus and acquired immune deficiency syndrome. AIDS-related hearing disorders. Journal of the American Academy of Audiology 6: 358–64.

Maestas Y, Moores J (1980) Early language environment: Interactions of deaf parents and their infants. Sign Language Studies 26: 1–13.

Magliulo G, Cristofari P, Terranova, G (1996) Glomus tumor in pediatric age. International Journal of Pediatric Otorhinolaryngology 38: 77–80.

Magnusson L, Borjesson E, Axelsson AC (1997) Visual reinforcement audiometry. Comparison of loudspeaker arrangements. Scandinavian Audiology 26: 247–51.

Mahshie S (1995) Educating Deaf Children Bilingually. Washington, DC: Pre-College Programs, Gallaudet University DC.

Makhdoum MJ, Snik AF, Van den Broek P (1997) Cochlear implantation: A review of the literature and the Nijmegen results. Journal of Laryngology and Otology. 111: 1008–17.

Maliszewski SJ (1988) The impact of a child's hearing impairment on the family: A parent's perspective. In Bess FH (ed.) Hearing Impairment in Children. Parkton, MD: York Press.

Mallo M, Gridley T (1996) Development of the mammalian ear: Co-ordinate regulation of formation of the tympanic ring and the external acoustic meatus. Development 122: 173–9.

Mandell EM, Rockette HE, Bluestone CD et al. (1992) Efficacy of myringotomy with and without tympanostomy tubes. Tympanostomy tubes for chronic otitis media with effusion. Pediatric Infectious Disease Journal 11: 270–7.

Mangat KS, Morrison GAJ, Daniwalla TM (1993) T-tubes: A retrospective review of 1,274 insertions over a 4-year period. International Journal of Pediatric Otorhinolaryngology 25: 119–25.

Mansfield JD, Baghurst PA, Newton VE (1999) Otoacoustic emissions in 28 young adults exposed to amplified music. British Journal of Audiology 33: 211–22.

Mansour SL, Goddard JM, Capecchi MR (1993) Mice homozygous for a targeted disruption of the proto-oncogene int-2 have developmental defects of the tail and inner ear. Development 117: 13–28.

Margolis RH, Rykken JR, Hunter LL, Giebink GS (1993) Effects of otitis media on extended high frequency hearing in children. Annals of Otology, Rhinology and Laryngology 102: 1–5.

Margolis RH, Saly GL, Hunter LL (2000) High frequency hearing loss and wideband middle ear impedance in children with otitis media histories. Ear and Hearing 21: 206–11.

Markides A (1986) Age of fitting hearing aids and speech intelligibility. British Journal of Audiology 20: 165–8.

Markides A (1988) Speech intelligibility: Auditory-oral approach versus total communication. Journal of the British Association of Teachers of the Deaf 12: 136–41.

Marlin S, Denoyelle F, Garabedian EN, Petit C (1998) Etiological diagnosis of sensorineural deafness in children: A year-long review of genetic counseling for deaf people. (French). Annals of Oto-Laryngologie et de Chirurgie Cervico-Faciale 115: 3–8.

Marlow ES, Hunt LP, Marlow N (2000) Sensorineural hearing loss and prematurity. Archives of Disease in Childhood. Fetal Neonatal Edition 82: 141–4.

Marra CM, Longstreth WT, Hunter Handsfield H et al. (1996) Neurological manifestations of HIV infection without AIDS: Follow up of a cohort of homosexual and bisexual men. Journal of Neuro-AIDS 1: 41–65.

Marres HA, van Ewijk M, Heygen P et al. (1997) Inherited non-syndromic hearing loss. An audio vestibular study in a large family with autosomal dominant progressive hearing loss related to DFNA2. Archives of Otolaryngology, Head and Neck Surgery 123: 573–7.

Marres HA, Cremers CW, Dixon MJ et al. (1995a) The Treacher Collins syndrome. A clinical, radiological, and genetic linkage study on two pedigrees. Archives of Otolaryngology, Head and Neck Surgery 121: 509–14.

Marres HA, Cremers CW, Marres EH (1995b) Treacher-Collins syndrome. Management of major and minor anomalies of the ear. Reviews of Laryngology Otology Rhinology (Bord) 116: 105–8.

Marres HA, Cremers CW (1991) Congenital conductive or mixed deafness, pre-auricular sinus, external ear anomaly and commissural lip pits: An autosomal dominant inherited syndrome. Annals of Otology, Rhinology and Laryngology 100: 928–32.

Marres HA, Cremers CW, Huygen PL, Joosten FB (1994) The deafness, pre-auricular sinus, external ear anomalies and commissural lip pits syndrome. Otological, vestibular and radiological findings. Journal of Laryngology and Otology 108: 13–18.

Marschark M (1993) Psychological Development of Deaf Children. Buckingham: Open University Press.

Marschark, M (1997) Raising and Educating a Deaf Child. Buckingham: Open University Press.

Marschark, M (1998) Psychological Perspectives on Deafness. Mahwah, NJ: LEA.

Marshall JD, Ludman MD, Shea SE et al. (1997) Genealogy, natural history and phenotype of Alstrom syndrome in a large Acadian kindred and three additional families. American Journal of Medical Genetics 73: 150–61.

Martin J, Bentzen O, Colley J et al. (1981) Childhood deafness in the European Community. Scandinavian Audiology 10: 165–74.

Martin J, Hennebert D, Bentzen O et al. (1979) Childhood Deafness in the European Community. Brussels: Commission of the European Communities.

Martin JAM (1982) Aetiological factors relating to childhood deafness in the European Community. Audiology 21: 149–58.

Martin KS, Snashall S (1994) Children presenting with tinnitus: A retrospective study. British Journal of Audiology 28: 111–15.

Martinez A, Esteban AI, Castro A et al. (1999) Novel potential agents for human cytomegalovirus infection: Synthesis and antiviral activity evaluation of benzothiadiazine dioxide acyclonucleosides. Journal of Medicinal Chemistry 42: 1145–50.

Martini A, Prosser A, Mazzoli M, Rosignoli M (1996) Contribution of age-related factors to the progression of non-syndromic hereditary hearing impairment. Journal of Audiological Medicine 5: 141–56.

Mason S, Davis A, Wood S, Farnsworth A (1998) Field sensitivity of targeted neonatal hearing screening using the Nottingham ABR screener. Ear and Hearing 19: 91–102.

Matkin ND (1984) Early recognition and referral of hearing impaired children. Pediatrics in Review 6: 151–6.

Matkin ND (1988) Re-evaluating our approach to evaluation: Demographics are changing – are we? In: Bess F (ed.) Hearing Impairment in Children. Parkton, MD: York Press.

Mauk GW, White KR, Mortenson LB, Behrens TR (1991) The effectiveness of screening programs based on high-risk characteristics in early identification of hearing impairment. Ear and Hearing 12: 312–18.

Maw A (1995) Glue Ear in Childhood. Clinics in Developmental Medicine No 135. London: MacKeith Press.

Maw OR, Bawden R (1993) Spontaneous resolution of severe chronic glue ear in children and the effect of adenoidectomy, tonsillectomy, and insertion of ventilation tubes (grommets). British Medical Journal 306: 756–60.

Maw AR, Bawden R (1994) The long-term outcome of secretory otitis media in children and the effects of surgical treatment: A 10-year study. Acta Otorhinolaryngologica (Belgium) 48: 317–24.

McCracken W, Laoide-Kemp S (eds) (1998) Audiology in Education. London: Whurr Publishers Ltd.

McCormick B (1977) The Toy Discrimination Test: An aid for screening the hearing of children above a mental age of 2 years. Public Health 91: 67–9.

McCormick B (1983) Hearing screening by Health Visitors: A critical appraisal of the distraction test. Health Visitor 56: 449–51.

McCormick B (ed.) (1988) Paediatric Audiology: 0 – 5 years. London: Taylor & Francis.

McCormick B (1990) Commentary on early identification of hearing loss: Screening and surveillance methods. Archives of Disease in Childhood 65: 484–5.

McCormick B (2000) Managing the transition to Universal Neonatal Hearing Screening – the missing link. (letter) British Journal of Audiology 34: 67–70.

McCormick B, Curnock DA, Spavins F (1984) Auditory screening of special care neonates using the Auditory Response Cradle. Archives of Disease in Childhood 59: 1168–72.

McCroskey RL (1986) Wichitab Auditory Fusion Test. Tulsa, OL: Modern Educational Corporation.

McCroskey RL, Keith RW (1996) The Auditory Fusion Test-Revised. St Louis, MO: Auditec.

McCroskey RL, Pavlovic D, Allen M et al. (1981) Auditory fusion procedures assess reverberation in a theater. Sound and Vibration 15: 24–6.

McGregor JA, French JI (1997) Preterm Birth: The role of infection and inflammation. Medscape Womens Health 2: 1–10.

McIntyre PB, Berkey CS, King SM et al. (1997) Dexamethasone as adjunctive therapy in bacterial meningitis. A meta-analysis of randomised clinical trials since 1988. Journal of American Medical Association 278: 925–31.

McKusick V (1988) Mendelian Inheritance in Man. 8 edn. Baltimore, MD: John Hopkins University Press.

McKusick VA, Francomano CA, Antonorakis SE, Pearson P (1994) Mendelian Inheritance in Man, a Catalog of Human Genes and Genetic Disorders. Baltimore, MD: John Hopkins University Press.

McLachlan J (1994) Medical Embryology. London: Addison Wesley.

McLeod RP, Bently PC (1996) Understanding deafness as a culture with a unique language and not a disability. Advanced Practice Nursing Quarterly 2: 50–8.

McPhee JR, Van de Water TR (1986) Epithelial-mesenchymal tissue interactions guiding otic capsule formation: The role of the otocyst. Journal of Embryology and Experimental Morphology 97: 1–24.

McPherson DL (ed.) (1996) Late Potentials of the Auditory System. San Diego, CA: Singular Publishing Group.

Meador KJ (1982) Self-heard venous bruit due to increased intracranial pressure. Lancet 1: 391.

Meadow KP, Greenberg MT, Erting C, Carmichael H (1981) Interactions of deaf mothers and deaf preschool children: Comparisons with three other groups of deaf and hearing dyads. American Annals of the Deaf 126: 454–68.

Meadow-Orlans KP (1997) Effects of mother and infant hearing status on interactions at twelve and eighteen months. Journal of Deaf Studies and Deaf Education 2: 26–36.

Meadow-Orlans KF (1995) Sources of stress for mothers and fathers of deaf and hard of hearing infants. American Annals of the Deaf 140: 352–7.

Meier S (1978a) Development of the embryonic chick otic placode. 2. Light microscopic analysis. Anatomical Record 191: 447–58.

Meier S (1978b) Development of the embryonic chick otic placode. 1. Electron microscopic analysis. Anatomical Record 191: 459–78.

Melnick M, Bixler D, Nance WE, Yune H (1976) Familial branchio-oto-renal dysplasia: A new addition to the branchial arch syndromes. Clinical Genetics 9: 25–34.

Melville-Jones G (1974) Functional significance of semicircular canal size. In Kornhuber HH (ed.) Handbook of Sensory Physiology. VI/I. Berlin: Springer-Verlag.

Melville- Jones G, Milsum JH (1971) Frequency-response analysis of central vestibular unit activity resulting from rotational stimulation of the semicircular canals. Journal of Physiology 219: 191–215.

Mencher GT (2000) Challenge of epidemiological research in the developing world: Overview. Audiology 39: 178–83.

Ménière P (1861) Pathologie auriculaire: memoire sur des lesions de l'oreille interne donnant lieu des symptomes de congestion cerebrale apoplectiforme. Gazette Medicale de Paris 38: 597–601.

Menser MA, Forrest JM, Bransby RD (1978) Rubella infection and diabetes mellitus. Lancet 1: 57–60.

Menyuk P (1992) Relationship of otitis media to speech processing and language development. In Katz J, Stecker N, Henderson H (eds) Central Auditory Processing: A transdisciplinary view. St. Louis, MO: Mosby Year Book.

Merzenich M, Jenkins W, Johnston P et al. (1996) Temporal processing deficits of language-learning impaired children ameliorated by training. Science 271: 77–81.

Merzenich MM, Roth GL, Anderson RA et al. (1977) Some basic features of the organisation of the central nervous system. In Evans EF, Wilson PJ (eds) Psychophysics and Physiology of Hearing. London: Academic Press.

Messer D (1978) The integration of mother's referential speech with joint play. Child Development 49: 781–7.

Meyer C, Witte J, Hildmann A et al. (1999) Neonatal screening for hearing disorders in infants at risk: Incidence, risk factors and follow-up. Pediatrics 104: 900–4.

Meyerhoff WL, Paparella MN, Shea D (1978) Ménière's disease in children. Laryngoscope 88: 1504—11.

Middelweed M (1990) Difficulties with speech intelligibility in noise in spite of a normal pure-tone audiogram. Audiology 29: 1–7.

Millay K, Roeser RJ, Godfrey TJ (1977) Reliability of performance for dichotic listening using two response modes. Journal of Speech and Hearing Research 20: 510–18.

Miller E, Cradock-Watson JE, Pollock TM (1982) Consequences of confirmed maternal rubella at successive stages of pregnancy. Lancet 2: 781–4.

Miller P (1997) The effect of communication mode on the development of phonemic awareness in prelingually deaf students. Journal of Speech, Language and Hearing Research 40: 1151–63.

Millman B, Giddings NA, Cole JM (1996) Long-term follow-up of stapedectomy in children and adolescents. Otolaryngology Head and Neck Surgery 115: 78–81.

Mills RP, Albert DM, Brain CE (1986) Tinnitus in childhood. Clinical Otolaryngology 11: 431–4.

Mills RP, Cherry JR (1984) Subjective tinnitus in children with otological disorders. International Journal of Pediatric Otorhinolaryngology 7: 21–7.

Mindel ED, Vernon M (1971) They Grow in Silence. Silver Spring, MD: National Association of the Deaf.

Miyamoto RT, Osberger MJ, Robbin AM et al. (1992) Longitudinal evaluation of communication skills of children with single- or multi-channel cochlear implants. American Journal of Otology 13: 215–22.

Miyamoto RT, Kirk KI, Renshaw J, Hussain D (2000) Cochlear implantation in auditory neuropathy. Laryngoscope 109: 181–5.

MMWR (Morbidity and Mortality Report) (1999) Congenital Syphilis - United States (1998) Morbidity and Mortality Weekly Report 48: 757–61.

Mogford K (1988) Oral language acquisition in the prelingually deaf. In Bishop D, Mogford K (eds) Language Development in Unexceptional Circumstances. London: Churchill Livingstone.

Moller A (1985) Physiology of the ascending auditory pathway with special reference to the auditory brainstem response (ABR) in central auditory dysfunction. In Pinheiro M, Musiek F (eds) Assessment of Central Auditory Dysfunction. Baltimore, MD: Williams & Wilkins.

Möller C (1996) Balance function and hearing loss. In Martini A, Read AP, Stephens SDG (eds) Genetics and Hearing Impairment. London: Whurr Publishers.

Möller C, Kimberling W, Davenport S et al. (1989) Usher syndrome: An otoneurologic study. Laryngoscope 99: 73–9.

Moncur J, Dirks D (1967) Binaural and monaural speech intelligibility in reverberation. Journal of Speech and Hearing Research 10: 186–95.

Moncur JP (1968) Judgement reliability in infant testing. Journal of Speech and Hearing Research 11: 348–57.

Mondini C (1791) Anatomica surdi nati section. Bononiensi scientarium et artium instituto atque academic commentarii. Bononiae VII: 419–28.

Moore KJ (1995) Insight into the micropthalmia gene. Trends in Genetics 11: 442–8.

Moores DF (1996) Educating the Deaf. 4 edn. Boston, MA: Houghton Mifflin Company.

Morgan JL, Demuth K (eds) (1996) Signal to Syntax. Mahwah, NJ: Lawrence Erlbaum Associates.

Morton NE (1991) Genetic epidemiology of hearing impairment. Annals of the New York Academy of Science 630: 16–31.

Mosavy SH, Shafegh F (1976) Cardio-auditory syndrome of Jervell and Lange-Nielsen. Audiology 27: 535–8.

Moscicki RA, San Martin JE, Quintero CH et al. (1994) Serum antibody to inner ear proteins in patients with progressive hearing loss, correlation with disease activity and response to cortico steroid treatment. Journal of the American Medical Association 272: 611–16.

Muchner G (1981) Inner ear hearing loss in acute and chronic otitis media. Advances in Otorhinolaryngology 27: 138–43.

Mueller HG, Hall JW (1999) The Audiologists' Desk Reference, Volume II: Audiologic management, rehabilitation and terminology. San Diego, CA: Singular Publishing Group.

Mueller RF (1996) Genetic counselling for hearing impairment. In Martini A, Read A, Stephens D (eds) Genetics and Hearing Impairment. London: Whurr Publishers.

Mueller RF, Nehammer A, Middleton A et al. (1999) Congenital non-syndromal sensorineural hearing impairment due to connexin 26 gene mutations – molecular and audiological findings. International Journal of Pediatric Otorhinolaryngology 50: 3–13.

Murai K, Tyler RS, Harker LA, Stouffer JL (1992) Review of pharmacologic treatment of tinnitus. American Journal of Otology 13: 454–64.

Murray NM, Byrne D (1986) Performance of hearing-impaired and normal hearing listeners with various high frequency cut-off in hearing aids. Australian Journal of Audiology 8: 21–8.

Musiek F, Baron J, Pinherio M (eds) (1994) CAPD in Children and Adults with Learning Disabilities. Neuroaudiology Case studies. San Diego, CA: Singular Publishing Group.

Musiek FE, Baran JA, Pinheiro ML et al. (1990) Duration pattern recognition in normal subjects and patients with cerebral and cochlear lesions. Audiology 29: 304–13.

Musiek FE, Gollegly KM, Kibbe KS et al. (1991) Proposed screening test for central auditory disorders: Follow-up on the Dichotic Digits Test. American Journal of Otology 12: 109–13.

Musselman C, Kircaali-Iftar G (1996) The development of spoken language in deaf children: Explaining the unexplained variance. Journal of Deaf Studies and Deaf Education 1: 108–21.

Musselman CR, Wilson AK, Lindsay PH (1989) Factors affecting the placement of preschool-aged deaf children. American Annals of the Deaf 134: 9–13.

Mustapha M, Chardenoux S, Nieder A et al. (1998) A sensorineural progressive autosomal recessive form of isolated deafness, DFNB13, maps to chromosome 7q34-q36. European Journal of Human Genetics 6: 245–50.

Myer CM, Farrer SM, Drake AF, Cotton RT (1989) Perilymphatic fistulas in children: Rationale for therapy. Ear and Hearing 10: 112–16.

Myers EN, Stool S (1968) Cytomegalic inclusion disease of the inner ear. Laryngoscope 78: 1904–15.

Myklebust HR (1954) Auditory Disorders in Children: A manual for differential diagnosis. New York: Grune & Stratton.

Mylanus EAM, Pouw van der CTM, Snik AFM, Cremers CWRJ (1998) An intraindividual comparison of the BAHA and air-conduction hearing aids. Archives of Otolaryngology, Head and Neck Surgery 124: 271–6.

Naarden Kvan, Decoufle (1999) Relative and attributable risks for moderate to profound bilateral sensorineural hearing impairment associated with lower birthweight in children 3 to 10 years old. Pediatrics 104: 905–10.

Naclerio OR, Nealy JG, Alford BR (1981) A retrospective analysis of the intact canal wall tympanoplasty with mastoidectomy. American Journal of Otology 2: 315–18.

Nadol JB (1978) Hearing loss as a sequela of meningitis. Laryngoscope 88: 739–55.

Nager FR, DeReynier JP (1948) Das Gehörorgan bei den angeborenen kopfmissbildungen. Pract Oto-Rhino-Laryngol (Basel) (Suppl.10) 1–128.

NDCS (1994) Quality Standards in Paediatric Audiology, Vol I: guidelines for the early identification of hearing impairment. London: National Deaf Children's Society.

NDCS (1996) Quality Standards in Paediatric Audiology, Vol II: the audiological management of the child with permanent hearing loss. London: National Deaf Children's Society.

NDCS (1998) Quality Standards Initiative. London: National Deaf Children's Society.

NDCS (1999) Quality Standards in Education in Britain. London: National Deaf Children's Society.

NIH (National Institutes of Health) Consensus Conference Statement (1993) Identification of hearing impairment in infants and young children, Volume 11, Number 1. Bethesda, MD: National Institutes of Health.

Neilsen SE, Olsen SO (1997) Validation of play-conditioned audiometry in a clinical setting. Scandinavian Audiology 26: 187–91.

Nelson K, Loncke F, Camarata S (1993) Implications of research on deaf and hearing children's language learning. In Marschark M, Clark D (eds) Psychological Perspectives on Deafness. Hillsdale, NJ: Lawrence Erlbaum Associates.

Nelson KB , Ellenberg JH (1986) Antecedents of cerebral palsy. Multivariant analysis of risk. The New England Journal of Medicine 315: 81–6.

Newby HA (1964) Audiology. 2 edn. New York: Appleton-Century-Crofts.

Newman CW, Sandridge SA (1998) Benefit from, satisfaction with and cost-effectiveness of three different hearing aid technologies. American Journal of Audiology 7: 115–28.

Newton L (1985) Linguistic environment of the deaf child: A focus on teachers' use of non-literal language. Journal of Speech and Hearing Research 28: 336–64.

Newton VE (1983) Sound localization in children with a severe unilateral hearing loss. Audiology 22: 189–98.

Newton VE (1985) Aetiology of bilateral sensori-neural hearing loss in young children. The Journal of Laryngology and Otology (Suppl. 10): 1–57.

Newton VE, Rowson VJ (1988) Progressive sensorineural hearing loss in childhood. British Journal of Audiology 22: 287–95.

Nicholas JG, Geers AE (1997) Communication of oral deaf and normally hearing children at 36 months of age. Journal of Speech Language and Hearing Research 40: 1314–27.

Nield TA, Schrier S, Ramos AD et al. (1986) Unexpected hearing loss in high risk infants. Pediatrics 78: 417–21.

Niskar AS, Kieszak SM, Holmes A et al. (1998) Prevalence of hearing loss among children 6 to 19 years of age. Journal of the American Medical Association 279: 1071–5.

Ng M, Linthicum FH (1998) Morphology of the developing human endolymphatic sac. Laryngoscope 108: 190–4.

Nober LW, Nober EH (1975) Auditory discrimination of learning disabled children in quiet and classroom noise. Journal of Learning Disabilities 8: 656–773.

Nodar R (1972) Tinnitus aurium in school age children: A survey. Journal of Auditory Research 12: 133–5.

Nodar RH, Graham JT (1965) An investigation of frequency characteristics of tinnitus associated with Ménière's disease. Archives of Otolaryngology 82: 28–31.

Nodar RH, LeZak MHW (1981) Pediatric tinnitus (a thesis revisited). Journal of Laryngology and Otology (Suppl. 9): 234–5.

Nolan M, Tucker IG (1981) Functional hearing loss in children. Journal of British Association of Teachers of the Deaf 5: 2–10.

Norlund B, Fritzell N (1963) The influence of azimuth on speech signals. Acta Otolaryngologica 56: 1–11.

Nornes HO, Dressler GR, Knapik EW et al. (1990) Spatially and temporally restricted expression of Pax 2 during murine neurogenesis. Development 109: 797–809.

North KN, Wu BL, Cao BN et al. (1995) CHARGE association in a child with de novo inverted duplication (14) (q22–q24.3). American Journal of Medical Genetics 57: 610–14.

Northern JL (1992) Introduction to computerised probe-microphone real ear measurements in hearing aid evaluation procedures In Mueller HG, Hawkins DB, Northern JL (eds) Probe Microphone Measurements: Hearing aid selection and assessment, San Diego, CA: Singular Publishing Group.

Northern JL, Downs MP (1991) Hearing in Children. 4 edn. Baltimore, MD: Williams & Wilkins.

Notoya M, Suzuki S, Furukawa M (1994) Effects of early manual instruction on the oral-language development of two deaf children. American Annals of the Deaf 139: 348–51.

Notoya M, Suzuki S, Furukawa M (1996) Long term progress in reading abilities in hearing impaired children trained by the Kanazawa method. Auris Nasus Larynx. 23: 43–7.

Nozza R (1998) Thresholds are not enough: Understanding how infants process speech has a role in how we manage hearing loss. Presented at the International Conference: A Sound Foundation through Early Amplification, October, Chicago, IL.

Nozza R J, Rossman RNF, Bond LC (1991) Infant-adult differences in unmasked thresholds for the discrimination of CV syllable pairs. Audiology 30: 102–12.

Nozza RJ, Rossman RNF, Bond LC, Miller SL (1990) Infant speech-sound discrimination in noise. Journal of the Acoustical Society of America 87: 339–50.

Nwaesei CG, van Aerde J, Boyden M, Periman M (1984) Changes in auditory brainstem responses in hyperbilirubinemic infants before and after exchange transfusion. Pediatrics 74: 800–3.

Obrzut JE, Hynd GW, Obrzut A et al. (1981) Effect of directed attention on cerebral asymmetries in normal and learning-disabled children. Developmental Psychology 17: 118–25.

Oda K, Oki S, Tsumura N et al. (1995) Detection of cytomegalovirus DNA in urine from newborns in NICU using a polymerase chain reaction. The Kurume Medical Journal 42: 39–44.

Odio CM, Faingezicht I, Paris M et al. (1991) The beneficial effects of early dexamethasone administration in infants and children with bacterial meningitis. New England Journal of Medicine 324: 1525–31.

Okamoto M, Shitara T, Nakayama M et al. (1994) Sudden deafness accompanied by asymptomatic mumps. Acta Otolaryngologica (Suppl. 514): 45–8.

Oller DK, Eilers RE (1988) The role of audition in infant babbling. Child Development 59: 441–9.

Olsen WO (1991) Special auditory tests: A historical perspective. In Jacobson J, Northern J (eds) Diagnostic Audiology. Austin, Tx: Pro–Ed.

Olsen WO, Noffsinger D (1976) Masking level differences for cochlear and brain stem lesions. Annals of Otolology, Rhinology and Laryngology 86: 820–5.

O Mahoney CF, Luxon LM, Chew SL, Wass J (1996) When the triad of congenital hearing loss, goitre and perchlorate positive is not Pendred syndrome. Journal of Audiological Medicine 5: 157–65.

OMIM: Online Mendelian Inheritance in Man. Internet database freely accessible at http: //www.ncbi.nlm.nih.gov/Omim/ or at http: //www.hgmp.mrc.ac.uk/omim/

O'Rahilly R (1963) The early development of the otic vesicle in staged human embryos. Journal of Embryology and Experimental Morphology 11: 741-55.

O'Rahilly R, Muller F (1987) Developmental Stages in Human Embryos. Washington, DC: Carnegie Institution of Washington Publication 637.

Osberger MJ, Robbins AM, Todd SL et al. (1994) Speech production skills of children with multichannel cochlear implants. In Hochmair-Desoyer IJ, Hochmair ES (eds) Advances in Cochlear Implants. Vienna: Manz.

Osborne MP, Comis SD, Tarlow MJ, Stephen J (1995) The cochlear lesion in experimental bacterial meningitis of the rabbit. International Journal of Experimental Pathology 76: 317–30.

Osen KK , Roth K (1969) Histochemical localisation of cholinesterases in the cochlear nuclei of the cat with notes on the origin of acetycholinesterase – positive afferent to superior olive. Brain Research 16: 165–85.

Osterhammel P, Shallop J (1985) The effect of sleep on the auditory brainstem response (ABR) and the middle latency response (MLR). Scandinavian Audiology 14: 47–50.

Ostehammel PA, Shallop JK, Terkilson K (1985) The effect of sleep on the auditory brainstem response (ABR) and the middle latency response (MLR). Scandinavian Audiology 14: 47–50.

Oti-Boateng P, Seshadri R, Petrick S et al. (1998) Iron status and dietary iron intake of 6–24 month old children in Adelaide. Journal of Paediatrics and Child Health 34: 250–3.

Ousey J, Sheppard S, Twomey T, Palmer AR (1989) The IHR-McCormick Toy Discrimination Test – description and initial evaluation. British Journal of Audiology 23: 245–9.

Oyler RF, Matkin ND (1991) Unilateral hearing loss; demographics and educational impact. Language, Speech and Hearing Services in the Schools 19: 201–9.

Ozdamar O, Kraus N (1983) Auditory brainstem response in infants recovering from bacterial meningitis. Neurological Assessment. Archives of Neurology 40.

Pabla H, McCormick B, Gibbin, K (1991) Retrospective study of the prevalence of bilateral sensorineural deafness in childhood. International Journal of Pediatric Otorhinolarygology 22: 161–5.

Paget J (1877) Cases of branchial fistulae on the external ears. Lancet ii: 804.

Paget J (1878) Cases of branchial fistulae in the external ears. Medical and Chirurgical Transactions 61: 41–50.

Pagon RA, Graham JM, Zonana J, Yong SL (1981) Coloboma, congenital heart disease and choanal atresia with multiple anomalies: CHARGE association. Journal of Pediatrics 99: 223–7.

Pakarinen L, Karjalainen S, Simola KO et al. (1995) Usher's Syndrome type 3 in Finland. Laryngoscope 105: 613–17.

Palmer AR (1987) Physiology of the cochlear nerve and cochlear nucleus. British Medical Bulletin 43: 838–55.

Palmer AR (1995) Neural signal processing. In Moore BCJ (ed.) Hearing. Handbook of Perception and Cognition. 2 edn. London: Academic Press.

Pandya A, Xia X-J, Erdenetungalag R et al. (1999) Heterogeneous point mutations in the mitochondrial tRNASer(UCN) precursor coexisting with the A1555G mutation in deaf students from Mongolia. American Journal of Human Genetics 65: 1803–6.

Paparella MM, Jung TK (1984) Intact bridge mastoidectomy. Otolaryngology, Head and Neck Surgery 92: 334–8.

Paparella MM, Bluestone CD, Arnold W et al. (1985) Definition and classification of otitis media. Annals of Otology, Rhinology and Laryngology 94 (Suppl. 116).

Paparella M, Monzono T, Le CT et al. (1984) Sensorineural hearing loss in otitis media. Annals of Otology, Rhinology and Laryngology 93: 623–9.

Paparella M, Sugiura S, Hoshino T(1969) Familial progressive sensorineural deafness. Annals of Otolaryngology 90: 44–51.

Paradise JL, Elster BA, Tan L (1994) Evidence in infants with cleft palate that breast milk protects against otitis media. Pediatrics 94: 853–60.

Parker G, Webb H, Stevens J (1997) Outcome of infants with TEOAEs present and a high ABR threshold at birth. Paper presented at the British Society of Audiology Annual Conference.

Parker G, Webb H, Stevens J (1999) Outcome of infants with TEOAEs present and a high ABR threshold. European Federation of Audiology Societies International Conference Oulu 1999.

Parker MJ, Fortnum H, Young ID, Davis AC (1999) Variations in genetic assessment and recurrence risks quoted for childhood deafness: A survey of clinical geneticists. Journal of Medical Genetics 36: 126–30.

Parker W (1989) Migraine and the vestibular system in childhood and adolescence. American Journal of Otology 10: 364–71.

Parnes LS, McCabe BF (1987) Perilymph fistula: An important cause of deafness and dizziness in children. Pediatrics 80: 524–8.

Parving A (1976) Ménière's disease in childhood. Journal of Laryngology and Otology 90: 817–21.

Parving A (1983) Epidemiology of hearing loss and aetiological diagnosis of hearing impairment in childhood. International Journal of Pediaric Otorhinolaryngology 5: 151–65.

Parving A (1984) Early detection and identification of congenital early acquired hearing disability – who takes the initative? International Journal of Pediatric Otorhinolaryngology 7: 107–17.

Parving A (1985) Hearing disorders in childhood, some procedures for detection, identification and diagnostic evaluation. International Journal of Pediatric Otorhinolaryngology 9: 31–57.

Parving A (1988) Longitudinal study of hearing-disabled children. A follow-up investigation. International Journal of Pediatric Otorhinolaryngology 15: 233–44.

Parving A (1993) Epidemiology of hearing loss and aetiological diagnosis of hearing impairment in childhood. International Journal of Pediatric Otorhinolaryngology 5: 151–65.

Parving A (1996) Study group in the epidemiology of genetic hearing impairment. HEAR Infoletter, (2) November: 18–22.

Parving A, Hauch A (1994) The causes of profound hearing impairment in schools for the deaf – a longitudinal study. British Journal of Audiology 28: 63–9.

Parving A, Newton V (1995) Editorial: Guidelines for description on inherited hearing loss. Journal of Audiological Medicine. 4: ii–v.

Pascoe DP (1988) Clinical measurements of the auditory dynamic range and their relation to formulae for hearing aid gain. In Jensen JH (ed.) Hearing Aid Fitting: Theoretical and practical views. Copenhagen: Stougaard.

Patten BM (1953) Human Embryology. London: Churchill.

Patuzzi R (1996) Cochlear micromechanics and macromechanics. In Popper AN, Fay RR (eds) The Cochlea: Springer Handbook of Auditory Research. New York: Springer.

Patuzzi RB, Yates GK, Johnstone BM (1989a) Outer hair cell receptor current and sensorineural hearing loss. Hearing Research 39: 189–202.

Patuzzi RB, Yates GK, Johnstone BM (1989b) The origin of the low-frequency microphonic in the first cochlear turn of guinea pig. Hearing Research 39: 177–88.

Pearson A, Jacobson A, Van Calcar R, Sauter R (1973) The development of the ear. American Academy of Ophthalmology and Otolaryngology. Rochester, MN.

Peckham C (1986) Hearing Impairment in Childhood. British Medical Bulletin 42: 145–9.

Peckham CS (1972) Clinical and laboratory study of children exposed in utero to maternal rubella. Archives of Disease of Childhood 47: 571–7.

Peckham CS (1989) Cytomegalovirus in the neonate. Journal of Antimicrobial Chemotherapy 23 (Suppl. E): 17–21.

Peckham CS, Stark O, Dudgeon JA et al. (1987) Congenital cytomegalovirus infection: A cause of sensorineural hearing loss. Archives of Disease of Childhood 62: 1233–7.

Pederson U (1984) Hearing loss in patients with osteogenesis imperfecta. Scandinavian Audiology 13: 67–74.

Perry B, Gantz BJ (2000) Medical and surgical evaluation and management. In Tyler RS (ed.) Handbook on Tinnitus. San Diego, CA: Singular Publishing Group.

Peter G, Nelson JS (1978) Factors affecting neonatal E.coli K1 rectal colonisation. Journal of Paediatrics 93: 866–9.

Peters K, Ornitz D, Werner S, Williams L (1993) Unique expression of the FGF receptor 3 during mouse organogenesis. Developmental Biology 155: 423–40.

Peterson C, Seigal M (1995) Deafness, conservation and theory of mind. Journal of Child Psychology and Psychiatry 36: 359–75.

Petit C (1996) Genes responsible for human deafness: Symphony of a thousand. Nature Genetics 14: 395–91.

Petitto LA, Marentette PF (1991) Babbling in the manual mode: Evidence in the manual mode. Science 251: 1493–6.

Phelps PD (1986) Congenital cerebrospinal fluid fistulae of the petrous temporal bone. Clinical Otolaryngology 11: 79–92.

Phelps PD (1994) Historical article: Ear dysplasia after Mondini. Journal of Laryngology and Otology 108: 461–5.

Phelps PD, Coffey RA, Trembath RC et al. (1998) Radiological malformations of the ear in Pendred Syndrome. Clinical Radiology 53: 268–73.

Phelps PD, Lloyd GAS, Poswillo DE (1983) Journal of Laryngology and Otology 47: 995–1005.

Phelps PD, O'Mahoney CF, Luxon LM. (1997) Large endolymphatic sac. A congenital deformity of the inner ear shown by magnetic resonance imaging. Journal of Laryngology and Otology 111: 754– 6.

Phelps PD, Poswillo D, Lloyd GAS (1981) The ear deformities in mandibulofacial dysostosis (Treacher Collins Syndrome). Clinical Otolaryngology 6: 15–28.

Phelps PD, Reardon W, Pembrey M et al. (1991) X-linked deafness, stapes gushers and a distinctive defect of the inner ear. Neuroradiology 33: 326–30.

Phillips DP, Farmer ME (1990) Acquired word deafness, and the temporal grain of sound representation in the primary auditory cortex. Behavioral Brain Research 15: 85–94.

Philips SG, Miyamoto RT (1986) Congenital conductive hearing loss in Apert syndrome. Otolaryngology, Head and Neck Surgery 95: 429–33.

PHLS (1999) Sexually transmitted diseases quarterly report: syphilis – national and international epidemiology. Communicable Disease Report 9: 38–9.

Phrintzen RJ, Croft C, Berkman MD, Rakoff SJ (1979) Pharyngeal hypoplasia in Treacher Collins syndrome. Archives of Otolaryngology 105: 127–31.

Piaget J (1964) Six Psychological Studies. New York: Basic Books.

Picard A, Cheliot Heraut F, Bouskraoui M et al. (1998) Sleep EEG and developmental dysphasia. Developmental Medicine and Child Neurology 40: 595–9.

Pickersgill M (1997) Towards a model of bilingual education for deaf children. Deafness and Education 21: 10–19.

Pickles JO (1988) An Introduction to the Physiology of Hearing. London: Academic Press.

Pickles JO, Comis SD, Osborne MP (1984) Cross-links between stereocilia in the guinea pig organ of Corti, and their possible relation to sensory transduction. Hearing Research 15: 103–12.

Pinheiro ML, Musiek FE (1985) Sequencing and temporal ordering in the auditory system in central auditory dysfunction. In Pinheiro M, Musiek F (eds) Assessment of Central Auditory Dysfunction. Baltimore, MD: Williams & Wilkins.

Plante E (1996) Phenotypic Variability in brain-behaviour studies of specific language impairment. In Rice ML (ed.) Towards a Genetics of Language. Mahwah, NJ: Lawrence Erlbaum Associates.

Pollitt RJ, Green A, McCabe CJ et al. (1997) Neonatal screening for inborn errors of metabolism: Cost, yield and outcome. Health Technology Assessment 1 (7): i–iv, 1–202.

Power D, Wood D, Wood H (1990) Conversational strategies of teachers using three methods of communication with deaf children. American Annals of the Deaf 135: 9–13.

Powers S (1996) Deaf pupils' achievement in ordinary schools in 1996. Journal of the British Association of Teachers of the Deaf 20: 111–23.

Powers S (1998) An analysis of deaf pupils' exam results in ordinary schools in 1996. Journal of the British Association of Teachers of the Deaf 22: 30–6.

Prensky A, Sommer D (1979) Diagnosis and treatment of migraine in children. Neurology 29: 506–9.

Prezant TR, Agapian JV, Bohlman MC et al. (1993) Mitochondrial ribosomal RNA mutation associated with both antibiotic-induced and non-syndromic deafness. Nature Genetics 4: 289–94.

Prezbindowski AK, Adamson LB, Lederberg AR (1998) Joint attention in deaf and hearing children and their hearing mothers. Journal of Applied Developmental Psychology 19: 377–87.

Prieve BA, Gorga MP, Neely ST (1991) Otoacoustic emissions in an adult with severe hearing loss. Journal of Speech and Hearing Research 24: 379–85.

Primus MA (1992) The role of localisation in visual reinforcement audiometry. Journal of Speech and Hearing Research 35: 1137–41.

Primus MA, Thompson G (1985) Response strength of young children in operant audiometry. Journal of Speech and Hearing Research 28: 539–47.

Psarommatis IM, Tsakanikos MD, Kontorgiaani AD et al. (1997) Profound hearing loss and presence of click-evoked otoacoustic emissions in the neonate: A report of two cases. International Journal of Pediatric Otorhinolaryngology 39: 237–43.

Pye A, Collins P (1991) Interaction between sound and gentamycin: Immediate threshold and stereociliary changes. British Journal of Audiology 25: 381–90.

Pye C (1986) Quiché Mayan speech to children. Journal of Child Language 13: 85–100.

Quarry JG (1972) Unilateral objective tinnitus. Archives of Otolaryngology 96: 252–3.

Quigley SP (1978) Effects of hearing-impairment on normal language development. In Martin FN (ed.) Paediatric Audiology. Englewood Cliffs, NJ: Prentice-Hall.

Qiu WW, Yin SS, Stucker FJ(1998) Audiologic manifestations of Noonan's syndrome. Otolaryngology, Head and Neck Surgery 118: 319–23.

Qiu WW, Yin S, Stucker FJ (1999) Critical evaluation of deafness. Ausis Nasus Larynx 26: 269–76.

Raglan E, Prasher DK, Trinder E, Rudge P (1987) Auditory function in hereditary motor and sensory neuropathy (Charcot Marie Tooth Disease). Acta Otolaryngologica (Stockholm) 103: 50–5.

Raine C, Ajayi F, Cruikshank H et al. (1997) Relationship of intraoperative stapedial reflex thresholds and programming thresholds and comfort levels. In Clark GM (ed.) Cochlear Implants. XVI World Congress of Otolaryngology Head and Neck Surgery, Sydney, Australia 2–7 March 1997. Bologna, Italy: Monduzzi Editore.

Rajput K, Phelps PD, Alles R et al. (1999) Congenital middle-ear cholesteatoma in branchio-oto-renal syndrome. Journal of Audiological Medicine 8: 30–7.

Ramkalawan TW, Davis AC (1992) The effects of hearing loss and age intervention on some language metrics in young hearing impaired children. British Journal of Audiology 26: 97–107.

Rance G, Beer DE, Cone-Wesson B (1999) Clinical findings for a group of infants and young children with auditory neuropathy. Ear and Hearing 20: 238–52.

Rapin I, Allen DA (1987) Developmental dysphasia and autism in pre-school children: Characteristics and subtypes. Proceedings of the first International Symposium on specific speech and language disorders in children. London: Association for all Speech Impaired Children.

Rarey KE, Davis LE (1993) Temporal bone histopathology 14 years after cytomegalic inclusion disease: A case study. Laryngoscope 103: 904–9.

Rasmussen GL (1940) Studies of the VIII cranial nerve. Laryngoscope 50: 67–83.

Rasmussen N, Johnsen NJ, Bohr VA (1991) Otologic sequelae after pneumococcal meningitis: A survey of 164 consecutive cases with a follow-up of 94 survivors. Laryngoscope 101: 876–82.

Rauch SD, Xu W-Z, Nadol JB Jr. (1993) High jugular bulb: implications for posterior fossa neurotologic and cranial base surgery. Annals of Otology, Rhinology and Laryngology 102: 100–7.

Rauschecker JP (1998) Parallel processing in the auditory cortex of primates. Audiology and Neuro-otology 3: 86–103.

Razi MS, Das VK (1994) Effects of adverse perinatal events on hearing. International Journal of Pediatric Otorhinolaryngology 30: 29–40.

Read AP, Newton VE (1997) Syndrome of the Month: Waardenburg Syndrome. Journal of Medical Genetics 34: 656–65.

Reardon W (1992) Genetics of deafness: Clinical aspects. British Journal of Hospital Medicine 47: 507–11.

Reardon W, Coffey R, Pembrey M et al. (1997) Pitfalls in practice – diagnosis and misdiagnosis in Pendred Syndrome. Journal of Audiological Medicine 6: 1–9.

Reardon W, Harding AE (1995) Mitochondrial genetics and deafness. Journal of Audiological Medicine 4: 40–51.

Reardon W, Pembrey M (1990) The genetics of deafness. Archives of Disease in Childhood 65: 1196–7.

Reilly KM, Owens E, Uken D et al. (1981) Progressive hearing loss in children: Hearing aids and other factors. Journal of Speech and Hearing Disorders 46: 328–34.

Requejo AM, Navia B, Ortega RM et al. (1999) The age at which meat is first included in the diet affects the incidence of iron deficiency and ferropenic anaemia in a group of pre-school children from Madrid. International Journal of Vitamin and Nutritional Research 69: 127–31.

Reron E, Turowski G, Olszewski E (1995) Ubiquitin biotherapy in sensorineural hearing loss in children. International Journal of Thymology 3: 288–93.

Rescorla L, Schwartz E (1990) Outcome of toddlers with specific expressive language delay. Applied Psycholinguistics 11: 393–407.

Revello MG, Furione M, Zavattoni M, Gerna G (1994) Human cytomegalovirus infection: Diagnosis by antigen and DNA detection. Reviews in Medical Microbiology 5: 265–76.

Reynell J (1977) Reynell Developmental Language Scales (revised). Windsor: NFER.

Rice M, Buhr J, Nemeth M (1990) Fast mapping word-learning abilities of language delayed preschoolers. Journal of Speech and Hearing Disorders 55: 33–42.

Rice M, Hadley P, Alexander A (1993) Social biases toward children with speech and language impairments: A correlative causative model of language limitation. Applied Linguistics 14: 445–71.

Rice ML (1997) Specific language impairments: In search of diagnostic markers and genetic contributions. Mental Retardation and Developmental Disabilities Research Reviews 3: 350–7.

Richards BJ (1994) Child-directed speech and influences on language acquisition: Methodology and interpretation. In Gallaway C, Richards BJ (eds) Input and Interaction in Language Acquisition. Cambridge: Cambridge University Press.

Richardson MP, Reid A, Tarlow MJ, Rudd PT (1997) Hearing loss during bacterial meningitis. Archives of Diseases of Childhood 76: 134–8.

Rickards FW, Tan LE, Cohen LT et al. (1994) Auditory steady state evoked potentials in newborns. British Journal of Audiology 28: 327–37.

Ridgeway S (1998) Deaf People and Psychological Health. Manchester: Manchester University (PhD thesis).

Rittenhouse R, Kenyon P (1996) Conservation and metaphor acquisition in hearing impaired children. American Annals of the Deaf 136: 313–20.

Robbins AM, Renshaw JJ, Berry SW (1991) Evaluating meaningful auditory integration in profoundly hearing-impaired children. American Journal of Otology (Suppl. 12): 144–50.

Robbins AM, Svirsky M, Kirk KI (1997) Children with implants can speak, but can they communicate? Otolaryngology, Head and Neck Surgery 117: 155–60.

Robert-Gangneux F, Gavinet MF, Ancelle T et al. (1999) Value of prenatal diagnosis and early postnatal diagnosis of congenital toxoplasmosis: Retrospective study of 110 cases. Journal of Clinical Microbiology 37: 2893–8.

Roberts F, Boyer K, McLeod R (1998) Toxoplasmosis. In Katz SL, Gershon AA, Hotez PJ (eds) Krugman's Infectious Diseases of Children. 10 edn. London and New York: Mosby Press.

Roberts J, Wallace I, Hendersen F (eds) (1997) Otitis Media in Young Children. Medical, Developmental and Educational Considerations. Baltimore, MD: Paul Brookes.

Robertson CM, Finer NN, Grace MG (1989) School performance of survivors of neonatal encephalopathy associated with birth asphyxia at term.

Robertson SE, Cutts FT, Samuel R, Diaz Ortega JL (1997) Control of rubella and congenital rubella syndrome (CRS) in developing countries. 2. Vaccination against rubella. Bulletin of the World Health Organization 75: 69–80.

Robinshaw H (1992) Communication and language development in deaf and hearing infants. Unpublished PhD thesis, University of Cambridge.

Robinshaw HM (1995) Early intervention for hearing impairment: Differences in the timing of communicative and linguistic development. British Journal of Audiology 29: 315–34.

Robinson DA (1976) Adaptive gain control of vestibuloocular reflex by the cerebellum. Journal of Neurophysiology 39: 954–69.

Robinson DO, Sterling GR (1980) Hearing aids and children in school: A follow-up study. Volta Review 82: 229–35.

Robinson M (1983) Juvenile otosclerosis. A 20-year study. Annals of Otology, Rhinology and Laryngology 92: 561–5.

Robinson RJ (1987) Introduction and overview. In Proceedings of the First International Symposium on Specific Speech and Language Disorders in Children. London: AFASIC.

Rodgers GK, Telischi FF (1997) Ménière's disease in children. Otolaryngologic Clinics of North America 30: 1101–4.

Rodriguez GP, DiSamon J, Hardiman CJ (1990) Central auditory processing in normal-hearing elderly adults. Audiology 29: 85–92.

Roizen NJ (1999) Etiology of hearing loss in children: Nongenetic causes. Pediatric Clinics of North America 46: 49–64.

Roizen NJ, Wolters C, Nicol T, Blondis TA (1993) Hearing loss in children with Downs syndrome. Journal of Pediatrics 123: S9–12.

Rolfs RT (1995) Treatment of syphilis, 1993. Clinical Infectious Diseases (Suppl. 20): S23–38.

Rose JE, Brugge JF, Anderson DJ, Hind JE (1967) Phase locked response to low-frequency tones in single auditory nerve fibers of the squirrel monkey. Journal of Neurophysiology 30: 769–93.

Rose SP, Conneally PM, Nance WE (1977) Genetic analysis of childhood deafness. In Bess FH (ed.) Childhood Deafness. New York: Grune & Stratton.

Rosenberg PE (1978) Case history. The first test. In Katz J (ed.) Handbook of Clinical Audiology. 2 edn. Baltimore, MD: Williams & Wilkins Co.

Rosenhall U, Kankunnen A (1981) Hearing alterations following meningitis 2. Variable hearing. Ear and Hearing 2: 170–6.

Ross M (1981) Personal versus group amplification: The consistency versus inconsistency debate. In Bess FH, Freeman BA, Sinclair JS (eds) Amplification in Education. Washington, DC: AG Bell Association.

Ross M (1990) Hearing-impaired Children in the Mainstream. Parkton, MD: York Press.

Ross M (1992) Implications of audiologic success. Journal of American Academy of Audiology 3: 1–4.

Ross M (1997) A retrospective look at the future of aural rehabilitation. Journal of the Academy of Rehabilitative Audiology 30: 11–26.

Ross M, Giolas TG (1971) Effect of three classroom listening conditions on speech intelligibility. American Annals of the Deaf 116: 580–4.

Ross M, Giolas TG, Carver PW (1973) Effect of classroom listening conditions on speech intelligibility. Language, Speech and Hearing Services in the School 4: 72–5.

Rothenberg R (1979) Syphilitic hearing loss. Southern Medicine 72: 118–20.

Rowson KEK, Hinchcliffe R, Gamble DR (1975) A virological and epidemiological study of patients with acute hearing loss. Lancet 1: 471–3.

Ruben RJ (1990) Diseases of the inner ear and sensorineural deafness. In Bluestone CD, Stool SE, Scheetz MD (eds) Pediatric Otolaryngology, Vol. 1. Philadelphia, PA: WB Saunders.

Russell IJ, Sellick PM (1978) Intracellular studies of hair cells in the mammalian cochlea. Journal of Physiology 284: 261–90.

Rutter M, Mahwood L (1991) The long-term psychological sequelae of specific developmental disorders of speech and language. In Rutter M, Casaer P (eds) Biological Risk Factors for Psychosocial Disorders. Cambridge: Cambridge University Press.

Ryan AF (1997) Transcription factors and the control of inner ear development. Seminars in Cell and Developmental Biology 8: 249–56.

Rybak LP, Whitworth C, Scott V, Weberg A (1991) Ototoxicity of furosemide during development. Laryngoscope 101: 1167–74.

Sabin AB (1941) Toxoplasmic encephalitis in children. Journal of the American Medical Association 116: 801–7.

Sachs J (1997) Communication development in infancy. In Berko Gleason J (ed.) The Development of Language. 4 edn. Boston, MA: Allyn & Bacon.

Salamy A, Eldredge L, Tooley WH (1989) Neonatal status and hearing loss in high-risk infants. Journal of Pediatrics 114: 847–52.

Sancho J, Hughes E, Davis A, Haggard M (1988) Epidemiological basis for screening hearing. In McCormick B (ed.) Paediatric Audiology, 0–5 years. London: Taylor & Francis.

Sandberg L, Terkildsen K (1965) Caloric tests in deaf children. Archives of Otolaryngology 81: 352–4.

Sandridge SA, Boothroyd A (1996) Using naturally produced speech to elicit the mismatch negativity. Journal of the American Academy of Audiology.

Sassen ML, Brand H, Grote JJ (1977) Risk factors for otitis media with effusion in children aged 0–2 years. American Journal of Otolaryngology 18: 324–30.

Satz P (1976) Cerebral dominance and reading disability: An old problem revisited. In Knights RM, Bakker DJ (eds) The Neuropsychology of Learning Disorders: Theoretical Approaches. Baltimore, MD: University Park Press.

Saunders J (1965) Noise conditions in normal school classrooms. Exceptional Child 31: 344–53.

Saunders J, Field A, Haggard M et al. (1992) A clinical test battery for obscure auditory dysfunction. British Journal of Audiology 26: 33–42.

Savastano M, Savini M, Andreoli C (1993) Idiopathic progressive sensorineural hearing loss in children. International Journal of Pediatric Otorhinolaryngology 26: 225–33.

Saxton M (1997) The contrast theory of negative input. Journal of Child Language 24: 139–62.

Saxton M, Gallaway C (1998) Acquiring the grammatical system: How do children recover from their errors? Deafness and Education International 22: 16–23.

Schacht J (1993) Biochemical basis if aminoglycoside ototoxicity. Otolaryngological Clinics of North America 26: 845–56.

Scharf, B (1968) Binaural loudness summation as a function of bandwidth. Reports of the International Congress on Acoustics 25–8.

Schildroth A, Hotto S (1991) Annual survey of hearing-impaired children and youth: 1989–90 school year. American Annals of the Deaf 138: 46–54.

Schildroth AN (1994) Congenital cytomegalovirus and deafness. American Journal of Audiology 3: 27–38.

Schlesinger H, Meadow K (1972) Sound and Sign. Berkeley, CA: University of California Press.

Schluter WW, Reef SE, Redd SC, Dykewicz CA (1998) Changing epidemiology of congenital rubella syndrome in the United States. Journal of Infectious Diseases 178: 636–64.

Schreiner CE, Langner G (1988) Periodicity coding in the inferior colliculus of the cat. II. Topographical organisation. Journal of Neurophysiology 60: 1823–40.

Schwartz D, Lyregaard PE, Lundh P (1988) Hearing aid selection for severe/profound hearing losses. Hearing Journal 41: 13–17.

Schwartz DM, Larson VD (1977) A comparison of three hearing aid evaluation procedures for young children. Archives of Otolaryngology 103: 401–6.

Sculerati N, Ledesma-Medina J, Finegold DN, Stool SE (1990) Otitis media and hearing loss in Turner syndrome. Archives of Otolaryngology, Head and Neck Surgery 116: 704–7.

Sculerati N, Oddoux C, Clayton CM et al. (1996) Hearing loss in Turner syndrome. Laryngoscope 106: 992.

Sebag J, Albert DM, Craft JL (1984) The Alstrom syndrome: Ophthalmic histopathology and retinal ultra structure. British Journal of Ophthalmology 68, 7: 494–501.

Seewald RC (1992) The desired sensation level method for fitting children: Version 3.0. Hearing Journal 45: 36–41.

Seewald RC (1998) Infants are not average adults: Clinical procedures for individualising the fitting of amplification in infants and toddlers. Presented at the International Conference: A Sound Foundation through Early Amplification, October, Chicago, IL.

Seewald RC, Ramji KV, Sinclair ST et al. (1993) Computer-assisted Implementation of the Desired Sensation Level Method for Electroacoustic Selection and Fitting in Children: User's Manual. London, Ontario: University of Western Ontario.

Seewald RC, Ross M, Stelmachowicz PG (1987) Selecting and verifying hearing aid performance characteristics for young children. Journal of the Academy of Rehabilitative Audiology 20: 25–37.

Seewald RC, Sinclair S, Moodie KS (1994) Predictive accuracy of a procedure for electroacoustic fitting in young children. Presented at the Twenty-second International Congress on Audiology, July, Halifax.

Seki A, Nishino I, Goto Y, Maegaki Y, Koeda T (1997) Mitochondrial encephalomyopathy with 15915 mutation. Clinical report. Pediatric Neurology 17: 161–4.

Semel E, Wiig EH, Secord W, Sabers D (1987) CELF-R. New York: Harcourt, Brace Jovanovich Inc.

Shambaugh G (1930) Statistical studies of children in public schools for deaf. Archives of Otolaryngology 12: 190–245.

Shapiro JR, Pikus A, Weiss G, Rowe D (1982) Hearing and middle ear function in osteogenesis imperfecta. Journal of the American Medical Association 247: 2120–6.

Shaw EAG (1974) The external ear. In Keidel WD, Neff WD (eds) Handbook of Sensory Physiology. Berlin: Springer.

Shaw P (1997) The Parrot Speech Discrimination Test. British Society of Audiology News 20: 44–5.

Shenoi PM (1972) Wildervanck's syndrome. Journal of Laryngology and Otology 86: 1121–35.

Sheridan MD (1964) Final report of a prospective study of children whose mothers had rubella in early pregnancy. British Medical Journal 2: 536–9.

Shriberg L, Tomblin B (1999) Prevalence of speech delay and comorbidity with language impairment. Poster presented at Afasic Symposium.

Shui J, Purvis M, Sutton G (1996). Detection of childhood hearing impairment in the Oxford Region. Report of the Regional Audit Project. Oxford: Oxfordshire RHA.

Siatkowski RM, Flynn, JT Hodges AB, Balkany TJ (1994) Ophthalmologic abnormalities in the pediatric cochlear implant population. American Journal of Ophthalmology 118: 70–6.

Siger LP (1978) That deaf child and you: A forensic approach to the problems of hearing and speech. Journal of Communication Disorders 11: 149–58.

Silva P (1987) Epidemiology, longitudinal course and some associated factors: Annual update. In Yule W, Rutter M (eds) Language Development and Disorders. Clinics in Developmental Medicine. London: MacKeith Press.

Silver S, Kapitulnik J, Sohmer H (1995) Contribution of asphyxia to the induction of hearing impairment in jaundiced Gunn rats. Pediatrics 95: 579–83.

Simmons FB, Russ FN (1974) Automated newborn hearing screening, the crib-o-gram. Archives of Otolaryngology 100: 1–7.

Simonton KM (1940) Ménière's symptom complex: Review of the literature. Annals of Otology 60: 610.

Singer DB (1991) The haematopoietic system. In Wigglesworth J, Singer DB (eds) Textbook of Fetal and Perinatal Pathology. Oxford: Blackwell Scientific Publishers.

Sininger Y, Hood LH, Starr A et al. (1995) Hearing loss due to auditory neuropathy. Audiology Today 7: 10–13.

Sirimanna T, Stephens D (1997) Hearing loss in Alport syndrome. Journal of Audiological Medicine 6: 71–8.

Skolnik PR, Nadol JB Jr, Baker AS (1986) Tuberculosis of the middle ear: Review of the literature with an instructive case report. Review of Infectious Diseases 8: 403–10.

Slack RWT, Phelps PD (1985) Familial mixed deafness with branchial arch defects (earpits-deafness syndrome). Clinical Otolaryngology 10: 271–7.

Sloan C (1986) Treating Auditory Processing Difficulties in Children. San Diego, CA: College-Hill Press.

Smacchia C, Parolin A, DiPerri G et al.(1998) Syphilis in prostitutes from Eastern Europe. Lancet 351(9102): 572.

Smith PA, Evans PIP (2000) Hearing assessment in general practice, schools and health clinics: Guidelines for professionals who are not qualified audiologists. British Journal of Audiology 34: 57–61.

Smith RL (1979) Adaptation, saturation and physiological masking in single auditory nerve fibers. Journal of Acoustical Society of America 65: 166–78.

Smith S (1996) Adult-child interaction in a BSL nursery getting their attention! In Knight P, Swanwick R (eds) Bilingualism and the education of deaf children: Advances in practice. Conference Proceedings, University of Leeds.

Smoski WJ, Brunt MA, Tannahill JC et al. (1992) Listening characteristics of children with central auditory processing disorders. Language Speech and Hearing Services in the Schools, ASHA 23: 145–52.

Snik AFM, Van den Borne S, Brokx JPL, Hoekstra C (1995) Hearing aid fitting in profoundly hearing-impaired children: Comparison of prescription rules. Scandinavian Audiology 24: 225–30.

Snik AFM, Vermeulen AM, Brokx JPL et al. (1997) Speech perception performance of children with cochlear implant compared to that of children with conventional aids. I: The equivalent hearing loss concept. Acta Otolaryngologica (Stockholm) 117: 750–4.

Snow CE (1994) Beginning from Baby Talk: Twenty years of research on input in interaction. In Gallaway C, Richards BJ (eds) Input and Interaction in Language Acquisition. Cambridge: Cambridge University Press.

Snow CE (1995) Issues in the study of input: Fine-tuning, universality, individual and developmental differences and necessary causes. In Fletcher P, MacWhinney B (eds) The Handbook of Child Language. Oxford: Blackwell.

Snow CE, Ferguson CA (eds) (1977) Talking to Children: Language input and acquisition. Cambridge: Cambridge University Press.

Snowling M, Bishop DVM, Stothard SE (2000) Is pre-school language impairment a risk factor for dyslexia in adolescence? Journal of Child Psychology and Psychiatry 14: 587–600.

Solc CF, Derfler BH, Duyk GM, Corey DP (1995) Molecular cloning of myosins from the bullfrog saccular macula: A candidate for the hair cell adaptation motor. Auditory Neuroscience 1: 63–76.

Song BB, Sha SH, Schacht J (1998) Ironchelators protect from aminoglycoside-induced cochleo-and vestibulo-toxicity. Free Radical Biology and Medicine 25: 189–95.

Soucek S, Stephens SDG, Limburg CM, Kastein TE (1985) Betahistine dihydrochloride in patients with idiopathic progressive sensorineural hearing loss. IRCA Medical Science 13: 70–1.

Spencer P, Gutfeund M (1990) Characteristics of dialogues between mothers and prelinguistic hearing impaired and normally hearing children. Volta Review 97: 351–60.

Spencer P, Stafford L, Meadow-Orlans K (1994) Communicative interactions of deaf and hearing children in a day care centre: An exploratory study. American Annals of the Deaf 139: 512–18.

Spencer PE (1993) Communication behaviors of infants with hearing loss and their mothers. Journal of Speech and Hearing Research 36: 311–21.

Sperber D, Wilson D (1986) Relevance, Communication and Cognition. Oxford: Blackwell.

Sperry JL, Wiley TL, Chial MR et al. (1997) Word recognition performance in various background competitors. Journal of the American Academy of Audiology 8: 71–80.

Spitzer MW, Semple MN (1993) Responses of inferior colliculus neurons to time-varying interaural phase disparity: Effects of shifting the locus of virtual motion. Journal of Neurophysiology 69: 1245–63.

Spoendlin H (1966) Ultrastructure of the vestibular sense organ. In Robert J Wolfson (ed.) The Vestibular System and its Diseases: Transactions of the International Vestibular Symposium of the Graduate School of Medicine of the University of Pennsylvania. Philadelphia, PA: University of Pennsylvania Press.

Spoendlin H (1972) Innervation densities of the cochlea. Acta Otolaryngologica 73: 235–48.

Stackhouse J (1992) Developmental verbal dyspraxia: A review and a critique. European Journal of Disorders of Communication 27: 19–35.

Stackhouse J, Wells B (1993) Psycholinguistic assessment of developmental speech disorders. European Journal of Disorders of Communication 28: 331–49.

Stagno S (1995) Cytomegalovirus. In Remington JS, Klein JO (eds) Infectious Diseases of the Fetus and Newborn Infant. 4 edn. Philadelphia, PA: WB Saunders.

Stagno S, Pass RF, Dworsky ME et al. (1982) Congenital cytomegalovirus infection: The relative importance of primary and recurrent maternal infection. New England Journal of Medicine 306: 945–9.

Stagno S, Pass RF, Dworsky ME, Alford CA (1983) Congenital and perinatal cytomegalovirus infections. Seminars in Perinatology 7: 31–42.

Stagno S, Reynolds DW, Amos CS et al. (1977) Auditory and visual defects resulting from symptomatic and sub-clinical congenital cytomegalovirus and toxoplasma infections. Pediatrics 59: 669–78.

Stagno S, Reynolds DW, Pass RF, Alford CA (1980) Breast milk and the risk of cytomegalovirus infection. New England Journal of Medicine 302: 1073–6.

Stapells DR, Oats P (1997) Estimation of the pure tone audiogram by the auditory brainstem response: A review. Audiology and Neuro-otology 2: 257–80.

Starr A, Picton TW, Sininger Y et al. (1996) Auditory neuropathy. Brain 119: 741–53.

Starr A, Sininger Y, Winter M et al. (1998) Transient deafness due to temperature-sensitive auditory neuropathy. Ear and Hearing 19: 169–79.

Steckelberg JM, McDonald TJ (1984) Otologic involvement in late syphilis. Laryngoscope 94: 753–7.

Steel KP (1995) Inherited hearing defects in mice. Annual Review of Genetics 29: 675–701.

Stein L, Clark S, Kraus N (1983) The hearing impaired infant: Patterns of identification and habilitation. Ear and Hearing 4: 232–6.

Stein L, Kraus N (1988) Auditory evoked potentials with special populations. Seminars in Hearing 9: 35–46.

Stein L, Tremblay K, Pasterak J et al. (1996) Brainstem abnormalities in neonates with normal otoacoustic emissions. Seminars in Hearing 17: 197–213.

Stelmachowicz PG, Lewis D (1988) Some theoretical considerations concerning the relationship between functional gain and insertion gain. Journal of Speech and Hearing Research 31: 491–6.

Stenberg AE, Nylen O, Windh M, Hultcrantz M (1998) Otological problems in children with Turner's syndrome. Hearing Research 124: 85–90.

Stengerup SE, Sederberg-Olssen JF, Balle V (1992) Auto-inflation as a treatment of secretory otitis media. A randomized controlled study. Archives of Otolaryngology, Head and Neck Surgery 118: 149–52.

Stengstrom RJ, Bernard PAM, Feldman W et al. (1996) Long-term sequelae of ventilation tube insertion for the treatment of otitis media with effusion and recurrent acute otitis media. In Lim DJ, Bluestone CD, Castlebrant MD, Klein JO, Ogra PL (eds) Proceedings of the 6th International Symposium on Recent Advances in Otitis Media. Hamilton, Canada: BC Decker, Inc.

Stenström C, Ingvarsson L (1997) Otitis-prone children and controls: A study of possible predisposing factors. One hereditary, family background and perinatal period. Acta Otolaryngologica (Stockholm) 117: 696–703.

Stern, R (1995) Models of binaural processing. In Moore BCJ (ed.) Handbook of Perception and Cognition: Hearing. San Diego, CA: Academic Press.

Stevens JC, Webb HD (1997) The Sheffield targeted neonatal hearing study. Neonatal TEOAE, ABR and 8 month testing as predictors of hearing impairment at age 5 years. European Federation of Audiological Societies. Prague. May 1997.

Stevens JC, Webb HD et al. (1991) Evaluation of click-evoked oto-acoustic emissions in the newborn. British Journal of Audiology 25: 11–14.

Stevens JC, Hall DMB, Davis A et al. (1998) The costs of early hearing screening in England and Wales. Archives of Disease in Childhood 78: 14–19.

Stevens JC, Elliott C, Lightfoot G et al. (1999) Auditory brainstem response testing in babies – a recommended test protocol. British Society of Audiology News. Issue 28.

Stevenson J, Richman N (1978) Behaviour, language and development in three year old children. Journal of Autism and Childhood Schizophrenia 8: 299–313.

Stewart D, Mehl A, Hall JW III et al. (1998) Newborn Hearing Screening with Automated Auditory Brainstem Response: A Multi-site Investigation. Paper presented at the American Academy of Pediatrics Annual Meeting, San Francisco, CA.

Stewart EJ, O'Reilly BF (1989) Klippel-Feil syndrome and conductive deafness. Journal of Laryngology and Otology 103: 947–9.

Stinckens C, Standaert L, Casselman JW et al. (2001) Branchio-oto-renal syndrome. Coincidence between a widened vestibular aqueduct and progressive sensorineural hearing loss. International Journal of Pediatric Otorhinolaryngology (submitted).

Stoel-Gammon C, Otomo K (1986) Babbling development of hearing impaired and normally-hearing subjects. Journal of Speech and Hearing Disorder 51: 33–40.

Stokes J, Bamford JM (1990) Transition from pre-linguistic to linguistic communication in hearing impaired infants. British Journal of Audiology 24: 217–22.

Stokoe W (1960) Sign Language Structure. Silver Spring, MD: Linstock Press.

Stone WL, Hoffman MD, Lewis SE, Ousley OY (1994) Early recognition of autism. Archives of Paediatric Adolescent Medicine 148: 174–9.

Stothard S, Snowling M, Bishop D et al. (1998) Language impaired preschoolers: A follow-up to adolescence. Journal of Speech, Language and Hearing Research 41: 407–18.

Stouffer JL, Tyler RS, Both JC, Buckrell B (1992) Tinnitus in normal-hearing and hearing-impaired children. In Aran J-M, Dauman R (eds) Tinnitus 91. Amsterdam/New York: Kugler.

Strachan T, Read AP (2000) Human Molecular Genetics. 2 edn. New York: Bios Scientific Publishers/John Wiley.

Strasnick B, Jacobson JT (1995) Teratogenic hearing loss. Journal of the American Academy of Audiology 6: 28–38.

Strauss M (1990) Human cytomegalovirus labyrinthitis. American Journal of Otolaryngology 11: 292–8.

Strauss M, Davis GL (1973) Viral disease of the labyrinth: I. Review of the literature and discussion of the role of cytomegalovirus in congenital deafness. Annals of Otology 82: 577–83.

Streeter GL (1918) The histogenesis and growth of the otic capsule and its contained periotic tissue spaces in the human embryo. Carnegie Contributions to Embryology 7: 7–54.

Streppel M, Betten T, Von-Wedel H et al. (1997) Progressive hearing loss in children treated with hearing aids. Laryngology, Rhinology, Otology 76: 123–6.

Strong M (1995) A review of bilingual/bicultural progress for deaf children in North America. American Annals of the Deaf 140: 84–94.

Strubbe EH, Cremers CWRJ, Willemson WNP et al. (1994) The Mayer Rokitansky Kuster Hauser (MRKH) syndrome without and with associated features: Two separate entities? Clinical Dysmorphology 3: 192–9.

Stuart A, Durieux-Smith A, Stenstrom R (1990) Critical differences in aided sound field thresholds in children. Journal of Speech and Hearing Research 33: 612–15.

Stuckless ER, Birch J (1966) The influence of early manual communication on the linguistic development of deaf children. American Annals of the Deaf 111: 452–60.

Studebaker GA (1985) Clinical Masking. In Rintelmann WF (ed.) Hearing Assessment. 2 edn. Baltimore, MD: University Park Press.

Suga N (1988) Auditory neuroethology and speech processing: Complex sound processing by combination sensitive neurons. In Edelman GM, Gall WE, Cowan WM (eds) Auditory Function. New York: Wiley.

Summerfield AQ, Marshall DH (1995) Cochlear implantation in the UK 1990–1994. Medical Research Council. Institute of Hearing Research. London: HMSO Books.

Sutton GJ, Rowe SJ (1997) Risk factors for childhood sensorineural hearing loss in the Oxford region. British Journal of Audiology 31: 39–54.

Sutton GJ, Scanlon PE (1999) Health Visitor screening versus vigilance: Outcomes of programmes for detecting permanent childhood hearing loss in West Berkshire. British Journal of Audiology 33: 145–56.

Sutton-Spence R, Woll B (1999) The Linguistics of British Sign Language: An introduction. Cambridge: Cambridge University Press.

Suzuki S, Hinokio Y, Ohtomo M et al. (1998) The effects of co-enzyme Q10 treatment on maternally inherited diabetes mellitus and deafness, and mitochondrial DNA 3243 (A - G) mutation. Diabetologia 41: 584–8.

Sweetow RW (1986) Cognitive aspects of tinnitus patient management. Ear and Hearing 7: 390–6.

Sweetow RW, Reddell RD (1978) The use of masking level differences in the identification of children with perceptual problems. Journal of American Auditory Society 4: 52–6.
Sweetow RW, Will TI (1993) Progression of hearing loss following the completion of chemotherapy and radiation therapy: Case report. Journal of the American Academy of Audiology 4: 360–3.
Swigonski N, Shallop J, Bull MJ, Lemons JA (1987) Hearing screening of high risk newborns. Ear and Hearing 8: 26–30.
Szentagothai J (1950) The elementary vestibulo-ocular reflex arc. Journal of Neurophysiology 13: 395–407.
Takasaka T (1993) The Cochlear Ultrastructure and its Micromechanics. Sendai, Japan: Printing and Publishing Co. Ltd.
Takasaka T, Ozawa K, Shoji S et al. (1996) Tympanostomy tube treatment in recurrent otitis media with effusion. In Lin DJ, Bluestone CD, Castlebrant M, Klein JO, Ogra PL (eds) Proceedings of the Sixth International Symposium on Recent Advances in Otitis Media. Hamilton, Canada: BC Decker, Inc.
Tallal P, Miller S, Fitch RH et al. (1993) Neurobiological basis of speech: A case for the pre-eminence of temporal processing. Annals of the New York Academy of Sciences 682: 27–46.
Tallal P, Miller SL, Bedi G et al. (1996) Language comprehension in language-learning impaired children improved with acoustically modified speech. Science 271: 77–80.
TamagawaY, Kitamura K, Ishida T et al. (1996) A gene for a dominant form of non-syndromic sensorineural deafness (DFNA11) maps within the region containing the DFNB2 deafness gene. Human Molecular Genetics 5: 849–52.
Tarkkanen J, Aho J (1966) Unilateral deafness in children. Archives of Otolaryngology 61: 270–8.
Tassabehji M, Read AP, Newton VE et al. (1992) Waardenburg's syndrome patients have mutations in the human homologue of the paired box gene. Nature 355: 635–6.
Teatini GP (1970) Sensitized Speech Tests: Results in normal subjects. Danavox Symposium, Odense, Denmark: Andelsbogtrykkeriet.
Terzic J, Muller C, Gajovic S, Saraga-Babic M (1998) Expression of PAX2 gene during human development. International Journal of Developmental Biology 42: 701–7.
Tewfik TL, Der Kaloustian VM (1997) Congenital Anomalies of the Ear, Nose and Throat. Oxford: Oxford University Press.
Thal D, Tobias S, Morrison D (1991) Language and gesture in late talkers: A 1 year follow up. Journal of Speech and Hearing Research 34: 604–12.
Tharpe AM, Bess FH (1991) Identification and management of children with minimal hearing loss. International Journal of Pediatric Otorhinolaryngology 21: 41–50.
Tharpe AM, Bess FH (1999) Minimal, progressive, and fluctuating hearing loss in children: Characteristics, identification, and management. Pediatric Clinics of North America 46: 65–78.
The Chipping Forecast. Nature Genetics (1999) (Suppl. 21).
Thiringer K, Kankkunen A, Liden G, Niklasson A (1984) Perinatal risk factors in the aetiology of hearing loss in preschool children. Developmental Medicine and Child Neurology 26: 799–907.
Thompson G, Folsom R (1981) Hearing assessment of at-risk infants: Current status of audiometry in young infants. Clinical Pediatrics 20: 257–61.

Thompson G, Thompson M, McCall A (1992) Strategies for increasing response behaviour of 1- and 2-year-old children during visual reinforcement audiometry. Ear and Hearing 13: 236–40.

Thompson JW, Cohen SR (1989) Management of bilateral carotid body tumors and a glomus jugular tumor in a child. International Journal of Pediatric Otorhinolaryngology 17: 75–87.

Thompson M, Thompson G, Vethivelu S (1989) A comparison of audiometric test methods for 2-year-old children. Journal of Speech and Hearing Disorders 54: 174–9.

Thompson ME, Abel SM (1992) Indices of hearing in patients with central auditory pathology. Scandinavian Audiology 21 (Suppl.) 35: 3–15.

Thornton AR, Raffin MJ (1978) Speech discrimination scores modelled as a binomial variable. Journal of Speech and Hearing Research 21: 497–506.

Thorogood PV (1987) Mechanisms of morphogenetic specification in skull development. In Wolff JR et al. (eds) Mesenchymal-epithelial Interactions in Neural Development (NATO ASI Series, Vol. H5). Berlin: Springer-Verlag.

Tillman TW, Kastin RN, Horner JS (1963) Effect of the head shadow effect on the reception of speech. ASHA 5: 778–9.

Toe DM (1998) The use of FM hearing aid systems by hearing impaired students in integrated settings. Unpublished doctoral dissertation, University of Melbourne.

Tomblin B, Smith E, Zhang X (1997) Epidemiology of specific language impairment: Prenatal and perinatal risk factors. Journal of Communication Disorders 30: 325–44.

Tomblin J, Sgriberg L, Nishimura C et al. (1999) Association of developmental language impairment with loci at 7Q3. Poster at Afasic Symposium.

Tookey P, Peckham CS (1996) Neonatal herpes simplex virus infection in the British Isles. Paediatric and Perinatal Epidemiology 10: 432–42.

Tookey PA, Peckham CS (1999) Surveillence of congenital rubella in Great Britain, 1971–96. British Medical Journal 318: 769–70.

Torres M, Gomez-Pardo E, Gruss P (1996) Pax2 contributes to inner ear patterning and optic nerve trajectory. Development 122: 3381–91.

Torroni A, Cruciani F, Rengo C et al. (1999) The A1555G mutation in the 12S RNA gene of human mtDNA: Recurrent origins and founder events in families affected by sensorineural deafness. American Journal of Human Genetics 65: 1349–58.

Toubi E, Ben-David J, Kessel A et al. (1997) Anticardiolipin antibodies. Lupus 6: 540–2.

Treacher Collins E (1900) Case with symmetrical congenital notches in the outer part of each lid and defective development of the malar bones. Transactions of the Ophthalmological Society of the UK 20: 190–2.

Tronick EZ, Ricks M, Cohn SF (1982) Maternal and infant affective exchange: Patterns of adaptation. In Field T, Fogel A (eds) Emotion and Early Interaction. Hillsdale, NJ: Lawrence Erlbaum Associates.

Tucker IG, Nolan M (1984) Educational Audiology. London: Croom Helm.

Tucker JB, Mogensen MT, Henderson CG et al. (1998) Nucleation and capture of large surface-associated microtubule arrays that are not located near centrosomes in certain cochlear epithelial cells. Journal of Anatomy 192: 119–30.

Tucker SM, Bhattacharya J (1992) Screening of hearing impairment in the newborn using the auditory response cradle. Archives of Disease in Childhood 67: 911–19.

Tuchman RF (1994) Epilepsy, language and behaviour: Clinical models in childhood. Journal of Child Neurology 9: 95–102.

Tyler RS (2000) Management of the tinnitus patient. In Luxon LM, Furman JM, Martini A, Stephens D (eds) Textbook of Audiological Medicine. Oxford: Isis Publications.

Tyler RS, Babin RW (1993) Tinnitus. In Cummings CW (ed.) Otolaryngology, Head and Neck Surgery. 2 edn. St Louis: Mosby.

Tyler RS, Bentler RA (1987) Tinnitus maskers and hearing aids for tinnitus. In Sweetow R (ed.) Seminars in Hearing. New York: Thieme Medical Publishers.

Tyler RS, Stouffer JL, Schum R (1989) Audiological rehabilitation of the tinnitus patient. Journal of the Academy of Rehabilitative Audiology 22: 30–42.

Tyler RS, Summerfield AQ (1996) Cochlear implantation: Relationships with research on auditory deprivation and acclimatisation. Ear and Hearing 17 (3 Suppl.): 38S–50S.

Unal M, Katircioglu S, Kataray MC et al. (1998) International Journal of Pediatric Otorhinolaryngology 45: 167–9.

UNESCO (1994) The Salamanca Statement and Framework for Action on Special Needs Education: World Conference on Special Needs Education: Access and Quality.

Updike CD (1994) Comparison of FM auditory trainers, CROS aids, and personal amplification in unilaterally hearing impaired children. Journal of American Academy of Audiology 5: 204–9.

Usami S, Abe S, Tono T et al. (1998) Isepamicin sulphate-induced sensorineural hearing loss in patients with the 1555A-G mitochondrial mutation. Otorhinolaryngology 60: 164–9.

Uus, K, Davis AC (2001) Epidemiology of permanent childhood hearing impairment in Estonia, 1985–90. Audiology 39: 192–7.

VACD (1992) Tonal and speech materials for auditory perceptual assessment. Long Beach, CA: Research and Development Service, Veterans' Administration Central Office.

Van Camp G, Willems PJ, Smith RJH (1997) Nonsyndromic hearing impairment: Unparalleled heterogeneity. American Journal of Human Genetics 60: 758–64.

Valvassori GE, Clemis JD (1978) The large vestibular aqueduct syndrome. Laryngoscope 88: 723–8.

Van de Bor M, Ens-Dokkum M, Schreuder AM et al. (1992) Hyperbilirubinaemia in low birthweight infants and outcome at five years of age. Pediatrics 89: 359–64.

Van der Hoeve J, De Kleyn A (1917) Blauwe sclera, broosheid van het beenstelsel en gehoorstoornissen. Ned Tijdschr Geneeskd 61: 1003–10.

Van de Water TR (1988) Tissue interactions and cell differentiation: Neurone-sensory cell interaction during otic development. Development (Suppl. 103): 185–93.

Van de Water TR, Frenz DA, Giraldez F et al. (1992) Growth factors and development of the stato-acoustic system. In Romand R (ed.) Development of Auditory and Vestibular Systems 2. New York: Academic Press.

Van Laer L, Van Camp G, Van Zuijen D et al. (1997) Refined mapping of a gene for autosomal dominant progressive sensorineural hearing loss (DFNA5) to a 2-cM region, and exclusion of a candidate gene that is expressed in the cochlea. European Journal of Human Genetics 5: 397–405.

Van Loon AM, Cleator GM, Klapper PE (1999) Herpesviruses. In Armstrong A, Cohen J (eds) Infectious Diseases. New York and London: Mosby Press.

Van Rijn PM (1990) Causes of Early Childhood Deafness. Thesis, Nijmegen University.

Van Rijin P, Cremers CWRJ (1991) Causes of childhood deafness at a Dutch school for the hearing impaired. Annals of Otology, Rhinology and Laryngology 100: 903–8.

Veen S, Sassen ML, Schreuder AM et al. (1993) Hearing loss in very preterm and very low birthweight infants at the age of 5 years in a nationwide cohort. International Journal of Pediatric Otorhinolaryngology 26: 11–28.

Veltri RW, Wilson WR, Sprinkle PM et al. (1981) The implication of viruses in idiopathic sudden hearing loss: Primary infection or reactivation of latent viruses? Otolaryngology, Head and Neck Surgery 89: 137–41.

Vernon JA (1998) Tinnitus: Treatment and relief. Needham Heights, MA: Allyn & Bacon.

Verwoerd CDA, van Oostrom CG, Verwoerd-Verhoef HL (1981) Otic placode and cephalic neural crest. Acta Otolaryngologica 91: 431–5.

Viani L (1989) Tinnitus in children with hearing loss. Journal of Laryngology and Otology 103: 1142–5.

Vienny H, Despland PA, Lutschg J et al. (1984) Early diagnosis and evolution of deafness in childhood bacterial meningitis: A study using brainstem auditory evoked potentials. Pediatrics 73: 586.

Vincent C, Kalatzis V, Abdelhak S et al. (1997) BOR and BO syndromes are allelic defects of EYA1. European Journal of Human Genetics 5: 242–6.

Vohr B, Carty LM, Moore PE, Letourneau K (1998) The Rhode Island Hearing Assessment Program: Experience with statewide hearing screening. Journal of Pediatrics 133: 353–7.

Volterra V, Beronesi S, Massoni P (1990) How does gestural communication become language? In Volterra V, Erting CJ (eds) From Gesture to Language in Hearing and Deaf Children. Heidelberg: Springer Verlag.

Volterra V, Taeschner T (1978) The acquisition and development of language by bilingual children. Journal of Child Language 5: 311–26.

Von Bekesy G (1960) Experiments in Hearing. New York: McGraw-Hill.

Von Graefe A (1858) Vereinzelte Beobachtungen und Bemerkungen. Exceptionelles Verhalten des Gesichtsfeldes bei Pigmententartung der Netzhaut. Albrecht von Graefes Arch Klin Ophthalmol 4: 250–352.

Walby AP, Barrera A, Schuknecht HF (1983) Cochlear function in chronic suppurative otitis media. American Journal of Otology, Rhinology, Laryngology 103 (Suppl) 1–19.

Walch C, Anderhuber W, Kole W, Berghold A (2000) Bilateral sensorineural hearing disorders in children: Etiology of deafness and evaluation of hearing tests. International Journal of Pediatric Otorhinolaryngology 53: 31–8.

Wald ER, Guerra N, Bayers C (1991) Upper respiratory tract infections in young children: Duration of and frequency of complications. Pediatrics 87: 129–33.

Wald ER, Kaplan SL, Mason EO Jr et al. (1995) Dexamethasone therapy for children with bacterial meningitis. Meningitis Study Group. Pediatrics 95: 21–8.

Walsh RM (1998) An In Vivo Study of Vestibular Sensory Hair-cell Degeneration and Regeneration in the Guinea Pig Inner Ear. MD Thesis, Trinity College, University of Dublin, Ireland.

Walton G, Bower N, Bower T (1992) Recognition of familiar faces by new borns. Infant Behaviour and Development 15: 265–9.

Waltzman SB, Cohen NL, Gomolin RH et al. (1997) Open-set speech perception in congenitally deaf children using cochlear implants. American Journal of Otology 18: 342–9.

Ward S (1992) The predictive validity and accuracy of a screening test for language delay and auditory perceptual disorder. European Journal of Disorders of Communication 27: 55–73.

Watkin P (1989) Otological disease in Turner's Syndrome. Journal of Laryngology and Otology 103: 731–8.

Watkin P, Baldwin M, Dixon R, Beckman A (1998) Maternal anxiety and attitudes to universal neonatal hearing screening British Journal of Audiology 32: 27–37.

Watkin, PM (1996) Outcomes of neonatal screening for hearing loss by otoacoustic emission. Archives of Disease in Childhood 75: 158–68.

Watkins S, Pittman P, Walden B (1998) The Deaf Mentor Experimental Project for young children who are deaf and their families. American Annals of the Deaf 143: 29–34.

Watson TJ (1957) Speech audiometry for children. In Ewing AWG (ed.) Educational Fuidance and the Deaf Child. Manchester: Manchester University Press.

Waxman RP, Spencer PE (1997) What mothers do to support infant visual attention: Sensitivities to age and hearing status. Journal of Deaf Studies and Deaf Education 2: 104–14.

Webb HD (1993) Auditory Screening in High Risk Neonates: An evaluation of the bone conduction auditory brainstem response test. M Med Science Thesis. University of Sheffield, UK.

Webster A, Wood D (1989) Children with Hearing Difficulties. London: Cassell.

Weisel A, Dromi E, Dor S (1990) Exploration of factors affecting attitudes towards sign language. Sign Language Studies 68: 257–76.

Weissman JL, Weber PC, Bluestone CD (1994) Congenital perilymphatic fistula: Computer tomography appearance of middle ear and inner ear anomalies. Otolaryngology, Head and Neck Surgery 11: 243–9.

Welling DB, Martyn MD, Miles BA et al. (1998) Endolymphic sac occlusion for the enlarged vestibular aqueduct syndrome. American Journal of Otology 19: 145–51.

Wessex Universal Neonatal Hearing Screening Trial Group (1998) Controlled trial of universal neonatal screening for early identification of permanent childhood hearing impairment. The Lancet 352: 1957– 64.

Wever EG, Vernon, JA (1955) The effects of the tympanic muscle reflexes upon sound transmission. Acta Otolaryngologica 45: 433–9.

White KR, Behrens TR (eds) (1993) The Rhode Island Hearing Assessment Project: Implications for Universal Newborn Hearing Screening. New York: Thieme Medical Publishers, vol. 14.

White KR, Vohr BR, Maxon AB et al. (1994) Screening all newborns for hearing-loss using transient evoked otoacoustic emissions. International Journal of Pediatric Otorhinolaryngology 29: 203–17.

Whitehurst GJ, Fischel JE (1994) Early developmental language delay: What, if anything, should the clinician do about it? Journal of Child Psychology and Psychiatry 35: 613–48.

Whitley RJ (1993) Neonatal herpes simplex virus infections. Journal of Medical Virology 1: 13–21.

Widdershoven J, Assman K, Monnens L, Cremers CWRJ (1983) Renal disorders in the branchio-oto-renal syndrome. Helv Paediatr Acta 38: 513–22.

Widen JE (1993) Adding objectivity to infant behavioral audiometry. Ear and Hearing 14: 49–57.

Wiedermann BL, Hawkins EP, Johnson GS et al. (1986) Pathogenesis of labyrinthitis associated with Haemophilus influenzae type b in experimental meningitis. Journal of Infectious Diseases 153: 27–32.

Wiener-Vacher SR, Amanou L, Denise P et al. (1999) Vestibular function in children with CHARGE-association. Archives of Otolaryngology 125: 342–7.

Wigney D, Ching TYC, Newall P (1997) Comparison of severely and profoundly hearing impaired children's amplification preferences with the NAL-RP and DSL 3.0 prescriptions. Scandinavian Audiology 26: 219–22.

Wild NJ, Sheppard S, Smithells RW et al. (1989) Onset and severity of hearing loss due to congenital rubella infection. Archives of Disease in Childhood 64: 1280–3.

Wild NJ, Sheppard S, Smithells RW et al. (1990) Delayed detection of congenital hearing loss in high risk infants. British Medical Journal 301: 903–4.

Wilichowski E, Gruters A, Kruse K et al. (1997) Hypoparathyroidism and deafness associated with pleioplasmic large scale rearrangements of the mitochondrial DNA: A clinical and molecular genetic study of four children with Kearns-Sayre Syndrome. Pediatric Research 41: 193–200.

Willeford J (1976) Central auditory function in children with learning disabilities. Audiology and Hearing Education 2: 12–20.

Williamson WD, Demmler GJ, Percy AK, Catlin FI (1992) Progressive hearing loss in infants with asymptomatic congenital cytomegalovirus. Pediatrics 90: 862–6.

Willis RW, Edwards JA (1996) A study of the comparative effectiveness of systematic desensitisation and implosive therapy. Behavior Research and Therapy 7: 387–95.

Wilson C, Grant CC, Wall CR (1999) Iron deficiency anaemia and adverse dietary habits in hospitalised children. New Zealand Medical Journal 112 (1089): 203–6.

Wilson DF, Hodgson RS, Talbot JM (1997) Endolymphatic sac obliteration for large vestibular aqueduct syndrome. American Journal of Otology 18: 101–6.

Wilson JMG, Junger G (1968) Principles and Practice for Screening of Disease. Geneva: World Health Organization.

Wilson PH, Henry JL (2000) Psychological management. In Tyler RS (ed.) Handbook on Tinnitus. San Diego, CA: Singular Publishing Group.

Wilson RH, Zizz CA, Sperry JL et al. (1994) Masking level difference for spondaic words in 2000-msec bursts of broadband noise. Journal of the American Academy of Audiology 5: 236–42.

Windle-Taylor PC, Emery PJ, Phelps PD (1981) Ear deformities associated with the Klippel-Feil syndrome. Annals of Otology, Rhinology and Laryngology 90: 210–46.

Wing L (1988) The continuum of autistic characteristics. In Schopler E, Mesibov GB (eds) Diagnosis and Assessment in Autism. New York: Plenum Press.

Winkel O, Mork Henson M, Kaaber K, Rozarth K (1978) A prospective study of gentamycin ototoxicity. Acta Otolaryngologica 86: 212–16.

Winston E (1990) English Use in the Deaf Community. Rochester, New York: International Congress of the Education of the Deaf.

Winter AJ, Comis SD, Osborne MP et al. (1998) Ototoxicity resulting from intraochlear perfusion of Streptococcus pneumoniae in the guinea pig is modified by cefotaxime or amoxycillin pretreatment. Journal of Infection 36: 71–7.

Wishart JH (1820) Case of tumours in the skull, dura mater and brain. Edinburgh Medical and Surgical Journal 18: 393–7.

Wolinsky JS (1996) Rubella. In Field BN, Knipe DM, Howley PM (eds) Fields Virology. 3 edn. Philadelphia, PA: Lippincott-Raven Publishers.

Woll B (1998) Development of signed and spoken languages. In Gregory S, Knight P, McCracken W, Powers S, Watson L (eds) Issues in Deaf Education. London: David Fulton Publishers Ltd.

Wood D (1996) Communication and cognition. American Annals of the Deaf 136: 247–51.

Wood D, Wood H (1992) Signed English in the classroom, IV. Aspects of children's speech and sign. First Language 12: 125–45.

Wood DJ (1982) The linguistic experiences of the prelingually hearing-impaired child. Journal of the British Association of Teachers of the Deaf 6: 86–93.

Wood DJ, Wood HA, Griffiths AJ, Howarth SP (1986) Teaching and Talking with Deaf Children. New York: John Wiley.

Wood S, Davis AC, McCormick B (1997) Changing performance of the Health Visitor Distraction Test when targeted neonatal screening is introduced into a Health District. British Journal of Audiology 31: 55–61.

Wood S, Farnsworth A, Davis A (1995) The identification and referral of babies with a family history of congenital hearing loss for hearing screening. Journal of Audiological Medicine: 4: 25–33.

Wood S, Mason A, Farnsworth A et al. (1998) Anomalous screening outcomes from click evoked otoacoustic emissions and auditory brainstem response test. British Journal of Audiology 32: 399–410.

Woodhouse W, Bailey A, Rutter M et al. (1996) Head circumference in autism and other pervasive developmental disorders. Journal of Child Psychology and Psychiatry 37: 665–72.

Woolley AL, Kirk KA, Neumann AM et al. (1999) Risk factors for hearing loss from meningitis in children. Archives of Otolaryngology, Head and Neck Surgery 125: 309–14.

Worley GA, Vats A, Harcourt J, Albert D (1999) Bilateral congenital cholesteatoma in branchio-oto-renal syndrome. Journal of Laryngology and Otology 113: 841–3.

Worthington D (1980) Quantifiable hearing and no ABR: Paradox or error? Ear and Hearing 1: 281.

Yang EY, Stuart A et al. (1993) Auditory brain stem responses to air- and bone-conducted clicks in the audiological assessment of at-risk infants. Ear and Hearing 14: 175–82.

Yassi A, Pollock N, Tran N, Cheang M (1993) Risks to hearing from a rock concert. Canadian Family Physician 39: 1045–50.

Yoshinaga-Itano C, Sedey AL, Coulter DK, Mehl AL (1998) Language of early- and later-identified children with hearing loss. Pediatrics 102: 1161–71.

Yost WA (1997) The cocktail party problem: Forty years later. In Gilkey RH, Anderson TR (eds) Binaural and Spatial Hearing in Real and Virtual Environments. Mahwah, NJ: Lawrence Erlbaum Associates.

Young AM (1997) Conceptualizing parents' sign language use in bilingual early intervention. Journal of Deaf Studies and Deaf Education 2: 264–76.

Zachmann M, Fuchs E, Prader A (1992) Progressive high frequency hearing loss: An additional feature in the syndrome of congenital adrenal hypoplasia and gonadotrophin deficiency. European Journal of Pediatrics 151: 167–9.

Zahr L, de Traversay J (1995) Premature infant responses to noise reduction by earmuffs: Effect on behavioural and physiologic measures. Journal of Perinatology 15: 448–55.

Zakrisson J-E, Borg E (1974) Stapedius reflex and auditory fatigue. Audiology 13: 231–5.

Zalzal GH, Tomaski SM, Vezina LG et al. (1995) Enlarged vestibular aqueduct and sensorineural hearing loss in childhood. Archives of Otolaryngology, Head and Neck Surgery 121: 23–8.

Zink GD (1972) Hearing aids children wear: A longitudinal study of performance. Volta Review 74: 41–52.

Zlotogora J, Sagi M, Schuper A et al. (1992) Variability of Stickler Syndrome. American Journal of Medical Genetics 42: 337–9.

Zori DT, Gray BA, Bent Williams A et al. (1993) Preaxial acrofacial dysostosis (Nager syndrome) associated with an inherited and apparently balanced X; 9 translocation. American Journal of Medicine 46: 379–83.

Index